Clinical Otology

Clinical Otology

Edited by Benjamin Davies

STATES
ACADEMIC PRESS
www.statesacademicpress.com

States Academic Press,
109 South 5th Street,
Brooklyn, NY 11249, USA

Visit us on the World Wide Web at:
www.statesacademicpress.com

ISBN: 978-1-63989-764-3

Cataloging-in-Publication Data

Clinical otology / edited by Benjamin Davies.
p. cm.
Includes bibliographical references and index.
ISBN 978-1-63989-764-3
1. Ear--Diseases. 2. Ear--Diseases--Diagnosis. 3. Ear--Surgery.
4. Otology. I. Davies, Benjamin.
RF121 .C55 2023
617.8--dc23

Table of Contents

Preface

Otology is a branch of otorhinolaryngology, which studies the physiology and pathology of the ear, its diseases, diagnosis and treatment. Trauma can affect the inner, external and middle ear structures individually or in combination, depending on the type and severity of the injury. The most frequent cause is a blunt head injury caused by a fall or road traffic accident (RTA). Such cases of head injury are usually associated with a temporal bone fracture combined with other injuries. Otologic trauma is classified into different types such as ossicular discontinuity, injuries of the external ear, concussive injuries to the structures of the inner ear, and disruptions of the tympanic membrane (TM). Patients with all types of traumatic conductive hearing loss can be treated using conservative methods such as watchful waiting and hearing aids. This book unravels the recent studies in the field of clinical otology. A number of latest researches have been included to keep the readers up-to-date with the global concepts in this area of medicine.

Various studies have approached the subject by analyzing it with a single perspective, but the present book provides diverse methodologies and techniques to address this field. This book contains theories and applications needed for understanding the subject from different perspectives. The aim is to keep the readers informed about the progresses in the field; therefore, the contributions were carefully examined to compile novel researches by specialists from across the globe.

Indeed, the job of the editor is the most crucial and challenging in compiling all chapters into a single book. In the end, I would extend my sincere thanks to the chapter authors for their profound work. I am also thankful for the support provided by my family and colleagues during the compilation of this book.

Editor

1

Macrophages Respond Rapidly to Ototoxic Injury of Lateral Line Hair Cells but are not Required for Hair Cell Regeneration

Mark E. Warchol[1,2]**, *Angela Schrader*[1] *and Lavinia Sheets*[1,3]

[1]*Department of Otolaryngology, Washington University School of Medicine, St. Louis, MO, United States,* [2]*Department of Neuroscience, Washington University School of Medicine, St. Louis, MO, United States,* [3]*Department of Developmental Biology, Washington University School of Medicine, St. Louis, MO, United States*

***Correspondence:**
Mark E. Warchol
mwarchol@wustl.edu

The sensory organs of the inner ear contain resident populations of macrophages, which are recruited to sites of cellular injury. Such macrophages are known to phagocytose the debris of dying cells but the full role of macrophages in otic pathology is not understood. Lateral line neuromasts of zebrafish contain hair cells that are nearly identical to those in the inner ear, and the optical clarity of larval zebrafish permits direct imaging of cellular interactions. In this study, we used larval zebrafish to characterize the response of macrophages to ototoxic injury of lateral line hair cells. Macrophages migrated into neuromasts within 20 min of exposure to the ototoxic antibiotic neomycin. The number of macrophages in the near vicinity of injured neuromasts was similar to that observed near uninjured neuromasts, suggesting that this early inflammatory response was mediated by "local" macrophages. Upon entering injured neuromasts, macrophages actively phagocytosed hair cell debris. The injury-evoked migration of macrophages was significantly reduced by inhibition of Src-family kinases. Using chemical-genetic ablation of macrophages before the ototoxic injury, we also examined whether macrophages were essential for the initiation of hair cell regeneration. Results revealed only minor differences in hair cell recovery in macrophage-depleted vs. control fish, suggesting that macrophages are not essential for the regeneration of lateral line hair cells.

Keywords: zebrafish, macrophage, lateral line, hair cell, regeneration, ototoxicity, inner ear

INTRODUCTION

Sensory hair cells of the vertebrate inner ear are mechanoreceptors that detect sound vibrations and head movements. Hair cells are also present in the lateral line systems of fish and amphibians, where they detect water motion along the external surface of the animal (Kindt and Sheets, 2018). Lateral line hair cells are contained in sensory organs known as neuromasts and are enclosed by an oval-shaped cluster of supporting cells. Because of their optical clarity and well-characterized genetics, the lateral line of larval zebrafish has become a commonly-studied model of hair cell development, pathology, and regeneration (e.g., Pickett and Raible, 2019).

Hair cells of the inner ear can be damaged or lost after noise exposure, ototoxicity, or as part of normal aging. Like their counterparts in the ear, lateral line hair cells can also be damaged by exposure to ototoxic drugs or by mechanical trauma (Harris et al., 2003; Hernández et al., 2006; Uribe et al., 2018; Holmgren et al., 2020). Many of the signaling pathways that mediate hair cell death have been identified (e.g., Wagner and Shin, 2019). However, the mammalian inner ear cannot regenerate hair cells after injury, and their loss typically results in sensorineural deafness and disequilibrium. In contrast, the ears of nonmammalian vertebrates can regenerate hair cells after acoustic trauma or ototoxic injury (e.g., Warchol, 2011), and a similar form of hair cell regeneration also occurs in lateral line neuromasts (e.g., Jones and Corwin, 1996; Harris et al., 2003; Denans et al., 2019). At present, the cellular mechanisms that underly hair cell regeneration in nonmammalian vertebrates are poorly understood.

Macrophages are key effector cells of the innate immune system and also contribute to debris clearance and cellular repair after tissue injury. The inner ears of birds and mammals contain resident populations of macrophages, which are recruited to sites of hair cell damage (Warchol, 1997; Bhave et al., 1998; Hirose et al., 2005; Warchol et al., 2012; Kaur et al., 2015a). Such macrophages have been shown to phagocytose dying hair cells (e.g., Kaur et al., 2015b), but the full role of macrophages in the process of otic pathology is not clear. Also, the signals that recruit macrophages toward sites of injury in the ear have not been identified (reviewed by Warchol, 2019). The mammalian inner ear is enclosed within the temporal bone of the skull, so it is not possible to directly image the interactions between macrophages and injured hair cells. Notably, however, macrophages are also activated after an injury to lateral line neuromasts of fish and salamanders, and their response can be directly imaged in living animals (e.g., Jones and Corwin, 1993, 1996; Hirose et al., 2017).

The present study used larval zebrafish to characterize the response of macrophages to ototoxic injury of lateral line hair cells. We show that posterior neuromasts typically possess 1–2 macrophages within a 25 μm radius. These macrophages quickly migrate into neuromasts during the early phases of ototoxic injury, where they contact and phagocytose the debris of dying hair cells. Ototoxicity also causes the swift externalization of phosphatidylserine on the apical surfaces of hair cells, which may target dying cells for removal. The signals that initiate macrophage migration are not known, but prior studies have shown that the Src kinase Lyn is a regulator of leukocyte response to injury (e.g., Yoo et al., 2011). Our experiments showed that macrophage entry into injured neuromasts was reduced after pharmacological inhibition of Src-family kinases. Zebrafish are also capable of regenerating hair cells after ototoxic injury, and we tested whether macrophages were essential for this regenerative response. We found that selective chemical-genetic elimination of macrophages did not affect the extent of the ototoxic injury and had only a minor impact on the numbers of regenerated hair cells. Together, these data suggest that macrophages serve as phagocytes after hair cell injury, but do not play a critical role in the initiation of hair cell regeneration.

MATERIALS AND METHODS

Ethics Statement

This study was performed with the approval of the Institutional Animal Care and Use Committee of Washington University School of Medicine in St. Louis and following NIH guidelines for use of zebrafish.

Zebrafish

Most experiments were performed using Tg(*mpeg1:yfp*) fish, which selectively express YFP under the regulation of the *Mpeg1* promoter (i.e., in macrophages and microglia—Ellett et al., 2011; Roca and Ramakrishnan, 2013; Svahn et al., 2013). Studies of hair cell regeneration used *Tg(mpeg1:Gal4FF/UAS:NTR-mCherry)* double transgenic fish, which express the Gal4 transcriptional activator driven by the macrophage-specific *Mpeg1* promoter and the gene for the bacterial enzyme nitroreductase fused to mCherry under the regulation of the Gal4-specific UAS enhancer sequence. Adult zebrafish were maintained at 27–29°C and housed in the Washington University Zebrafish Facility. Fertile eggs and larvae were maintained in embryo medium (EM: 15 mM NaCl, 0.5 mM KCl, 1 mM $CaCl_2$, 1 mM $MgSO_4$, 0.15 mM KH_2PO_4, 0.042 mM Na_2HPO_4, 0.714mM $NaHCO_3$; Westerfield, 2000) and, beginning at 5 days post-fertilization (dpf), were fed rotifers daily. At the end of the experiments, fish were euthanized by quick chilling to 4°C.

Ototoxic Ablation of Neuromast Hair Cells With Neomycin

Lateral line hair cells were lesioned by incubating fish in the ototoxic antibiotic neomycin (e.g., Harris et al., 2003). Groups of larval fish were placed in 25 mm "baskets" (Corning Cell Strainer, ~20–30 fish/basket) and transferred into 30 ml EM that contained 100 μM neomycin (Sigma–Aldrich). Depending on the specific experiment, fish were treated in neomycin for 90 s–30 min and were then either euthanized and fixed or rinsed 3× by immersion in 30 ml EM and maintained for an additional 1–48 h.

Annexin V Labeling

Dying cells transport phosphatidylserine (PtS) to their external membrane surfaces and such cells can be labeled by treatment with annexin V. Fish were incubated in EM that contained Alexa 555 conjugated annexin V (Thermo Fisher Scientific, diluted 1:100) and neomycin was added to the water for a final concentration of 100 μM. Fish were euthanized and fixed after 90 s–10 min of neomycin exposure and prepared for microscopy as described below.

Treatment With SFK Inhibitor

To examine the influence of inhibiting Src-family kinases on the macrophage response to ototoxic injury, fish were treated in PP2, an inhibitor of Src kinases (Caymen Chemical, 20 μM). A 20 mM stock solution was prepared in DMSO and diluted 1:1,000 in EM. Control specimens were maintained in parallel in 0.1% DMSO. Fish were treated in these media for 60 min (at 28.5°C) and then received 100 μM neomycin.

Selective Depletion of Macrophages

The influence of macrophages on hair cell regeneration was examined using *Tg(mpeg1:Gal4FF/UAS:NTR-mCherry)* transgenic fish. Macrophages were eliminated *via* incubation for 24 h in 10 mM metronidazole (MTZ, Sigma–Aldrich, with 0.1% DMSO). Controls in these studies were fish of the same genotype but incubated 24 h in 0.1% DMSO alone.

Immunohistochemical Labeling

Fish were fixed overnight in 4% paraformaldehyde (in 0.1 M phosphate buffer, pH = 7.4) at 4°C. The next day, fish were thoroughly rinsed in PBS, and nonspecific antibody binding was blocked by treatment for 2 h in 5% normal horse serum (NHS) in phosphate-buffered saline (PBS) with 1% Triton X-100. This was followed by incubation in primary antibodies, which were diluted in PBS, with 2% NHS and 1% Triton X-100. All specimens were treated in antibody solutions overnight, at room temperature, and with mild agitation. The next day, specimens were rinsed 3× in PBS and incubated for 2 h in secondary antibodies (anti-mouse IgG and anti-rabbit IgG, both raised in donkey) that were conjugated to Alexa-488 and Alexa-555, respectively (1:500, Invitrogen). The secondary solution also contained the nuclear dye DAPI. Following thorough rinsing in PBS, fish were mounted in glycerol:PBS (9:1) on microscope slides and coverslipped.

Primary Antibodies

Hair cells were labeled with HCS-1, which is specific for otoferlin (Goodyear et al., 2010). HCS-1 was developed by Jeffrey Corwin (University of Virginia) and obtained from the Developmental Studies Hybridoma Bank, created by the NICHD of the NIH, and maintained at the Department of Biology of the University of Iowa. HCS-1 was obtained as a purified concentrate and used at 1:500 dilution. The YFP or mCherry signals in macrophages were amplified by labeling with either anti-GFP or anti-mCherry (1:500; Thermo Fisher Scientific).

Confocal Imaging

Images of fixed samples were acquired using an LSM 700 laser scanning confocal microscope (Carl Zeiss). Confocal stacks of 15 μm depth were collected with a *z*-step of 1 μm. Regardless of the particular fluorophore expressed (YFP or mCherry), macrophages in all presented images were pseudo-colored green.

Confocal Image Processing and Analysis

Confocal image stacks were reconstructed and analyzed using Volocity software (Quorum Technologies). Intact hair cells were identified by the presence of a normal-appearing DAPI-stained nucleus that was surrounded by an uninterrupted region of otoferlin immunoreactivity. Pyknotic nuclei were identified as smaller bright puncta of DAPI labeling. Macrophage activity was quantified by scrolling through the 15 μm-depth image stacks (in the *z*-dimension) and counting: (1) the number of macrophages within a 25 μm radius of a neuromast (using a circle inscribed on the particular neuromast); (2) the number of macrophages directly contacting otoferlin-labeled hair cells; and (3) the number of macrophages that had internalized otoferlin-labeled material (hair cell debris). For each metric, the recorded number reflected the activity of a single macrophage, i.e., a macrophage that made contacts with multiple hair cells and/or had internalized debris from several hair cells was still classified as a single "event." For annexin V-labeled fish, the numbers of labeled stereocilia bundles were counted by scrolling through the individual *z*-sections of each confocal stack. Subsequent image processing for published figures was performed using Photoshop and Illustrator software (Adobe).

Statistical Analysis

Plotting and statistical analyses of data were performed using Prism 8 (Graphpad Software Incorporation). Statistical significance between two (parallel) data sets was determined *via* unpaired Student's *t*-test or Mann–Whitney *U* test, as appropriate. Statistical comparison of multiple parallel data sets was determined by one-way ANOVA or Kruskal–Wallis tests, with and appropriate *post hoc* tests. All plots show mean ± standard deviation.

RESULTS

Macrophages Reside Close to Lateral Line Neuromasts

Initial studies characterized the association of macrophages with lateral line neuromasts in untreated fish i.e., fish without neuromast injury. Confocal imaging of Tg(*mpeg1:yfp*) zebrafish at 6–7 days post-fertilization (dpf) revealed numerous macrophages distributed throughout the body of each fish. Quantification from low magnification images indicated that the posterior-most 500 μm of larval fish contained ~15 macrophages, many of which were located near neuromasts (**Figures 1A,A′**, arrows). Higher magnification images of individual neuromasts showed that most neuromast-associated macrophages possessed several processes (pseudopodia) that projected in various directions from the central cell body (**Figures 1B,B′**, arrows). We quantified macrophages located within a 25 μm radius of neuromasts L4 or L5 of the posterior lateral line (nomenclature described in Ledent, 2002; also see Kindt and Sheets, 2018). Data indicate that, at 6 dpf, neuromasts L4/5 normally possess 1.1 ± 0.7 nearby macrophages (n = 15 fish). These observations suggest macrophages may monitor posterior lateral line neuromasts, even in the absence of injury.

Macrophages Contact Hair Cells After Ototoxic Injury

In addition to their role in innate immunity, macrophages are also recruited to sites of tissue injury, where they remove the debris of dead cells and secrete bioactive factors that promote repair (e.g., Wynn and Vannella, 2016). We have previously shown that neomycin-induced hair cell death in the posterior-most ("terminal") neuromasts of larval zebrafish leads to macrophage entry and phagocytosis (Hirose et al., 2017). A comparable macrophage response was observed in neuromasts L4/5 after exposure to neomycin (**Figure 2**). Macrophages typically entered neuromasts within 10–20 min after the initiation of neomycin treatment, and confocal images frequently showed macrophages extending pseudopodial processes that

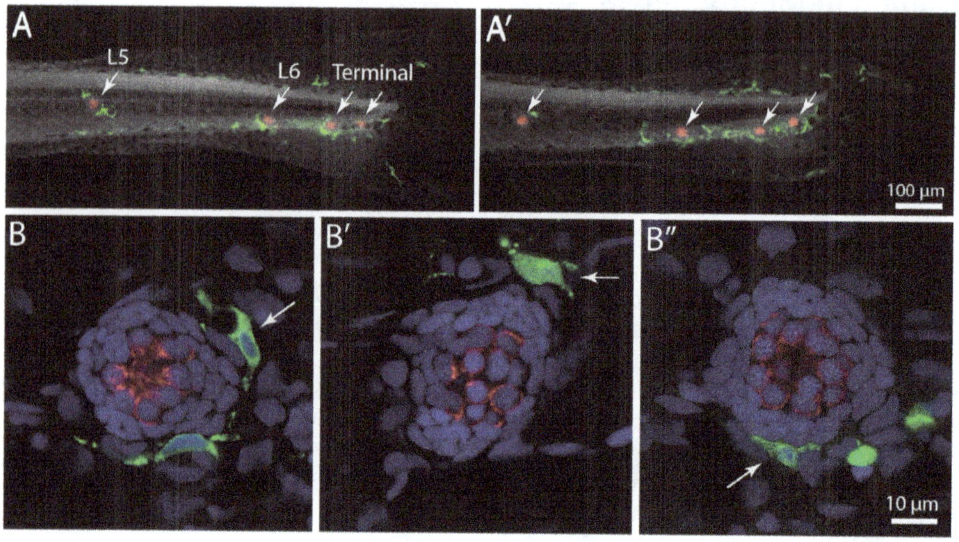

FIGURE 1 | Distribution of macrophages in the posterior lateral line of larval zebrafish. **(A,A′)** Tail regions of two Tg(*mpeg1:yfp*) zebrafish, fixed at 6 days post-fertilization (dpf). YFP in macrophages is shown in green, hair cells are labeled for otoferlin (red), and all nuclei are stained with DAPI (gray). Arrows show the four posterior-most neuromasts in each fish. Note that neuromasts possess 1–2 nearby macrophages. **(B,B′,B″)** High magnification views of neuromast L5 from three zebrafish. Arrows point to nearby macrophages.

contacted hair cells (**Figure 2**, arrow in 10 min image). Also, many macrophages had internalized otoferlin-labeled material (**Figure 2**, arrowhead in 20 min image), which was interpreted as evidence for macrophage phagocytosis of hair cell debris.

Macrophage Response Occurs Shortly After the Onset of Neomycin Exposure

In the mammalian cochlea, increased numbers of macrophages are observed within ~1–2 days of selective hair cell ablation (Kaur et al., 2015b). To characterize the latency of the macrophage response to the death of lateral line hair cells, we quantified macrophage activity at neuromasts L4/5 at various time points following the initiation of neomycin exposure (5, 10, 20, or 30 min) or after 30 min of neomycin exposure followed by 1 or 2 h recovery (**Figure 3**). Following immunohistochemical processing, data were derived from confocal images of neuromast L4 or L5 (one neuromast/fish, n = 13–26 fish/time point, data obtained from three separate trials). The numbers of pyknotic nuclei/neuromast began to increase after 10 min of neomycin exposure (**Figures 3A,D**, $p < 0.0001$, one-way ANOVA). Loss of otoferlin-labeled hair cells followed a similar time course (**Figures 3B,C**, $p = 0.019$, one-way ANOVA). The numbers of pyknotic nuclei peaked at 30 min of neomycin treatment and then declined, as dead hair cells were cleared from the neuromasts. Few hair cells (~1–2) were present 2 h after neomycin exposure (**Figures 3B,C**). Macrophages began to enter neuromasts and contact hair cells as early as 5 min into the neomycin treatment (**Figure 3B**), although such cases were rare. The increase in macrophage contacts with hair cells had significantly increased after 20 min of neomycin treatment and remained elevated until 60 min after treatment (**Figure 3E**, $p = 0.0038$, one-way ANOVA). The numbers of macrophages engaged in phagocytosis (as determined by internalization of either immunolabeled hair cell debris or pyknotic nuclei) also increased after 20 min of neomycin treatment (**Figure 3F**, $p = 0.0044$, one-way ANOVA). Despite these changes in macrophage localization and activity, the number of macrophages located within 25 μm of L4/5 at each time point ranged from 1.3 to 2.0, and did not differ significantly between time points or from controls ($p > 0.25$, one-way ANOVA). This observation suggests that the macrophage response to neomycin injury was mainly carried-out by nearby macrophages, rather than by macrophages recruited from more distant regions of the fish.

Neomycin Treatment Leads to Rapid Externalization of Phosphatidylserine

In many tissues, cells undergoing apoptosis are targeted for phagocytic removal *via* the presence of phosphatidylserine (PtS) on their external membrane surface (Fadok et al., 1992). A prior study has shown that short exposure to aminoglycoside antibiotics results in the translocation of PtS, from the inner to outer membrane leaflet, on the apical surfaces of mouse cochlear hair cells (Goodyear et al., 2008). To determine whether a similar response occurs in zebrafish hair cells, we treated fish in Alexa 555-conjugated annexin V, which binds to and labels externalized PtS (Koopman et al., 1994). Fish were preincubated for 10 min in DAPI (which passes through transduction channels and labels the nuclei of hair cells), and then transferred to embryo medium (EM) containing annexin V. Neomycin was added for a final concentration of 100 μM, and fish were removed, euthanized and fixed, beginning 90 s after the initiation of neomycin treatment and continuing until 10 min into the treatment. Control fish were treated for 10 min in annexin V but

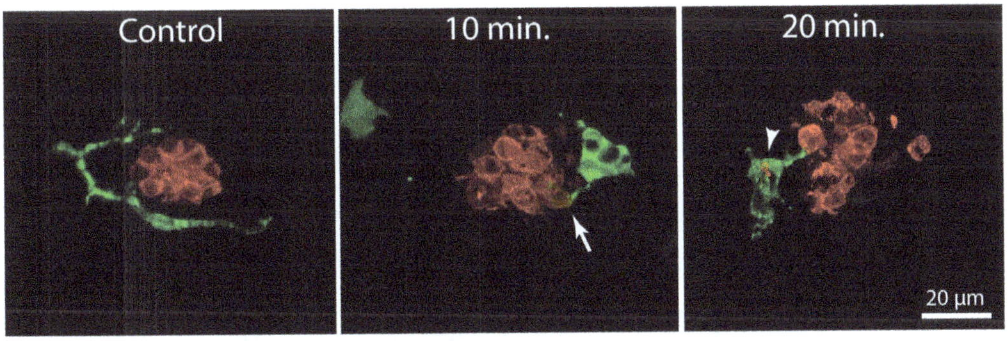

FIGURE 2 | Macrophage response to neomycin ototoxicity. Images are maximum-intensity projections of confocal z-stacks of 15 μm depth. Uninjured neuromasts ("Control") usually possess 1–2 adjacent macrophages (green). Macrophages enter the neuromasts in response to treatment in 100 μM neomycin. Images in the center and right show macrophages at 10 and 20 min of exposure to neomycin. Some macrophages (arrow, 10 min) extended processes that contact hair cells (red, otoferlin), while other macrophages had internalized the debris of dead hair cells (arrowhead, 20 min).

did not receive neomycin. Fluorescent labeling was observed on the apical surface (stereocilia bundles) of nearly all neomycin-treated fish (**Figure 4**, arrows, each labeled structure is a single stereocilia bundle). The numbers of annexin V-labeled hair cells increased during the 10 min exposure (data collected from L4/5; n = 17–40 neuromasts/time point). Reconstruction of high magnification images confirmed that the annexin-V label was confined to the stereocilia bundles on the apical surfaces of hair cells (**Figure 4**, "side view"). Quantification of the number of labeled hair cells revealed an increase with longer exposure times (see the plot in **Figure 4**). In contrast, we observed very few labeled hair cells in fish that were maintained for 10 min in annexin V but not exposed to neomycin (0.7 ± 1.4 HC/neuromast). Annexin V labeling was restricted to the apical (external) surface of hair cells and was not observed along their basal membranes (which are located beneath the epidermis). We also did not observe annexin V labeling in any cells within the body of any fish, suggesting that annexin V did not cross the epidermis.

Inhibition of Src-Family Kinases Reduces Macrophage Injury Response

The signals that trigger the macrophage response to hair cell injury are not known, but activation of Src-family kinases (SFKs) is an evolutionarily-conserved signal known to regulate the activity of phagocytes (Yoo et al., 2012; Freedman et al., 2015; Dwyer et al., 2016). To test whether SFK activation was necessary for macrophage entry into injured neuromasts, we treated fish with PP2, a specific inhibitor of SFKs (Zhu et al., 1999). In initial experiments, fish were treated for 1 h in either 20 μM PP2 (n = 14) or 0.1% DMSO (n = 10). Fish were then euthanized and processed for visualization of macrophages and hair cells. No differences were observed in either resident macrophages or hair cell numbers in the PP2-treated vs. control fish (**Figure 5A**, data not shown), suggesting that the association of macrophages with undamaged neuromasts (e.g., **Figure 1**) is not dependent on SFK signaling. We tested whether SFK signaling affected the macrophage response to hair cell injury by preincubating fish for 1 h in PP2 or DMSO, and then exposing both groups for 30 min to 100 μM neomycin (n = 34 fish/group). Exposure to PP2 did not affect the extent of the ototoxic lesion (2.7 ± 1.3 hair cells/neuromast in PP2-treated fish, vs. 3.4 ± 1.5 hair cells/neuromast in DMSO-treated fish, p = 0.08), or in the numbers of nearby macrophages (**Figure 5D**). However, PP2 treatment reduced macrophage contact with injured neuromasts following neomycin treatment (**Figures 5B,C,E**) and reduced the number of phagocytic events (**Figures 5B,C,F**). Together, these observations suggest that SFK signaling is involved in the macrophage response to hair cell injury.

Selective Depletion of Macrophages Has Minimal Effect on Hair Cell Regeneration

Lateral line neuromasts can quickly regenerate hair cells after ototoxic injury, but the biological basis of this regenerative process is not fully understood (Harris et al., 2003; Ma et al., 2008; Romero-Carvajal et al., 2015; Denans et al., 2019). Macrophages have been shown to play an important role in the initiation of regeneration in numerous other tissues and organ systems (reviewed by Keightley et al., 2014; Wynn and Vannella, 2016), and it has been suggested that macrophages may be one factor that stimulates the production of replacement hair cells in nonmammalian vertebrates (Corwin et al., 1991; Warchol, 1997; Carrillo et al., 2016; Denans et al., 2019). To evaluate the possible role of macrophages in the regeneration of lateral line hair cells, we quantified ototoxic injury and hair cell recovery in a transgenic fish line that permits the selective elimination of macrophages. *Tg(mpeg1:Gal4FF/UAS:NTR-mCherry)* double-transgenic fish expresses the gene for nitroreductase under the regulation of the macrophage-specific *Mpeg1* promoter (Davison et al., 2007; Ellett et al., 2011). Nitroreductase is a bacterial enzyme that generates a cytotoxin when exposed to the antibiotic metronidazole (MTZ). Incubation of these transgenic fish in MTZ results in selective elimination of macrophages and related cells, without other apparent pathology (Petrie et al., 2014). To verify macrophage depletion, we first treated transgenic fish for 24 h in 10 mM MTZ (n = 10) or in 0.1% DMSO (controls, n = 15), and then quantified fluorescently-labeled

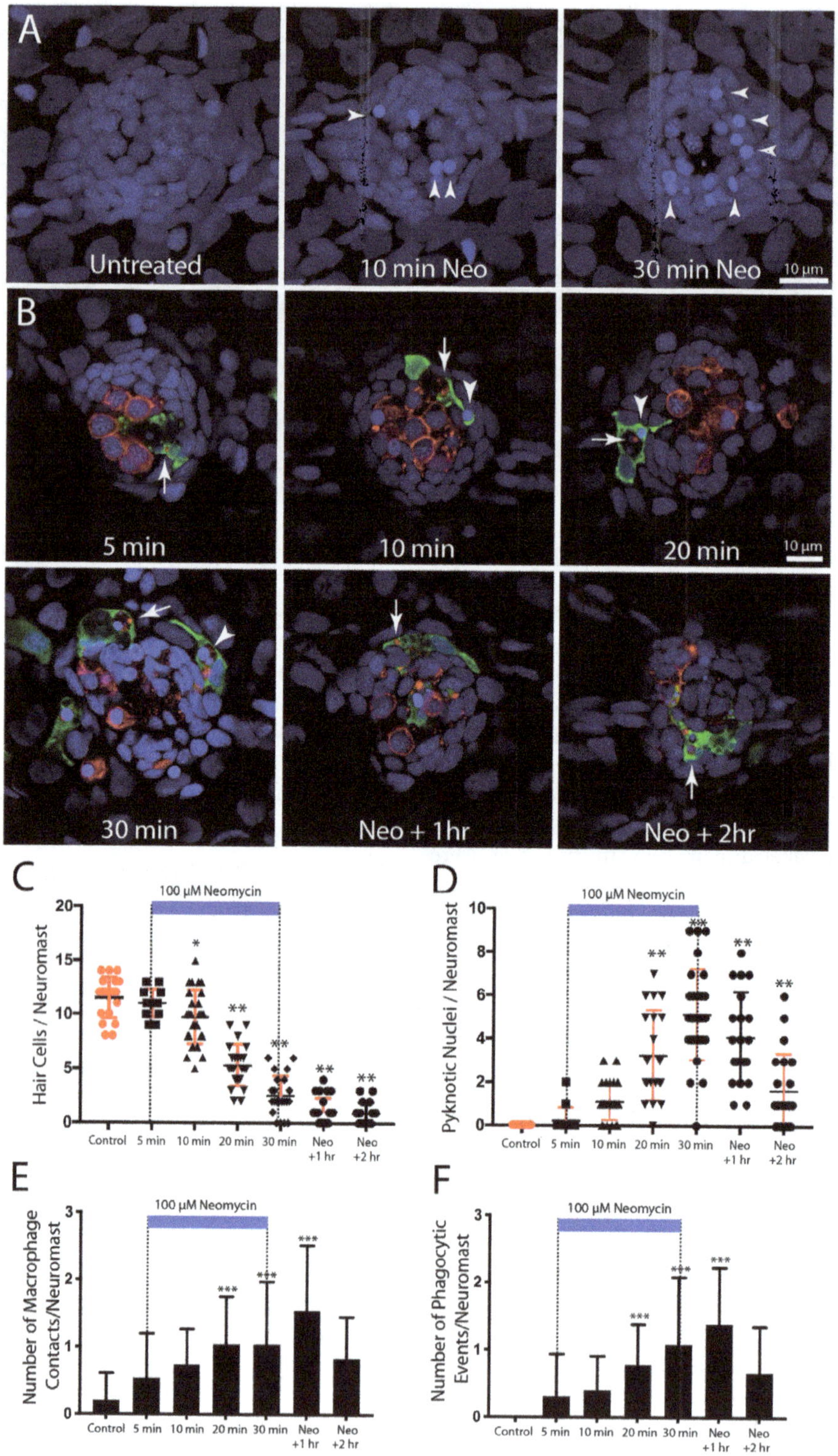

FIGURE 3 | Detailed time course of macrophage response to neomycin ototoxicity. Fish (6 dpf) were incubated in 100 µM neomycin. Some fish were fixed after 5, 10, 20, or 30 min of neomycin treatment, while other fish were removed from neomycin after 30 min, and rinsed and maintained in fresh embryo medium (EM) for 1 or 2 h. Fixed specimens were processed for immunolabeling of YFP-expressing macrophages (green) and hair cells (otoferlin, red), and nuclei were labeled with DAPI (blue). Images in panel **(A)** are maximum intensity projections, while images in panel **(B)** are single *z*-sections taken from 15 µm-depth confocal stacks. **(A)** Formation of pyknotic nuclei in response to neomycin treatment. Images show DAPI labeling in an untreated neuromast and in neuromasts that were exposed to neomycin for 10 and 30 min. Neomycin induces the formation of pyknotic nuclei (arrowheads), which are assumed to be dying hair cells. **(B)** Single *z*-stack sections at various

(*Continued*)

FIGURE 3 | Continued
time intervals after initiation of neomycin treatment. Arrows in all images indicate evidence for macrophage phagocytosis of dying hair cells. A few specimens displayed a macrophage response after only 5 min of neomycin exposure. Note that the macrophage in the 5 min image has internalized otoferlin-labeled debris (arrow). At later time points, macrophages had engulfed both otoferlin-labeled debris as well as pyknotic nuclei (arrowheads in 10, 20, and 30 min images). Also, beginning at 20 min of neomycin exposure, the number of otoferlin-labeled hair cells was significantly reduced. Neuromasts at 30 min exposure and 1 and 2 h recovery typically contained 0–3 surviving hair cells. **(C)** Surviving hair cells as a function of exposure/post-exposure time. Intact hair cells were identified by healthy nuclei that were completely enclosed by the otoferlin-labeled hair cell membrane. A significant decrease in hair cell numbers was observed, beginning after 10 min of neomycin exposure (***$p = 0.019$, **$p < 0.0001$, Tukey's multiple comparisons test). **(D)** Changes in the numbers of pyknotic nuclei plotted as a function of neomycin exposure/post-exposure time. The number of pyknotic nuclei/neuromast became significantly elevated after 20 min of neomycin exposure (**$p < 0.0001$). The time course of the neomycin-induced formation of pyknotic nuclei parallels the death of hair cells. **(E)** Contacts between macrophages and hair cells increased after 20 min of neomycin treatment (***$p = 0.0038$, one-way ANOVA) and remained elevated until 60 min after treatment. **(F)** Macrophage phagocytosis of hair cell debris (i.e., internalization of otoferlin-labeled material and/or pyknotic nuclei) was also increased, beginning after 20 min of neomycin treatment (***$p < 0.0044$, one-way ANOVA).

macrophages in the posterior-most 500 μm of all fish (**Figure 6**). Control fish contained 16.3 ± 4.9 macrophages in this region (**Figures 6A,C**), but the MTZ-treatment dramatically reduced the number of macrophages, to 0.8 ± 1.1. When MTZ-treated fish were allowed to recover for 48 h ($n = 14$), the tail contained 3.2 ± 2.2 macrophages ($p < 0.0001$, two-tailed t-test), indicating that significant macrophage depletion persists for (at least) 2 days. To verify that expression of the *Ntr* transgene did not affect the normal development of the lateral line, we also examined hair cell numbers in *Tg(mpeg1:Gal4FF/UAS:NTR-mCherry)* and sibling fish that lack the transgenes. Neuromast L5 of *Ntr*-expressing fish contained 10.1 ± 1.4 hair cells vs. 10.6 ± 1.2 hair cells in fish that lacked the *Ntr* transgene ($n = 10/15$, $p = 0.35$).

To determine whether the depletion of macrophages affected hair cell regeneration after ototoxic injury, *Tg(mpeg1:Gal4FF/UAS:NTR-mCherry)* fish were treated for 24 h with either 10 mM MTZ or 0.1% DMSO. All fish were then rinsed and: (1) exposed for 30 min to 100 μM neomycin; (2) thoroughly rinsed; and (3) returned to drug-free EM. Hair cells were quantified from neuromast L5 and the two most-posterior ("terminal") neuromasts at 2 and 48 h after neomycin treatment (examples shown in **Figures 7A,B**). At 2 h post-neomycin, the number of surviving hair cells was nearly identical in both MTZ-treated and control fish (**Figure 7C**; 1.1 ± 1.2 vs. 0.9 ± 1.0; $n = 30/40$; $p = 0.32$), suggesting that macrophage depletion did not affect ototoxicity. Hair cell regeneration was evident in both MTZ-treated and control fish at 48 h after neomycin treatment. Neuromast L5 of MTZ-treated fish contained 6.7 ± 2.2 hair cells, while L5 of DMSO-treated fish contained 7.7 ± 2.0 hair cells ($n = 19$/group, $p = 0.19$). In the two terminal neuromasts, the number of regenerated hair cells in MTZ-treated fish was 5.6 ± 1.5 vs. 6.9 ± 1.8 in DMSO-treated fish (**Figure 7D**, $n = 44/38$; $p = 0.0012$). Together, these observations suggest that depletion of macrophages had only a small effect on hair cell regeneration after neomycin ototoxicity.

DISCUSSION

Macrophages are a type of leukocyte that recognize, engulf, and neutralize invading pathogens and are also actively involved in tissue homeostasis and injury response (e.g., Gordon and Plüddemann, 2018). Macrophages are recruited to tissue lesion sites, where they remove the debris of dead cells and release extracellular matrix constituents and growth factors that promote repair and regeneration. The inner ears of birds and mammals contain resident macrophages which are activated by hair cell injury (Warchol, 1997; Bhave et al., 1998; Hirose et al., 2005; Warchol et al., 2012). Prior studies have shown that otic macrophages remove cellular debris after noise trauma or ototoxicity (Kaur et al., 2015a, 2018). It should be noted, however, that macrophages are not the only resident phagocyte in the inner ear. The supporting cells of the sensory epithelium can also act as "amateur phagocytes," by forming multi-cellular complexes that engulf dying cells (Bird et al., 2010; Anttonen et al., 2014; Monzack et al., 2015; Bucks et al., 2017)

Our data suggest that the interactions between macrophages and lateral line hair cells are similar to those that occur in the inner ear. As noted, the uninjured cochlea and vestibular organs possess resident populations of macrophages (Warchol, 1997; Hirose et al., 2005; Kaur et al., 2015a), and our data indicate that 1–2 macrophages are typically present within a 25 μm radius of uninjured neuromasts (**Figure 1**; also see Herbomel et al., 1999). The signals responsible for the association between macrophages and hair cell epithelia are not known, but our data are consistent with the notion that a chemoattractant may be released from uninjured neuromasts, to maintain a nearby "resident" population. Our data further show that the numbers of macrophages present at injured neuromasts are comparable to the numbers observed at undamaged neuromasts. This result, which is consistent with previous data (Hirose et al., 2017), suggests that the initial macrophage response to hair cell injury is mediated by "local" macrophages.

Studies of the mammalian ear indicate that hair cell death alone—without any accompanying damage to other cells or tissues—is sufficient to recruit macrophages into the sensory regions of the cochlea and utricle (Kaur et al., 2015a,b). The signals that evoke this response have not been identified. Our data show that neomycin-induced hair cell death causes macrophages to enter lateral line neuromasts, and the rapid nature of this response suggests that hair cells (or perhaps supporting cells) release a chemotactic signal early in the ototoxic process. The macrophage response to hair cell injury occurs more quickly in zebrafish than in mammals. In part, this is due to the very fast process of neomycin-induced hair cell death (~20–30 min; **Figure 3**). Also, macrophages are usually present immediately outside the borders of lateral line neuromasts, so they can quickly detect and respond to a hypothetical injury signal from dying hair cells. Numerous signals have

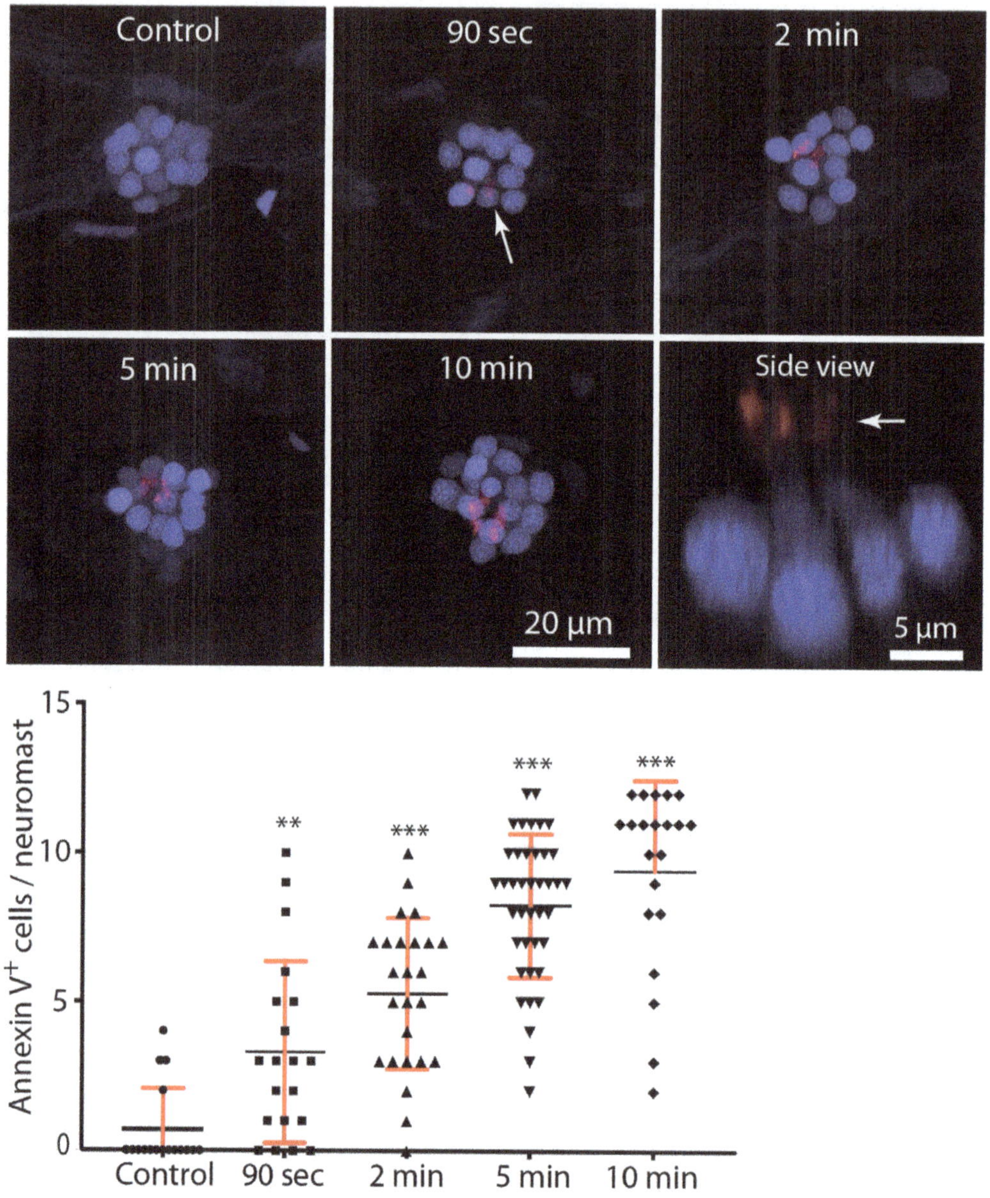

FIGURE 4 | Rapid externalization of phosphatidylserine (PtS) in response to neomycin treatment. Larval zebrafish (6 dpf) were incubated in Alexa 555-conjugated annexin V and neomycin was added to the water, for a final concentration of 100 μM. Fish were euthanized and fixed after 90 s, 2, 5, or 10 min of exposure to neomycin. Annexin V labeling was observed on the stereocilia bundles of most neomycin-treated fish (e.g., arrow, 90-s image, each red structure represents a single stereocilia bundle), and indicates the presence of PtS on the outer membrane surface. We observed annexin V binding as early as 90 s after the initiation of neomycin treatment (** $p = 0.0045$, one-way ANOVA), and the number of annexin V-labeled cells increased with longer exposure times (*** $p < 0.0001$, one-way ANOVA). Annexin V labeling was limited to the apical (external) surface of hair cells, as confirmed by side view reconstruction of confocal stacks (arrow, "side view"). We observed no labeling on the basal hair cell surface, which is located within the epidermal barrier of the fish. We also did not observe annexin V binding on any other cells within the body of the fish, suggesting that annexin V does not become internalized. Plotted data were collected from neuromasts L4/5, for a total of 17–40 neuromasts/time point.

been shown to recruit macrophages to injury sites in other tissues. These include the pannexin-mediated release of ATP (Adamson and Leitinger, 2014), the generation and release of reactive oxygen species (ROS) such as H_2O_2 (Tauzin et al., 2014), and the release of certain chemokines (Gillitzer and Goebeler, 2001). It is further notable that both ATP and ROS are known to be produced or released during ototoxic injury and hair cell death (e.g., Gale et al., 2004; Lahne and Gale, 2010; Esterberg et al., 2016), making them ideal candidates for future studies of hair cell-macrophage interactions. The rapid macrophage response reported here suggests that the zebrafish lateral line may be an advantageous model system in which to identify the signals that attract macrophages to injured hair cells.

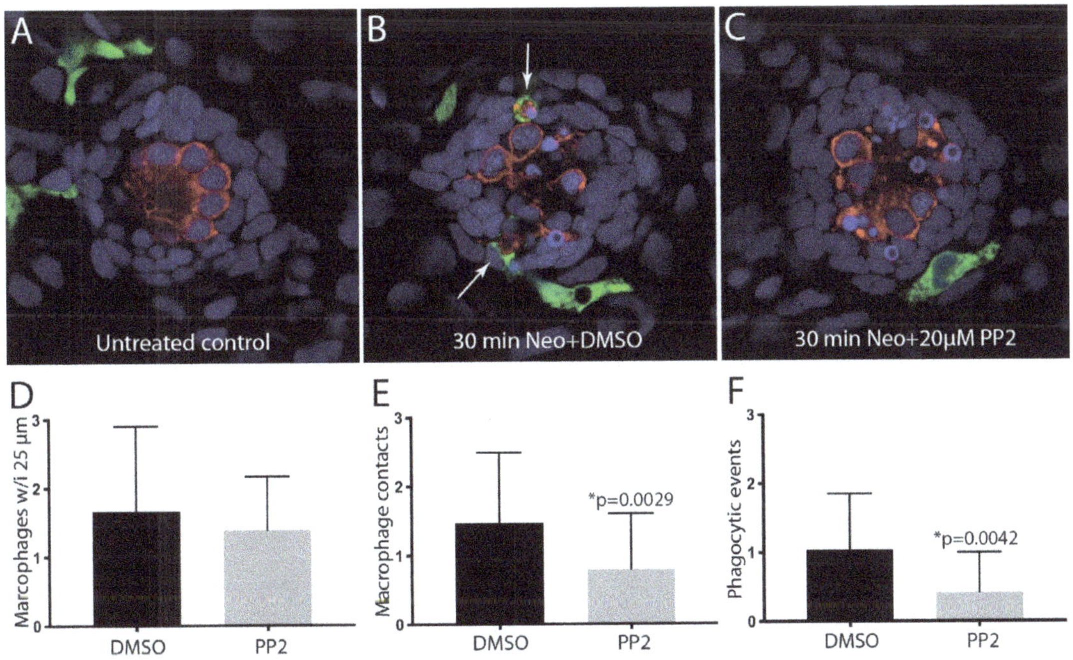

FIGURE 5 | Inhibition of Src-family kinases reduced macrophage entry into injured neuromasts. Larval zebrafish were treated in 20 μM PP2, an inhibitor of several Src kinases. Control fish were treated in parallel with 0.1% DMSO. After 1 h pretreatment, neomycin was added to the water of both treatment groups (for a final concentration of 100 μM), and all specimens were euthanized and fixed after 30 min of neomycin exposure. **(A–C)** Single *z*-section images taken from 15 μm-depth confocal stacks. Arrows in panel **(B)** indicate macrophage phagocytosis of dying hair cells. **(D–F)** Quantification of macrophage activity. Normal numbers of macrophages were present near neuromasts L4/5 in all fish **(D)**. Fish that were treated with 0.1% DMSO displayed a normal macrophage response to neomycin injury, but pretreatment with PP2 resulted in fewer macrophage contacts with dying hair cells **(E)** and reduced numbers of phagocytic events **(F)**. Data were obtained from 34 fish for each treatment group/time point.

The signals that target dying hair cells for phagocytosis are also not known. One common "eat me" signal displayed by dying cells is the presence of phosphatidylserine (PtS) on the external membrane surface. Healthy cells possess asymmetrical localization of phospholipids on the inner and outer membrane leaflets, with PtS present on the inner leaflet and phosphatidylcholine exposed on the outer leaflet (Nagata, 2018). This distribution pattern is maintained by ATP-dependent transporters ("flippases"). In contrast, dying cells are characterized by the presence of PtS on the outer membrane leaflet. The internal-to-external translocation of PtS on injured cells is mediated *via* two distinct mechanisms: (1) Ca^{2+} -dependent activation of the TMEM16 transporter and (2) caspase-dependent activation of the XKR8 "scramblase." Externalized PtS is a highly-conserved signal that is recognized by phagocytes and leads to the engulfment and removal of apoptotic cells (reviewed by Klöditz et al., 2017). The present study used Alexa 555-conjugated Annexin V to examine PtS externalization in hair cells after exposure to neomycin. We found that very few hair cells in normal (control) fish possessed external PtS. However, enhanced levels of externalized PtS were observed on the apical surfaces of lateral line hair cells after only 90 s of neomycin treatment, and the number of such PtS-expressing cells increased with longer exposure times. These observations are very similar to those reported in studies of the mammalian cochlea (Goodyear et al., 2008), and suggest that neomycin induces very rapid changes in hair cell homeostasis. The timing is also consistent with the notion that externalized PtS may target injured hair cells for phagocytic removal. One complication with this suggestion is that macrophages are likely to detect PtS on the basal (internal) surfaces of hair cells, while we observed annexin V labeling only on the apical (external) surface. Given that larval fish are likely to contain numerous cells undergoing developmental apoptosis (e.g., Shklover et al., 2015), we speculate that the lack of internal annexin V labeling is a consequence of the inability of annexin V to cross the epidermal barrier. We cannot, however, rule out the possibility that externalized PtS is not present on the basal surfaces of injured hair cells.

Our data further suggest that activation of Src family kinases is involved in the entry of macrophages into injured neuromasts and the subsequent phagocytosis of hair cell debris. The Src family consists of nine nonreceptor tyrosine kinases that serve diverse roles in cell signaling. Macrophages express several SFK's (e.g., Fgr, Fyn, Hck, Lyn), which are activated downstream of toll-like receptors and regulate macrophage response to pathogens (reviewed by Byeon et al., 2012). Also, Lyn can be directly activated by diffusible H_2O_2, which functions as a leukocyte chemoattractant (Yoo et al., 2011; 2012). A prior study has shown that ROS are generated by zebrafish hair cells within 5–10 min of exposure to neomycin (Esterberg et al., 2016), raising the possibility that such hair cells may release H_2O_2, which then recruits macrophages into neuromasts in a Lyn-dependent

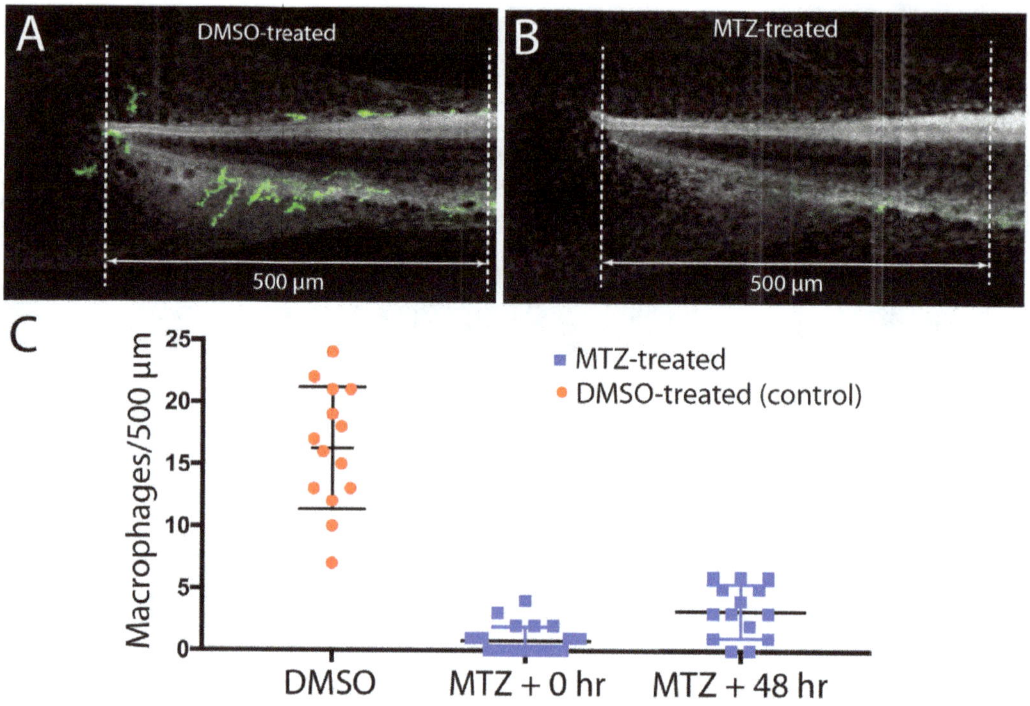

FIGURE 6 | Selective depletion of macrophages in *Tg(mpeg1:Gal4FF/UAS:NTR-mCherry)* fish. Experiments utilized a transgenic fish line that expresses the bacterial enzyme NTR under the regulation of the *Mpeg1* promoter (i.e., selectively in macrophages and microglia). Treatment of these fish with 0.1% DMSO did not affect the numbers of macrophages distributed within the posterior-most 500 µm of the spinal column **(A,C)**. However, treatment for 24 h in 10 mM MTZ resulted in the nearly complete elimination of macrophages from this same region **(B,C)**. Macrophage numbers remained low after 48 h recovery from MTZ treatment **(C)**. Data obtained from 10 to 15 fish/treatment group.

fashion. Generation of ROS also occurs in mammalian hair cells after noise trauma or ototoxic injury (reviewed by Fetoni et al., 2019) and it conceivable that extracellular release of ROS may also promote macrophage migration towards the injured organ of Corti. In future studies, the possible involvement of Lyn activation and SFK signaling in hair cell-macrophage interactions in the mammalian ear can be tested using genetic knockout animals (e.g., Chan et al., 1997).

Finally, our experiments tested the possible role of macrophages in the process of hair cell regeneration. Nonmammalian vertebrates can regenerate hair cells after injury, resulting in the restoration of sensory function. Such regeneration is mediated by nonsensory supporting cells, which surround hair cells in their native epithelia and are involved in homeostasis and regulation of the ionic environment. Hair cell death in nonmammals triggers supporting cells to either divide or undergo phenotypic conversion, leading to the production of replacement hair cells (reviewed by Warchol, 2011; Denans et al., 2019). The biological signals responsible for hair cell regeneration are largely unidentified. Given that macrophages have been shown to promote regeneration in many injured tissues (e.g., Theret et al., 2019), it has been proposed that recruited macrophages may also help initiate hair cell regeneration (e.g., Corwin et al., 1991; Warchol, 1997, 1999). The time course of macrophage recruitment is consistent with this notion since macrophages migrate to sites of hair cell injury before the onset of regenerative proliferation or phenotypic conversion (Warchol, 1997; Hirose et al., 2017). However, a more recent study of regeneration in the avian cochlea found that the selective macrophage depletion had no impact on either supporting cell proliferation or hair cell replacement (Warchol et al., 2012). The data presented here further indicate that macrophages are not essential for hair cell regeneration. Macrophages quickly entered injured neuromasts and phagocytosed dying cells, but chemical-genetic depletion of macrophages had very little impact on the level of hair cell regeneration after neomycin injury. Also, macrophage depletion did not affect the number of surviving hair cells or the extent of ototoxic injury. It should be noted that Warchol et al. (2012) found that depletion of macrophages caused a reduction in proliferation of some mesenchymal cells that reside outside of the sensory epithelium, so it is still possible that macrophages may be involved in the maintenance and repair of nonsensory structures within the inner ear.

A prior study has also examined the contribution of macrophages to hair cell regeneration in larval zebrafish (Carrillo et al., 2016). Macrophage depletion was induced by local injections of liposomally-encapsulated clodronate, which reduced macrophage numbers in the vicinity of identified neuromasts. These interventions appeared to cause a slight reduction in the number of regenerated hair cells/neuromast

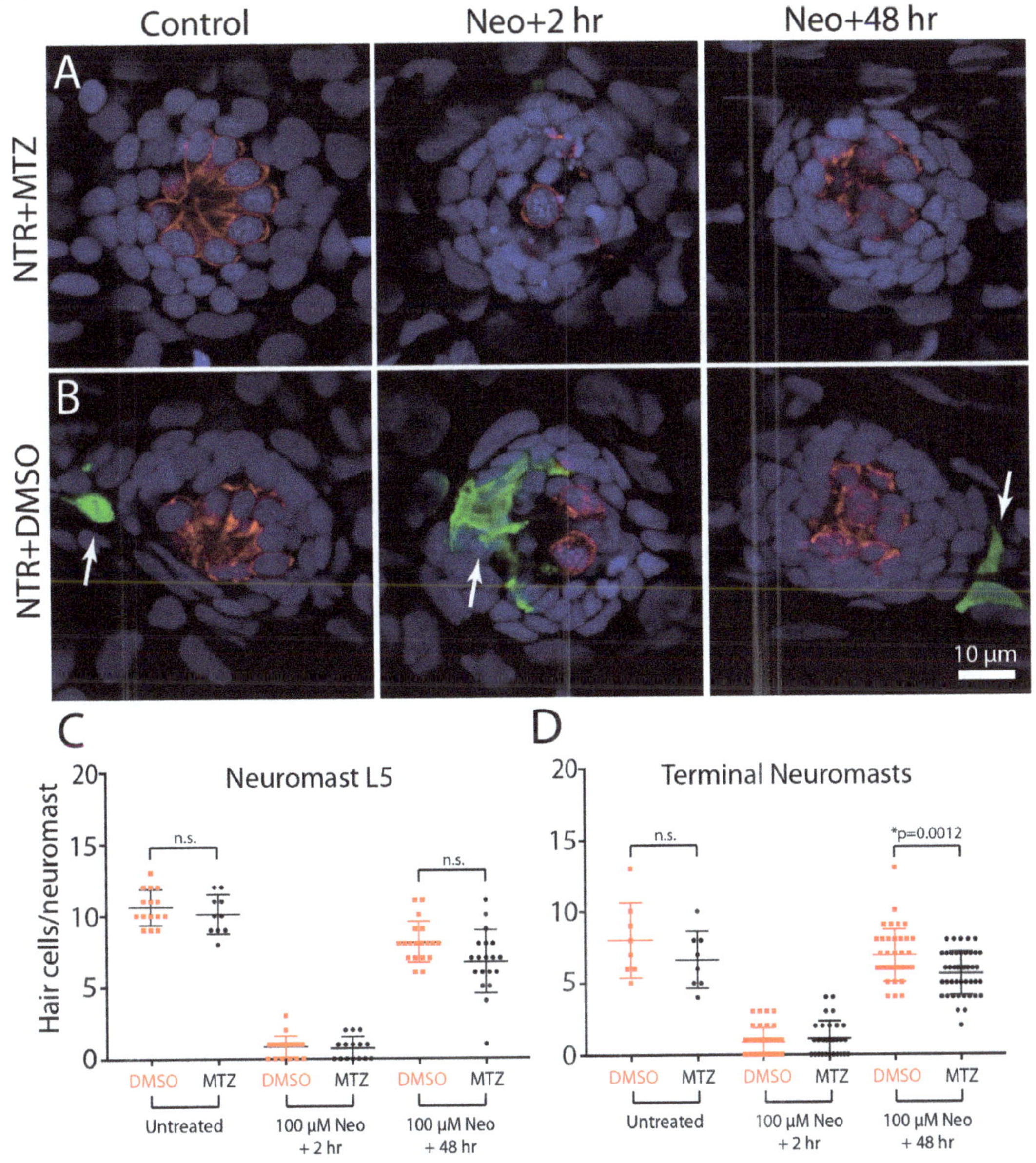

FIGURE 7 | Depletion of macrophages had minimal impact on hair cell regeneration. *Tg(mpeg1:Gal4FF/UAS:NTR-mCherry)* fish were treated for 24 h in either 10 mM MTZ or 0.1% DMSO. All fish were then rinsed and incubated for 30 min in 100 μM neomycin. Fish were rinsed again and maintained for an additional 2 h or 48 h. Hair cells and macrophages were immunolabeled and hair cell numbers were quantified from neuromast L5 and the two terminal neuromasts. Images from MTZ-treated fish **(A)** show the absence of macrophages, but otherwise normal levels of neomycin injury and subsequent regeneration. **(B)** Normal ototoxicity, macrophage recruitment (arrows), and regeneration in DMSO-treated fish. Quantitative data **(C,D)** show that hair cell injury and regeneration were nearly-identical in normal and macrophage-depleted fish, although the number of regenerated hair cells in the two terminal neuromasts of MTZ-treated was slightly reduced when compared to DMSO-treated controls (*$p = 0.0012$; n.s.–$p > 0.05$).

at 24 h recovery (~4 HCs in clodronate-treated vs. ~5 HCs in controls), but no difference in regeneration at 48 h recovery. The data reported by Carrillo et al. (2016) are generally consistent with those described reported here, i.e., we found that depleting macrophages caused a slight reduction in regeneration in the terminal neuromasts. However, the findings of both studies demonstrate that the presence of normal numbers of macrophages is not necessary for lateral line regeneration.

In summary, our results show that macrophages normally reside near lateral line neuromasts and are recruited into neuromasts during the early stages of ototoxic injury. Such macrophages quickly engulf the debris of dying hair cells. Our data further suggest that activation of Src-family kinases is required for normal macrophage recruitment and that dying hair cells possess externalized PtS, a signal that targets other types of apoptotic cells for phagocytic removal. However, our data indicate that selective elimination of macrophages had a very minimal effect on hair cell recovery after ototoxic injury, suggesting that macrophages do not serve an essential role in the process of hair cell regeneration. The molecules that mediate signaling between sensory hair cells and macrophages are currently not known, but our findings suggest that the zebrafish lateral line may be an advantageous model system in which to study hair cell-immune interactions.

AUTHOR CONTRIBUTIONS

MW designed the study. MW and AS performed the experimental work. MW and LS assessed the data and wrote the manuscript. All authors contributed to the article and approved the submitted version.

ACKNOWLEDGMENTS

Transgenic fish lines were provided by Drs. David Raible and Lalita Ramakrishnan. This manuscript has been released as a pre-print at bioRxiv (Warchol et al., 2020).

REFERENCES

Adamson, S. E., and Leitinger, N. (2014). The role of pannexin1 in the induction and resolution of inflammation. *FEBS Lett.* 588, 1416–1422. doi: 10.1016/j.febslet.2014.03.009

Anttonen, T., Belevich, I., Kirjavainen, A., Laos, M., Brakebusch, C., Jokitalo, E., et al. (2014). How to bury the dead: elimination of apoptotic hair cells from the hearing organ of the mouse. *J. Assoc. Res. Otolaryngol.* 15, 975–992. doi: 10.1007/s10162-014-0480-x

Bhave, S. A., Oesterle, E. C., and Coltrera, M. D. (1998). Macrophage and microglia-like cells in the avian inner ear. *J. Comp. Neurol.* 398, 241–256. doi: 10.1002/(sici)1096-9861(19980824)398:2<241::aid-cne6>3.0.co;2-0

Bird, J. E., Daudet, N., Warchol, M. E., and Gale, J. E. (2010). Supporting cells eliminate dying sensory hair cells to maintain epithelial integrity in the avian inner ear. *J. Neurosci.* 30, 12545–12556. doi: 10.1523/JNEUROSCI.3042-10.2010

Bucks, S. A., Cox, B. C., Vlosich, B. A., Manning, J. P., Nguyen, T. B., and Stone, J. S. (2017). Supporting cells remove and replace sensory receptor hair cells in a balance organ of adult mice. *eLife* 6:e18128. doi: 10.7554/eLife.18128

Byeon, S. E., Yi, Y. S., Oh, J., Yoo, B. C., Hong, S., and Cho, J. Y. (2012). The role of Src kinase in macrophage-mediated inflammatory responses. *Mediators Inflamm.* 2012:512926. doi: 10.1155/2012/512926

Carrillo, S. A., Anguita-Salinas, C., Peña, O. A., Morales, R. A., Muñoz-Sánchez, S., Muñoz-Montecinos, C., et al. (2016). Macrophage recruitment contributes to regeneration of mechanosensory hair cells in the zebrafish lateral line. *J. Cell. Biochem.* 117, 1880–1889. doi: 10.1002/jcb.25487

Chan, V. W., Meng, F., Soriano, P., DeFranco, A. L., and Lowell, C. A. (1997). Characterization of the B lymphocyte populations in Lyn-deficient mice and the role of Lyn in signal initiation and down-regulation. *Immunity* 7, 69–81. doi: 10.1016/s1074-7613(00)80511-7

Corwin, J. T., Jones, J. E., Katayama, A., Kelley, M. W., and Warchol, M. E. (1991). Hair cell regeneration: the identities of progenitor cells, potential triggers and instructive cues. *Ciba Found. Symp.* 160, 103–120; discussion 120–130. doi: 10.1002/9780470514122.ch6

Denans, N., Baek, S., and Piotrowski, T. (2019). Comparing sensory organs to define the path for hair cell regeneration. *Ann. Rev. Cell Dev. Biol.* 35, 567–589. doi: 10.1146/annurev-cellbio-100818-125503

Davison, J. M., Akitake, C. M., Goll, M. G., Rhee, J. M., Gosse, N., Baier, H., et al. (2007). Transactivation from Gal4-VP16 transgenic insertions for tissue-specific cell labeling and ablation in zebrafish. *Dev. Biol.* 304, 811–824. doi: 10.1016/j.ydbio.2007.01.033

Dwyer, A. R., Mouchemore, K. A., Steer, J. H., Sunderland, A. J., Sampaio, N. G., Greenland, E. L., et al. (2016). Src family kinase expression and subcellular localization in macrophages: implications for their role in CSF-1-induced macrophage migration. *J. Leukoc. Biol.* 100, 163–175. doi: 10.1189/jlb.2A0815-344RR

Ellett, F., Pase, L., Hayman, J. W., Andrianopoulos, A., and Lieschke, G. J. (2011). mpeg1 Promoter transgenes direct macrophage-lineage expression in zebrafish. *Blood* 117, e49–e56. doi: 10.1182/blood-2010-10-314120

Esterberg, R., Linbo, T., Pickett, S. B., Wu, P., Ou, H. C., Rubel, E. W., et al. (2016). Mitochondrial calcium uptake underlies ROS generation during aminoglycoside-induced hair cell death. *J. Clin. Invest.* 126, 3556–3566. doi: 10.1172/JCI84939

Fadok, V. A., Voelker, D. R., Campbell, P. A., Cohen, J. J., Bratton, D. L., and Henson, P. M. (1992). Exposure of phosphatidylserine on the surface of apoptotic lymphocytes triggers specific recognition and removal by macrophages. *J. Immunol.* 148, 2207–2216.

Fetoni, A. R., Paciello, F., Rolesi, R., Paludetti, G., and Troiani, D. (2019). Targeting dysregulation of redox homeostasis in noise-induced hearing loss: oxidative stress and ROS signaling. *Free Radic. Biol. Med.* 135, 46–59. doi: 10.1016/j.freeradbiomed.2019.02.022

Freedman, T. S., Tan, Y. X., Skrzypczynska, K. M., Manz, B. N., Sjaastad, F. V., Goodridge, H. S., et al. (2015). LynA regulates an inflammation-sensitive signaling checkpoint in macrophages. *eLife* 4:e09183. doi: 10.7554/eLife.09183

Gale, J. E., Piazza, V., Ciubotaru, C. D., and Mammano, F. (2004). A mechanism for sensing noise damage in the inner ear. *Curr. Biol.* 14, 526–529. doi: 10.1016/j.cub.2004.03.002

Gillitzer, R., and Goebeler, M. (2001). Chemokines in cutaneous wound healing. *J. Leukoc. Biol.* 69, 513–521.

Goodyear, R. J., Gale, J. E., Ranatunga, K. M., Kros, C. J., and Richardson, G. P. (2008). Aminoglycoside-induced phosphatidylserine externalization in sensory hair cells is regionally restricted, rapid and reversible. Version 2. *J. Neurosci.* 28, 9939–9952. doi: 10.1523/JNEUROSCI.1124-08.2008

Goodyear, R. J., Legan, P. K., Christiansen, J. R., Xia, B., Korchagina, J., Gale, J. E., et al. (2010). Identification of the hair cell soma-1 antigen, HCS-1, as otoferlin. *J. Assoc. Res. Otolaryngol.* 11, 573–586. doi: 10.1007/s10162-010-0231-6

Gordon, S., and Plüddemann, A. (2018). Macrophage clearance of apoptotic cells: a critical assessment. *Front. Immunol.* 9:127. doi: 10.3389/fimmu.2018.00127

Harris, J. A., Cheng, A. G., Cunningham, L. L., MacDonald, G., Raible, D. W., and Rubel, E. W. (2003). Neomycin-induced hair cell death and rapid regeneration in the lateral line of zebrafish (*Danio rerio*). *J. Assoc. Res. Otolaryngol.* 4, 219–234. doi: 10.1007/s10162-002-3022-x

Herbomel, P., Thisse, B., and Thisse, C. (1999). Ontogeny and behaviour of early macrophages in the zebrafish embryo. *Development* 126, 3735–3745.

Hernández, P. P., Moreno, V., Olivari, F. A., and Allende, M. L. (2006). Sub-lethal concentrations of waterborne copper are toxic to lateral line neuromasts in zebrafish (*Danio rerio*). *Hear. Res.* 213, 1–10. doi: 10.1016/j.heares.2005.10.015

Hirose, K., Discolo, C. M., Keasler, J. R., and Ransohoff, R. (2005). Mononuclear phagocytes migrate into the murine cochlea after acoustic trauma. *J. Comp. Neurol.* 489, 180–194. doi: 10.1002/cne.20619

Hirose, K., Rutherford, M. A., and Warchol, M. E. (2017). Two cell populations participate in clearance of damaged hair cells from the sensory epithelia of the inner ear. *Hear. Res.* 352, 70–81. doi: 10.1016/j.heares.2017.04.006

Holmgren, M., Ravicz, M. E., Hancock, K. E., Strelkova, O., Indzhykulian, A. A., Warchol, M. E., et al. (2020). Mechanical overstimulation causes acute injury followed by fast recovery in lateral line neuromasts of larval zebrafish. *BioRxiv* [Preprint]. doi: 10.1101/2020.07.15.205492

Jones, J. E., and Corwin, J. T. (1993). Replacement of lateral line sensory organs during tail regeneration in salamanders: identification of progenitor cells and analysis of leukocyte activity. *J. Neurosci.* 13, 1022–1034. doi: 10.1523/JNEUROSCI.13-03-01022.1993

Jones, J. E., and Corwin, J. T. (1996). Regeneration of sensory cells after laser ablation in the lateral line system: hair cell lineage and macrophage behavior revealed by time-lapse video microscopy. *J. Neurosci.* 16, 649–662. doi: 10.1523/JNEUROSCI.16-02-00649.1996

Kaur, T., Ohlemiller, K. K., and Warchol, M. E. (2018). Genetic disruption of fractalkine signaling leads to enhanced loss of cochlear afferents following ototoxic or acoustic injury. *J. Comp. Neurol.* 526, 824–835. doi: 10.1002/cne.24369

Kaur, T., Hirose, K., Rubel, E. W., and Warchol, M. E. (2015a). Macrophage recruitment and epithelial repair following hair cell injury in the mouse utricle. *Front. Cell. Neurosci.* 9:150. doi: 10.3389/fncel.2015.00150

Kaur, T., Zamani, D., Tong, L., Rubel, E. W., Ohlemiller, K. K., Hirose, K., et al. (2015b). Fractalkine signaling regulates macrophage recruitment into the cochlea and promotes the survival of spiral ganglion neurons after selective hair cell lesion. *J. Neurosci.* 35, 15050–15061. doi: 10.1523/JNEUROSCI.2325-15.2015

Keightley, M. C., Wang, C. H., Pazhakh, V., and Lieschke, G. J. (2014). Delineating the roles of neutrophils and macrophages in zebrafish regeneration models. *Int. J. Biochem. Cell Biol.* 56, 92–106. doi: 10.1016/j.biocel.2014.07.010

Kindt, K. S., and Sheets, L. (2018). Transmission disrupted: modeling auditory synaptopathy in zebrafish. *Front. Cell Dev. Biol.* 6:114. doi: 10.3389/fcell.2018.00114

Klöditz, K., Chen, Y. Z., Xue, D., and Fadeel, B. (2017). Programmed cell clearance: from nematodes to humans. *Biochem. Biophys. Res. Commun.* 482, 491–497. doi: 10.1016/j.bbrc.2016.12.005

Koopman, G., Reutelingsperger, C. P., Kuijten, G. A., Keehnen, R. M., Pals, S. T., and van Oers, M. H. (1994). Annexin V for flow cytometric detection of phosphatidylserine expression on B cells undergoing apoptosis. *Blood* 84, 1415–1420.

Lahne, M., and Gale, J. E. (2010). Damage-induced cell-cell communication in different cochlear cell types *via* two distinct ATP-dependent Ca waves. *Purinergic Signal.* 6, 189–200. doi: 10.1007/s11302-010-9193-8

Ledent, V. (2002). Postembryonic development of the posterior lateral line in zebrafish. *Development* 129, 597–604.

Ma, E. Y., Rubel, E. W., and Raible, D. W. (2008). Notch signaling regulates the extent of hair cell regeneration in the zebrafish lateral line. *J. Neurosci.* 28, 2261–2273. doi: 10.1523/JNEUROSCI.4372-07.2008

Monzack, E. L., May, L. A., Roy, S., Gale, J. E., and Cunningham, L. L. (2015). Live imaging the phagocytic activity of inner ear supporting cells in response to hair cell death. *Cell Death Differ.* 22, 1995–2005. doi: 10.1038/cdd.2015.48

Nagata, S. (2018). Apoptosis and clearance of apoptotic cells. *Annu. Rev. Immunol.* 36, 489–517. doi: 10.1146/annurev-immunol-042617-053010

Petrie, T. A., Strand, N. S., Yang, C. T., Rabinowitz, J. S., and Moon, R. T. (2014).Macrophages modulate adult zebrafish tail fin regeneration. *Development* 141, 2581–2591. doi: 10.1242/dev.098459

Pickett, S. B., and Raible, D. W. (2019). Water waves to sound waves: using zebrafish to explore hair cell biology. *J. Assoc. Res. Otolaryngol.* 20, 1–19. doi: 10.1007/s10162-018-00711-1

Roca, F. J., and Ramakrishnan, L. (2013). TNF dually mediates resistance and susceptibility to mycobacteria *via* mitochondrial reactive oxygen species. *Cell* 153, 521–534. doi: 10.1016/j.cell.2013.03.022

Romero-Carvajal, A., Navajas Acedo, J., Jiang, L., Kozlovskaja-Gumbrienė, A., Alexander, R., Li, H., et al. (2015). Regeneration of sensory hair cells requires localized interactions between the Notch and Wnt pathways. *Dev. Cell* 34, 267–282. doi: 10.1016/j.devcel.2015.05.025

Shklover, J., Levy-Adam, F., and Kurant, E. (2015). Apoptotic cell clearance in development. *Curr. Top. Dev. Biol.* 114, 297–334. doi: 10.1016/bs.ctdb.2015.07.024

Svahn, A. J., Graeber, M. B., Ellett, F., Lieschke, G. J., Rinkwitz, S., Bennett, M. R., et al. (2013). Development of ramified microglia from early macrophages in the zebrafish optic tectum. *Dev. Neurobiol.* 73, 60–71. doi: 10.1002/dneu.22039

Tauzin, S., Starnes, T. W., Becker, F. B., Lam, P. Y., and Huttenlocher, A. (2014). Redox and Src family kinase signaling control leukocyte wound attraction and neutrophil reverse migration. *J. Cell Biol.* 207, 589–598. doi: 10.1083/jcb.201408090

Theret, M., Mounier, R., and Rossi, F. (2019). The origins and non-canonical functions of macrophages in development and regeneration. *Development* 146:dev156000. doi: 10.1242/dev.156000

Uribe, P. M., Villapando, B. K., Lawton, K. J., Fang, Z., Gritsenko, D., Bhandiwad, A., et al. (2018). Larval zebrafish lateral line as a model for acoustic trauma. *eNeuro* 5:ENEURO.0206-18.2018. doi: 10.1523/ENEURO.0206-18.2018

Wagner, E. L., and Shin, J. B. (2019). Mechanisms of hair cell damage and repair. *Trends Neurosci.* 42, 414–424. doi: 10.1016/j.tins.2019.03.006

Warchol, M. E. (1997). Macrophage activity in organ cultures of the avian cochlea: demonstration of a resident population and recruitment to sites of hair cell lesions. *J. Neurobiol.* 33, 724–734.

Warchol, M. E. (1999). Immune cytokines and dexamethasone influence sensory regeneration in the avian vestibular periphery. *J Neurocytol.* 28, 889–900. doi: 10.1023/a:1007026306730

Warchol, M. E. (2019). Interactions between macrophages and the sensory cells of the inner ear. *Cold Spring Harb. Perspect. Med.* 9:a033555. doi: 10.1101/cshperspect.a033555

Warchol, M. E. (2011). Sensory regeneration in the vertebrate inner ear: differences at the levels of cells and species. *Hear. Res.* 273, 72–79. doi: 10.1016/j.heares.2010.05.004

Warchol, M. E., Schwendener, R. A., and Hirose, K. (2012). Depletion of resident macrophages does not alter sensory regeneration in the avian cochlea. *PLoS One* 7:e51574. doi: 10.1371/journal.pone.0051574

Warchol, M. E., Schrader, A., and Sheets, L. (2020). Macrophages respond rapidly to ototoxic injury of lateral line hair cells but are not required for hair cell regeneration. *BioRxiv.* [Preprint]. doi: 10.1101/2020.09.28.314922

Westerfield, M. (2000). *The Zebrafish Book. A Guide for the Laboratory Use of Zebrafish (Danio rerio).* 4th Edn. Eugene: University of Oregon Press.

Wynn, T. A., and Vannella, K. M. (2016). Macrophages in tissue repair, regeneration and fibrosis. *Immunity* 44, 450–462. doi: 10.1016/j.immuni.2016.02.015

Yoo, S. K., Starnes, T. W., Deng, Q., and Huttenlocher, A. (2011). Lyn is a redox sensor that mediates leukocyte wound attraction *in vivo*. *Nature* 480, 109–112. doi: 10.1038/nature10632

Yoo, S. K., Freisinger, C. M., LeBert, D. C., and Huttenlocher, A. (2012). Early redox, Src family kinase and calcium signaling integrate wound responses and tissue regeneration in zebrafish. *J. Cell Biol.* 199, 225–234. doi: 10.1083/jcb.201203154

Zhu, X., Kim, J. L., Newcomb, J. R., Rose, P. E., Stover, D. R., Toledo, L. M., et al. (1999). Structural analysis of the lymphocyte-specific

2

Rapamycin Added to Diet in Late Mid-Life Delays Age-Related Hearing Loss in UMHET4 Mice

Richard A. Altschuler[1,2,3], Lisa Kabara[1], Catherine Martin[1], Ariane Kanicki[1], Courtney E. Stewart[1,2], David C. Kohrman[1] and David F. Dolan[1]*

[1] Kresge Hearing Research Institute, Department of Otolaryngology, Head and Neck Surgery, University of Michigan, Ann Arbor, MI, United States, [2] VA Ann Arbor Health Care System, Ann Arbor, MI, United States, [3] Department of Cell and Developmental Biology, University of Michigan, Ann Arbor, MI, United States

Correspondence:
Richard A. Altschuler
shuler@umich.edu

Our previous study demonstrated rapamycin added to diet at 4 months of age had significantly less age-related outer hair cell loss in the basal half of the cochlea at 22 months of age compared to mice without rapamycin. The present study tested adding rapamycin to diet later in life, at 14 months of age, and added a longitudinal assessment of auditory brain stem response (ABR). The present study used UMHET4 mice, a 4 way cross in which all grandparental strains lack the Cdh23^{753A} allele that predisposes to early onset, progressive hearing loss. UMHET4 mice typically have normal hearing until 16–17 months, then exhibit threshold shifts at low frequencies/apical cochlea and later in more basal high frequency regions. ABR thresholds at 4, 12, 24, and 48 kHz were assessed at 12, 18, and 24 months of age and compared to baseline ABR thresholds acquired at 5 months of age to determine threshold shifts (TS). There was no TS at 12 months of age at any frequency tested. At 18 months of age mice with rapamycin added to diet at 14 months had a significantly lower mean TS at 4 and 12 kHz compared to mice on control diet with no significant difference at 24 and 48 kHz. At 24 months of age, the mean 4 kHz TS in rapamycin diet group was no longer significantly lower than the control diet group, while the 12 kHz mean remained significantly lower. Mean TS at 24 and 48 kHz in the rapamycin diet group became significantly lower than in the control diet group at 24 months. Hair cell counts at 24 months showed large loss in the apical half of most rapamycin and control diet mice cochleae with no significant difference between groups. There was only mild outer hair cell loss in the basal half of rapamycin and control diet mice cochleae with no significant difference between groups. The results show that a later life addition of rapamycin can decrease age-related hearing loss in the mouse model, however, it also suggests that this decrease is a delay/deceleration rather than a complete prevention.

Keywords: rapamycin, age-related hearing loss, aging, auditory, cochlea, deafness

INTRODUCTION

Age-related hearing loss (ARHL) occurs in approximately one-third of people in the United States over the age of 65 increasing to approximately half of those over the age of 75 (e.g., Gates, 2006; Gates et al., 2010). ARHL can reduce ability to communicate, quality of life and social integration and has been identified as a major risk factor for depression and dementia (e.g., Gates et al., 2010; Lin et al., 2011; Davis and Smith, 2013). One major cause of ARHL is an age-related loss of sensory hair cells, predominantly outer hair cells, and an accompanying decrease in auditory sensitivity as measured by threshold shifts (TS) in auditory brain stem response (ABR) in animal models and audiometric thresholds in people. The underlying mechanisms responsible for age-related hair cell loss remain unknown and there are no treatments currently being clinically applied to prevent or reduce this pathology.

The National Institute on Aging Intervention Testing Program (NIA-ITP) tests for treatments that can be added to diet to increase lifespan, using UMHET3 mice, a four-way cross, as a model. Four-way cross mice (from four different grandparent strains) provide for genetic heterogeneity and reduce strain specific effects. Among several effective treatments identified through NIA-ITP, addition of rapamycin to diet at 9 months of age was found to increase life span by 26% in male mice and 23% in female mice (Miller et al., 2014). We hypothesized that ARHL might share underlying mechanisms, such that treatments that enhance life span could also reduce and/or delay ARHL. This is consistent with studies that demonstrate the positive effects of rapamycin on age-related disorders in animal models, including decreases in cardiac pathology (Dai et al., 2014); muscle weakness (Bitto et al., 2016), cancer incidence (Anisimov et al., 2011), and cognitive decline (Halloran Hussong et al., 2012; Majumder et al., 2012).

In a previous study (Altschuler et al., 2018) we evaluated cochleae from 22 months old UMHET3 mice that had rapamycin added to their diet at 4 months of age as well as from control littermates with normal diet. The 22 months old rapamycin-treated mice had significantly less loss of outer hair cells in the basal half of the cochlea compared to the untreated controls. This sparing of hair cell loss was restricted to the basal half of the cochleae, while the apical half of the cochleae exhibited equivalently large losses of outer hair cells in both rapamycin-fed and normal diet controls (Altschuler et al., 2018).

These results showing rapamycin could reduce or delay age-related hair cell loss in the basal half of the cochlea at 22 months of age raised two pertinent issues. First, the apparent limitation of the treatment effect of rapamycin to the basal half of the cochlea could reflect differences in mechanisms underlying hair cell loss along the cochlear spiral. Alternatively, the effect of rapamycin treatment could be due to delaying rather than preventing age-related hair cell loss. Hair cell loss occurs earlier in apical vs. basal cochlea in most mouse strains (for reviews; Gratton and Vazquez, 2003; Ohlemiller, 2006). If the effect of rapamycin is to "delay" rather than prevent age-related hair cell loss, a treatment induced difference in apical cochleae might also have been present at an earlier time, but by 22 months of age the delay was over and the hair cell loss had equilibrated. The current study was designed to address these points by generating a longitudinal assessment of auditory brain stem response (ABR) thresholds at 4, 12, 24, and 48 kHz in individual mice at 5, 12, 18, and 24 months of age. The current study also addressed a second question of whether beginning rapamycin treatment at a more clinically relevant later age would still be effective in reducing or delaying ARHL. Recent studies have shown that rapamycin can extend life span in mice even when added to diet at 19–20 months of age (Harrison et al., 2009; Zhang et al., 2014) and can also reduce age-related pathologies such as cancer incidence and decreased muscle (Zhang et al., 2014) and cardiac function (Quarles and Rabinovitch, 2020) with late life application. We therefore chose to add rapamycin at a later time but prior to the first appearance of ARHL. Three of the four "grandparent strains" of the UMHET3 mice carry homozygous *ahl* alleles ($Cdh23^{753A}$) that predispose to early onset, hair cell loss and progressive deafness in mice, thus restricting the progeny that can be used in auditory aging studies and decreasing the utility of this four way cross for auditory aging studies (Noben-Trauth et al., 2003; Mianné et al., 2016). For this reason, earlier studies from our group (Schacht et al., 2012; Altschuler et al., 2015) developed a different four-way cross, UMHET4, in which the grandparent strains lack the *ahl* predisposing $Cdh23^{753A}$ alleles. We returned to use of UMHET4 mice in the current study so that all of the progeny could be used. Our previous studies using UMHET4 mice (Schacht et al., 2012; Altschuler et al., 2015) and pilot animals in the current study showed that UMHET4 mice generally have a later appearing ARHL than UMHET3 mice and that ABR TS do not commonly initiate until around 18 months of age. The current study therefore tested the influence of adding rapamycin to mouse diet at 14 months of age.

STUDY DESIGN

UMHET4 mice were entered into the study sequentially as they reached appropriate age points and tested for ABR as they reached 5 months of age. Mice with ABR thresholds more than three standard deviations from the mean at any of the four frequencies (4, 12, 24, and 48 kHz) assessed were excluded from the study. The ABR thresholds at 5 months of age served as individual and group mean baselines and the basis for determining TS at later ages. Mice received a second ABR at 12 months of age and any mice with greater than 10 dB SPL TS at any frequency tested were excluded from the study. At 14 months of age, eligible male and female mice were randomly placed into one of two groups, either a rapamycin diet group or a control diet group. Rapamycin was given encapsulated in the food (pelleted chow) to the mice in the rapamycin treatment group at a dose of 42 mg kg^{-1}, the dose found most effective in increasing lifespan by Miller et al. (2014). Both groups had diet changed at 14 months of age, from standard chow to either rapamycin diet or control diet without rapamycin (but containing the other additions to the rapamycin chow that allowed the rapamycin to be encapsulated). Longitudinal ABR measures from mice in both groups were continued at 18 and 24 months of age and TS (from 5 months old baseline) determined. The control diet group started with 37 mice with 29 surviving until euthanasia at 24 months of age and the rapamycin diet group started with 29 mice with 24 surviving until the 24 months old end point. Animals were euthanized within eight days after the 24 months old ABR measure. The left cochleae were used for hair cell count evaluations (cytocochleograms) and the right cochleae were processed and saved for future gene expression studies.

Breeding

The UM-HET4 mice were generated as described previously (Schacht et al., 2012) by a four-way cross between MOLF/EiJ (Jackson Laboratory stock #000550) × 129S1/SvImJ F1 (Jackson Laboratory stock #002448) female mice and C3H/HeJ (Jackson Laboratory stock #000659) × FVB/NJ F1 (Jackson Laboratory stock #001800) male mice. All of the four grandparental strains lack the *ahl* allele that typically leads to hearing loss appearing at 2–4 months of age (Johnson et al., 2006, for review). Each mouse in the tested UM-HET4 population inherits 25% of its genome from each of the four distinct inbred grandparental stocks and is genetically unique, but shares 50% of its alleles with every other mouse in the tested population. The UM-HET4 mice exhibit variability in their ARHL hearing loss that was correlated with polymorphisms in specific genetic loci (Schacht et al., 2012).

Auditory Brain Stem Response (ABR)

Animals were anesthetized with ketamine (65 mg/kg), xylazine (7 mg/kg), and acepromazine (2 mg/kg). Body temperature was maintained with water circulating heating pads and heat lamps. Additional anesthetic (ketamine and xylazine) was administered when needed to maintain anesthesia depth sufficient to insure immobilization and relaxation. ABRs were then recorded in an electrically and acoustically shielded chamber (Acoustic Systems, Austin, TX, USA). Needle electrodes were placed at vertex (active), the test ear (reference) and the contralateral ear (ground) pinnae. Tucker Davis Technologies (TDT) System III hardware and SigGen/BioSig software (TDT, Alachua, FL, USA) were used to present the stimulus and record responses. Tones were delivered through a EC1 sound driver (TDT) with the speculum placed just inside the tragus. Stimulus presentation used 15 ms tone bursts, with 1 ms rise/fall times, presented 10 per second.

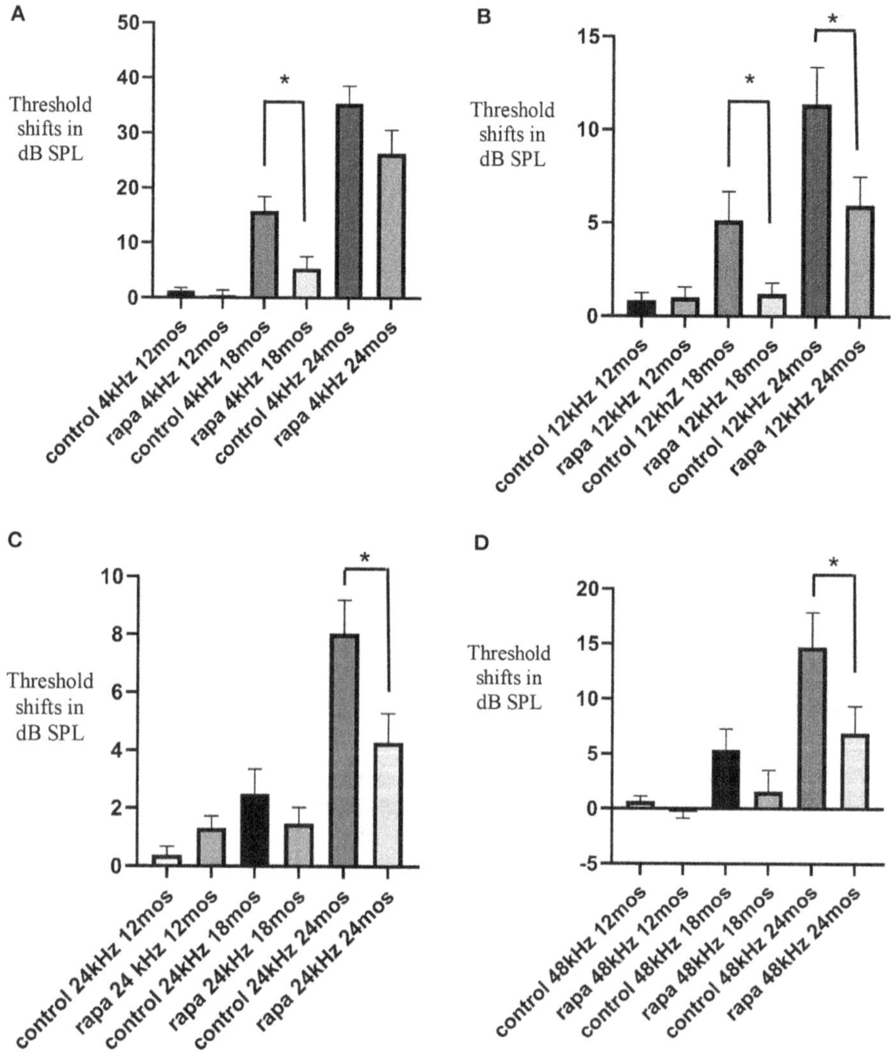

FIGURE 1 | Comparison of mean auditory brain stem response threshold shifts (compared to 5 months of age) in the group with rapamycin added to diet at 14 months of age (rapa) vs. the group on control diet without rapamycin (control) at 12, 18, and 24 months of age at 4 kHz **(A)**, 12 kHz **(B)**, 24 kHz **(C)** and 48 kHz **(D)**. Asterisks indicate significant differences. Please note differences between A, B, C, and D in scale bars for dB SPL on the "y" axis.

Up to 1,024 responses were averaged for each stimulus level. Responses were collected for stimulus levels in 10 dB steps at higher stimulus levels, with additional 5 dB steps near threshold. Thresholds were interpolated between the lowest stimulus level where a response is observed, and 5 dB lower, where no response is observed. The frequencies tested were 4, 12, 24, and 48 kHz.

Histology

Mice were euthanized by intraperitoneal injection of Sodium Pentobarbital (Fatal Plus) followed by decapitation. Cochleae were rapidly removed and middle ears assessed for signs of middle ear infection under a dissection microscope. An opening made through the otic capsule in the apex of the left cochleae and fixative (4% paraformaldehyde in phosphate buffer) was slowly infused into the cochlear fluids. The cochleae were then immersed in fixative for 2–6 h at room temperature on a rotator and rinsed in phosphate buffered saline (PBS) before a 16–24 h decalcification in 5% EDTA at room temperature. This was followed by removal of the otic capsule and tectorial membrane. Cochleae were then stained with 1% Phalloidin- Alexa Fluor 568 in PBS and then micro dissected into three segments, apex, base, and hook. Each segment was mounted separately as a surface preparation on a glass slide with Prolong Gold as mounting media. Slides were stored at 4°C before examination and viewing.

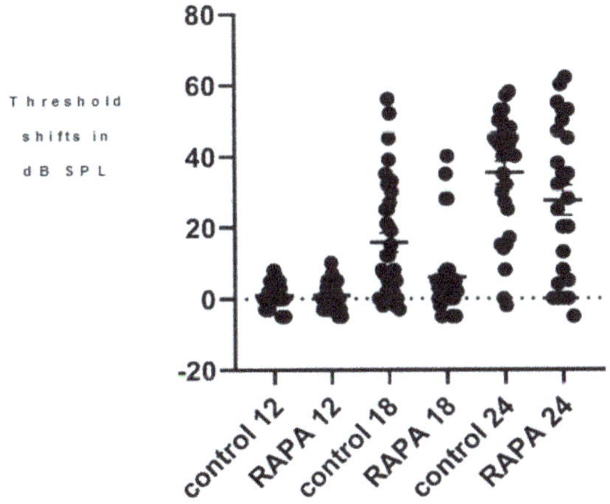

FIGURE 2 | A scatter plot of the 4 kHz auditory brain stem response threshold shifts (compared to 5 months of age) at 12, 18, and 24 months of age in the control diet group (without rapamycin) and in the group with rapamycin added to diet at 14 months of age. There is little variability in either group at 12 months of age. At 18 months of age more variability is seen in the control diet group (control 18) while the rapamycin treatment group (RAPA18) remains more skewed toward little threshold shift. At 24 months of age there is less variability in the control group (control 24) now skewed toward large threshold shifts while the rapamycin treatment group (RAPA24) has more distribution across the range of threshold shifts.

Hair Cell Assessment

Phalloidin labeling of hair cells was used to identify presence or absence of hair cells. Hair cells were counted under epifluorescence optics on a Leica fluorescent microscope under double blind conditions. The number of inner hair cells and outer hair cells (OHC) that were present or absent for each 0.19 mm reticule length was entered into a cytocochleogram program starting at the apex and moving basally until the entire length of the cochlear spiral had been assessed. The program compares hair cell numbers to a normal data base. The program can generate a graph of hair cell loss by position along the cochlear spiral for each cochlea (cytocochleogram), can provide the analysis in absolute numbers, as the total percent of hair cells lost in each animal assessed and can be used to generate means for groups.

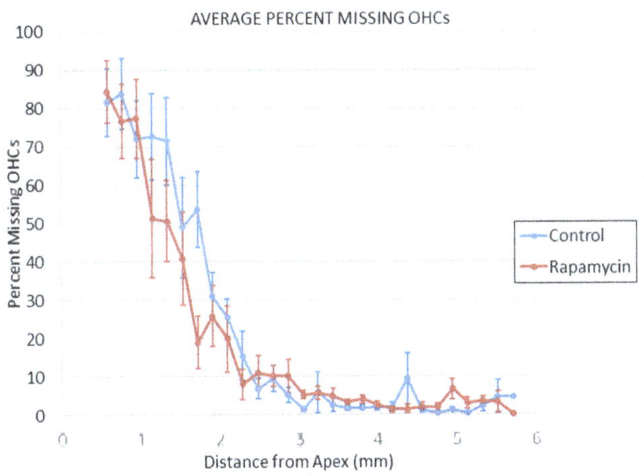

FIGURE 3 | Cytochleograms comparing the mean outer hair cell loss across the cochlea spiral at 24 months of age in mice from the group that had rapamycin added to diet at 14 months of age (red line) vs. the control diet group without rapamycin added to diet (blue line). Apical cochlea is to the left and base to the right, the transition from apical turn to basal turn is ~1.75 mm from the apex and the transition from basal turn to the hook is at ~3.9 mm from apex. There is large loss of outer hair cells in the apical third of the cochlea in both groups and minimal loss in the remaining cochlea (including hook) in both groups.

Statistics

Significance for ABR threshold changes was tested using an unpaired "t" test with Welch's correction and the non-parametric Mann–Whitney test with Bonferroni adjustment. Significance was considered at both $p < 0.01$ and $p < 0.05$ levels. There was no significant difference in the mean ABR thresholds or TS between male and females within the rapamycin diet or within the diet control group at any age and so males and females were combined when testing for significance. Means are given in text plus/minus the standard error of the mean (SEM).

RESULTS

Auditory Brain Stem Response

There was no significant difference in the mean ABR thresholds or TS between male and females in either control diet or rapamycin diet groups at any age for any of the frequencies assessed and males and females were therefore combined for comparisons. At 12 months of age there were no animals with TS above 10 dB SPL at any frequency in animals to be assigned to either group. The progression of ABR TS in the control diet group

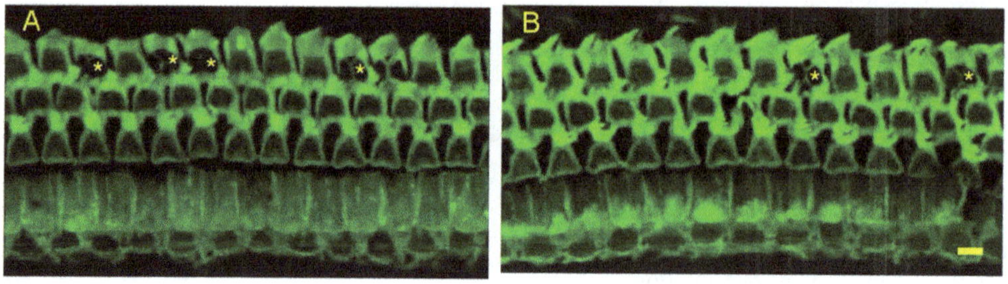

FIGURE 4 | Representative photomicrographs from surface preparations of organ of Corti from a 24 months old Control Diet mouse **(A)** and a 24 months old mouse on the Rapamycin Diet **(B)** Both have outer hair cell loss in the third row, with scars marked by asterisks. Bar = 10 μ.

was consistent with the pattern we have previously reported in UMHET4 mice with significant TS first appearing at low frequencies and later at higher frequencies (Schacht et al., 2012; Altschuler et al., 2015) (**Figures 1A–D**). There was variability across animals in the timing of their progression of hearing loss (e.g., **Figure 2** for 4 kHz) with a few mice (3–29) in the control diet group retaining normal hearing thresholds across all frequencies even at the latest 24 months of age ABR assessment time, also consistent with what we have previously observed in UMHET4 mice (Schacht et al., 2012; Altschuler et al., 2015).

Threshold Shifts at 18 Months of Age

At 18 months of age, the mean ABR TS at 4 kHz in the rapamycin diet group was 5.5 ± 2.2 dB SPL compared to a 15.8 ± 2.7 dB SPL mean in the control diet group, this difference was significant ($p < 0.01$) (**Figure 1A**). This was a consequence of a larger number of animals (17–37) showing 4 kHz ABR TS over 10 dB in the control diet group compared to 5–29 in the rapamycin diet group. Variability among mice in timing of TS and rapamycin treatment effect is shown in a scatter plot at 4 kHz in **Figure 2**. At 12 kHz the mean TS in the rapamycin diet group was 1.2 ± 0.6 dB SPL compared to a 5.1 ± 1/6 dB SPL in the control diet group, this difference was also significant ($p < 0.05$). There were no significant differences in 24 or 48 kHz TS means between rapamycin and control diet groups (**Figures 1C,D**). One mouse in the rapamycin diet group was an outlier with a large (53 dB SPL) TS at 48 kHz without a TS at 4 kHz.

Threshold Shifts at 24 Months of Age

At 24 months of age there was no longer a significant difference ($p = 01.4$) in the mean 4 kHz TS between the rapamycin diet (27.2 ± 4.5 dB SPL) and the control diet (35.3 ± 3.2 dB SPL) groups (**Figure 1A**). The difference in mean 12 kHz TS between rapamycin diet (5.9 ± 1.5 dB SPL) and control diet (11.4 ± 2.0 dB SPL) groups remained significant ($p < 0.05$) (**Figure 1B**). Differences now appeared at higher frequencies, with a significant difference ($p < 0.05$) in mean TS between rapamycin and control diet groups for both 24 kHz (rapamycin = 4.2 ± 1.0 dB SPL; control = 8.0 ± 1.2 dB SPL) and 48 kHz (rapamycin = 6.9 ± 2.5 dB SPL; control = 14.7 ± 3.2 dB SPL) assessments (**Figures 1C,D**).

Histology and Hair Cell Assessment

There were no signs of middle ear infection in the cochleae of any mice in the study. At 24 months of age there was large outer hair cell loss in the apical half of cochlea of most mice in both control diet mice and rapamycin diet groups (**Figure 4**), with no significant difference in the mean loss between these groups. There was only minimal outer hair cell loss in the basal half of the cochlea of most mice in both groups with mean outer hair cell loss well under 10% in both groups (**Figures 3, 4**) despite ABR threshold shifts.

DISCUSSION

The results of the present study extend results of our previous study (Altschuler et al., 2018) that found rapamycin added to diet at 4 months of age reduced outer hair cell loss in the basal half but not apical half of the cochleae of 22 months old UMHET3 mice. The present study used longitudinal measure of ABR to show rapamycin added to diet reduced mean threshold shifts at 4 and 12 kHz in 18 months old UMHET4 mice, largely by reducing the percent of mice showing TS. It is not well understood why hair cell loss occurs first in apical regions, then in basal regions in most mouse models and it has been suggested that different mechanisms could be influencing basal vs. apical age-related hearing loss (e.g., Schulte and Schmiedt, 1992; Dubno et al., 2013; Wu et al., 2020). Since 4 kHz is processed in the apical half of the mouse cochlea, ~1.25 mm from apex (Viberg and Canlon, 2004), the results of the present study show that the influence of rapamycin is not restricted to the basal half of the cochlea. This provides indirect evidence that at least some components underlying age-related hearing loss (those that can be influenced by rapamycin) are present in both basal and apical cochleae. Rapamycin acts on mammalian-target-of-rapamycin (mTOR) pathways (both mTORC1 and mTORC2). These pathways are multifaceted and in turn act on other functional signaling pathways including those associated with metabolism, proliferation, immune response and cell survival (Inoki et al., 2005a,b; Perl, 2015 for reviews; Wataya-Kaneda, 2015). The mTORC1 pathway can influence endoplasmic reticulum (ER) stress and the unfolded protein response (UPR) (e.g., Ye et al., 2015). ER stress-related factors have been shown to increase in the cochleae of aged mice

(Wang et al., 2015) and ER stress-mediated apoptosis has been associated with noise-induced, ototoxic drug-induced and age-related hearing losses (Oishi et al., 2015; Wang et al., 2015; Hu et al., 2016; Mahdi et al., 2016). ER stress pathways could therefore be a target of the rapamycin effect on ARHL. Rapamycin could also stimulate the survival pathway of p-Akt (S473) via mTOR2 signaling, including reducing mitochondrial stress. Rapamycin could also act through its influence on the inflammatory response or through inhibition of oxidative stress pathways previously implicated in hair cell pathology (Yamasoba et al., 2013, for review). Future studies will be necessary to identify the specific target or targets and pathways underlying the treatment effect seen in the current study.

Another important result is that the rapamycin treatment-related sparing of 4 kHz hearing loss at 18 months is no longer present at 24 months of age and there is an associated large hair cell loss in the apical cochlea of most rapamycin diet and control diet mice at 24 months of age, with no difference between the groups. This suggests that rapamycin treatment delays but does not prevent hearing loss. It would be valuable to identify the specific mechanisms by which rapamycin delays hair cell loss, not only to increase understanding of general mechanisms underlying ARHL but to determine if the delay could be extended and even turned into prevention. The timing of the last ABR and terminal euthanasia in the present study was before large TS generally occurs at higher frequencies in the UMHET4 mouse model. A greater rapamycin induced sparing of hair cell loss and TS than observed in the current study might therefore be found at a later age when greater hair cell loss is occurring, as observed in the previous study in UMHET3 mice where ARHL occurs more rapidly. The lack of correlation between ABR TS and OHC loss in the more basal cochlea at 24 months of age is consistent with reports of age-related reduction or loss in OHC function with reduced distortion product otoacoustic emissions (DPOAE) appearing before age-related OHC loss (e.g., Syka, 2010, for review). One explanation is an age-related disruption of prestin in morphologically intact OHC (Chen et al., 2009; Syka, 2010). It would be valuable to examine the influence of rapamycin treatment on age-related decrements in DPOAE. The variability in the progression and extent of ARHL seen in the control diet UMHET4 mice may reflect their genetic diversity and we have previously shown this variability can be correlated with polymorphisms in specific genetic loci (Schacht et al., 2012). The variability seen in the treatment effect of rapamycin in the rapamycin diet group might also reflect UMHET4 genetic diversity and it would be interesting to identify such differences in future studies.

The present study also addressed the question of whether beginning rapamycin treatment later in life than the 4 months of age used in Altschuler et al. (2018) would be effective. The results show beginning treatment later in life, at 14 months of age is still effective. This is consistent with studies showing late life rapamycin delivery also enhances life span and delays/reduces age-related declines in cardiac, muscle and cognitive functions (Quarles and Rabinovitch, 2020, for review). The literature also suggests that late life intermittent administration of rapamycin and rapamycin-like compounds ("rapalogs") with less side-effects in people, can also increase life span and decrease age-related declines (Anisimov et al., 2011; Arriola Apelo et al., 2016; Shavlakadze et al., 2018; Quarles and Rabinovitch, 2020). It would therefore be valuable to test late-life intermittent treatment effects of rapamycin and rapalogs on ARHL.

AUTHOR CONTRIBUTIONS

RA, DD, and DK: contributed to the study in design: LK, AK, and CM: carrying out studies and measures: RA, DD, DK, CM, and CS: analysis of results and their impact. All authors contributed to the article and approved the submitted version.

REFERENCES

Altschuler, R. A., Kanicki, A., Martin, C., Kohrman, D., and Miller, R. A. (2018). Rapamycin but not acarbose decreases age-related loss of outer hair cells in the mouse Cochlea, Hearing *Reserarch* 370, 11–15. doi: 10.1016/j.heares.2018.09.003

Altschuler, R. A., Zabezhinski, M. A., Popovich, I. G., Piskunova, T. S, Semenchenko, A. V., Tyndyk, M. L., et al. (2015). Age-related changes in auditory nerve—inner hair cell connections, hair cell numbers, auditory brain stem response and gap detection in UM-HET4 mice, *Neuroscience* 292, 22–33. doi: 10.1016/j.neuroscience.2015.01.068

Anisimov, V. N., Zabezhinski, M. A., Popovich, I. G., Piskunova, T. S., Semenchenko, A. V., Tyndyk, M. L., et al. (2011). Rapamycin increases lifespan and inhibits spontaneous tumorigenesis in inbred female mice. *Cell Cycle* 10, 4230–4236. doi: 10.4161/cc.10.24.18486

Arriola Apelo, S. I., Pumper, C. P., Baar, E. L., Cummings, N. E., and Lamming, D. W. (2016). Intermittent administration of rapamycin extends the life span of female C57BL/6J Mice. *J Gerontol A Biol Sci Med Sci.* 71, 876–881. doi: 10.1093/gerona/glw064

Bitto, A., Ito, T. K., Pineda, V. V., LeTexier, N. J., Huang, H. Z., Sutlief, E., Tung, H., et al. (2016). Transient rapamycin treatment can increase lifespan and healthspan in middle-aged mice. *elife* 5:e16351. doi: 10.7554/eLife.16351

Chen, G.-D., Li, M., Tanaka, C., Bielefeld, E. C., Hu, B. H., Kermany, M. H., et al. (2009). Aging outer hair cells (OHC) in the Fischer 344 rat cochlea: function and morphology. *Hear. Res.* 248, 39–47. doi: 10.1016/j.heares.2008.11.010

Dai, D. F., Karunadharma, P. P., Chiao Y. A., Basisty, N., Crispin, D., and Hsieh, E. J., (2014). Altered proteome turnover and remodeling by short-term caloric restriction or rapamycin rejuvenate the aging heart. *Aging Cell* 13, 529–539. doi: 10.1111/acel.12203

Davis, A., and Smith, P. (2013). Adult hearing screening: health policy issues-what happens next. *Am. J. Audiol.* 22, 167–170. doi: 10.1044/1059-0889(2013/12-0062)

Dubno, J. R., Eckert, M. A., Lee, F.-S., Matthews, L. J., and Schmiedt, R. A. (2013). Classifying human audiometric phenotypes of age-related hearing loss from animal models. *J. Assoc. Res. Otolaryngol.* 14, 687–701. doi: 10.1007/s10162-013-0396-x

Gates, G. A. (2006). The effect of noise on cochlear aging. *Ear Hear.* 27:91. doi: 10.1097/01.aud.0000194512.51849.ab

Gates, G. A., Gibbons, L. E., McCurry, S. M., Crane, P. K., Feeney, M. P., and Larson, E. B. (2010). Executive dysfunction and presbycusis in older persons with and without memory loss and dementia. *Cogn. Behav. Neurol.* 23, 218–223. doi: 10.1097/WNN.0b013e3181d748d7

Gratton, M. A., and Vazquez, A. E. (2003). Age-related hearing loss: current research. *Curr. Opin. Otolaryngol. Head Neck Surg.* 11, 367–371. doi: 10.1097/00020840-200310000-00010

Halloran Hussong, S. A., Burbank, R., Podlutskaya, N., Fischer, K. E., and Sloane, L. B. (2012). Chronic inhibition of mammalian target of rapamycin by rapamycin modulates cognitive and non-cognitive components of behavior throughout lifespan in mice. *Neuroscience* 223:102–13. doi: 10.1016/j.neuroscience.2012.06.054

Harrison, D. E., Strong, R., Sharp, Z. D., James, F., Nelson, C. M. and Kevin, A. (2009). Rapamycin fed late in life extends lifespan in genetically heterogeneous mice. *Nature* 460, 392–395. doi: 10.1038/nature08221

Hu, J., Li, B., Apisa, L., Yu, H., Entenman, S., Xu, M., Stepanyan, R., et al. (2016). ER stress inhibitor attenuates hearing loss and hair cell death inCdh23erl/erlmutant mice. *Cell Death Dis.* 7:e2485doi: 10.1038/cddis.2016.386

Inoki, K., Corradetti, M. N., and Guan, K. L. (2005b). Dysregulation of the TSC-mTOR pathway in human disease. *Nat. Genet.* 37, 19–24. doi: 10.1038/ng1494

Inoki, K., Ouyang, H., Li, Y., and Guan, K. L. (2005a). Signaling by target of rapamycin proteins in cell growth control. *Microbiol. Mol. Bio.l Rev.* 69, 79–100. doi: 10.1128/MMBR.69.1.79-100.2005

Johnson, K. R., Zheng, Q. Y., and Noben-Trauth, K. (2006). Strain background effects and genetic modifiers of hearing in mice. *Brain Res.*1091, 79–88. doi: 10.1016/j.brainres.2006.02.021

Lin, F. R., Ferrucci, L., Metter, E. J., An, Y., Zonderman, A. B., and Resnick, S. M. (2011). Hearing loss and cognition in the Baltimore Longitudinal Study of Aging. *Neuropsychology*. 25, 763–770. doi: 10.1037/a0024238

Mahdi, A. A., Rizvi, S. H. M., and Parveen, A. (2016). Role of endoplasmic reticulum stress and unfolded protein responses in health and diseases. *Ind. J. Clin.l Biochem. IJCB* 31, 127. doi: 10.1007/s12291-015-0502-4

Majumder, S., Caccamo, A., Medina, D. X., Benavides, A. D., Javors, M. A., Kraig, E, Strong, R., et al. (2012). Lifelong rapamycin administration ameliorates age-dependent cognitive deficits by reducing IL-1beta and enhancing NMDA signaling. *Aging Cell* 11, 326–335. doi: 10.1111/j.1474-9726.2011.00791.x

Mianné, J., Chessum, L, Kumar, S., Aguilar, C., Codner, G., Hutchison, M., et al. (2016). Correction of the auditory phenotype in C57BL/6N mice via CRISPR/Cas9-mediated homology directed repair Genome *Medicine* 8:16. doi: 10.1186/s13073-016-0273-4

Miller, R. A., Harrison, D. E., Astle, C. M., Fernandez, E., Flurkey, K., Han, M., et al. (2014). Rapamycin-mediated lifespan increase in mice is dose and sex dependent and metabolically distinct from dietary restriction. *Aging Cell.* 13, 468–477. doi: 10.1111/acel.12194

Noben-Trauth, K., Zheng, Q. Y., and Johnson, K. R. (2003). Association of cadherin 23 with polygenic inheritance and genetic modification of sensorineural hearing loss. *Nat. Genet.* 345, 21–23. doi: 10.1038/ng1226

Ohlemiller, K. K. (2006). Contributions of mouse models to understanding age- and noise-related hearing loss. *Brain Res.* 109, 189–102. doi: 10.1016/j.brainres.2006.03.017

Oishi, N., Duscha, S., Boukari, H., Meyer, M., Xie, J., Wei, G., et al. (2015). XBP1 mitigates aminoglycoside-induced endoplasmic reticulum stress and neuronal cell death. *Cell Death Dis.* 6:e1763. doi: 10.1038/cddis.2015.108

Perl, A. (2015). mTOR activation is a biomarker and a central pathway to autoimmune disorders, cancer, obesity, and aging. *Ann N Y Acad Sci.* 1346, 33–44. doi: 10.1111/nyas.12756

Quarles, E., and Rabinovitch, P. S. (2020). Transient and later-life rapamycin for healthspan extension, *Aging* 12, 4050–4051. doi: 10.18632/aging.102947

Schacht, J., Altschuler, R. A., Burke, D. T., Chen, S., Dolan, D., Galecki, A. T., et al. (2012). Alleles that modulate late life hearing in genetically heterogeneous mice. *Neurobiol. Aging*, 1842. 15–29. doi: 10.1016/j.neurobiolaging.2011.12.034

Schulte, B. A., and Schmiedt, R. A. (1992). Lateral wall Na,K-ATPase and endocochlear potentials decline with age in quiet-reared gerbils. *Hear Res.* 61, 35–46. doi: 10.1016/0378-5955(92)90034-K

Shavlakadze, T., Zhu, J., Wang, S., Zhou, W., Morin, B., Egerman, M. A. et al., (2018). Short-term low-dose mTORC1 inhibition in aged rats counter-regulates age-related gene changes and blocks age-related kidney pathology. *J Gerontol A Biol Sci Med Sci.* 73, 845–852. doi: 10.1093/gerona/glx249

Syka, J. (2010). The Fischer 344 rat as a model of presbycusis. *Hear. Res.* 264, 70–78. doi: 10.1016/j.heares.2009.11.003

Viberg, A., and Canlon, B. (2004). The guide to plotting a cytocochleogram, *Hear Res.* 197, 1–10. doi: 10.1016/j.heares.2004.04.016

Wang, W., Sun, Y., Chen, S., Zhou, X., Wu, X., Kong, W., and Kong, W. (2015). Impaired unfolded protein response in the degeneration of cochlea cells in a mouse model of age-related hearing loss. *Exp. Gerontol*, 70, 61–70. doi: 10.1016/j.exger.2015.07.003

Wataya-Kaneda, M. (2015). Mammalian target of rapamycin and tuberous sclerosis complex. *J. Dermatol. Sci.* 79, 93–100. doi: 10.1016/j.jdermsci.2015.04.005

Wu, P. Z., O'Malley, J. T., de Gruttola, V., and Liberman, M. C. (2020). Age-related hearing loss is dominated by damage to inner ear sensory cells, not the cellular battery that powers them. *J. Neurosci.* 40, 6357–6366. doi: 10.1523/JNEUROSCI.0937-20.2020

Yamasoba, T., Lin, F. R., Someya, S., Kashio, A., Sakamoto, T., and Kondo, K. (2013). Current concepts in age-related hearing loss: epidemiology and mechanistic pathways. *Hear. Res*, 303, 30–38. doi: 10.1016/j.heares.2013.01.021

Ye, X., Luo, H., Chen, Y., Wu, Q., Xiong, Y., Zhu, J., et al. (2015). MicroRNAs 99b-5p/100-5p regulated by endoplasmic reticulum stress are involved in abeta-induced pathologies. *Front. Aging Neurosci.* 7:210. doi: 10.3389/fnagi.2015.00210

Zhang, Y., Bokov, A., Gelfond, J., Soto, V., Ikeno, Y., and Hubbard, G. (2014) Rapamycin extends life and health in C57BL/6 mice. *J. Gerontol. A Biol. Sci. Med. Sci.* 69, 119–130. doi: 10.1093/gerona/glt056

3

Use of Radical Oxygen Species Scavenger Nitrones to Treat Oxidative Stress-Mediated Hearing Loss: State of the Art and Challenges

Isabel Varela-Nieto[1,2,3]*, Silvia Murillo-Cuesta*[1,2,3]*, Lourdes Rodríguez-de la Rosa*[1,2,3]*, María Jesús Oset-Gasque*[4,5] *and José Marco-Contelles*[6]*

[1] *Institute for Biomedical Research "Alberto Sols," Spanish National Research Council (CSIC)-Autonomous University of Madrid, Madrid, Spain,* [2] *Biomedical Research Networking Center on Rare Diseases (CIBERER), Institute of Health Carlos III, Madrid, Spain,* [3] *Hospital La Paz Institute for Health Research, Madrid, Spain,* [4] *Department of Biochemistry and Molecular Biology, School of Pharmacy, Complutense University of Madrid, Madrid, Spain,* [5] *Institute of Neurochemistry Research, Complutense University of Madrid, Madrid, Spain,* [6] *Laboratory of Medicinal Chemistry, Institute of General Organic Chemistry, CSIC, Madrid, Spain*

***Correspondence:**
José Marco-Contelles
iqoc21@iqog.csic.es

Nitrones are potent antioxidant molecules able to reduce oxidative stress by trapping reactive oxygen and nitrogen species. The antioxidant potential of nitrones has been extensively tested in multiple models of human diseases. Sensorineural hearing loss has a heterogeneous etiology, genetic alterations, aging, toxins or exposure to noise can cause damage to hair cells at the organ of Corti, the hearing receptor. Noxious stimuli share a battery of common mechanisms by which they cause hair cell injury, including oxidative stress, the generation of free radicals and redox imbalance. Therefore, targeting oxidative stress-mediated hearing loss has been the subject of much attention. Here we review the chemistry of nitrones, the existing literature on their use as antioxidants and the general state of the art of antioxidant treatments for hearing loss.

Keywords: antioxidants, free radicals, sensorineural hearing loss, *N*-acetyl-L-cysteine, NXY-059, 4-OHPBN, PBN

INTRODUCTION

Nitrones are organic molecules able to trap reactive oxygen and nitrogen species (ROS, RNS) (Rosselin et al., 2017). Thus, nitrones constitute potent antioxidant molecules able to reduce oxidative stress (Firuzi et al., 2011). Nitrones power to scavenge free radicals derives from its activated carbon nitrogen double bond (**Figure 1A**) that prompts easy free radical attack leading to less reactive and harmful nitroxide species for biomolecules (Oliveira et al., 2018). However, the fact that the doses used for spin trapping experiments are 1,000-fold higher than those usually applied in the *in vitro* neuroprotection assays (10–50 μM), and that the amounts of nitrones used *in vivo* are currently under 50 μM, clearly insufficient to trap ROS/RNS, suggest that other mechanisms are responsible for nitrones scavenging capacity (Rosselin et al., 2017). Nitrones also suppress signal transduction processes with significant anti-inflammatory, anti-apoptotic (Floyd et al., 2008) and NO-releasing properties (Croitoru et al., 2011). These actions together with ROS and RNS scavenging may account for the antioxidant/neuroprotective profile exhibited by nitrones (Villamena et al., 2012).

Nitrone derivatives have been extensively used in both preclinical models and clinical assays as therapeutics to reduce oxidative stress in several pathologies, mainly stroke (Marco-Contelles, 2020), neurodegenerative disorders (Cancela et al., 2020) and cancer (Thomas et al., 2020). Oxidative stress is also considered a major pathological mechanism in several auditory pathologies, including ototoxicity, noise-induced hearing loss (NIHL) and presbycusis (Bermúdez-Muñoz et al., 2020, 2021; Varela-Nieto et al., 2020).

Thus, the purpose of this minireview is to discuss how the antioxidant properties of selected nitrones, such as alpha-phenyl-tert-butylnitrone (PBN), 4-hydroxy PBN (4-OHPBN), disufenton sodium (NXY-059, also referred to as HPN-07) (**Figure 1B**), have been explored as potential therapeutic small molecules for the treatment of hearing loss of different etiologies and to identify the current challenges to translate these results into the clinical practice.

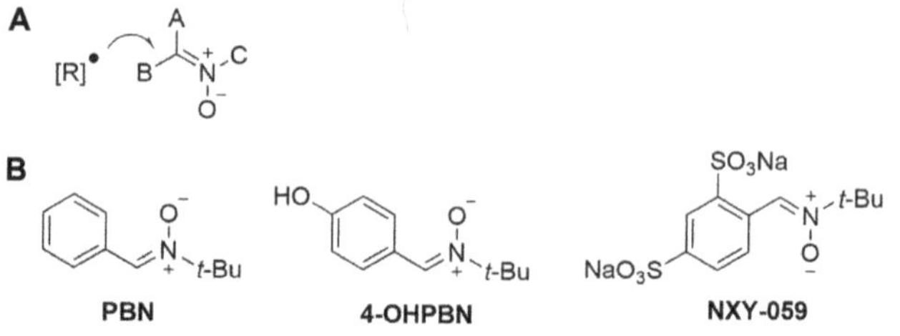

FIGURE 1 | (A) Reaction of a free radical [R]• with a nitrone. **(B)** Structures of nitrones PBN, 4-OHPBN and NXY-059.

NITRONES AS THERAPEUTIC AGENTS FOR SENSORINEURAL HEARING LOSS

Sensorineural hearing loss (SNHL) is the most common sensory deficit in adults, and is associated with normal aging. SNHL is intensified due to the exposure to pollutants such as carbon monoxide (CO) (Marcano Acuña et al., 2019), hydrogen cyanide (Fechter et al., 2002), trimethyltin (Yu et al., 2016) and acrylonitrile, as well as by the combination of high levels of noise and these toxins (Fechter et al., 2004; Pouyatos et al., 2009). SNHL is also caused by drugs such as aminoglycosides and cisplatin (Kros and Steyger, 2019; Murillo-Cuesta et al., 2021). Although the underlying mechanisms of age- or environmental toxins-mediated SNHL are still unknown, there is large consensus in that free radical processes are effectively involved (Fechter et al., 2004; Wang et al., 2007; Fetoni et al., 2019; Varela-Nieto et al., 2020).

Oxidative stress plays a key role in the induction of cochlear injury after noise exposure (Wang et al., 2007; Varela-Nieto et al., 2020). Very interestingly, one of the consequences of the oxidative stress induced by excessive noise is the onset of apoptosis linked to mitochondrial release of cytochrome C, activation of caspases and the N-terminal-c-JUN kinase pathway (Wang et al., 2007).

The key role of oxidative stress in producing cochlear injury is supported by the positive therapeutic effect shown by antioxidants in preclinical studies carried out in animal models. Furthermore, deletion of antioxidant enzymes like *Gpx1* (glutathione-peroxidase1) results in NIHL and loss of hair cells in mice (Ohlemiller et al., 2000). Accordingly, the organoselenium compound Ebselen, which mimic GPX1 activity, prevents outer hair cells loss in rats after oral treatment, before and immediately after noise exposure (Kil et al., 2007). Ebselen has also shown a moderate effect in clinical trials for NIHL (Kil et al., 2017). Also, adenoviral-mediated antioxidant gene therapy to overexpress human catalase and superoxide dismutases (SOD1 and SOD2) has been used to prevent aminoglycoside ototoxic trauma in the guinea pig cochlea (Kawamoto et al., 2004). **Supplementary Table 1A** summarizes main published data studying antioxidants, such as acetyl-*L*-carnitine (ALCAR), *N*-acetyl-L-cysteine (NAC) or Ebselen, among others. NAC and ALCAR are known to efficiently reduce NIHL (Choi, 2011; Varela-Nieto et al., 2020) and aminoglycoside ototoxicity (Somdas et al., 2015; García-Alcántara et al., 2018). Furthermore, NAC also reduces oxidative stress, inflammation and protects hearing (Bermúdez-Muñoz et al., 2021) in a genetic model of early onset age-related hearing loss (Celaya et al., 2019). More recently, researchers have tested HK-2, a multifunctional antioxidant, which has been shown to protect against NIHL and hair cell loss administered orally in rats before and after noise (Chen et al., 2020).

Despite their potent antioxidant power, nitrones have been poorly studied as a therapy for SNHL. Alone or in combination with other well-known antioxidant agents, such as NAC (Kopke et al., 2007, 2015), nitrones have been reported to be effective in the prevention and treatment of NIHL (Kopke et al., 2005; Ewert et al., 2017) or CO ototoxicity (Fechter et al., 1997).

Here we will discuss in detail the reported actions of free radical scavenger nitrones PBN, 4-OHPBN and NXY-059 (**Figure 1B**) in SNHL protection.

PBN

Phenyl-tert-butylnitrone (**Figure 1B**) has been shown to be effective in mitigating the SNHL that occurs in Long Evans hooded rats exposed to CO (Rao and Fechter, 2000) or to acrylonitrile (Fechter et al., 2004), plus exposure to high level noise. Acrylonitrile when associated with acoustic overexposure increased hearing loss, implying that the mechanism of the potentiation of NIHL by these compounds involved enhancing cochlear oxidative stress (Pouyatos et al., 2005). Rao and Fechter observed that PBN given before and after high-level steady-state noise decreased CO-mediated potentiation of the noise-induced threshold shifts (Rao and Fechter, 2000). However, no statistically significant differences were found between animals only exposed to noise and untreated or treated with PBN (Rao and Fechter, 2000). The underlying mechanisms of PBN have not been studied in detail, but may involve the reduction of oxidative stress (Floyd, 1997). Indeed, PBN protects cochlear function from combined exposure to noise and CO by reducing the formation of ROS/RNS in the cochlea (Fechter et al., 2000). The otoprotection shown by PBN on acrylonitrile-induced damage seems due to oxidative stress reduction by preventing the depletion of glutathione caused by combined noise and acrylonitrile exposure and also reducing reactive epoxide binding to cytochrome C oxidase (Pouyatos et al., 2005). PBN was reported to have a potential key role in increasing the Cu/Zn form of superoxide dismutase in the cochlea (Pierson and Gray, 1982), which has been shown in other organs to restore the same type of antioxidant defense mechanisms associated with cochlear protection (Weisiger and Fridovich, 1973).

4-OHPBN

Nitrone 4-OHPBN (**Figure 1B**), a PBN derivative, and its major metabolite, has been reported to decrease permanent NIHL in chinchilla (Choi et al., 2008). This was very interesting because a previous report claimed that PBN was ineffective in reducing noise-induced auditory threshold shifts (Rao and Fechter, 2000). In fact, 4-OHPBN, administrated after 4 h of noise exposure, proved effective in the treatment of NIHL, and when administrated in combination (4-OHPBN + NAC, and 4-OHPBN + NAC + ALCAR) with other antioxidant drugs such as NAC or ALCAR, showed increased efficacy, since each antioxidant targeted different injury mechanisms (Choi et al., 2008). Choi et al. (2008) reported that animals exposed to a 105 dB octave-band noise for 6 h and then treated with 4-OHPBN drug combinations for 4 h increased the efficiency of the treatment, reducing the individual drug dose. The precise mechanisms by which 4-OHPBN reduces cochlear injury are still largely unknown; among the targets proposed by different authors we found free radical scavenging, inhibition of iNOS activation, suppression of ROS/RNS formation, decreased mitochondrial ROS production, reduced neuroinflammation and activation of MAP kinase cascades (Floyd, 1999; Du et al., 2011).

NXY-059

The potential therapeutic effect of nitrone NXY-059 (**Figure 1B**) and of its combination with NAC to treat permanent NIHL was explored in female chinchillas exposed to a 105 dB octave-band noise centered at 4 kHz, for 6 h, by starting treatment 4 h after noise exposure and continually injecting twice daily for the next 2 days (Choi, 2011). Results showed that the mean permanent hearing threshold of NXY-059 and NXY-059 + NAC treated groups was decreased compared to the noise exposed group. Furthermore, NXY-059 + NAC showed greater effects, demonstrating that this drug combination enhances the therapeutic effect (Choi, 2011). Indeed, the combination of antioxidants with different and complementary mechanisms of action has proven to be more effective than using just one drug (García-Alcántara et al., 2018). NXY-059 + NAC has been further evaluated as a therapeutic approach for NIHL in rats exposed to 115 dB octave-band noise (10–20 kHz) treated 1 h before and 1 h after noise exposure, and then for two consecutive days (Lu et al., 2014). Auditory brainstem response showed that this treatment significantly reduced the threshold shift across all tested frequencies along the 21 days studied. Reduced distortion product otoacoustic emission level shifts were also detected at 7 and 21 days following noise exposure of treated animals. Protection was associated to increased conservation of outer and inner hair cells in the organ of Corti. Treatment also significantly reduced the noise-induced expression of c-FOS in the cochlear nucleus neurons. These results indicated that NXY-059 + NAC is a promising pharmacological combination for NIHL therapy, as it decreases both temporary and permanent threshold shifts after intense noise exposure, protects cochlear sensory cells, and potentially afferent neurites, from the damaging effects of noise-induced oxidative stress. In addition, the drugs reduced aberrant activation of neurons in the central auditory regions of the brain following noise exposure (Lu et al., 2014). Finally, NXY-059 free radical spin trapping activity has been reported to protect the cochlea exposed to acute acoustic trauma (Ewert et al., 2017).

CONCLUSION AND FUTURE PERSPECTIVES

The pathophysiological response to oxidative stress has been a widely studied and is a well-established cochlear mechanism of injury leading to hearing loss (Choi and Choi, 2015; Wang and Puel, 2018; Bermúdez-Muñoz et al., 2020, 2021; Varela-Nieto et al., 2020). Oxidative stress occurs when cochlear cells show excessive amounts of oxidants or decreased levels of antioxidants and causes formation of free radicals. These free radicals can damage cellular DNA, proteins, lipids, and unregulated apoptotic pathways, causing cell death and irreversible damage to the cochlea (Kurabi et al., 2017). Secondary to oxidative stress, inflammation occurs and further expands cochlear injury leading to apoptotic cell death of the irreplaceable sensory hair cells and neurones (Perin et al., 2021). In this context, nitrones have been explored to prevent hearing loss rendering modest positive results, generally combined with NAC. The enormous potential of these molecules invites to study in depth their largely unknown biodistribution and pharmacokinetics when administered by different routes to the inner ear. Improving their solubility in biological membranes by means of medical chemistry strategies, the modification of their structure or their combination with biocompatible vehicles, could allow their local administration, which could eventually improve their preclinical results.

AUTHOR CONTRIBUTIONS

IV-N, SM-C, and JM-C wrote the manuscript. LR and MO-G revised the manuscript. All authors revised and approved the manuscript.

ACKNOWLEDGMENTS

We would like to thank our colleagues of the Neurobiology of Hearing Group for critical comments and sharing unpublished information.

REFERENCES

Bermúdez-Muñoz, J. M., Celaya, A. M., García-Mato, A., Muñoz-Espín, D., Rodríguez-de la Rosa, L., Serrano, M., et al. (2021). Dual-specificity phosphatase 1 (DUSP1) has a central role in redox homeostasis and inflammation in the mouse cochlea. *Antioxidants* in press.

Bermúdez-Muñoz, J. M., Celaya, A. M., Hijazo-Pechero, S., Wang, J., Serrano, M., and Varela-Nieto, I. (2020). G6PD overexpression protects from oxidative stress and age-related hearing loss. *Aging Cell* 19:e13275.

Cancela, S., Canclini, L., Mourglia-Ettlin, G., Hernández, P., and Merlino, A. (2020). Neuroprotective effects of novel nitrones: in vitro and in silico studies. *Eur. J. Pharmacol.* 871:172926. doi: 10.1016/j.ejphar.2020.172926

Celaya, A. M., Sánchez-Pérez, I., Bermúdez-Muñoz, J. M., Rodríguez-de la Rosa, L., Pintado-Berninches, L., Perona, R., et al. (2019). Deficit of mitogen-activated protein kinase phosphatase 1 (DUSP1) accelerates progressive hearing loss. *Elife* 8:e39159.

Chen, G. D., Daszynski, D. M., Ding, D., Jiang, H., Woolman, T., Blessing, K., et al. (2020). Novel oral multifunctional antioxidant prevents noise-induced hearing loss and hair cell loss. *Hear. Res.* 388:107880. doi: 10.1016/j.heares.2019.107880

Choi, C. H. (2011). Preliminary study of the therapeutic effect of a nitrone-based antioxidant drug (HPN-07) on acute acoustic trauma. *Korean J. Commun. Disord.* 16, 202–210.

Choi, C. H., Chen, K., Vasquez-Weldon, A., Jackson, R. L., Floyd, R. A., and Kopke, R. D. (2008). Effectiveness of 4-hydroxy phenyl N-tert-butylnitrone (4-OHPBN) alone and in combination with other antioxidant drugs in the treatment of acute acoustic trauma in chinchilla. *Free Radic. Biol. Med.* 44, 1772–1784. doi: 10.1016/j.freeradbiomed.2008.02.005

Choi, S. H., and Choi, C. H. (2015). Noise-induced neural degeneration and therapeutic effect of antioxidant drugs. *J. Audiol. Otol.* 19, 111–119. doi: 10.7874/jao.2015.19.3.111

Croitoru, M. D., Ibolya, F., Pop, M. C., Dergez, T., Mitroi, B., Dogaru, M. T., et al. (2011). Nitrones are able to release nitric oxide in aqueous environment under hydroxyl free radical attack. *Nitric Oxide* 25, 309–315. doi: 10.1016/j.niox.2011.05.007

Du, X., Choi, C. H., Chen, K., Cheng, W., Floyd, R. A., and Kopke, R. D. (2011). Reduced formation of oxidative stress biomarkers and migration of mononuclear phagocytes in the cochleae of chinchilla after antioxidant treatment in acute acoustic trauma. *Int. J. Otolaryngol.* 2011:612690.

Ewert, D., Hu, N., Du, X., Li, W., West, M. B., Choi, C. H., et al. (2017). HPN-07, a free radical spin trapping agent, protects against functional, cellular and electrophysiological changes in the cochlea induced by acute acoustic trauma. *PLoS One* 12:e0183089. doi: 10.1371/journal.pone.0183089

Fechter, L. D., Chen, G. D., and Johnson, D. L. (2002). Potentiation of noise-induced hearing loss by low concentrations of hydrogen cyanide in rats. *Toxicol. Sci.* 66, 131–138. doi: 10.1093/toxsci/66.1.131

Fechter, L. D., Chen, G.-D., Rao, D., and Larabee, J. (2000). Predicting exposure conditions that facilitate the potentiation of noise-induced hearing loss by carbon monoxide. *Toxicol. Sci.* 58, 315–323. doi: 10.1093/toxsci/58.2.315

Fechter, L. D., Gearhart, C., and Shirwany, N. A. (2004). Acrylonitrile potentiates noise-induced hearing loss in rat. *J. Assoc. Res. Otolaryngol.* 5, 90–98. doi: 10.1007/s10162-003-4028-8

Fechter, L. D., Liu, Y., and Pearce, T. A. (1997). Cochlear protection from carbon monoxide exposure by free radical blockers in the guinea pig. *Toxicol. Appl. Pharmacol.* 142, 47–55. doi: 10.1006/taap.1996.8027

Fetoni, A. R., Paciello, F., Rolesi, R., Paludetti, G., and Troiani, D. (2019). Targeting dysregulation of redox homeostasis in noise-induced hearing loss: oxidative stress and ROS signaling. *Free Radic. Biol. Med.* 135, 46–59. doi: 10.1016/j.freeradbiomed.2019.02.022

Firuzi, O., Miri, R., Tavakkoli, M., and Saso, L. (2011). Antioxidant therapy: current status and future prospects. *Curr. Med. Chem.* 18, 3871–3888. doi: 10.2174/092986711803414368

Floyd, R. A. (1997). Protective action of nitrone-based free radical traps against oxidative damage to the central nervous system. *Adv. Pharmacol.* 38, 361–378. doi: 10.1016/s1054-3589(08)60991-6

Floyd, R. A. (1999). Antioxidants, oxidative stress, and degenerative neurological disorders. *Proc. Soc. Exp. Biol. Med.* 222, 236–245. doi: 10.1046/j.1525-1373.1999.d01-140.x

Floyd, R. A., Kopke, R. D., Choi, C.-H., Foster, S. B., Doblas, S., and Towner, R. A. (2008). Nitrones as therapeutics. *Free Radic. Biol. Med.* 45, 1361–1374. doi: 10.1016/j.freeradbiomed.2008.08.017

García-Alcántara, F., Murillo-Cuesta, S., Pulido, S., Bermúdez-Muñoz, J. M., Martínez-Vega, R., Milo, M., et al. (2018). The expression of oxidative stress response genes is modulated by a combination of resveratrol and N-acetylcysteine to ameliorate ototoxicity in the rat cochlea. *Hear. Res.* 358, 10–21. doi: 10.1016/j.heares.2017.12.004

Kawamoto, K., Sha, S. H., Minoda, R., Izumikawa, M., Kuriyama, H., Schacht, J., et al. (2004). Antioxidant gene therapy can protect hearing and hair cells from ototoxicity. *Mol. Ther.* 9, 173–181. doi: 10.1016/j.ymthe.2003.11.020

Kil, J., Lobarinas, E., Spankovich, C., Griffiths, S. K., Antonelli, P. J., Lynch, E. D., et al. (2017). Safety and efficacy of Ebselen for the prevention of noise-induced hearing loss: a randomised, double-blind, placebo-controlled, phase 2 trial. *Lancet* 390, 969–979. doi: 10.1016/s0140-6736(17)31791-9

Kil, J., Pierce, C., Tran, H., Gu, R., and Lynch, E. D. (2007). Ebselen treatment reduces noise induced hearing loss *via* the mimicry and induction of glutathione peroxidase. *Hear. Res.* 226, 44–51. doi: 10.1016/j.heares.2006.08.006

Kopke, R., Bielefeld, E., Liu, J., Zheng, J., Jackson, R., Henderson, D., et al. (2005). Prevention of impulse noise-induced hearing loss with antioxidants. *Acta Otolaryngol.* 125, 235–243.

Kopke, R., Slade, M. D., Jackson, R., Hammill, T., Fausti, S., Lonsbury-Martin, B., et al. (2015). Efficacy and safety of N-acetylcysteine in prevention of noise induced hearing loss: a randomized clinical trial. *Hear. Res.* 323, 40–50. doi: 10.1016/j.heares.2015.01.002

Kopke, R. D., Jackson, R. L., Coleman, J. K., Liu, J., Bielefeld, E. C., and Balough, B. J. (2007). NAC for noise: from the bench top to the clinic. *Hear. Res.* 226, 114–125. doi: 10.1016/j.heares.2006.10.008

Kros, C. J., and Steyger, P. S. (2019). Aminoglycoside- and cisplatin-induced ototoxicity: mechanisms and otoprotective strategies. *Cold Spring Harb. Perspect. Med.* 9:a033548. doi: 10.1101/cshperspect.a033548

Kurabi, A., Keithley, E. M., Housley, G. D., Ryan, A. F., and Wong, A. C. (2017). Cellular mechanisms of noise-induced hearing loss. *Hear. Res.* 349, 129–137. doi: 10.1016/j.heares.2016.11.013

Lu, J., Li, W., Du, X., Ewert, D. L., West, M. B., Stewart, C., et al. (2014). Antioxidants reduce cellular and functional changes induced by intense noise in the inner ear and cochlear nucleus. *J. Ass. Res. Otolaryngol.* 15, 353–372. doi: 10.1007/s10162-014-0441-4

Marcano Acuña, M., Doménech Máñez, I., Llopis Llopis, F., and Salvador Marín, M. (2019). Reversible sensorineural hearing loss following carbon monoxide poisoning. *Acta Otorrinolaringol. Esp.* 70, 373–375. doi: 10.1016/j.otoeng.2018.06.005

Marco-Contelles, J. (2020). Recent advances on nitrones design for stroke treatment. *J. Med. Chem.* 63, 13413–13427. doi: 10.1021/acs.jmedchem.0c00976

Murillo-Cuesta, S., Celaya, A. M., Cervantes, B., Bermúdez-Muñoz, J. M., Rodríguez-de la Rosa, L., Contreras, J., et al. (2021). Therapeutic efficiency of the APAF-1 antagonist LPT99 in a rat model of cisplatin-induced hearing loss. *Clin. Transl. Med.* 11:e363.

Ohlemiller, K. K., McFadden, S. L., Ding, D. L., Lear, P. M., and Ho, Y. S. (2000). Targeted mutation of the gene for cellular glutathione peroxidase (Gpx1) increases noise-induced hearing loss in mice. *J. Assoc. Res. Otolaryngol.* 1, 243–254. doi: 10.1007/s101620010043

Oliveira, C., Benfeito, S., Fernandes, C., Cagide, F., Silva, T., and Borges, F. (2018). NO and HNO donors, nitrones, and nitroxides: past, present, and future. *Med. Res. Rev.* 38, 1159–1187. doi: 10.1002/med.21461

Perin, P., Marino, F., Varela-Nieto, I., and Szczepek, A. J. (2021). Editorial: neuroimmunology of the inner ear. *Front. Neurol.* 12:635359. doi: 10.3389/fneur.2021.635359

Pierson, M. G., and Gray, B. H. (1982). Superoxide dismutase activity in the cochlea. *Hear. Res.* 6, 141–151. doi: 10.1016/0378-5955(82)90050-8

Pouyatos, B., Gearhart, C. A., and Fechter, L. D. (2005). Acrylonitrile potentiates hearing loss and cochlear damage induced by moderate noise exposure in rats. *Toxicol. Appl. Pharmacol.* 204, 46–56. doi: 10.1016/j.taap.2004.08.015

Pouyatos, B., Gearhart, C. A., Nelson-Miller, A., Fulton, S., and Fechter, L. D. (2009). Selective vulnerability of the cochlear basal turn to acrylonitrile and noise. *J. Toxicol.* 2009:908596.

Rao, D., and Fechter, L. D. (2000). Protective effects of phenyl-N-tert-butylnitrone on the potentiation of noice-induced hearing loss by carbon monoxide. *Toxicol. Appl. Pharmacol.* 167, 125–131. doi: 10.1006/taap.2000.8995

Rosselin, M., Poeggeler, B., and Durand, G. (2017). Nitrone derivatives as therapeutics: from chemical modification to specific-targeting. *Curr. Top. Med. Chem.* 17, 2006–2022.

Somdas, M. A., Korkmaz, F., Gurgen, S. G., Sagit, M., and Akcadag, A. (2015). N-acetylcysteine prevents gentamicin ototoxicity in a rat model. *J. Int. Adv. Otol.* 11, 12–18. doi: 10.5152/iao.2015.650

Thomas, L., Smith, N., Saunders, D., Zalles, M., Gulej, R., Lerner, M., et al. (2020). Oklahoma Nitrone-007: novel treatment for diffuse intrinsic pontine glioma. *J. Transl. Med.* 18:424.

Varela-Nieto, I., Murillo-Cuesta, S., Calvino, M., Cediel, R., and Lassaletta, L. (2020). Drug development for noise-induced hearing loss. *Expert Opin. Drug Discov.* 15, 1457–1471.

Villamena, F. A., Das, A., and Nash, K. M. (2012). Potential Implication of the chemical properties and bioactivity of nitrone spin traps for therapeutics. *Future Med. Chem.* 4, 1171–1207. doi: 10.4155/fmc.12.74

Wang, J., Pignol, B., Chabrier, P. E., Saido, T., Lloyd, R., Tang, Y., et al. (2007). A novel dual inhibitor of calpains and lipid peroxidation (BN82270) rescues the cochlea from sound trauma. *Neuropharmacol.* 52, 1426–1437. doi: 10.1016/j.neuropharm.2007.02.007

Wang, J., and Puel, J. L. (2018). Toward cochlear therapies. *Physiol. Rev.* 98, 2477–2522. doi: 10.1152/physrev.00053.2017

Weisiger, R. A., and Fridovich, I. (1973). Superoxide dismutase. Organelle specificity. *J. Biol. Chem.* 248, 3528–3592.

Yu, J., Ding, D., Sun, H., Salvi, R., and Roth, J. A. (2016). Trimethyltin-induced cochlear degeneration in rat. *J. Otol.* 11, 118–126. doi: 10.1016/j.joto.2016.07.001

4

Antioxidants and Vasodilators for the Treatment of Noise-Induced Hearing Loss: Are they Really Effective?

Juan Carlos Alvarado [1], Verónica Fuentes-Santamaría [1] and José M. Juiz [1,2]*

[1]Facultad de Medicina, Instituto de Investigación en Discapacidades, Neurológicas (IDINE), Universidad de Castilla-La Mancha, Albacete, Spain, [2]Department of Otolaryngology, Hannover Medical School, NIFE-VIANNA, Cluster of Excellence Hearing4all-German Research Foundation, Hannover, Germany

***Correspondence:**
Juan Carlos Alvarado
juancarlos.alvarado@uclm.es

We live in a world continuously immersed in noise, an environmental, recreational, and occupational factor present in almost every daily human activity. Exposure to high-level noise could affect the auditory function of individuals at any age, resulting in a condition called noise-induced hearing loss (NIHL). Given that by 2018, more than 400 million people worldwide were suffering from disabling hearing loss and that about one-third involved noise over-exposure, which represents more than 100 million people, this hearing impairment represents a serious health problem. As of today, there are no therapeutic measures available to treat NIHL. Conventional preventive measures, including public awareness and education and physical barriers to noise, do not seem to suffice, as the population is still being affected by damaging noise levels. Therefore, it is necessary to develop or test pharmacological agents that may prevent and/or diminish the impact of noise on hearing. Data availability about the pathophysiological processes involved in triggering NIHL has allowed researchers to use compounds, that could act as effective therapies, by targeting specific mechanisms such as the excess generation of free radicals and blood flow restriction to the cochlea. In this review, we summarize the advantages/disadvantages of these therapeutic agents, providing a critical view of whether they could be effective in the human clinic.

Keywords: cochlear blood flow, deafness, magnesium, oxidative stress, sensorineural, vitamins

INTRODUCTION

Noise over-exposure is the major avoidable cause of permanent hearing loss (World Health Organization, 1997). As the second leading cause of adult-onset sensorineural deafness (Mathers et al., 2000), noise-induced hearing loss (NIHL) is a preventable condition that represents a large worldwide economic burden, as well as a health priority (World Health Organization, 1997, 2018; Mathers et al., 2000). It is well known that the main sources for excessive noise exposure, either alone or in combination are occupational, environmental, and recreational activities (World Health Organization, 1997, 2018; Hurtley, 2009). As far as the former is concerned, appropriate noise regulations and policies at workplaces are in effect. However, they have only been partially successful in reducing occupational-related NIHL (World Health Organization, 2018). Regarding environmental and recreational noise, the lack of awareness of the population about the hazard of over-exposure limits substantially the efficacy of regulatory measures (Śliwińska-Kowalska and Zaborowski, 2017; World Health Organization, 2018).

The importance of this issue is highlighted by the fact that the number of people exposed to noise is growing, while there is no actual medical treatment for NIHL, and conventional preventive measurements are not fully reaching their goals. There is overwhelming evidence that demonstrates that elevated calcium concentration, inflammation, increased oxidative stress, as well as a reduction in blood flow, are some of the pathophysiological mechanisms underlying NIHL (**Figure 1**; Lamm and Arnold, 1998; Henderson et al., 2006; Le Prell et al., 2007b; Shen et al., 2007; Bao et al., 2013; Fetoni et al., 2013; Altschuler and Dolan, 2015; Tan et al., 2016; Fuentes-Santamaría et al., 2017; Śliwińska-Kowalska and Zaborowski, 2017). It is worth noting, that at least the latter two cellular mechanisms seem to be part of a common pathogenic pathway that involves other sensorineural hearing loss conditions such as age-related hearing loss (ARHL) and drug-induced hearing loss (DIHL; Alvarado et al., 2015, 2018, 2019; Tavanai and Mohammadkhani, 2017). Therefore, therapies based on antioxidants and/or vasodilators have been postulated as strategies to prevent and/or reduce the progression of NIHL in several animal models and humans.

OXIDATIVE STRESS AND ANTIOXIDANTS

There is compelling evidence that suggests that noise over-exposure leads to an imbalance between excess free radical build-up, especially reactive oxygen, and nitrogen species (ROS and NRS), and its removal from cells in the auditory receptor. ROS build up in stressed mitochondria has been proposed as a major player at the origin of NIHL (Böttger and Schacht, 2013). This imbalance induces cell damage and ultimately, cell death in the organ of Corti (OC), the stria vascularis (SV) and the spiral ganglion (SG; Yamasoba et al., 1998; Henderson et al., 2006; Le Prell et al., 2007b; Fetoni et al., 2013; Altschuler and Dolan, 2015). Such reports support the hypothesis that therapeutic strategies targeting free radical overproduction are potentially useful to ameliorate the damaging effect of noise on hearing, which leads to cell death, mostly apoptotic (**Figure 2**). For instance, experimental studies that involve glutathione (Yamasoba et al., 1998; Ohinata et al., 2000; Hight et al., 2003; Henderson et al., 2006), N-acetylcysteine (Kopke et al., 2000, 2007), glutathione synthetic enzymes (Kil et al., 2007, 2017), multifunctional antioxidants (Chen et al., 2020) or micronutrients (Le Prell et al., 2007a,b) suggest attenuation of cochlear damage and/or reduction of the threshold shifts following noise exposure.

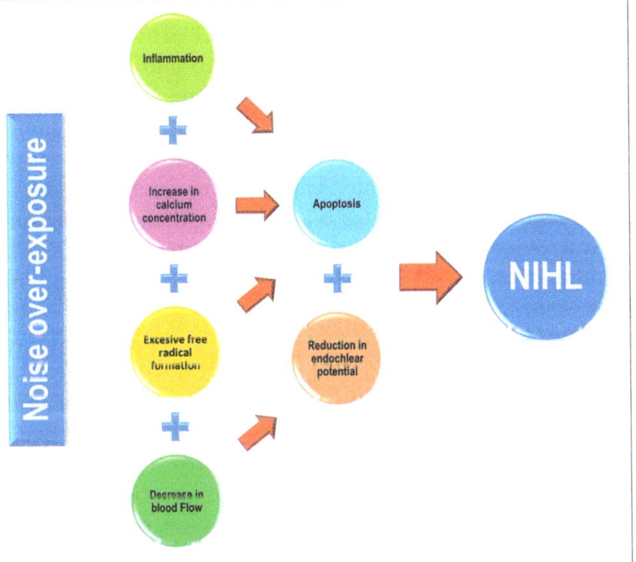

FIGURE 1 | Pathophysiological mechanisms involved in noise-induced hearing loss (NIHL). In response to noise over-exposure, a cascade of inflammatory-related events occurs in the exposed cochlea, leading to hair cell apoptosis and eventually, to hearing loss. Noise-induced cochlear increases in both calcium concentration and free radical production also activate sensory cell death processes that in turn, will cause hearing impairment. Additionally, noise triggers a direct and indirect (*via* calcium) vasoconstriction in the cochlea resulting in a decline in the endocochlear potential (EP), which correlates with impaired mechanotransduction in the organ of Corti (OC) and therefore, in hearing alterations.

Consistent with this idea, glutathione, a tripeptide molecule (cysteine, glutamic acid, and glycine) and the most abundant endogenous free radical scavenger in humans, was the first antioxidant evaluated for the treatment of NIHL (Yamasoba et al., 1998; Allen and Bradley, 2011; Schmitt et al., 2015). Glutathione is involved in many metabolic processes that include scavenging of free radicals and ROS, detoxification of several products such as lipid peroxides and xenobiotics, and it also plays a crucial role in the regeneration of ascorbate and tocopherol-based antioxidants (Yamasoba et al., 1998; Ohinata et al., 2000; Hight et al., 2003; Henderson et al., 2006; Allen and Bradley, 2011; Schmitt et al., 2015). Due to its wide distribution in the cochlea, preferentially in the SV and the spiral ligament (Yamasoba et al., 1998), therapeutic strategies aimed at increasing glutathione levels have been used as a proof of principle for the treatment of NIHL in rodent models. Increased glutathione levels in noise-exposed animal models have been associated with significantly smaller threshold shifts, due to reduced cochlear damage as compared to untreated animals (Yamasoba et al., 1998; Ohinata et al., 2000; Hight et al., 2003; Henderson et al., 2006). Conversely, reduced glutathione levels increase cochlear susceptibility to noise (Yamasoba et al., 1998; Ohlemiller et al., 2000). Despite these promising results, considerations regarding glutathione availability and administration route have precluded its use as a treatment for NIHL in humans. First, while oral administration of glutathione in experimental animals seems to be useful in increasing plasma levels, such oral supplementation in humans is controversial, as γ glutamyl transpeptidase, an intestinal enzyme, degrades exogenous glutathione before it could be absorbed (Allen and Bradley, 2011; Schmitt et al., 2015). Second, as glutathione in cells is mainly synthesized endogenously by its biochemical precursors, its parenteral administration may not result in a significant increase in the concentration of cellular glutathione levels (Hight et al., 2003).

N-acetylcysteine (NAC), a cysteine precursor, is an antioxidant molecule that enhances the production of

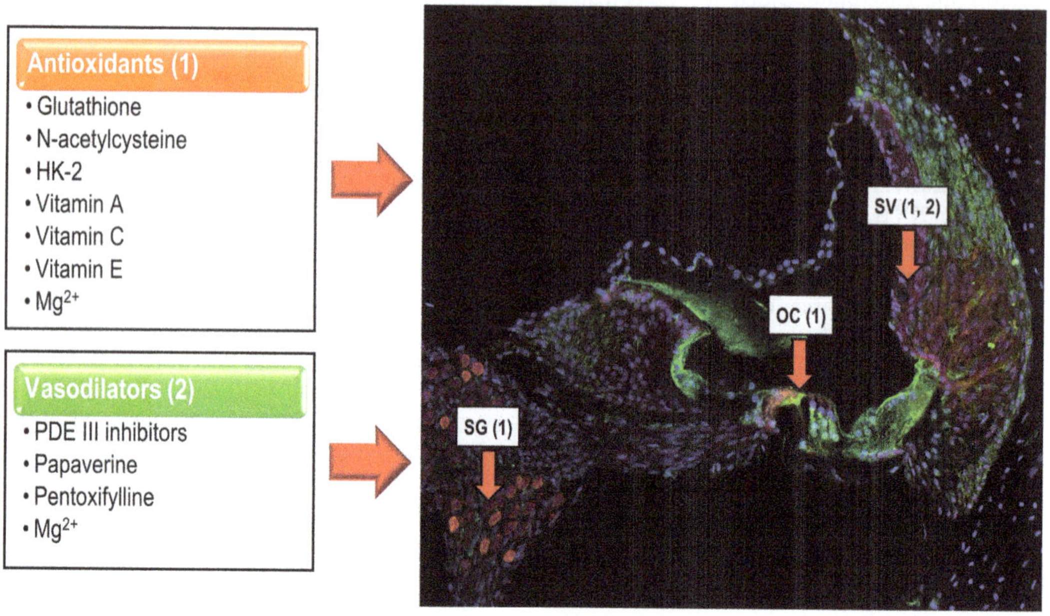

FIGURE 2 | Cochlear targets of antioxidants and vasodilators. Antioxidants (1) reduce the apoptotic cochlear damage that follows noise over-exposure, targeting hair cells in the OC, neurons of the spiral ganglion (SG) and stria vascularis (SV), exerting a protective effect over the cochlea and therefore, overhearing. Vasodilators (2), act mainly on the SV, minimizing noise-induced vasoconstriction, restoring the EP, and preserving auditory function.

glutathione (Kopke et al., 2000, 2007; Schmitt et al., 2015). Several studies in noise-exposed rats, chinchillas, and rabbits, have reported that the administration of NAC minimizes the progression of apoptosis in sensory hair cells and reduces significantly the auditory threshold shifts, at low and medium frequencies, as compared to untreated animals (Kopke et al., 2000; Mortazavi et al., 2010; Lu et al., 2014). In humans, the oral administration of NAC after noise exposure reduces significantly the incidence of temporary threshold shifts (TTS; Rosenhall et al., 2019) and when compared with glutathione, it has the advantage of better intestinal absorption. Thus, the available data largely support the notion that NAC could be used orally, increasing plasma levels of glutathione and acting as **a** replenisher of this endogenous scavenger (Kopke et al., 2007; Mortazavi et al., 2010; Schmitt et al., 2015). However, preliminary results suggest that high doses of NAC, still within therapeutic margins, do not limit but increase oxidative stress in the cochlea after treatment with ototoxic drugs, which share oxidative stress-related pathogenic pathways with NIHL. This finding highlights the notion that therapeutic margins for NAC, and maybe other antioxidants administered alone or in combinations, are relatively narrow and may limit synergistic interactions. It should be kept in mind that free radicals, like ROS, maybe "foes or friends." There are physiological ROS levels that are needed for biological redox reactions to proceed in a balanced manner (Ray et al., 2012). If treatments, for instance with NAC, bring ROS levels below a threshold, redox imbalances may lead to "paradoxical" oxidative damage. Also, since glutathione synthesis is reduced with aging, the effectiveness of administered NAC decreases as subjects age (Schmitt et al., 2015). An alternative approach to potentiate glutathione-mediated mechanisms involves priming enzymatic synthesis routes. Glutathione-peroxidase1 (Gpx1) is primarily involved in glutathione synthesis in the cochlea, and reduced activity has been linked to NIHL (Ohlemiller et al., 2000; Kil et al., 2007). Ebselen, a selenium-based organic compound, mimics and potentiates Gpx1 activity, and it has been shown to reduce auditory thresholds and hair cell death when administered parenterally to rats immediately before or after NIHL (Kil et al., 2007). More recently, safety and limited but significant efficacy of Ebselen has been shown in humans (Kil et al., 2017), supporting interventions on enzymatic activities in glutathione metabolic routes as a promising therapeutic avenue.

Interestingly, recent evidence suggests that HK-2, a multifunctional antioxidant with a metal chelator and free radical scavenger properties (Kawada and Kador, 2015; Kawada et al., 2015; Chen et al., 2020), is effective in treating NIHL. Oral administration of HK-2 to Sprague-Dawley rats 10 days before noise over-exposure exerts a significant protective effect in the cochlea, not only enhancing hair cell survival but also reducing the auditory threshold shifts when compared to untreated rats. While oral intake 10 days after noise exposure did not improve overall cell survival, it still preserved auditory function (Chen et al., 2020), suggesting a mild protective effect of HK-2 when taken several days after the exposure. Given that HK-2 is efficient at reducing noise-induced cell damage, it could be administered orally and it shows no side effects, at least in rats, it has been suggested as a new treatment option for NIHL (Chen et al., 2020). However, further studies will be needed to confirm that HK-2 is a valid therapeutic alternative without adverse side effects on humans.

Several micronutrients such as vitamins A, C, and E show antioxidant properties and have been used either individually or combined as experimental treatments for NIHL. The antioxidant mechanisms of vitamins are diverse. For instance, vitamin A (an *in vivo* product derived mainly from β-carotene) is an excellent scavenger of singlet oxygen, blocking and/or reverting lipid peroxidation in the plasma membrane (Sies and Stahl, 1995; Le Prell et al., 2007a; Alvarado et al., 2015, 2018). Experimentally, when retinoic acid, the most active metabolite of vitamin A, is administered in noise-exposed mice, it protects the cochlea by reducing significantly the apoptosis of hair cells and consequently, inducing a faster recovery of the auditory thresholds when compared to untreated animals (Ahn et al., 2005, 2013; Prasad and Bondy, 2020). Vitamin E is one of the main radical scavengers of the cell membrane as it blocks and/or reverts lipid peroxidation, by reacting with, and reducing peroxyl radicals (Sies and Stahl, 1995; Le Prell et al., 2007a; Alvarado et al., 2015, 2018). Vitamin E also has a protective effect in the cochlea by reducing cell death and cellular damage in guinea pigs (Hou et al., 2003; Fetoni et al., 2008), and by diminishing the auditory threshold shifts following noise over-exposure in guinea pigs (Hou et al., 2003; Fetoni et al., 2008) and humans (Kapoor et al., 2011). Vitamin C, a water-soluble molecule, is considered a primary extracellular antioxidant and it is extremely effective in blocking and/or reverting lipid peroxidation in the plasma membrane (Sies and Stahl, 1995; Le Prell et al., 2007a; Alvarado et al., 2015, 2018). Additionally, this vitamin also protects the cell membrane by regenerating vitamin E from its oxidized form. Therefore, the oxidative functions of both vitamin C and E are coupled (Sies and Stahl, 1995; Le Prell et al., 2007a; Alvarado et al., 2015, 2018). Regarding vitamin C, its administration before noise over-exposure diminishes significantly the TTS in rats (Loukzadeh et al., 2015) and the permanent threshold shifts (PTS) in guinea pigs (McFadden et al., 2005). Interestingly, the combination of vitamins A, C, and E administered orally to patients did not show any effect over music-induced TTS (Le Prell et al., 2016). In this latter report, the authors stated that three possible explanations may account for these negative results, including participant compliance, as only one of the six doses was administered under supervision; the bioavailability of orally administered vitamins and the possible degradation of the components during the shipping process (Le Prell et al., 2016). As there are no known disadvantages associated with the oral intake of the above-mentioned antioxidant vitamins, the main advantage lays in the fact that they present good safety profiles and are free from harmful side effects (Diplock, 1995; Hathcock, 1997). Nevertheless, additional studies will be required to ascertain whether these micronutrients are beneficial for treating NIHL in humans.

REDUCTION OF THE COCHLEAR BLOOD FLOW AND VASODILATORS

Exposure to loud noise, in addition to inducing oxidative stress, also diminishes cochlear blood flow by reducing blood vessel diameter and erythrocyte velocity in the basilar membrane, the spiral ligament and the SV (Sendowski, 2006; Le Prell et al., 2007a,b; Alvarado et al., 2015; Shin et al., 2019). Morphologic alterations in the SV, a key structure for producing and maintaining the endocochlear potential (EP), decrease the EP and consequently, affect the cochlear amplification of acoustic signals leading to an increase in auditory thresholds, even in the absence of hair cell death (Gates and Mills, 2005; Sendowski, 2006; Schmiedt, 2010; Alvarado et al., 2015). Therefore, it is expected that therapeutic agents that improve cochlear blood flow, would also reduce auditory thresholds in NIHL, with potentially beneficial effects in patients that suffer from this condition. This is the rationale for using vasodilator drugs such as phosphodiesterase (PDE) III inhibitors, papaverine, and pentoxifylline or micronutrients like magnesium (Mg^{2+}) which seem to have protective effects in the noise-exposed cochlea (**Figure 2**).

Accordingly, administration of milrinone, a PDE III inhibitor, to Wistar rats before noise over-exposure, ameliorates vacuolization, inflammation, and apoptotic processes in the sensory epithelium and the SV as compared to untreated rats (Ceylan et al., 2019). Although milrinone could be given orally as well as parenterally, it should be done under medical monitoring as one of its main side effects is dose-dependent cardiac arrhythmias (Davidenko and Antzelevitch, 1984; Ceylan et al., 2019). Regarding papaverine, a direct-acting vasodilator, when injected intraperitoneally in noise-exposed Wistar rats significantly decreases the apoptotic death of hair cells resulting in significantly smaller threshold shifts when compared to noise-exposed untreated animals (Kum et al., 2018). As a pharmacological agent, papaverine is not exempt from adverse effects including endothelium damage, epileptic seizures, transient neurological dysfunction, and hemodynamic changes, among others (Dipp et al., 2001; Chadwick et al., 2008). Pentoxifylline, another vasodilator compound used as a possible treatment for NIHL, has been reported to have no beneficial effects in noise-exposed guinea pigs, even though it improved the blood supply to the cochlea when administered parenterally (Lamm and Arnold, 1999). However, another study also in guinea pigs demonstrated that pentoxifylline reduced both cochlear damage and threshold shifts to values similar to untreated animals (Kansu et al., 2011; Sakat et al., 2016). Another observation to take into account is that, although pentoxifylline is a well-tolerated drug, it has several dose-related adverse effects including diarrhea, dyspepsia, constipation, confusion, seizures, hypotension, anaphylactoid reaction and hemorrhage (Tanikella et al., 2008; Hassan et al., 2014)

The micronutrient Mg^{2+} also has been proposed as a treatment for NIHL, not only for its function as a potential cochlear vasodilator but for other pharmacological properties, which include modulation of NMDA glutamate receptors and the regulation of calcium influx into hair cells, preventing or reducing apoptosis (Cevette et al., 2003; Sendowski, 2006; Le Prell et al., 2007a; Alvarado et al., 2015; Sakat et al., 2016). Further evidence supporting this idea comes from studies demonstrating that the subcutaneous injection of Mg^{2+} for one month enhanced hair cell survival and reduced significantly the auditory threshold shift in noise-exposed guinea pigs (Abaamrane et al., 2009). Similarly, the oral administration of salts of this cation, two weeks before high-level impulse-noise exposure significantly reduced the rate of acoustic trauma in guinea pigs (Scheibe et al., 2000).

However, parenteral administration of Mg^{2+} alone 1 h before and up to 5 days after noise stimulation in guinea pigs, did not show reliable effects over noise over-exposure. When Mg2+ was administered combined with vitamins A, C, and E there was a substantial protective effect reflected in increased hair cell survival and decreased auditory threshold shifts (Le Prell et al., 2007a). In noise-exposed mice, a similar combination of Mg^{2+} plus vitamins A, C and E partially recovers PTS, along with a significant reduction of type II fibrocytes in the cochlear lateral wall (Le Prell et al., 2011). In humans, it has been observed that the oral administration of Mg^{2+} significantly reduced PTS (Attias et al., 1994) and TTS (Attias et al., 2004), without any notable side effect, when compared to untreated subjects. Overall, Mg^{2+} is well-tolerated although there are some dose-dependent side effects such as nausea, diarrhea, stomachache, headache, tinnitus, and dizziness, which appear when used at high concentrations (Attias et al., 1994; Sendowski, 2006; Coates, 2010).

CONCLUSIONS

In light of new evidence about the etiopathogenic and pathophysiological mechanisms underlying NIHL, it becomes a priority to develop new therapeutic strategies that help to improve the quality of life of millions of people affected by this condition. The above-presented body of literature in this review strongly supports the fact that there are several pharmacologic agents available to prevent, at least in part, this disability. Acting preventively either on the excessive production of free radicals in the noise-exposed cochlea and/or on noise-induced cochlear vasoconstriction, they may help to ease the consequences of NIHL. It is important to keep in mind, however, that some of these substances may have pharmacological limitations, including the mechanism of drug action, administration route, tolerability, side effects, and proven efficacy, that should be considered before they could be approved for its use in this pathology. The most successful therapy, besides being efficient in reducing noise-induced cochlear damage, should be easy to administer (preferably orally), have a good safety profile, reduced drug acquisition costs, and few or no side effects. Antioxidants such as N-acetylcysteine, HK-2, vitamins A, C, and E and the vasodilator Mg^{2+} meet all these requirements acting either in different etiopathogenic pathways or on the same pathway through different targets. Therefore, it seems plausible to expect that a combination with some or all of them produces synergism and/or redundancy in their mechanisms of action, potentiating the beneficial effect over noise over-exposure. Even though these otoprotective agents represent a promising new therapeutic strategy for ameliorating, delaying, or even preventing the impact of noise on hearing, finding the ideal therapeutic agent will remain a challenging topic for the future.

AUTHOR CONTRIBUTIONS

JA and VF-S: drafting of the manuscript and design of figures. JA, VF-S, and JJ: critical revision of the manuscript for important intellectual content.

REFERENCES

Abaamrane, L., Raffin, F., Gal, M., Avan, P., and Sendowski, I. (2009). Long-term administration of magnesium after acoustic trauma caused by gunshot noise in guinea pigs. *Hear. Res.* 247, 137–145. doi: 10.1016/j.heares.2008.11.005

Ahn, J. H., Kang, H. H., Kim, Y.-J., and Chung, J. W. (2005). Anti-apoptotic role of retinoic acid in the inner ear of noise-exposed mice. *Biochem. Biophys. Res. Commun.* 335, 485–490. doi: 10.1016/j.bbrc.2005.07.114

Ahn, J. H., Shin, J.-E., Chung, B. Y., Lee, H. M., Kang, H. H., Chung, J. W., et al. (2013). Involvement of retinoic acid-induced peroxiredoxin 6 expression in recovery of noise-induced temporary hearing threshold shifts. *Environ. Toxicol. Pharmacol.* 36, 463–471. doi: 10.1016/j.etap.2013.05.012

Allen, J., and Bradley, R. D. (2011). Effects of oral glutathione supplementation on systemic oxidative stress biomarkers in human volunteers. *J. Altern. Complement. Med.* 17, 827–833. doi: 10.1089/acm.2010.0716

Altschuler, R. A., and Dolan, D. (2015). "Basic mechanisms underlying noise-induced hearing loss," in *Free Radicals in ENT Pathology*, eds J. M. Miller, C. G. Le Prell and L. Rybak (Cham: Springer International Publishing), 129–146.

Alvarado, J. C., Fuentes-Santamaría, V., Gabaldón-Ull, M. C., and Juiz, J. M. (2018). An oral combination of vitamins A, C, E, and Mg++ improves auditory thresholds in age-related hearing loss. *Front. Neurosci.* 12:527. doi: 10.3389/fnins.2018.0052

Alvarado, J. C., Fuentes-Santamaría, V., Gabaldón-Ull, M. C., and Juiz, J. M. (2019). Age-related hearing loss is accelerated by repeated short-duration loud sound stimulation. *Front. Neurosci.* 13:77. doi: 10.3389/fnins.2019.00077

Alvarado, J. C., Fuentes-Santamaría, V., Melgar-Rojas, P., Valero, M. L., Gabaldón-Ull, M. C., Miller, J. M., et al. (2015). Synergistic effects of free radical scavengers and cochlear vasodilators: a new otoprotective strategy for age-related hearing loss. *Front. Aging Neurosci.* 7:86. doi: 10.3389/fnagi.2015.00086

Attias, J., Sapir, S., Bresloff, I., Reshef-Haran, I., and Ising, H. (2004). Reduction in noise-induced temporary threshold shift in humans following oral magnesium intake. *Clin. Otolaryngol. Allied Sci.* 29, 635–641. doi: 10.1111/j.1365-2273.2004.00866.x

Attias, J., Weisz, G., Almog, S., Shahar, A., Wiener, M., Joachims, Z., et al. (1994). Oral magnesium intake reduces permanent hearing loss induced by noise exposure. *Am. J. Otolaryngol.* 15, 26–32. doi: 10.1016/0196-0709(94)90036-1

Bao, J., Hungerford, M., Luxmore, R., Ding, D., Qiu, Z., Lei, D., et al. (2013). Prophylactic and therapeutic functions of drug combinations against noise-induced hearing loss. *Hear. Res.* 304, 33–40. doi: 10.1016/j.heares.2013.06.004

Böttger, E. C., and Schacht, J. (2013). The mitochondrion: a perpetrator of acquired hearing loss. *Hear. Res.* 303, 12–19. doi: 10.1016/j.heares.2013.01.006

Cevette, M. J., Vormann, J., and Franz, K. (2003). Magnesium and hearing. *J. Am. Acad. Audiol.* 14, 202–212. Available online at: https://audiology.org/sites/default/files/journal/JAAA_14_04_04.pdf.

Ceylan, S. M., Uysal, E., Altinay, S., Sezgin, E., Bilal, N., Petekkaya, E., et al. (2019). Protective and therapeutic effects of milrinone on acoustic trauma in rat cochlea. *Eur. Arch. Otorhinolaryngol.* 276, 1921–1931. doi: 10.1007/s00405-019-05417-5

Chadwick, G. M., Asher, A. L., Van Der Veer, C. A., and Pollard, R. J. (2008). Adverse effects of topical papaverine on auditory nerve function. *Acta Neurochir.* 150, 901–909. doi: 10.1007/s00701-008-0004-8

Chen, G. D., Daszynski, D. M., Ding, D., Jiang, H., Woolman, T., Blessing, K., et al. (2020). Novel oral multifunctional antioxidant prevents noise-induced hearing loss and hair cell loss. *Hear. Res.* 388:107880. doi: 10.1016/j.heares.2019.107880

Coates, L. (2010). The effects of magnesium supplementation on sensorineural hearing damage: a critical review of the literature. *Univ. West. Ont. Sch. Commun. Sci. Disord.* Available online at https://www.uwo.ca/fhs/csd/ebp/reviews/2009-10/Coates.pdf.

Davidenko, J. M., and Antzelevitch, C. (1984). The effects of milrinone on conduction, reflection, and automaticity in canine Purkinje fibers. *Circulation* 69, 1026–1035. doi: 10.1161/01.cir.69.5.1026

Diplock, A. T. (1995). Safety of antioxidant vitamins and beta-carotene. *Am. J. Clin. Nutr.* 62, 1510S–1516S. doi: 10.1093/ajcn/62.6.1510S

Dipp, M. A., Nye, P. C. G., and Taggart, D. P. (2001). Phenoxybenzamine is more effective and less harmful than papaverine in the prevention of radial artery vasospasm. *Eur. J. Cardiothorac. Surg.* 19, 482–486. doi: 10.1016/s1010-7940(01)00598-x

Fetoni, A. R., De Bartolo, P., Eramo, S. L. M., Rolesi, R., Paciello, F., Bergamini, C., et al. (2013). Noise-induced hearing loss (NIHL) as a target of oxidative stress-mediated damage: cochlear and cortical responses after an increase in antioxidant defense. *J. Neurosci.* 33, 4011–4023. doi: 10.1523/JNEUROSCI.2282-12.2013

Fetoni, A. R., Ferraresi, A., Greca, C. L., Rizzo, D., Sergi, B., Tringali, G., et al. (2008). Antioxidant protection against acoustic trauma by coadministration of idebenone and vitamin E:. *NeuroReport* 19, 277–281. doi: 10.1097/WNR.0b013e3282f50c66

Fuentes-Santamaría, V., Alvarado, J. C., Melgar-Rojas, P., Gabaldón-Ull, M. C., Miller, J. M., and Juiz, J. M. (2017). The role of glia in the peripheral and central auditory system following noise overexposure: contribution of TNF-α and IL-1β to the pathogenesis of hearing loss. *Front. Neuroanat.* 11:9. doi: 10.3389/fnana.2017.00009

Gates, G. A., and Mills, J. H. (2005). Presbycusis. *Lancet* 366, 1111–1120. doi: 10.1016/S0140-6736(05)67423-5

Hassan, I., Dorjay, K., and Anwar, P. (2014). Pentoxifylline and its applications in dermatology. *Indian Dermatol. Online J.* 5:510. doi: 10.4103/2229-5178.142528

Hathcock, J. N. (1997). Vitamins and minerals: efficacy and safety. *Am. J. Clin. Nutr.* 66, 427–437. doi: 10.1093/ajcn/66.2.427

Henderson, D., Bielefeld, E. C., Harris, K. C., and Hu, B. H. (2006). The role of oxidative stress in noise-induced hearing loss. *Ear Hear.* 27, 1–19. doi: 10.1097/01.aud.0000191942.36672.f3

Hight, N. G., McFadden, S. L., Henderson, D., Burkard, R. F., and Nicotera, T. (2003). Noise-induced hearing loss in chinchillas pre-treated with glutathione monoethylester and R-PIA. *Hear. Res.* 179, 21–32. doi: 10.1016/s0378-5955(03)00067-4

Hou, F., Wang, S., Zhai, S., Hu, Y., Yang, W., and He, L. (2003). Effects of α-tocopherol on noise-induced hearing loss in guinea pigs. *Hear. Res.* 179, 1–8. doi: 10.1016/s0378-5955(03)00065-0

Hurtley, C., and World Health Organization (2009). *Night Noise Guidelines for Europe.* Copenhagen, Denmark: World Health Organization Europe.

Kansu, L., Ozkarakas, H., Efendi, H., and Okar, I. (2011). Protective effects of pentoxifylline and nimodipine on acoustic trauma in guinea pig cochlea. *Otol. Neurotol.* 32, 919–925. doi: 10.1097/MAO.0b013e3182267e06

Kapoor, N., Shyam, R., Singh, A., Mani, K., Sharma, R., and Selvamurthy, W. (2011). Effect of vitamin E supplementation on carbogen-induced amelioration of noise induced hearing loss in man. *Noise Health* 13:452. doi: 10.4103/1463-1741.90327

Kawada, H., Blessing, K., Kiyota, T., Woolman, T., Winchester, L., and Kador, P. F. (2015). Effects of multifunctional antioxidants on mitochondrial dysfunction and amyloid-β metal dyshomeostasis. *J. Alzheimers Dis.* 44, 297–307. doi: 10.3233/JAD-132471

Kawada, H., and Kador, P. F. (2015). Orally bioavailable metal chelators and radical scavengers: multifunctional antioxidants for the coadjutant treatment of neurodegenerative diseases. *J. Med. Chem.* 58, 8796–8805. doi: 10.1021/acs.jmedchem.5b00272

Kil, J., Lobarinas, E., Spankovich, C., Griffiths, S. K., Antonelli, P. J., Lynch, E. D., et al. (2017). Safety and efficacy of ebselen for the prevention of noise-induced hearing loss: a randomised, double-blind, placebo-controlled, phase 2 trial. *Lancet* 390, 969–979. doi: 10.1016/S0140-6736(17)31791-9

Kil, J., Pierce, C., Tran, H., Gu, R., and Lynch, E. D. (2007). Ebselen treatment reduces noise induced hearing loss *via* the mimicry and induction of glutathione peroxidase. *Hear. Res.* 226, 44–51. doi: 10.1016/j.heares.2006.08.006

Kopke, R. D., Jackson, R. L., Coleman, J. K. M., Liu, J., Bielefeld, E. C., and Balough, B. J. (2007). NAC for noise: From the bench top to the clinic. *Hear. Res.* 226, 114–125. doi: 10.1016/j.heares.2006.10.008

Kopke, R. D., Weisskopf, P. A., Boone, J. L., Jackson, R. L., Wester, D. C., Hoffer, M. E., et al. (2000). Reduction of noise-induced hearing loss using L-NAC and salicylate in the chinchilla. *Hear. Res.* 149, 138–146. doi: 10.1016/s0378-5955(00)00176-3

Kum, N. Y., Yilmaz, Y. F., Gurgen, S. G., Kum, R. O., Ozcan, M., and Unal, A. (2018). Effects of parenteral papaverine and piracetam administration on cochlea following acoustic trauma. *Noise Health* 20, 47–52. doi: 10.4103/nah.NAH_31_17

Lamm, K., and Arnold, W. (1998). The effect of prednisolone and non-steroidal anti-inflammatory agents on the normal and noise-damaged guinea pig inner ear. *Hear. Res.* 115, 149–161. doi: 10.1016/s0378-5955(97)00186-x

Lamm, K., and Arnold, W. (1999). Successful treatment of noise-induced cochlear ischemia, hypoxia and hearing loss. *Ann. N Y Acad. Sci.* 884, 233–248. doi: 10.1111/j.1749-6632.1999.tb08645.x

Le Prell, C. G., Dolan, D. F., Bennett, D. C., and Boxer, P. A. (2011). Nutrient plasma levels achieved during treatment that reduces noise-induced hearing loss. *Transl. Res.* 158, 54–70. doi: 10.1016/j.trsl.2011.02.003

Le Prell, C. G., Fulbright, A., Spankovich, C., Griffiths, S. K., Lobarinas, E., Campbell, K. C. M., et al. (2016). Dietary supplement comprised of β-carotene, vitamin C, vitamin E and magnesium: failure to prevent music-induced temporary threshold shift. *Audiol. Neurotol. Extra* 6, 20–39. doi: 10.1159/000446600

Le Prell, C. G., Hughes, L., and Miller, J. M. (2007a). Free radical scavengers vitamins A, C and E plus magnesium reduce noise trauma. *Free Radic. Biol. Med.* 42, 1454–1463. doi: 10.1016/j.freeradbiomed.2007.02.008

Le Prell, C. G., Yamashita, D., Minami, S. B., Yamasoba, T., and Miller, J. M. (2007b). Mechanisms of noise-induced hearing loss indicate multiple methods of prevention. *Hear. Res.* 226, 22–43. doi: 10.1016/j.heares.2006.10.006

Loukzadeh, Z., Hakimi, A., Esmailidehaj, M., and Mehrparvar, A. H. (2015). Effect of ascorbic acid on noise induced hearing loss in rats. *Iran. J. Otorhinolaryngol.* 27, 267–272. Available online at: https://www.ncbi.nlm.nih.gov/pmc/articles/PMC4710878/pdf/ijo-27-267.pdf.

Lu, J., Li, W., Du, X., Ewert, D. L., West, M. B., Stewart, C., et al. (2014). Antioxidants reduce cellular and functional changes induced by intense noise in the inner ear and cochlear nucleus. *J. Assoc. Res. Otolaryngol.* 15, 353–372. doi: 10.1007/s10162-014-0441-4

Mathers, C., Smith, A., and Concha, M. (2000). Global burden of hearing loss in the year 2000. *Glob. Burd. Dis.* 18, 1–30. doi: 10.1097/mao.0000000000001630

McFadden, S. L., Woo, J. M., Michalak, N., and Ding, D. (2005). Dietary vitamin C supplementation reduces noise-induced hearing loss in guinea pigs. *Hear. Res.* 202, 200–208. doi: 10.1016/j.heares.2004.10.011

Mortazavi, S., Kashani, M. M., Khavanin, A., Alameh, A., Mirzaee, R., and Akbari, M. (2010). Effects of N-acetylcysteine on auditory brainstem response threshold shift in rabbits exposed to noise and carbon monoxide. *Am. J. Appl. Sci.* 7, 201–207. doi: 10.3844/ajassp.2010.201.207

Ohinata, Y., Yamasoba, T., Schacht, J., and Miller, J. M. (2000). Glutathione limits noise-induced hearing loss. *Hear. Res.* 146, 28–34. doi: 10.1016/s0378-5955(00)00096-4

Ohlemiller, K. K., McFadden, S. L., Ding, D. L., Lear, P. M., and Ho, Y. S. (2000). Targeted mutation of the gene for cellular glutathione peroxidase (Gpx1) increases noise-induced hearing loss in mice. *J. Assoc. Res. Otolaryngol.* 1, 243–254. doi: 10.1007/s101620010043

Prasad, K. N., and Bondy, S. C. (2020). Increased oxidative stress, inflammation and glutamate: Potential preventive and therapeutic targets for hearing disorders. *Mech. Ageing Dev.* 185:111191. doi: 10.1016/j.mad.2019.111191

Ray, P. D., Huang, B.-W., and Tsuji, Y. (2012). Reactive oxygen species (ROS) homeostasis and redox regulation in cellular signaling. *Cell. Signal.* 24, 981–990. doi: 10.1016/j.cellsig.2012.01.008

Rosenhall, U., Skoog, B., and Muhr, P. (2019). Treatment of military acoustic accidents with N-Acetyl-L-cysteine (NAC). *Int. J. Audiol.* 58, 151–157. doi: 10.1080/14992027.2018.1543961

Sakat, M. S., Kilic, K., and Bercin, S. (2016). Pharmacological agents used for treatment and prevention in noise-induced hearing loss. *Eur. Arch. Otorhinolaryngol.* 273, 4089–4101. doi: 10.1007/s00405-016-3936-2

Scheibe, F., Haupt, H., and Ising, H. (2000). Preventive effect of magnesium supplement on noise-induced hearing loss in the guinea pig. *Eur. Arch. Otorhinolaryngol.* 257, 10–16. doi: 10.1007/pl00007505

Schmiedt, R. A. (2010). "The physiology of cochlear presbycusis," in *The Aging Auditory System*, eds S. Gordon-Salant, R. D. Frisina, A. N. Popper and R. R. Fay (New York, NY: Springer), 9–38.

Schmitt, B., Vicenzi, M., Garrel, C., and Denis, F. M. (2015). Effects of N-acetylcysteine, oral glutathione (GSH) and a novel sublingual form of GSH on oxidative stress markers: A comparative crossover study. *Redox Biol.* 6, 198–205. doi: 10.1016/j.redox.2015.07.012

Sendowski, I. (2006). Magnesium therapy in acoustic trauma. *Magnes. Res.* 19, 244–254. Available online at: https://pdfs.semanticscholar.org/8adf/e95647ac1465e8ee5f917a7a370af24b9f25.pdf?_ga=2.41126436.760994297.1593958950-2089061770.1587115630.

Shen, H., Zhang, B., Shin, J.-H., Lei, D., Du, Y., Gao, X., et al. (2007). Prophylactic and therapeutic functions of T-type calcium blockers against noise-induced hearing loss. *Hear. Res.* 226, 52–60. doi: 10.1016/j.heares.2006.12.011

Shin, S.-A., Lyu, A.-R., Jeong, S.-H., Kim, T. H., Park, M. J., and Park, Y.-H. (2019). Acoustic trauma modulates cochlear blood flow and vasoactive factors in a rodent model of noise-induced hearing loss. *Int. J. Mol. Sci.* 20:5316. doi: 10.3390/ijms20215316

Sies, H., and Stahl, W. (1995). Vitamins E and C, beta-carotene and other carotenoids as antioxidants. *Am. J. Clin. Nutr.* 62, 1315S–1321S. doi: 10.1093/ajcn/62.6.1315S

Śliwińska-Kowalska, M., and Zaborowski, K. (2017). WHO environmental noise guidelines for the european region: a systematic review on environmental noise and permanent hearing loss and tinnitus. *Int. J. Environ. Res. Public. Health* 14:1139. doi: 10.3390/ijerph14101139

Tan, W. J. T., Thorne, P. R., and Vlajkovic, S. M. (2016). Characterisation of cochlear inflammation in mice following acute and chronic noise exposure. *Histochem. Cell Biol.* 146, 219–230. doi: 10.1007/s00418-016-1436-5

Tanikella, R., Philips, G. M., Faulk, D. K., Kawut, S. M., and Fallon, M. B. (2008). Pilot study of pentoxifylline in hepatopulmonary syndrome. *Liver Transpl.* 14, 1199–1203. doi: 10.1002/lt.21482

Tavanai, E., and Mohammadkhani, G. (2017). Role of antioxidants in prevention of age-related hearing loss: a review of literature. *Eur. Arch. Otorhinolaryngol.* 274, 1821–1834. doi: 10.1007/s00405-016-4378-6

World Health Organization. (1997). *Prevention of Noise-Induced Hearing Loss.* Available online at: http://apps.who.int/iris/bitstream/handle/10665/65390/WHO_PDH_98.5.pdf?sequence=1andisAllowed=y. Accessed October 28, 1997.

World Health Organization. (2018). *Addressing the Rising Prevalence of Hearing Loss.* World Health Organization. Available online at: http://apps.who.int/iris/handle/10665/260336. Accessed November 29, 2018.

Yamasoba, T., Nuttall, A. L., Harris, C., Raphael, Y., and Miller, J. M. (1998). Role of glutathione in protection against noise-induced hearing loss. *Brain Res.* 784, 82–90. doi: 10.1016/s0006-8993(97)01156-6

5

Spike Generators and Cell Signaling in the Human Auditory Nerve: An Ultrastructural, Super-Resolution and Gene Hybridization Study

Wei Liu[1]*, Maria Luque*[2]*, Hao Li*[1]*, Anneliese Schrott-Fischer*[2]*, Rudolf Glueckert*[2]*, Sven Tylstedt*[3]*, Gunesh Rajan*[4,5]*, Hanif Ladak*[6]*, Sumit Agrawal*[7] *and Helge Rask-Andersen*[1]*

[1] Section of Otolaryngology, Department of Surgical Sciences, Head and Neck Surgery, Uppsala University Hospital, Uppsala, Sweden, [2] Department of Otorhinolaryngology, Medical University of Innsbruck, Innsbruck, Austria, [3] Department of Olaryngology, Västerviks Hospital, Västervik, Sweden, [4] Department of Otolaryngology, Head & Neck Surgery, Luzerner Kantonsspital, Luzern, Switzerland, [5] Department of Otolaryngology, Head & Neck Surgery, Division of Surgery, Medical School, University of Western Australia, Perth, WA, Australia, [6] Department of Otolaryngology-Head and Neck Surgery, Department of Medical Biophysics and Department of Electrical and Computer Engineering, Western University, London, ON, Canada, [7] Department of Otolaryngology-Head and Neck Surgery, Western University, London, ON, Canada

***Correspondence:**
Helge Rask-Andersen
helge.rask-andersen@surgsci.uu.se
orcid.org/0000-0002-2552-5001

Background: The human auditory nerve contains 30,000 nerve fibers (NFs) that relay complex speech information to the brain with spectacular acuity. How speech is coded and influenced by various conditions is not known. It is also uncertain whether human nerve signaling involves exclusive proteins and gene manifestations compared with that of other species. Such information is difficult to determine due to the vulnerable, "esoteric," and encapsulated human ear surrounded by the hardest bone in the body. We collected human inner ear material for nanoscale visualization combining transmission electron microscopy (TEM), super-resolution structured illumination microscopy (SR-SIM), and RNA-scope analysis for the first time. Our aim was to gain information about the molecular instruments in human auditory nerve processing and deviations, and ways to perform electric modeling of prosthetic devices.

Material and Methods: Human tissue was collected during trans-cochlear procedures to remove petro-clival meningioma after ethical permission. Cochlear neurons were processed for electron microscopy, confocal microscopy (CM), SR-SIM, and high-sensitive *in situ* hybridization for labeling single mRNA transcripts to detect ion channel and transporter proteins associated with nerve signal initiation and conductance.

Results: Transport proteins and RNA transcripts were localized at the subcellular level. Hemi-nodal proteins were identified beneath the inner hair cells (IHCs). Voltage-gated ion channels (VGICs) were expressed in the spiral ganglion (SG) and axonal initial segments (AISs). Nodes of Ranvier (NR) expressed Nav1.6 proteins, and encoding genes critical for inter-cellular coupling were disclosed.

Discussion: Our results suggest that initial spike generators are located beneath the IHCs in humans. The first NRs appear at different places. Additional spike generators and transcellular communication may boost, sharpen, and synchronize afferent signals by cell clusters at different frequency bands. These instruments may be essential for the filtering of complex sounds and may be challenged by various pathological conditions.

Keywords: human, auditory nerve, gene expression, structured illumination microscopy, spike generation

INTRODUCTION

Human Speech—Reception and Spike Generation

Humans have developed sophisticated abilities to produce and perceive oral speech. This involves particular anatomy, complex neural circuits in the brain, and a perceptual apparatus that deciphers "multifaceted" air-borne signals (Hockett et al., 1964). How this cladistics took place is fiercely discussed among linguistic anthropologists. Its components, such as morphology, phonetics, and semantics, may have been shaped by several environmental factors (Wiener, 1984). In all cases, the human auditory nerve relays intricate speech-coded information to the brain that depends on an unbroken signal acuity to the central nervous system (CNS). The established signals are vulnerable, and their conservation is essential for proper decrypting. They are not readily restored centrally once distorted by tumor compression or deficient conversion at the inner hair cell (IHC) ribbon synapse. Gene mutations (FOXP2) have been associated with abnormal development of neural structures important for human speech and language (Lai et al., 2001), and the locus on chromosome 16 has been associated with specific language impairment (Newbury et al., 2005), a more or less central deficiency in perception of speech (Bishop et al., 2007).

It remains unclear how speech is coded in the auditory nerve, but it has been studied in animal models (Kiang, 1980, Khanna and Teich, 1989). Even though potentials recorded from the cochlea and auditory nerve are similar for most mammals, different species have developed arrangements to optimally process sound most relevant for their survival (Theunissen and Elie, 2014). Evolutionary adaptation may include modifications of inherent molecular systems. Since there are substantial anatomical differences between humans and other species (Kimura et al., 1979; Ota and Kimura, 1980; Arnold, 1987; Spoendlin and Schrott, 1988; Tylstedt and Rask-Andersen, 2001; Liu et al., 2015), distinct features may have developed and been reflected in the morphology, distribution of coding proteins, excitation pattern, and nerve conductivity. Researchers have indicated that frequency resolution relevant for speech development is higher in humans than in laboratory animals (Shera et al., 2010; Sumner et al., 2018). Nonetheless, this remains controversial (Ruggero and Temchin, 2005; Lopez-Poveda and Eustaquio-Martin, 2013), and studies have claimed that sharpness of tuning is similar in all mammals and birds.

It is undetermined how and where action potentials (APs) are generated in the human auditory nerve. Possible sites are the (1) nerve-receptor junction, (2) spiral ganglion (SG), (3) axonal initial segments (AISs), and (4) Nodes of Ranvier (NR). Studies of voltage-gated ion channels (VGICs) were performed in several non-human species with variable results (Mo and Davis, 1997; Adamson et al., 2002; Hossain et al., 2005; Fryatt et al., 2009; McLean et al., 2009; Smith et al., 2015; Kim and Rutherford, 2016). A multitude of voltage-gated K^+ channels with various gating kinetics were discovered in the auditory pathway (Liu Q, et al., 2014), and literature reviews on these have been presented (Oak and Yi, 2014; Reijntjes and Pyott, 2016). RNA sequencing and single molecule *in situ* hybridization mapped transcripts encoding potassium channels were found to be essential for normal auditory function (Reijntjes et al., 2019). Different K^+-channels are thought to contribute to individual neuronal coding frequencies in the auditory system (Adamson et al., 2002). Single-cell RNA sequencing demonstrated that type I SG neurons (SGNs) are molecularly diverse and identified three subclasses of type I neurons. They were subdivided into six classes based on the genetic framework defining intensity coding properties in a transcriptional catalog of the murine cochlea (Petitpré et al., 2018; Sun et al., 2018). Surprisingly, disruption of IHC signaling before hearing onset was found to influence spontaneous activity and molecular diversification of type I cells (SGNs) (Sun et al., 2018).

A remarkable outcome of speech recognition is gained in the severely hearing impaired by today's auditory electric prostheses, even in patients lacking peripheral dendrites. This suggests that electrically evoked speech signals may be relayed centrally

Abbreviations: ABR, auditory brain stem response; AIS, axonal initial segment; AP, action potential; BK-channel, Big potassium or (calcium-activated potassium channel KCa1.1); Caspr1, contactin-associated protein 1; CI, cochlear implant; CM, confocal microscopy; CNS, central nervous system; Cx30, connexin30; DAPI, 4′, 6-diamidino-2-phenylindole dihydro-chloride; diceCT, diffusible iodine-based contrast-enhanced computed tomography; EDTA, ethylene-diamine-tetra-acetic acid; EPSP, excitatory post-synaptic potential; GFAP, glia fibrillary acidic protein; GJ, gap junction; HCN, hyperpolarization-activated cyclic nucleotide-gated channels; HP, habenular perforata; IAC, internal acoustic canal; IGSB, intra-ganglionic spiral bundle; IHC, inner hair cell; Kv, voltage-gated potassium channel; LGC, large ganglion cell; LOC, lateral olive-cochlear; LW, lateral wall; MBP, myelin basic protein; MOC, medial olivo-cochlear; Micro-CT, micro-computerized tomography; Na/K-ATPase, sodium potassium adenosine-tri-phosphatase; Nav, voltage-gated sodium channel; NF, nerve fiber; NR, node of Ranvier; OC, organ of Corti; OHC, outer hair cell; PBS, phosphate buffered saline; PFD, paraformaldehyde; RC, Rosenthal's canal; RNA scope, ribonucleic acid detection device; RT-PCR, reverse transcription polymerase chain reaction; SEM, scanning electron microscopy; SG, spiral ganglion; SGCs, satellite glia cells; SGN, spiral ganglion neuron; SNHL, severe sensorineural hearing loss; SR-SIM, super-resolution structured illumination microscopy; TEM, transmission electron microscope/microscopy; TUJ1, tubulin-1; Type I cells, large spiral ganglion neurons (~95% of total numbers); Type II cells, small spiral ganglion neurons (~5% of total numbers); VGIC, voltage-gated ion channel; VGSC, voltage-gated sodium channel.

without peripheral or electro-phonic hair cell stimulation. How this happens is virtually unknown.

Goals of the Present Investigation

We aimed to further analyze and review the micro-anatomy of the human cochlea and auditory nerve using transmission and scanning electron microscopy and 3D imaging. In addition, efforts were made to localize VGICs, their associated proteins and ion transporter Na/K-ATPase and their isoforms using immunohistochemistry and high-resolution structured illumination microscopy (SR-SIM) and confocal microscopy (CM). A first attempt was made to use *in situ* RNA hybridization to detect mRNA transcripts. For this, tissue was harvested in connection with surgeries for life-threatening petro-clival meningioma where the cochlea had to be sacrificed. Ethical permission and patient consent were obtained. Since cochlear function was preserved, it offered unique possibilities to study some of the molecular organization under "near-normal" settings. Besides, we searched for alternate cellular communication pathways capable of synchronized firing that could be essential for processing complex sounds in humans. One donated human temporal bone was analyzed using micro-computerized tomography (MicroCT) and soft tissue staining. Hopefully, the results may bring further elucidation on spike generation and signal characteristics in the human auditory nerve. It may provide information on how and where electric prostheses target stimulation of the human nerve. Due to the limited amount of tissue that can be collected at surgery, a quantitative display and gradient molecular expression of VGICs along the entire cochlear spiral is not possible at this stage.

MATERIALS AND METHODS

Ethical Statements

The study of human cochleae was approved by the local ethics committee (Etikprövningsnämnden Uppsala, no. 99398, 22/9 1999, cont, 2003, no. C254/4; C209/10, no. C45/7 2007, Dnr. 2013/190), and patient consent was obtained. Ethics approval for the microCT project was obtained from the University of Western Australia (UWA, RA/4/1/5210), and the human temporal bones were provided by the Department of Anatomy at UWA. The study adhered to the rules of the Declaration of Helsinki.

Tissue Sampling

The surgical specimens were from patients suffering from life-threatening posterior cranial fossa meningioma compressing the brain stem (Rask-Andersen et al., 1997). Human cochleae were harvested at major trans-cochlear skull base surgeries, including facial nerve rerouting. The operations were performed at Uppsala University Hospital by a team of neurosurgeons and oto-neuro-surgeons. Five cochleae were dissected out using diamond drills of various sizes (**Table 1**). Six Dunkin Hartley guinea pigs were processed and underwent similar fixation and immunohistochemistry.

Immunohistochemistry

Immunohistochemistry procedures on human cochlear sections were described in previous publications (Liu et al., 2009, 2020). In short, tissue was fixed in a solution of 4% (or 2% for sodium channels) paraformaldehyde (PFD) phosphate buffer solution (PBS). Different fixation durations are determined by channel types detected, ranging from 45 min to hours. After fixation, the fixative was replaced with 0.1 M PBS, and cochleae were decalcified in 10% ethylene-diamine-tetra-acetic acid (EDTA) solution at pH 7.2 for 4 weeks. The cochleae were embedded in Tissue-Tek OCT embedding compound (Polysciences, Inc., Warrington, PA, USA), rapidly frozen, and sectioned at 8–10 µm using a cryostat microtome. Sections were incubated with an antibody solution under a humidified atmosphere at 4°C for 20 h. Sections were incubated with secondary antibodies conjugated to Alexa Fluor (Thermo Fisher Scientific, Uppsala) counterstained with the nuclear stain 4′,6-diamidino-2-phenylindole dihydro-chloride (DAPI), mounted with ProLong® Gold Antifade Mountant (Thermo Fisher Scientific, Uppsala, Catalog number: P10144), and then covered with the specified cover glass compatible with both confocal and super-resolution microscopes. Primary and secondary antibody controls and labeling controls were used to exclude endogenous labeling or reaction products (Burry, 2011). The antibodies used for immunohistochemistry are shown in **Table 2**.

Stained sections were first investigated with an inverted fluorescence microscope (TE2000; Nikon, Tokyo, Japan) equipped with a spot digital camera with three filters (for emission spectra maxima at 358, 461, and 555 nm). Image-processing software (NIS Element BR-3.2; Nikon), including image merging and a fluorescence intensity analyzer, was installed on a computer system connected to the microscope. For laser CM, we used the same microscope equipped with a three-channel laser emission system. SR-SIM was performed (Gustafsson et al., 2008) using a Zeiss Elyra S.1 SIM system and a 63×/1.4 oil Plan-Apochromat objective (Zeiss, Oberkochen, Germany), sCMOS camera (PCO Edge), and ZEN 2012 software (Carl Zeiss Microscope). The resolution of the SR-SIM system at BioVis, Uppsala University, was 107 nm in the X–Y plane and 394 nm in the Z plane. The following laser and filter setup was as follows: 405 nm laser of excitation coupled with BP 420–480 + LP 750 filter, 488 nm laser of excitation with BP 495–550 + LP750 filter, 561 nm laser of excitation with BP 570–620 + LP 750 filter, and 647 nm laser of excitation with LP 655 filter. From the SR-SIM dataset, 3D reconstruction was done with Imaris 8.2 (Bitplane, Zürich, Switzerland). A bright-field channel was able to merge fluorescence channels to visualize cell/tissue borders.

RNA-Scope Protocol

Fixed-frozen human tissue sections underwent pretreatment with H_2O_2 (10 min, RT) and protease III (30 min, 40°C). After protease III incubation, the sections were subjected to RNA-scope hybridization assay. The probes were designed and produced by BioTechne depending on targets' gene ID. To start the hybridization, the RNA probe(s) (in our study, a fluid mixture of probes named C1, C2, and C3 channels) was added to the

TABLE 1 | Patient data and functioning of their cochleae used for IHC and RNA-scope.

Age	Gender	PTT/SD	Analysis
43	Female	50 dB (1–8 kHz)	IHC
51	Male	Normal	IHC
72	Male	50 dB (2–4 kHz)	IHC
67	Female	Normal	IHC
67	Female	SD 85%	IHC, RNA-scope

TEM and SEM data were obtained from archival material as described in papers (Tylstedt et al., 1997; Rask-Andersen et al., 2012; Liu W, et al., 2014). PTT, pure tone thresholds; SD, speech discrimination. The specimens were from persons without any known hearing impairment and were obtained at surgery for removal of large, life-threatening petroclival meningioma where the cochlea hade to be sacrificed during trans-cochlear surgery. Re-routing of the facial nerve is performed routinely at this type of surgery.

slide with sections. Incubation was going on in a HybEZ™ Oven (Bio-Techne co.) for 2 h at 40°C. After hybridization incubation, the slides were washed using 1× RNA-scope® Wash Buffer. Then the sections were incubated with RNA-scope® Multiplex FL v2 Amp 1, 2, and 3 (for 30 min/30 min/15 min, respectively) sequentially at 40°C to amplify the signal. For signal development, RNAscope® Multiplex FL v2 HRP-C1, HRP-C2 and HRP-C3 were added to the sections sequentially (incubation time 15 min) in our RNA-scope® Multiplex study. For revealing signals, TSA-diluted Opal™ 520, 570, and 690 fluorophores were added to sections after HRP-C1, C2, and C3, incubating the sections for 30 min each at 40°C. When the three Opal fluorophores were assigned to each channel, in our experiment, three channels C1, C2, and C3 were assigned to Na/K-ATP1A1, Na/K-ATP1B1, and Na/K-ATP1B3 or Cx probes (Ref: 567981 RNAscope probe Hs-GJD2, Ref: 541391 RNAscope probe Hs-GJB6, Ref: 539891 RNAscope probe Hs-ATPase alpha 1, Ref: 568261 RNAscope probe Hs-ATPase Beta 1) (**Table 3**). After each fluorophore incubation and rinse with 1× RNA-scope® Wash Buffer, RNA-scope® Multiplex FL v2 HRP blocker was added and incubated in oven for 15 min at 40°C. Finally the sections were counterstained with DAPI and the slides cover-slipped with ProLong® Glass Antifade Mountant (Thermo fisher Scientific). RNA-scope ISH produces puncta of signal that represent a single mRNA transcript (Grabinski et al., 2015).

TABLE 2 | Antibodies used in the present investigation.

Antibody	Type	Host	Cat#	Company
ATPase (α1)	Monoclonal (m)	Mouse (m)	NB300-146	Novus
ATPase (α2)	Polyclonal (p)	Rabbit (r)	AP5828c-ev	Nordic BioSite
ATPase (α3)	m	m	MA3-915	Thermo Fisher
ATPase (β1)	m	m	Ma3-930	Abcam
ATPase (β2)	p	r	PA5-26279	Invitrogen
NKCC1	p	r	ab59791	Abcam
Laminin β2	m	r	05-206	Millipore
Cx30	p	r	71-2200	Invitrogen
Cx26	m	m	33-5800	Invitrogen
Cx26	p	r	ACC-2121	Alomone
Cx36	m	m	37-4600	Invitrogen
Cx43	p	r	71-0700	Invitrogen
Cx43	m	m	MAB3068	Millipore
KCa1.1	p	r	APC-107	Alomone
Collagen II	m	m	CP18	Millipore
Collagen IV	p	goat	AB769	Millipore
MBP	m	r	#AB980,	Millipore
S-100	p	r	Z 0311	Dako
Tuj-1	m	m	MAB1637	Millipore
Parvalb.	m	m	MAB1572	Chemicon
Tuj-1	p	r	#04-1049	Millipore
Laminin β2	m	r	#05-206	Millipore
GFAP	p	r	AB5804	Chemicon
GFAP	m	m	MAB360	Millipore
CGRP	p	r	Ab71225	Abcam
Kv1.1	p	r	APC-161	Alomone Labs
Kv1.2	p	r	APC-010	Alomone Labs
Kv3.1	p	r	APC-014	Alomone Labs
Kv7.1	p	r	APC-022	Alomone Labs
Ankyrin G	m	m	NBP2-59310	Novus
Caspr-1	m	m	SMC-370D	Nordic BioSite
Pan-Nav	p	r	ASC-003	Alomone Labs
Nav1.1	m	m	S74-71	Novus
Nav1.3	p	r	ASC-004	Alomone Labs
Nav1.6	m	m	SMC-378D	Nordic BioSite
Nav1.7	p	r	ASC-008	Alomone Labs
Nav1.8	p	r	ASC-016	Alomone Labs
Nav1.9	p	r	ASC-017	Alomone Labs

MicroCT

MicroCT was used to analyze the 3D anatomy of the nerves in the internal acoustic meatus. We used a diffusible iodine-based technique to enhance contrast of soft tissues for diffusible iodine-based contrast-enhanced computed tomography (diceCT). Increased time penetration of Lugol's iodine (aqueous I2KI, 1% I_2, 2% KI) offers possibilities to visualize between and within soft tissue structures (Camilieri-Asch et al., 2020). The temporal bone was fixed in a modified Karnovsky's fixative solution of 2.5% glutaraldehyde, 1% paraformaldehyde, 4% sucrose, and 1% dimethyl sulfoxide in 0.13 M of Sorensen's phosphate buffer. Soft tissue contrast was achieved by staining the sample for 14 days as described by Culling (Culling, 1974). X-ray microCT was conducted using a Versa 520 XRM (Zeiss, Pleasanton, CA, USA) running Scout and Scan software (v11.1.5707.17179). Scans were conducted at a voltage of 80 kV and 87 μA, using the LE4 filter under 0.4× optical magnification and a camera binning of 2. Source and detector positions were adjusted to deliver an isotropic voxel size of 23 μm. A total of 2,501 projections were collected over 360°, each with an exposure time of 1 s. Raw projection data were reconstructed using XM Reconstructor software (v10.7.3679.13921; Zeiss) following a standard center shift and beam hardening (0.1) correction. The standard 0.7 kernel size recon filter setting was also used (Culling, 1974). Images were imported into the 3D Slicer program (Slicer 4.6; www.slicer.org), an open-source software platform for medical image informatics, image processing, and 3D visualization. Images were resized at a scale of 4:1, and opacity and gray scale values were adjusted during volume rendering. The technique allows reconstruction in three dimensions, and bones were made transparent and cropped.

Transmission and Scanning Electron Microscopy (TEM and SEM)

Four archival specimens collected during surgery were analyzed in Uppsala and Innsbruck; the technique used was previously described (Tylstedt and Rask-Andersen, 2001). Briefly, specimens were fixed in 3% phosphate-buffered glutaraldehyde, pH 7.4, and rinsed in 0.1 M cacodylate buffer, and then immersed in 1% osmium tetroxide at 4°C for 4 h. The specimens were dehydrated and infiltrated with Epon resin in a vacuum chamber for 4 h. Sections were viewed in a JEOL 100 SX electron microscope in Uppsala. For SEM, specimens were placed in 3% sodium phosphate buffered glutaraldehyde and perfused through the oval and round windows. Specimens were coated with a 10 to 15 nm layer of gold-palladium in a BALTECH® MED 020 Coating System and observed with a ZEISS® DSM 982 Gemini Field Emission Electron Microscope operating at 4 to 5 kV (Rask-Andersen et al., 2012).

RESULTS

SEM of a hemi-sectioned human cochlea and organ of Corti (OC) is shown in **Figure 1**. Higher magnification of the organ of Corti shows the multicellular acoustic crest with sensory hair cells and surrounding supporting cells (**Figure 1B**) and innervation pathway (**Figure 1C**).

The nerve and vascular supply to the human hearing organ is demonstrated using microCT. It reproduced both the afferent and efferent nerve supply within the internal acoustic meatus. 3D modeling demonstrates the vestibular-cochlear anastomosis of Oort and blood vessels in a right ear in **Figure 2**. Several efferent bundles leave the inferior vestibular nerve to reach the cochlea 3–4 mm from its basal end. At surgery it was also possible to remove and directly fix a human cochlear nerve for LM and TEM as well as for immunohistochemistry (**Figures 3B–E, 4**). Cross-sections at different levels show the nerve both near the fundus and at the transitional zone after glutaraldehyde fixation and osmium staining. The transitional zone contained a central lucent part with glia and astrocyte tissue projecting peripherally into the nerve. It was surrounded by a part with Schwann cells (**Figures 3C–E**). Immune staining of a cross-sectioned human auditory nerve near the fundus is shown in **Figure 4A** and shows that nerve fibers express the myelin marker MBP and neuron marker TUJ1. Only a few single fibers were unmyelinated and are believed to represent NRs. Though, peripherin antibody staining was not performed so it cannot be excluded entirely that they represent type II afferent fibers originating from the small ganglion cells passing to the brain. At the transitional zone astrocytes stained positive for GFAP and Cx43 (**Figure 4B** and inset). Surprisingly, a few Nav1.6-positive ganglion cells were occasionally found in the distal part of the IAC along nerve fascicles (not shown here). Their axonal initial segments (AISs) express Nav1.6.

The Spiral Ganglion and Expression of Nav, Kv, Caspr1, and Ankyrin G

The SG is located in a 13–14 mm long bony canal in the modiolus called Rosenthal's canal (RC) (Ariyasu et al., 1989; Stakhovskaya et al., 2007; Li et al., 2018). It is well-defined in the basal turn only. It contains afferent large ganglion cells (LGCs) or type I cells (87–97%) innervating the IHCs and small ganglion cells (SGCs) or type II cells (3–13%) that innervate the outer hair cells (OHCs) (Arnold et al., 1980; Arnold, 1987; Spoendlin and Schrott, 1989; Rosbe et al., 1996). Large or type I spiral ganglion cell soma are surrounded by non-myelinating satellite glial cells (SGCs) and lack expression of MBP. In the apex, SGCs form a more or less complete honeycomb layer. SGCs were surrounded by a basal lamina expressing lamininβ2 and collagen IV and were connected by gap junctions (GJs) expressing Cx43. Expression of voltage-gated sodium channels is summarized in **Table 4**. Large and small spiral ganglion cell bodies expressed Pan Nav, Nav1.6, and TUJ1 with no particular concentration in the plasmalemma (**Figures 5A,B**). Large ganglion cell bodies also expressed Nav1.2, 1.7, 1.8, and 1.9 but were not present in NRs (**Figures 5C–F**). The intensity of Nav staining varied among cell bodies. There was no expression of Nav1.1 and 1.3. Type I spiral ganglion cell bodies expressed calcium-activated potassium channels (BK-channel) (**Figure 5F**).

Several RN/para-nodes were identified in RC and a cross-sectioned RN can be seen with TEM in **Figure 6A**. Radially oriented arrays of Schwann cell microvilli can be seen to contact the axolemma (**Figure 6B**). The microvilli are known to contribute to and maintain Nav channel clustering in NRs (Gatto et al., 2003; Zuo et al., 2008). A thick coat beneath the plasma membrane forms assembly of cytoskeletal proteins. If the PFA concentration was lowered to 2%, Nav1.6 plasmalemma staining increased and in the AIS, but at the same time cell preservation weakened (**Figures 6C,D,H**). Nerve terminals and varicosities on small ganglion cell bodies expressed Nav1.6 (**Figure 6D**). The NRs expressed Nav1.6 and was limited by contactin-associated protein 1 (Caspr1) at the paranodal region (**Figures 6E–G**). "Double" NRs were noted in the RC (**Figures 6F,G**). Ankyrin G was expressed around the LGC bodies (**Figures 6I,J**). Including a fourth channel showed that Ankyrin G co-expressed with the basal lamina protein lamininβ2. The basal lamina was often crumpled at axon hillock regions where both laminin β2 and ankyrin G were expressed. Ankyrin G was also expressed in NFs at the habenula perforata (HP) (**Figure 6K**). HP also strongly expressed Caspr1 beneath the basilar membrane (**Figures 6L,M**). Several first NRs were found beneath the basilar membrane that expressed Caspr1 while staining of Nav1.6 was generally faint. Unmyelinated efferent nerve fibers belonging to the intra-ganglionic spiral bundle (IGSB) also expressed Kv1.2 and Nav1.6 (**Figure 6N**). Kv7.1 (KCNQ1) was discretely expressed in the LGCs (not shown), while Kv1.2 labeled their plasmalemma (**Figure 6O**). If the ganglion cell bodies expressed also Kv1.1 could not be settled with certainty.

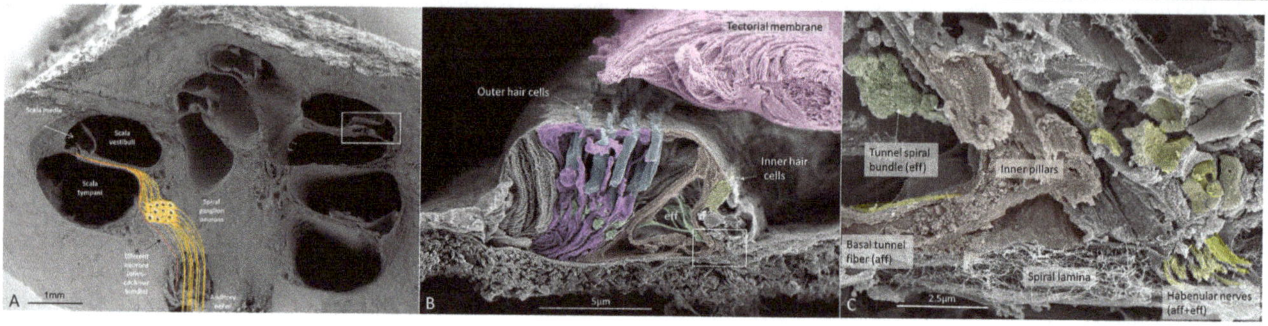

FIGURE 1 | (A) SEM of a decalcified hemi-sectioned human cochlea. Framed area shows the OC. The SG (yellow) contains two types of afferent neurons: one innervating outer (5%) and one IHCs (95%). In total, there are about 30,000 nerve fibers (NFs). Efferent NFs (red) also reach and interact with SG cell bodies, IHC nerve terminals, and outer hair cells OHCs. Printed with permission from Hearing, Balance, and Communication 2020.
(B) SEM of a human OC. There are four rows of OHCs and one row of IHCs. Efferent NFs are colored green. **(C)** Higher magnification of framed area in **(B)**. A basal afferent tunnel fiber runs in the inner pillar cell foot. It is an afferent fiber innervating OHCs. IHC afferent terminals are swollen. A similar, but not identical, image was earlier published in Anatomical Record 2012 (Rask-Andersen et al., 2012).

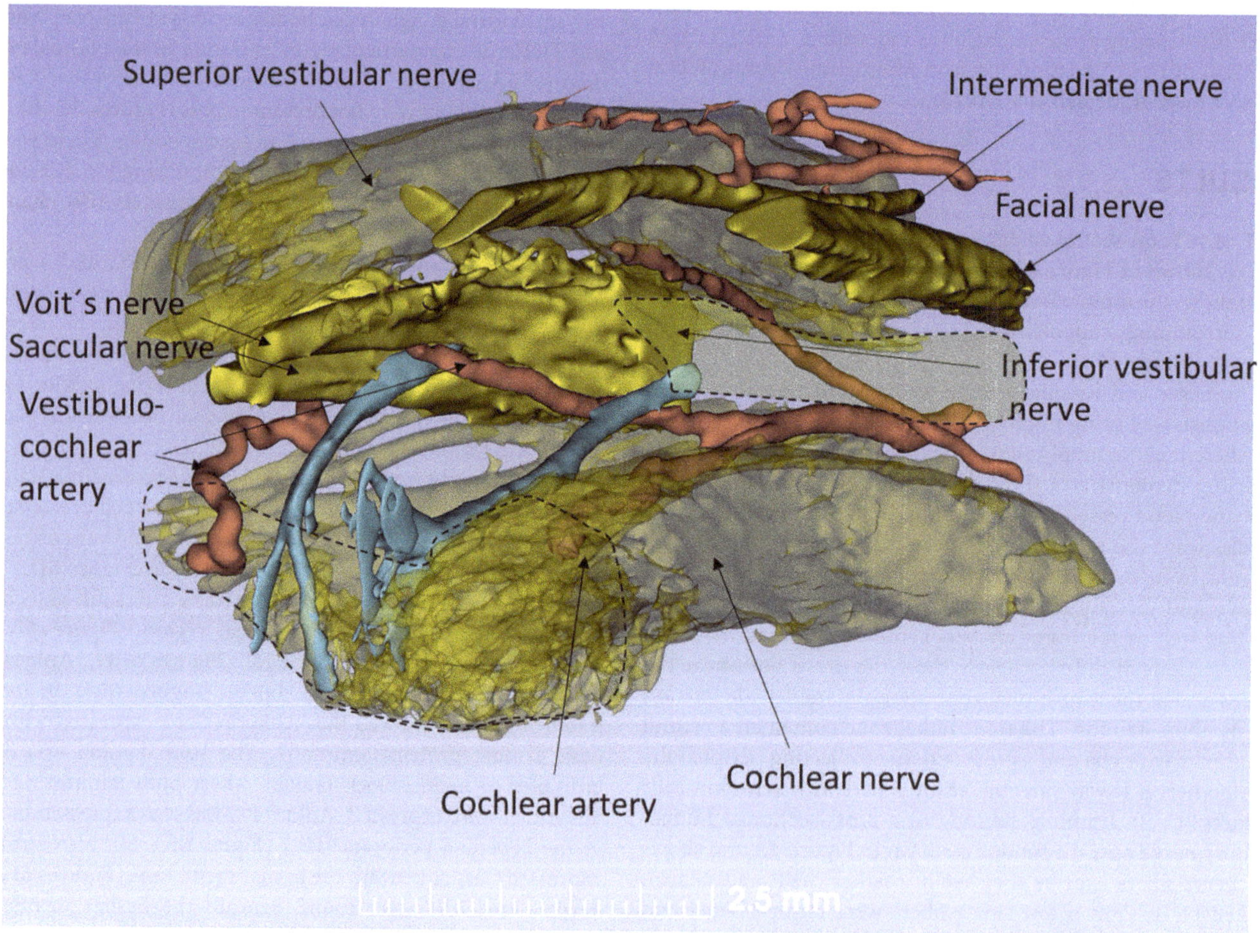

FIGURE 2 | Human efferent innervation. MicroCT, 3D reconstruction and modeling of soft tissue in a right human IAC (anterior-medial view, broken line represents cochlear nerve at fundus). For clarity, some nerves are semi-transparent. An efferent cochlear nerve supply is mediated via the vestibular-cochlear anastomosis of Oort (blue). NFs exit from the inferior vestibular and saccular nerves and reach the cochlea and SG ~3–4 mm from its basal end. Their role in signal modulation, protection, and spatial hearing is still unclear.

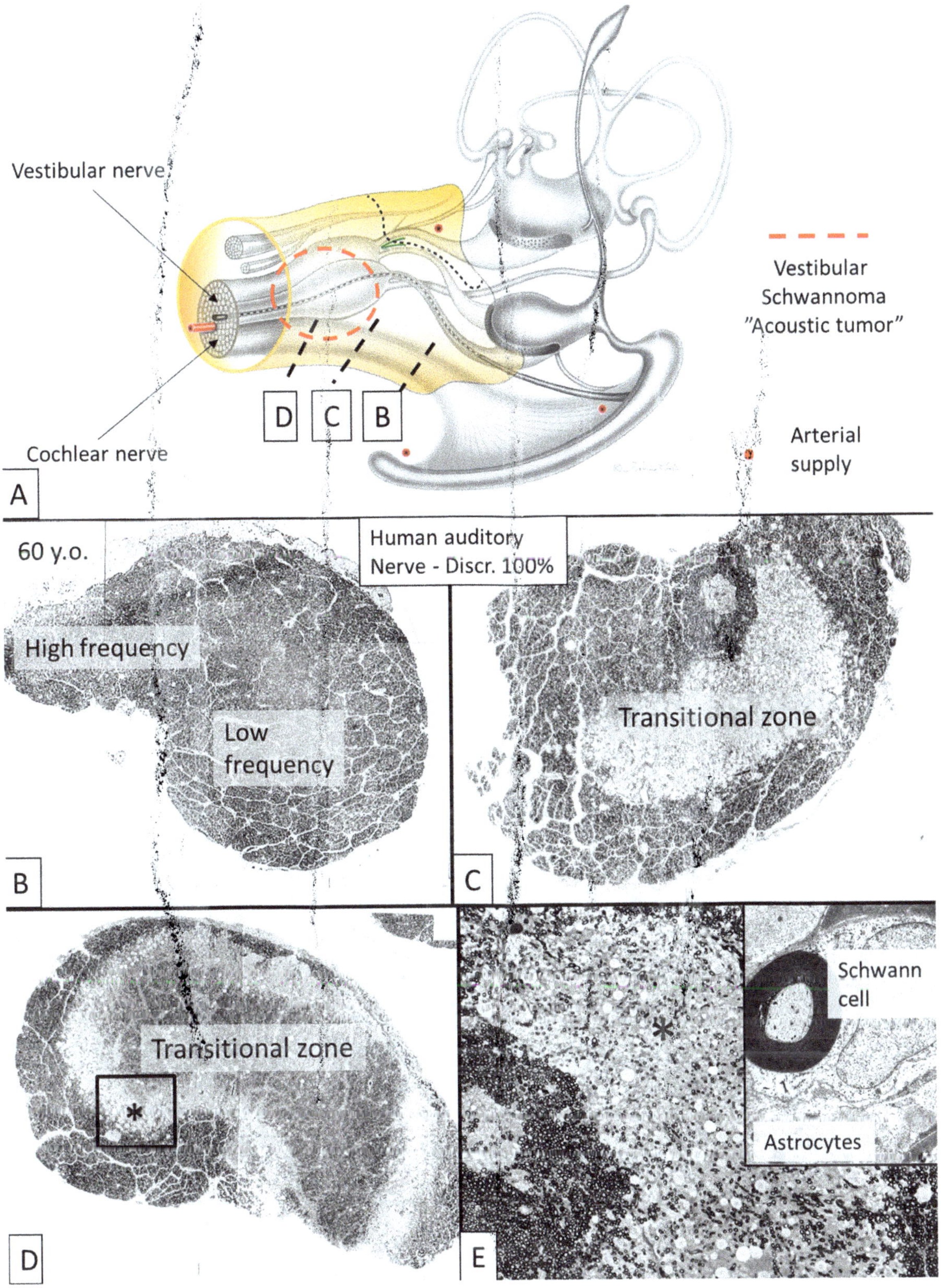

FIGURE 3 | Cross-sectioned human auditory nerve at different levels shown in **(A)**. **(B)** The nerve near the fundus. **(C,D)** A transitional zone with central glia and astrocyte tissue project into the nerve (lucent part). It is surrounded by the peripheral component containing Schwann cells. **(E)** Higher magnification of framed area shown in **(D)**. Inset shows TEM image at the transitional zone with astrocyte tissue (asterisk). Tissue was fixed immediately in 3% buffered glutaraldehyde and post-stained in 1% osmium tetroxide.

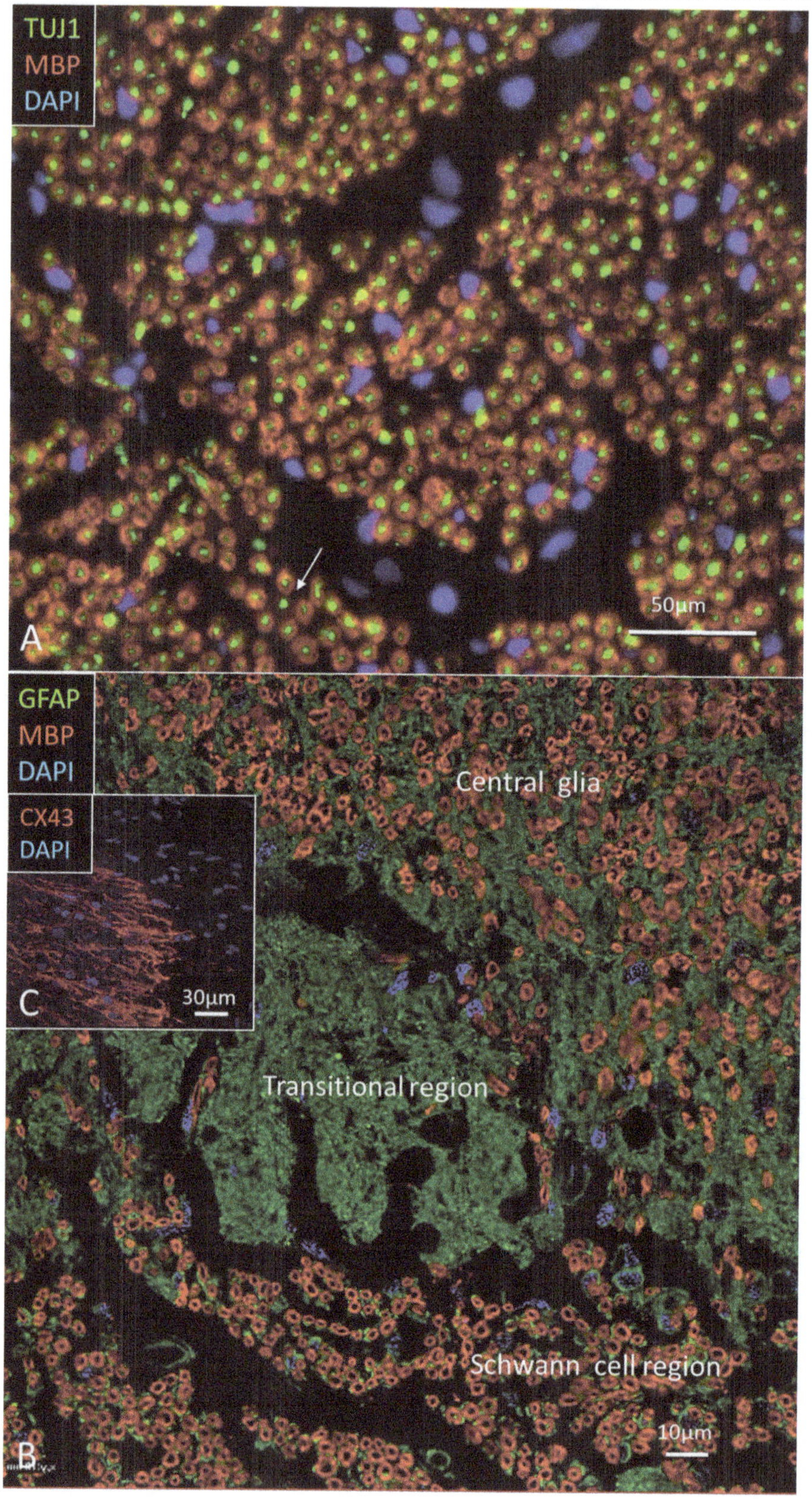

FIGURE 4 | (A) Immune staining of a cross-sectioned human auditory nerve corresponding to the level shown in **Figure 3B**. **(A)** Nerve fibers express the myelin marker MBP and neuron marker TUJ1. Few fibers are unmyelinated (arrow) and may represent NRs. **(B)** Cochlear nerve at the transitional zone (corresponding to level shown in **C**). Astrocytes stain positive for GFAP (green) and Cx43 (inset). MBP, myelin basic protein; TUJ1, tubulin-1; GFAP, glia-fibrillary acidic protein; Cx43, connexin43.

TABLE 3 | RNA probes used in the present investigation.

Gene	Species	Gene ID	Chromosome location	Cat#	Company
GJD2	Human (h)	57369	15q14	567981	BioTechne (b)
GJB6	h	10804	13q12.11	541391	b
Na/K-ATPase β1	h	481	1q24.2	568261	b
Na/K-ATPase β3	h	483	3q23	568271	b
Na/K-ATPase α1	h	476	1p13.1	539891	b

TABLE 4 | Immunohistochemical expression of Nav channels.

Channel type /Location	Nav1.1	Nav1.2	Nav1.3	Nav1.6	Nav1.7	Nav1.8	Nav1.9
Hair cells	N/A	N/A	N/A	+(OHCs)	N/A	N/A	N/A
SG cell body	–	+	–	+	+	+	+
Dendrites	–	+	–	–	–	–	–
Axons	–	+	–	–	–	–	–

N/A; not analyzed. +; positive expression. –; no expression.

Immunohistochemistry and TEM of the Spiral Lamina and Habenular Canal

In the spiral lamina fibers, the NRs and juxta-para-nodes expressed Kv1.1 margined by Caspr1 as can be seen in **Figures 7A,B**. The radial myelinated afferent fibers were Nav1.6-negative, except at the NR. Their fiber diameter was around 2 μm. The spiral lamina also contained groups of very thin myelinated and unmyelinated fibers running spirally. They strongly expressed TUJ1 and Nav1.6. These neurons are thought to represent efferent fibers and were earlier shown to be synaptophysin-positive (Khalifa et al., 2003). They also enter the OC through the foramina nervosa. Single radial unmyelinated fibers can also be seen to run in the spiral lamina using SEM (not shown here). They have a diameter of less than 0.5μm. Whether they express Na1.6 could not be established with certainty. Immunohistochemistry of the spiral lamina beneath the HP is shown in **Figure 7C**. At this region the afferent NFs lose myelin and coalesce into bundles embedded in S-100 positive glial cells that follow the fibers through the canal. It could not be established with certainty if the NFs beneath the HP expressed Kv1.1 and Kv1.2. Radial sectioning with TEM showed the afferent NFs beneath the HP which were rich on mitochondria and surrounded by glial cells and a thin basal lamina expressing laminin β2 (**Figures 7C,D**). The lamina tapered the inner wall of the habenular canal. The length of the canal was 10–15 microns. The length of the unmyelinated region was ~20–30 μm with fibers having a diameter around 1μm. The fibers were rich in mitochondria, and a blood capillary was typically situated where the nerves enter the canal. In the canal, the neurite diameter diminished to around 0.5 μm (**Figure 7D**). The diameter of the habenular canal varied and was around 6 × 4 microns (area 20–40 μm²). NFs almost completely filled the canal and were surrounded by a thin glial sheet into the OC. Type II afferents and efferents could not be separated in the habenular canal.

Expression of Na/K-ATPase in the Human Auditory Nerve

The expression of Na/K-ATPase in the human cochlea was recently presented in a separate study (Liu et al., 2019). **Table 5** summarizes the expression of various isoforms in the human cochlea. Na/K-ATPase β1 subunit was heavily expressed generally in the human cochlea, mostly combined with the α1 isoform. Neurons, however, expressed the β1 subunit combined with α3, while SGCs expressed the α1 isoform. LGC plasmalemma strongly expressed Na/K-ATPase α3/β1. The central and peripheral myelinated axons stained positive for Na/K-ATPase α3/β1 isoforms all the way (**Figures 8A–C**). The groups of small spirally running myelinated and unmyelinated lamina fibers strongly expressed Na/K-ATPase α3/β1 (not shown) and also Nav1.6 (**Figures 8D,E**).

In the organ of Corti, both afferent and efferent nerve terminals strongly expressed Na/K-ATPase α3/β1 (**Figure 9**). Nav1.6 co-expressed with Na/K-ATPase β1 in inner, outer, tunnel spiral bundles, and tunnel crossing fibers. The highest activity of Na/K-ATPase β1 in the OC was at the IHC/nerve junction, inner and outer spiral bundles, Hensen cells, marginal cells, type II fibrocytes and spiral prominence. RNA-scope hybridization confirmed gene transcripts of Na/K-ATPase ATP1B1 and even ATP1B3 in LGC bodies. The ATP1B1 was confined to the cell periphery, while ATP1B3 transcripts were distributed more evenly in the cytoplasm and cell nuclei. The localization of ATP1B1 and ATP1B3 encoding Na/K-ATPaseβ1 and β3 in human large, type I SG cell bodies are seen in **Figure 12**. ATPB1 gene expression is concentrated near the cell membrane while ATP1B3 is mostly expressed in the cell nuclei. SR-SIM shows intense expression of the Na/K-ATPaseβ1 in the plasmalemma of large ganglion cells lying closely together. SR-SIM verified both genes encoding β1 and β3 Na/K-ATPase isoforms in the same cell.

TEM of Human Organ of Corti

The basal lamina accompanied neurites for a short distance inside the OC, with "entrance gate." Thereafter, the basal lamina turned back and followed the basal region of the organ. Neurites contained several mitochondria, while surrounding glial cells showed electron-dense bodies, rER, and glycogen granules. Each nerve fiber entered the organ of Corti through minor openings in the surrounding glial cell layer. Ribbon synapses occurred in both IHCs and OHCs, and not infrequently, several ribbons were found against the same nerve terminal in both IHCs and OHCs. TEM images of a well-preserved human IHC with numerous afferent and efferent nerve terminals located at the basal pole are shown in **Figure 10**. Afferent boutons are shown to have different morphology with multiple synaptic plaques. Typically is the large numbers of mitochondria in the basal cytoplasm of the IHC synaptic

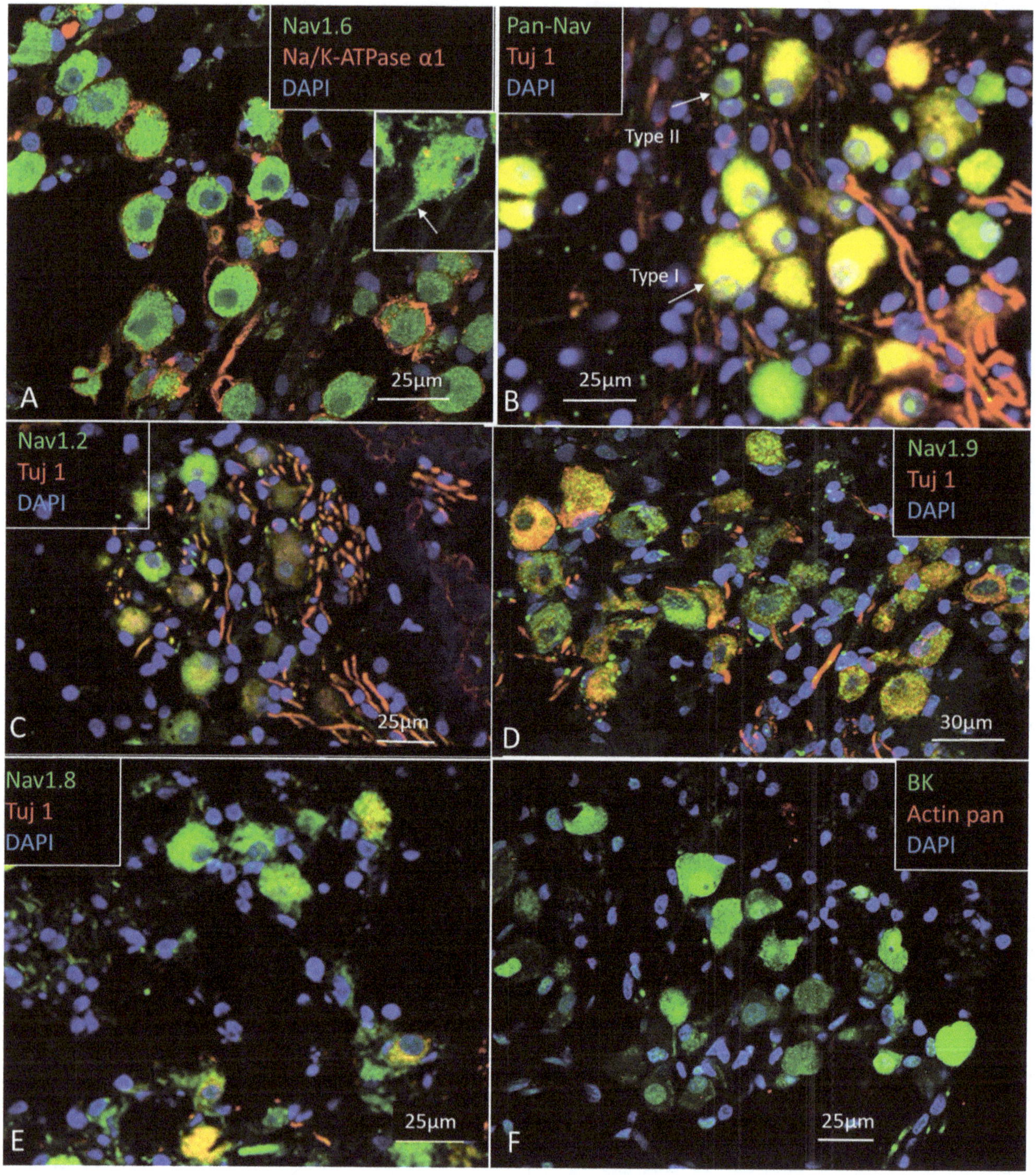

FIGURE 5 | (A–E) Expression of Nav, and TUJ1 in the human SG. The large cell bodies show various expression of Nav channels, mostly restricted to the cell bodies and the AIS. **(F)** Spiral ganglion cell bodies also expressed calcium-activated potassium channel (BK channel). Fixation in 4% PFA.

region. Efferent axo-synaptic contact show multiple synaptic vesicles and large dense-core vesicles. A systematic study of the ultrastructure of the IHC receptor-neural junction is under way.

TEM and Connexin30 in Human Spiral Ganglion Cells

Large ganglion cell bodies surprisingly expressed Cx30. Cell bodies had a "mulberry-like" appearance at immunofluorescence

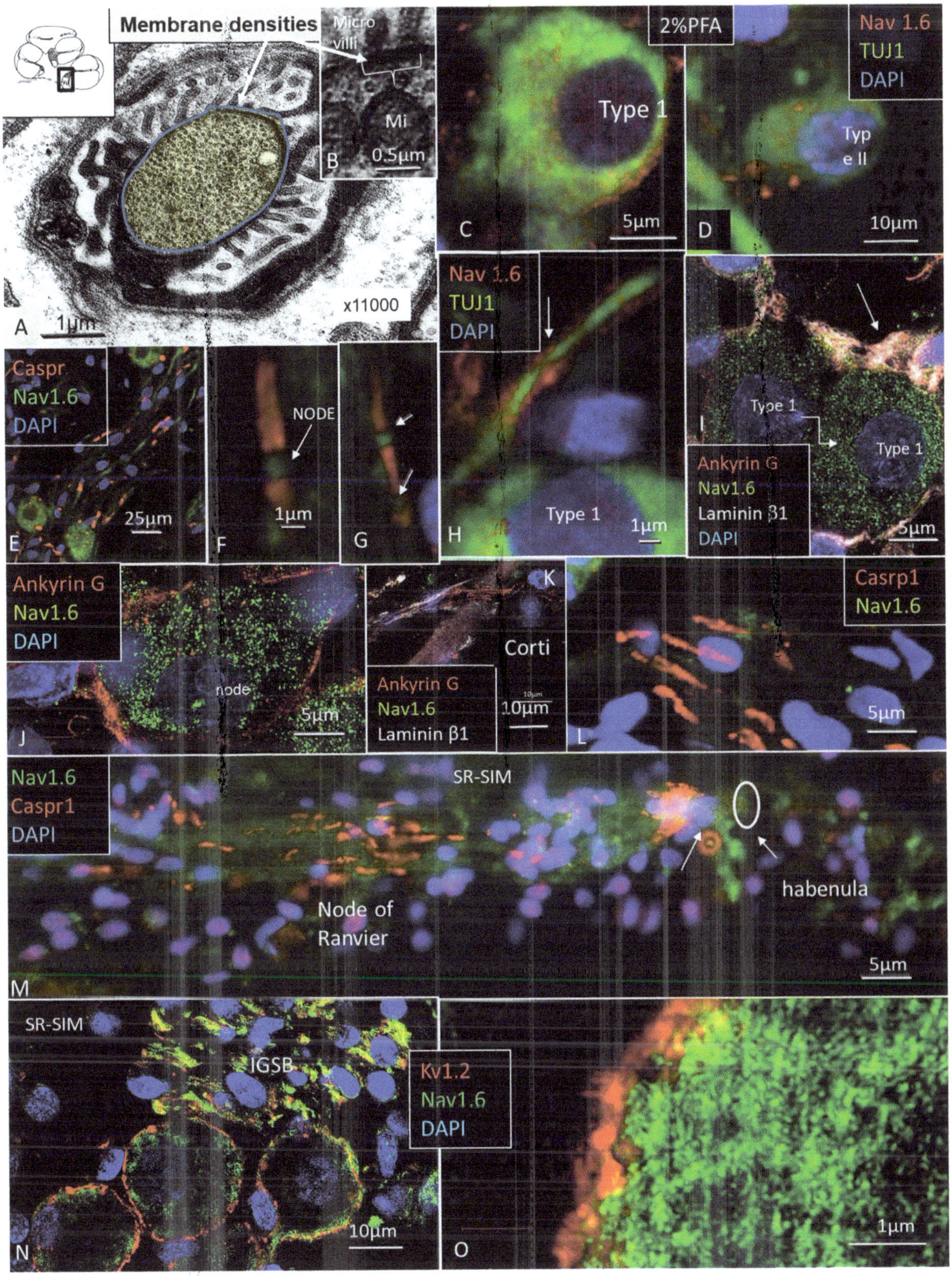

FIGURE 6 | (A,B) TEM of a cross-sectioned node/paranode in the basal RC. Axoplasm is stained yellow. Radially oriented arrays of Schwann cell microvilli contact the axolemma **(B)**. Mi, mitochondria. **(C)** Co-expression of Nav1.6 and TUJ1 in a large type I cell after fixation in 2% PFA. **(D)** Small type II cell with adjoining Nav1.6-positive fibers fixed in 2% PFA. **(E,F)** Nav1.6 expression in NRs. **(G)** A double NR (arrows). **(H)** Type I AIS (arrow) expresses Nav1.6. **(I,J)** Ankyrin G expression in Type I cell axon hillock (arrow) and plasmalemma. **(K)** Ankyrin G expressed in neurons at the HP. **(L)** Caspr1 is expressed in neurons beneath the HP. **(M)** Radial NFs express Caspr1 beneath the HP (arrows) and at NRs. **(N)** Expression of Kv1.2 and Nav1.6 in type I SGNs. Efferent fibers in the IGSB also express Nav1.6. **(O)** Higher magnification shows expression of Kv1.2 in the type I SGN plasmalemma.

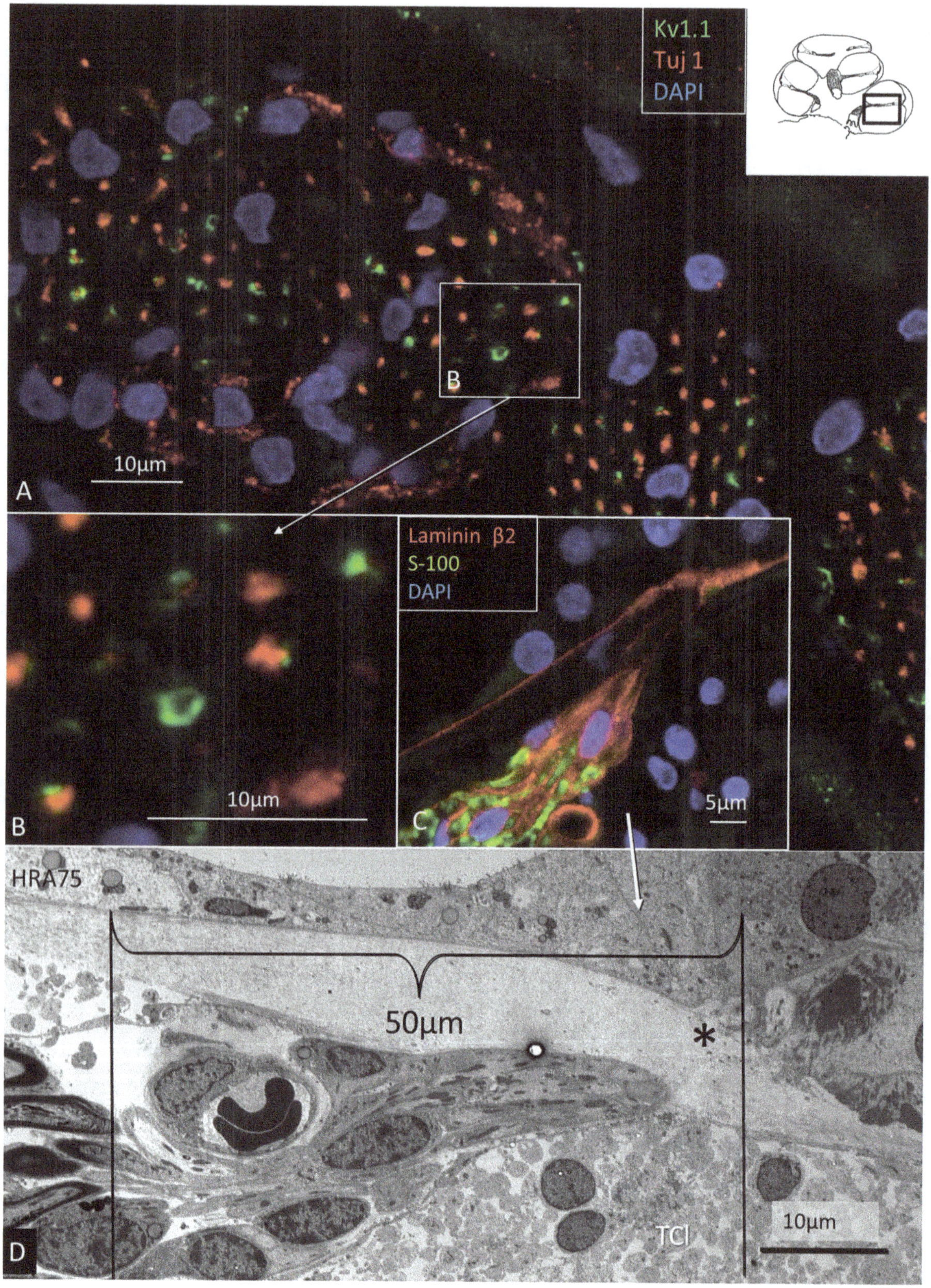

FIGURE 7 | Immunohistochemistry **(A–C)** and TEM **(D)** of spiral lamina NFs in a human cochlea. **(A)** Double-labeling of TUJ1 and Kv1.1. Framed area is magnified in **(B)**. **(C)** Radial section at the HP with a fiber bundle expressing lamininβ2 and S-100. **(D)** TEM of radial NFs beneath the HP (asterisk). The length of the unmyelinated region is around 50 µm. The unmyelinated NFs are rich in mitochondria. A blood capillary is located typically near the nerve bundle. The basal lamina is folded at the habenular opening. TCL, tympanic covering layer.

TABLE 5 | Immunohistochemical expression of Na/K-ATPase isoforms.

SGN-p (Type I)	ATPase α1 -	ATPase β1 +(RNA-scope +)	ATPase α2 -	ATPase β2 -	ATPase α3 +	ATPase β3 N/A (RNA-scope +)
SGCs	+	–	–	?	–	N/A
Axons	–	+	–	–	+	N/A
Dendrites	–	+	–	–	+	N/A
Nerve endings	–	+	–	–	+	N/A
ISB	–	+	–	–	+	N/A
OSB	–	+	–	–	+	N/A
TCF	–	+	–	–	+	N/A
TBF	–	+	–	–	+	N/A
SGN (Type II)	–	?	–	–	+	N/A

SGN-p, Large type I spiral ganglion neuron perikarya; SGC, Satellite glial cells; Axons and Dendrites are large SGN's neurites; Nerve endings, SGN terminal fibers, and nerve endings inside OC are unmyelinated. OSB; outer spiral bundle. ISB; inner spiral bundle. TCF; tunnel crossing fibers (efferents). TBF; tunnel basal fibers; afferents Type II fibers. N/A: not analyzed. +; positive expression. –; no expression.

(**Figures 11A–D**). Laser CM and SR-SIM with 3D reconstructions demonstrated both neural markers TUJ1 and Cx30. An elaborate network of Cx30 protein extended between the nuclear envelope and cell periphery (**Figures 11C,D**). A rich network of rough endoplasmic reticulum (rER) was observed with TEM (**Figures 12C,D,G**). RNA-scope hybridization confirmed gene transcripts of GJB6 in LGC bodies (**Figure 12B**). Cx36 could not be verified with RNA-ISH. Human IHC and OHCs and neurons heavily expressed parvalbumin but there was no co-expression with Cx30 (**Figure 11E**). Likewise, SR-SIM demonstrated no co-expression of Cx30 and TUJ1 in nerve elements beneath the OHCs (**Figure 11F**). Cx30 could be demonstrated in the OC, spiral limbus, and lateral cochlear wall in guinea pigs and pig but not in the SGNs (**Supplementary Figure 1**, **Supplementary Video 1**). The rich expression of Cx26 and Cx30 in the human OC is demonstrated in **Supplementary Figure 2A** and **Supplementary Video 2**.

DISCUSSION

This study presents some information on the anatomy of the human auditory nerve including its molecular constituents. Results suggest that initial spike generators are located beneath the IHCs in humans. However, additional mechanisms seem to be essential for the filtering of complex sounds that may be challenged by various pathological conditions. The cochlear nerve relays acoustic information to the brain along homogenously sized myelinated fibers. The retro-cochlear meatal part contains a highly vulnerable transitional zone where synchronized nerve signaling may be compromised by external influences. Efferent nerve fibers from the vestibular nerve reach the cochlear nerve at its entrance near bony perforations of the fundus. Micro-CT results herein and synchrotron phase-contrast imaging (Mei et al., 2020) expose the 3D anatomy of the associated arteries extending from the cranium. Despite the obvious difficulties in studying well preserved human material, these emerging molecular analyses show the specific distribution of VGICs and expression of connecting proteins among physically interacting ganglion cell bodies. It seems to suggest that human acoustic nerve signaling may be partly different from most laboratory animals.

Human Receptor-Neural Segment—An Intriguing Spike Generator

The innervation pattern points to the IHC system is the main transfer of acoustic information to the CNS, while the OHCs provide hair cell-based amplification to increase auditory sensitivity and frequency selectivity (Rhode, 1971; Kemp, 1979; Flock et al., 1986). A detailed examination of the human receptor-neural complex is challenging due to its extraordinary anoxia-sensitivity and nerve terminal swelling. Therefore, studies of transduction channels and excitatory activity in human sensory cells are challenging. The human cochlea contains 3,400 IHC receptors that relay acoustic information to the brain via 30,000 nerve fibers (Retzius, 1884; Guild et al., 1931; Wright et al., 1987). Graded transduction currents and voltage-gated Ca^{2+} channels activate a sublime system of multi-vesicular ribbon synapses releasing hundreds of quantized transmitter vesicles per second to glutamate/AMPA-receptors in each nerve terminal with remarkable endurance (Moser and Beutner, 2000; Glowatzki and Fuchs, 2002; Grant et al., 2010). Modulated synchronized release produces excitatory postsynaptic potentials (EPSPs) (Geisler, 1981; Siegel and Dallos, 1986; Moser and Beutner, 2000; Nouvian et al., 2006; Safieddine et al., 2012), and APs are generated to transfer sound features as phasic, fast adapting signals with extraordinary temporal and spectral resolution (Siegel, 1992; Fuchs, 2005; Rutherford et al., 2012). Remarkably, human IHC afferent boutons were associated with more than one synaptic ribbon, contrary to most laboratory animals where each fiber seems to make only one contact with the IHC (Nadol, 1988; Kantardzhieva et al., 2013). In humans, one terminal can make multiple synaptic contacts with a single IHC or two adjacent IHCs (Nadol, 1983). Bodian (1978) though, found dual ribbon synapses in non-human primates (Bodian, 1978). In turtles and frogs, hair cell synapses have been extensively studied, and it was found that many ribbon

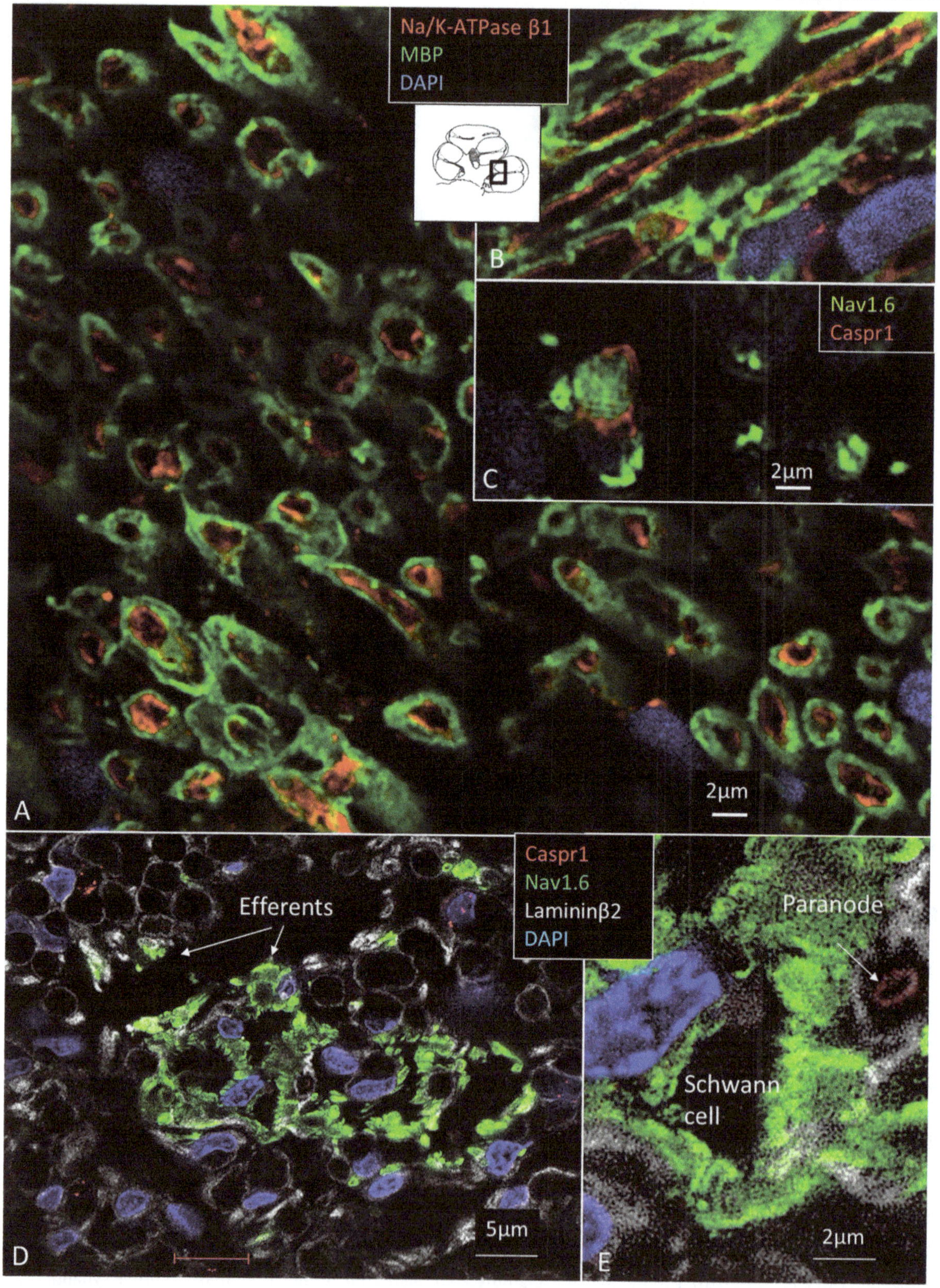

FIGURE 8 | (A) Spiral lamina NFs cross-sectioned and double-labeled with antibodies against MBP and Na/K-ATPase β1. **(B)** Longitudinal section. Axolemma expresses Na/K-ATPase β1 all the way. **(C)** Cross-sectioned axons labeled with antibodies against Nav1.6 and Caspr1 at and near a NR. **(D)** The spiral lamina contains bundles of thin NFs expressing Nav1.6 believed to represent efferent nerve fibers. The larger myelinated NFs are Nav1.6-negative. **(E)** Higher magnification of Nav1.6-positive NFs shown in **(D)**. A fourth channel (white) shows lamininβ2 expression in the basal lamina. MBP, myelin basic protein; Nav1.6, voltage-gated sodium channel 1.6; Caspr1, contactin-associated protein 1.

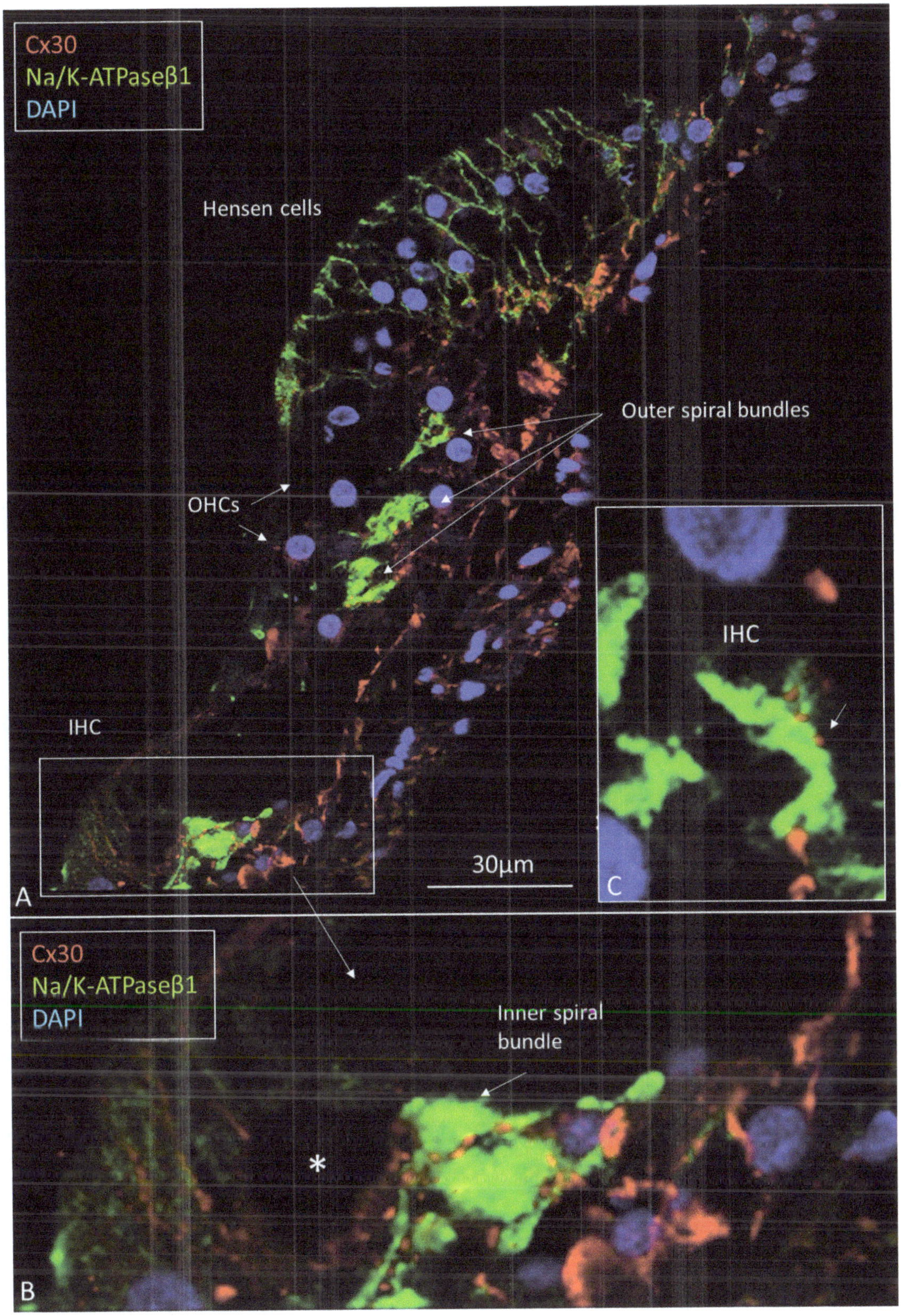

FIGURE 9 | (A) CM of the human OC double-labeled with antibodies against Na/K-ATPase β1 (green) and Cx30 (red). Inner and outer spiral bundles express Na/K-ATPase β1 with mostly separate Cx30 puncta **(B,C)**. *IHC nerve terminals are swollen.

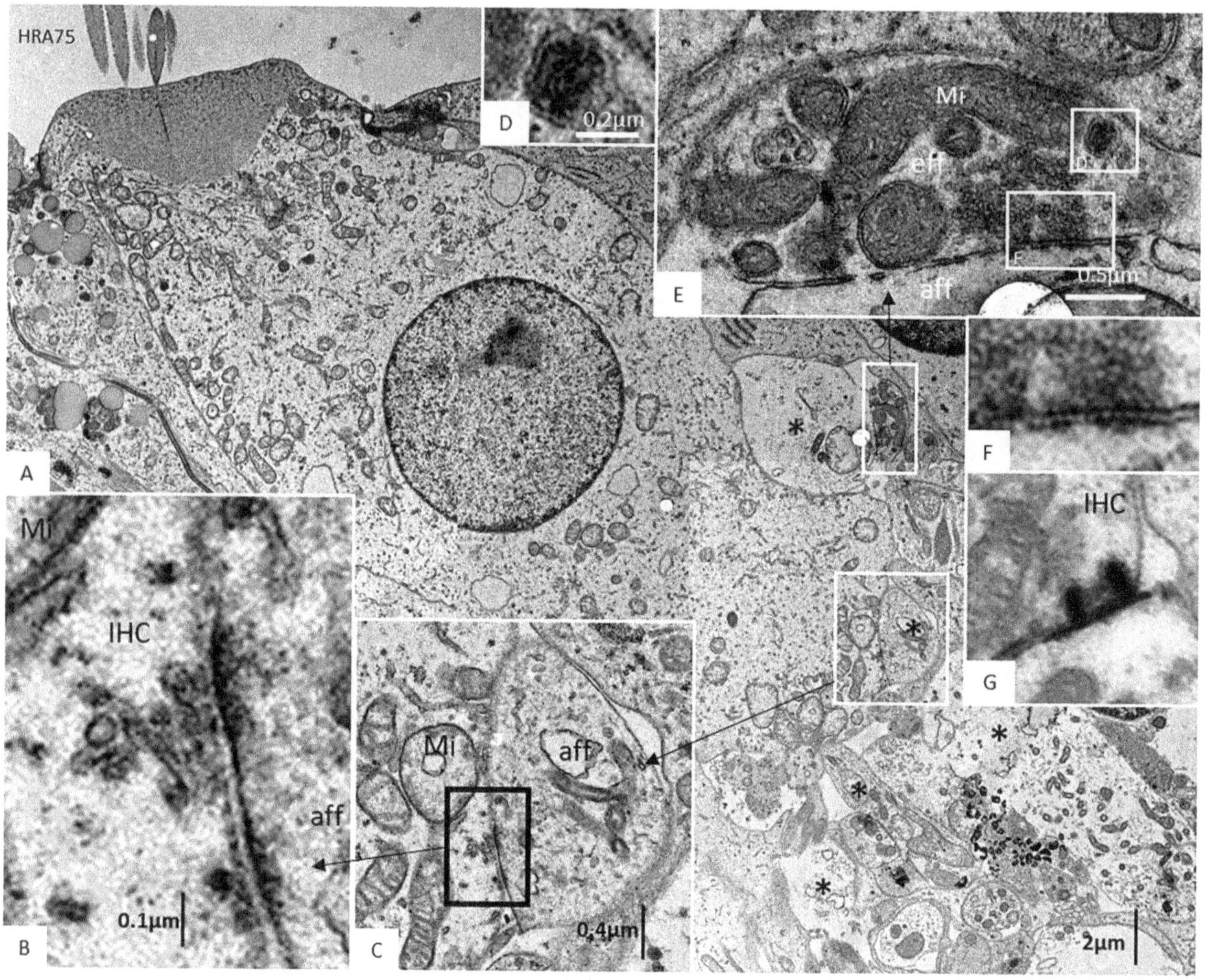

FIGURE 10 | (A) TEM image of a human IHC. A myriad of afferent (*) and efferent nerve terminals are located at the basal pole. **(B,C)** Afferent boutons (aff) have different morphology with multiple synaptic plaques. There are large numbers of mitochondria (Mi) in the IHC synaptic region. **(D–F)** An efferent axo-synaptic contact is shown with multiple synaptic vesicles, mitochondria, and large dense-core vesicles **(D)**. Some terminals face more than one ribbon synapse **(G)**. Fixation was done directly in the surgical room in oxygenated 3% buffered glutaraldehyde and then post-stained in 1% osmium tetroxide.

synapses converge on a single afferent, but each nerve fiber forms several synaptic terminals onto one to three hair cells (Keen and Hudspeth, 2006), and no synapses were associated with more than one synaptic thickening (Schnee et al., 2005). Presynaptic ribbons are also present in retinal photoreceptors where they exhibit sustained release of neurotransmitter activity that reaches several postsynaptic targets, such as horizontal cells and bipolar neurons at some distances (Matthews and Fuchs, 2010). Our results may suggest that signal transmission could be more "multifaceted" in humans and non-human primates, and whole-mount immunohistochemistry and SR-SIM can add new information about principal signaling and aberrations (Viana et al., 2015; Liu et al., 2019).

In human, we found a diversity of nerve terminals and neurites beneath the IHC. Afferent terminals and efferent fibers heavily expressed Na/K-ATPase $\alpha 3/\beta 1$, which is essential for repolarization after spike activation. Different sized afferents may represent those with variable thresholds and spontaneous rates (Nadol, 1983; Merchan-Perez and Liberman, 1996). Postsynaptic excitatory currents are known to arise within the OC (Grant et al., 2010) and may generate APs beneath the HP. Changes in the molecular machinery of ribbon synapses may lead to impaired speech perception, such as cochlear neuropathy (Roux et al., 2006; Safieddine et al., 2012). Injury caused by age or noise may result in "hidden hearing loss," (Schaette and McAlpine, 2011; Kujawa and Liberman, 2015) although conclusive evidence for noise-induced cochlear synaptopathy in humans remains elusive (Bramhall et al., 2019). Animal work may show that spontaneous rate and sensory coding of the type I afferents depends on the size of ribbon synapses and Ca-channels density (Sheets et al., 2017). Further studies of the human ribbon synapses and diversity of nerve terminals are needed along the cochlear spiral and are

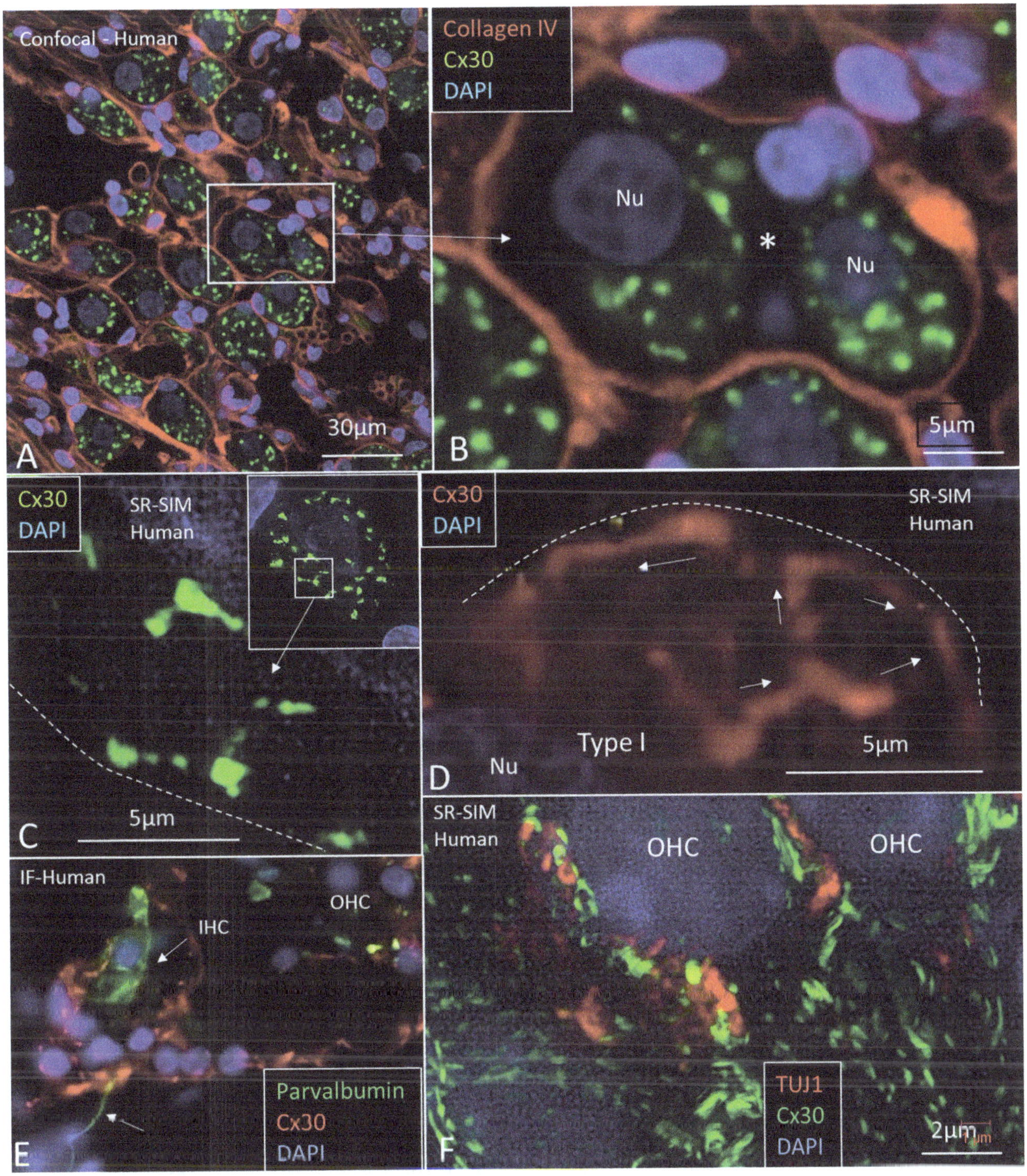

FIGURE 11 | CM and SR-SIM of human SG and OC. **(A)** Collagen IV and Cx30 co-staining shows a basal lamina "honeycomb" layer in the apical portion of the cochlea richly expressing Cx30. Framed area is magnified in **(B)**. **(B)** A SGC with no basal lamina is seen between the two large SG cell bodies (*). **(C,D)** SR-SIM shows labeled Cx30 near the plasmalemma (broken lines). **(E)** Inner hair cell with afferent (arrow) shows expression of parvalbumin but no Cx30. Surrounding cells heavily express Cx30. **(F)** SR-SIM at lower poles of OHCs. Neurons express TUJ1 but there is no co-expression with Cx30. Nu: nucleus.

underway at our laboratory. The organization of the human inner hair cell receptor-neural junction based on results obtained so far is given in **Figure 13**, **Supplementary Figure 3**.

Somatic sensory signaling is known to create receptor potentials and firing at hemi-nodes (Bewick and Banks, 2014; Carrasco et al., 2017) that open sodium channels to produce APs

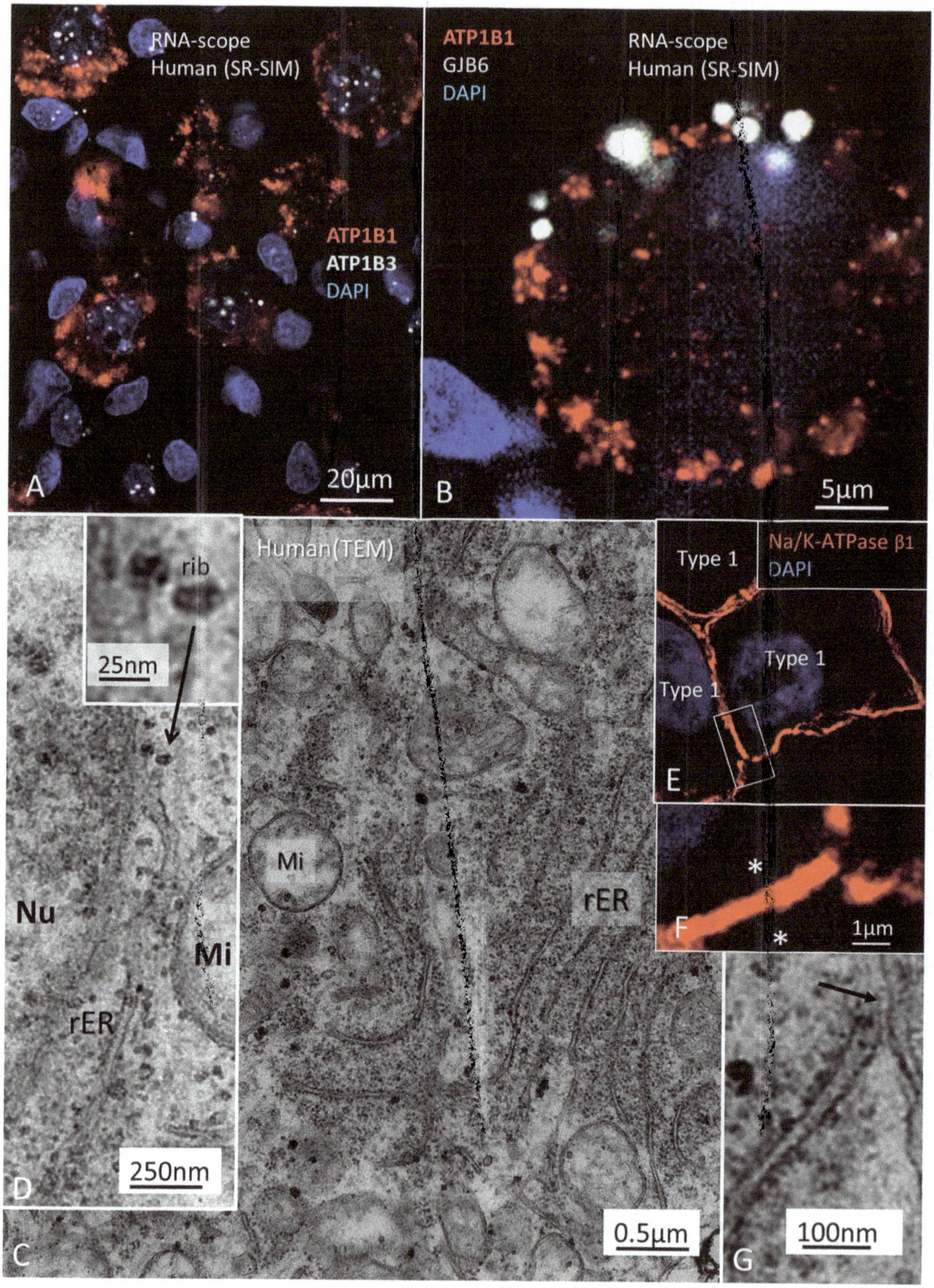

FIGURE 12 |

(Continued)

FIGURE 12 | (A) Localization of ATP1B1 and ATP1B3 in human large, type I SG cell bodies encoding Na/K-ATPaseβ1 and β3. ATPB1 gene expression is most concentrated at the periphery near the cell membrane while ATP1B3 is mostly expressed in the cell nuclei. **(B)** GJB6 encoding Cx30 protein is expressed near the plasmalemma of a type I ganglion cell. **(C)** TEM image of a type I ganglion cell shows many mitochondria (Mi) and extensive rough endoplasmic reticulum (rER) and free ribosomes in the cytoplasm. **(D)** Several ribosomes are located at the nuclear envelope. **(D)** shows ribosome (rib) in higher magnification. **(E)** A rER is closely associated with the plasmalemma (arrow). **(F)** SR-SIM shows expression of the Na/K-ATPaseβ1 protein in the plasmalemma of three large ganglion cells. The cell membranes lie close to each other (asterisks). Framed area is magnified in **(G)**. Nu; cell nucleus.

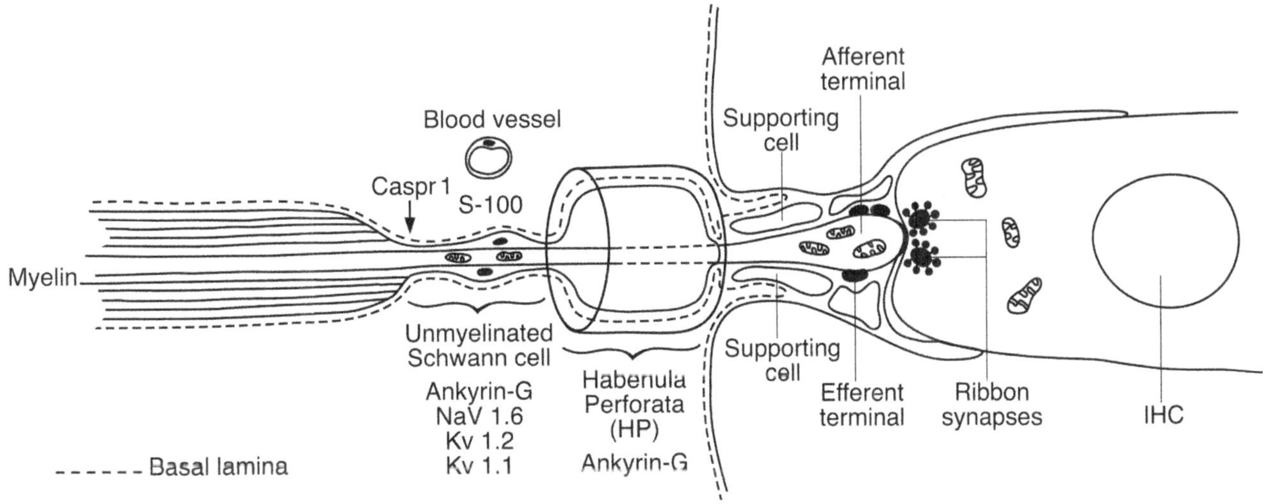

FIGURE 13 | Graphic illustration of the principal organization of the human inner hair cell receptor-neural junction. A basal lamina margins the neural pathway that coalesces with the organ of Corti. Action potentials are believed to be generated in the sub-receptor zone beneath the habenular canal. In rodents Nav1.6 is localized in a hemi-node consistent with the location of spike generation (Hossain et al., 2005). There are also low- and high-voltage activated potassium channels essential for adaptation and regulation of AP activity (Smith et al., 2015; Kim and Rutherford, 2016).

in the first NR (Loewenstein and Ishiko, 1960). Control of firing often occurs before myelination (Bender and Trussell, 2012). Each human IHC is innervated by ~10–15 afferent nerve fibers (Nadol, 1988) that pass through the foramina nervosa along a 34 mm long spiral. The present data point to the sub-habenular region as hemi-node and spike generator in humans. A limitation was that Nav1.6 could not be unequivocally established beneath the IHCs, but the scaffold proteins Caspr1 and Ankyrin G were identified. Ankyrin G-binding motifs are important for sodium channel clustering and targeting of Nav1.6, Kv7.2, and Kv7.3 as well as Na/K-ATPase and Na/Ca^{2+}-exchanger (JoséGarrido et al., 2003; Pan et al., 2006). The reason for the lack of detection of Nav1.6 in this region is not known at this stage. In the rat, this region clearly expresses Nav1.6 and low- and high-threshold voltage-gated potassium channels as well as Ankyrin G and Caspr1 (Lacas-Gervais et al., 2004; Smith et al., 2015; Kim and Rutherford, 2016). According to Kim and Rutherford Kv1.1 was present ubiquitously in axons and somas in the mature rat and enriched at juxta-para-nodes, Kv2.2 was expressed in internodes, Kv3.1 only in hemi-nodes and nodes and Kv7.2 and 7.3 in myelinated and unmyelinated segments in the osseous spiral lamina and beneath the IHCs. Nav1.6 was found to co-localize with Kv3.1b at hemi-nodes and nodes and Nav1.1 was located in hemi-nodes only (Kim and Rutherford, 2016). Hence, the visualization of VGIC may be influenced by the pattern of myelination and further analyses in man seem required. Hossain et al. showed that Nav1.6 channels in mice are located in afferent axons central to the HP and in unmyelinated afferents and terminals in the OC (Hossain et al., 2005). OHC afferents also expressed Nav1.6 channels. The spike generator was thought to reside near the postsynaptic bouton before axons myelinate. The unmyelinated efferent axons and endings on the inner and outer hair cells expressed Nav1.2 but never in the type II afferents running on the floor of the tunnel or in the outer spiral bundle or endings (Hossain et al., 2005). In human, the unmyelinated NFs beneath the HP displayed a large number of mitochondria constantly associated with a distinct vascular supply. It suggests that this is a metabolic "hot-spot" that could be consistent with its involvement in the generation of action potentials.

Can the Human Auditory Nerve Also Fire Through Electric Synapses?

The present findings raise queries as to whether IHC afferent activity can be modulated by mixed electric and chemical synapses. If so, cell coupling may play a role in short delay depolarization and fast signal conduction. Only a few GJ channels (which are morphologically undetectable) can drastically adjust electric transmission acting independent of the resting membrane potential (Bennett, 2009). Signaling through electric synapses is 10 times faster than chemical synapses (synaptic delay 0.2 ms), and Cx36 is the principal neuronal connexin in the mammalian CNS (Bennett, 2009). However, the gene transcript GJD1 could not be detected in our study. At double-labeling, Cx30 was not co-expressed with the TUJ1 or parvalbumin marker in the human OC. Double-labeling with Cx30 and Na/K-ATPaseβ1, however demonstrated Cx30 to be widely, but separately, expressed beneath OHCs and IHCs (**Figure 9**). Furthermore, there was no co-expression of parvalbumin and Cx30 or TUJ1 and CX30 in neurons beneath IHCs and OHCs (**Figures 11E,F**). The results give no evidence that electric synapses exist in the human organ of Corti.

Human SG—A Spike Generator and Acoustic Filter?

The human SG differs distinctly from other vertebrates, suggesting that electric activity is fundamentally different. Large or type I cell soma are unmyelinated and surrounded by SGCs (Kimura et al., 1979, 1980; Ota and Kimura, 1980; Spoendlin and Schrott, 1988; Tylstedt et al., 1997; Liu W, et al., 2014). These neurons terminate at the IHCs, while the small unmyelinated type II neurons innervate the OHCs (Spoendlin, 1972). Some authors have even suggested that the small neurons represent cholinergic parasympathetic fibers (Ross, 1969; Ross and Burkel, 1973). A third type was described in humans by Rosbe (Rosbe et al., 1996).

The percentage of compact myelination in large type I cells in different vertebrates is 85–100% (goldfish, rat, guinea pig, rabbit, and monkey), while in humans only 2–6% are myelinated, and mostly in older individuals (Arnold, 1987). The Ly5.1 mouse strain is the only rodent model reported to have "human-like spiral ganglion neurons" and may be useful for studying synchronous nerve activity (Jyothi et al., 2010). Myelination may secure a fast unbroken nerve conduction across the ganglion to the CNS. Signal speed may be slowed down, but the unmyelinated cell soma and pre- and post-soma segments expressing Nav1.6 may serve as additional spike generators modulated by voltage-gated potassium channels (Kv1.2) (Boulet et al., 2016). In humans, the proximal AISs are unmyelinated, often mitochondria-rich. In mice and other laboratory animals, impedance of the large cell body is thought to be compensated by the pattern of myelination of the cell bodies (Hossain et al., 2005). Hossain et al. (2005) found Nav1.6 expressed at the NRs flanked by Caspr at the para-nodal axoglial junctions, while the cell bodies lacked Nav immunoreactivity. Fryatt et al. used reverse transcription polymerase chain reaction (RT-PCR) and immunohistochemistry to study the distribution of Nav channels in rodent SG neurons (Fryatt et al., 2009). Nav1.1, Nav1.6, and Nav1.7 subunits were expressed in rat ganglion cells, and Nav1.1 and Nav1.6 were expressed in axonal processes suggesting that AIS plays a role in the extension of afferent signals across the SG cell soma. There was no difference in labeling between cell membrane and cytoplasm using RT-PCR. More Nav1.6 and Nav1.7 expressions were found in type I than in type II neurons. There was no expression of mRNA for Nav1.2, Nav1.3, Nav1.8 and Nav1.9 in the rat SGN. In a subsequent study Fryatt et al. showed modulation of VGSCs after noise and mild hearing loss with decreased Nav1.1 and Nav1.6 mRNA expression while Nav1.7 mRNA expression increased by ~20% when compared to control rats (Fryatt et al., 2011).

In the present study, ganglion cell bodies expressed Nav1.2, Nav1.6, Nav1.7, Nav1.8, and Nav1.9, suggesting considerable molecular diversity. Though, the pattern of staining of sodium channels seemed to be highly influenced by aldehyde concentration and cell preservation. The unmyelinated AIS also expressed Nav1.6, and "double nodes" of Ranvier were observed in the RC, suggesting additional modulation of saltatory conduction. Ankyrin G was expressed with laminin β2 and Kv1.2, indicating that electric impulses may be modulated with local voltage amplification to reach threshold (Bender and Trussell, 2012). Ankyrin G is known to gather cell adhesion molecules at the NR and AIS (Kordeli et al., 1995; Dzhashiashvili et al., 2007; Leterrier et al., 2017) and provide means for axon polarity and directional propagation (Rasband, 2010; Leterrier, 2016). Genetic aberrations can cause neuropathy and neural fatigue with enlarged ABR latency and fragmented Kv staining (Lacas-Gervais et al., 2004). Smith et al. found heteromeric Kv1.2 and Kv1.1 channels co-expressed in neurons that may control initiation and propagation of APs in the cochlea as well as Kv3.1b subunits in pre- and post-somatic NRs (Smith et al., 2015). We were not able to localize Kv3.1 or to establish if Kv1.1 and 1.2 were co-expressed.

Nerve fiber synapses were previously observed on the small SG cells in the human cochlea (Kimura et al., 1979; Rask-Andersen et al., 2000). LGC bodies also demonstrate synapse-like membrane specializations (Rask-Andersen et al., 1997; Tylstedt et al., 1997), including unique axo-somatic contacts (Tylstedt et al., 1997) otherwise not found in sensory ganglia (Pannese, 2020). Synaptic vesicles are lacking, but accretion of mitochondria suggests specialized neural interaction. These membrane densities are also present among clustered cell bodies where no separating glia layer exists, as demonstrated in **Figure 14**. This image shows a graphical 3D reconstruction from serial thin sections of membrane specializations between two human type I SG cell bodies in the apical turn of a human cochlea. Surrounding satellite cells show a "gap" in the interface between the two cells with several membrane specializations. These are both symmetrical and asymmetrical with different polarity. The findings may suggest that cell soma interaction is possible for processing of acoustic information. It may also infer a greater plasticity and complexity of cell signaling.

Similar asymmetric densities at opposing junctional membranes are found at synaptic junctions in OHC afferents in primates devoid of synaptic micro-vesicles (Bodian, 1978) and ribbons in the cat (Dunn and Morest, 1975). In these atypical synapses, transmitter vesicles were thought to play a minor role, and quantal chemical transmission was challenged. As in other sensory ganglia, our findings suggest that GJ proteins may be involved in nerve transmission even if electric synapses or GJ plaques were not identified. Moreover, the Cx30 protein was only verified in humans. RNA-scope demonstrated Cx30 gene transcripts confirming earlier Cx30 antibody labeling in the human LGCs (Liu et al., 2009). It suggests that Cx30 may play a role in inter-neuronal communication, seemingly associated with Na/K-ATPase. SR-SIM surprisingly labeled both the β1 and β3 subunits of Na/K-ATPase in the same cell (Liu et al., 2020) and in *in situ* hybridization RNA-scope also localized both genes. It was proposed that β-subunits may play a role in "gluing" cells

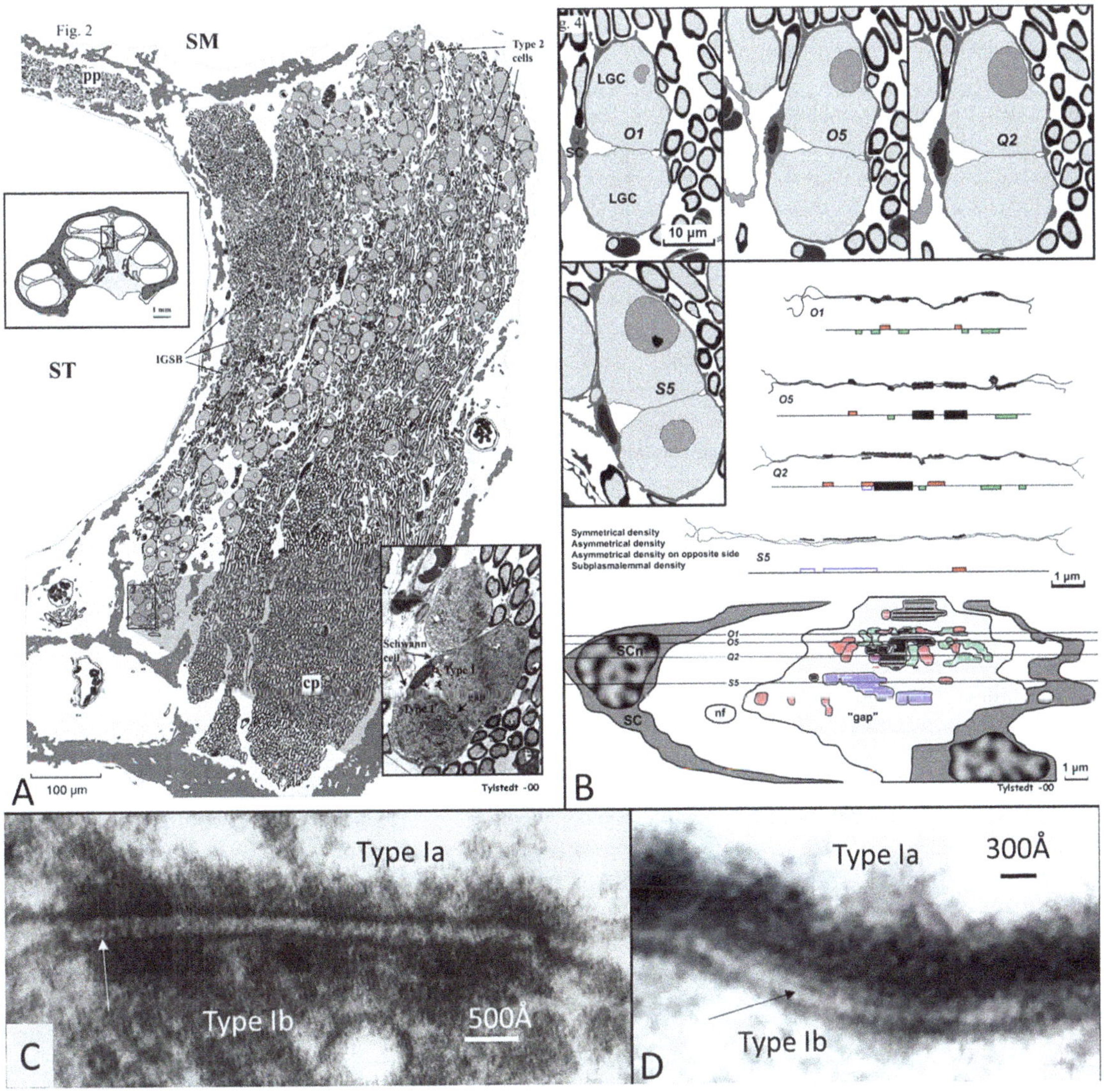

FIGURE 14 | (A) 3D model of membrane specializations between two human type I SG cell bodies in the apical turn of a human cochlea (voice fundamental frequency $F_0 \sim$ 100–250 Hz, 630–730°, normal subjective hearing). Two type I cells were serially sectioned and graphically reconstructed. Surrounding satellite cells (SCs) show a "gap" in the SC interface between the two cells with several membrane specializations. These are both symmetrical (black) and asymmetrical with different polarity (red and green). Some areas show sub-plasmalemmal densities (blue). **(C,D)** High-power TEM of somato somal membrane densities shown in **(B)**. Magnification ×160,000. Occasionally, a thin precipitous lamina is seen in the intercellular cleft (arrows). Fixed in oxygenated fluorocarbon containing 2% glutaraldehyde solution and 0.05 M sodium phosphate buffer (Tylstedt and Rask-Andersen, 2001).

together (Geering, 1991), essential for cell clustering. β1 was previously found to be co-expressed with α2 and β2 isoforms in the human brain (Tokhtaeva et al., 2012).

Notably, in a recent publication Luque et al. performed a comparative study of the distribution of the unique voltage-gated hyperpolarization-activated cyclic nucleotide-gated (HCN) channels among mammalian species (Luque et al., 2021). These channels have a reverse voltage-dependence activated by hyperpolarization and may generate "pacemaker currents" in heart muscle cells. They form homo- or hetero-tetramers and various subunits (HCN1-4) exist (Wahl-Schott and Biel, 2009). Besides in the OC, these channels were found in neuron clusters of the human SG suggesting a function of synchronization of timing cues. Particular intense staining of HCN 1, 2, and 4 was noted at adjoining cell membranes which may boost ephaptic coupling, synchronizing AP firing similar to that described earlier in the brain (Han et al., 2018).

Cochlear Injury and Spiral Ganglion Cell Signaling

In sensory ganglia, primary afferents do not seem to function independently but can depolarize via neighboring neurons, leading to cross-excitation through activity-dependent coupling (Amir and Devor, 1996). A critical role is played by the SGCs that are coupled by GJs (Hanani et al., 2002; Cherkas et al., 2004). GJs are also present in SGCs in the human SG and express Cx43 (Liu W, et al., 2014). Trans-cellular signaling among SGCs could partially explain remodeling and neural rescue and incomplete Wallerian degeneration following hair cell and dendrite loss, which are decisive in cochlear implantation. In dorsal root ganglia, cell injury increases neuronal coupling by upregulation of GJs and Cx43 so that adjacent neurons can activate together. SGCs may even proliferate (Hanani et al., 2002) together with activation of surrounding scavenger microglia also present in the human SG (Liu et al., 2018). This neuron-to-neuron communication was termed "crossed after-discharge" and does not seem to represent ephaptic crosstalk (Devor and Wall, 1990). Communication increases after axotomy and contributes to neuropathic pain, an analog to tinnitus (Kim et al., 2016). Inhibiting GJ-mediated coupling was proposed to be a way to relieve chronic pain. However, how neurons are connected was unclear, but Cx43 hemi-channels were suspected. Patch-clamp recordings, dye coupling, and Cx43CKO suggested that SGCs participate in coupled activation. GJs permit the spread of intercellular calcium waves important for signal transfer and induction of sensory disturbances (Dublin and Hanani, 2007). Thalakoti et al. (2007) verified for the first time neuron–glia signaling via GJs, and Damodaram et al. (2009) showed that GJs composed of Cx26 proteins likely mediate direct dye coupling of neurons and SGCs in the trigeminal ganglion. In this context, our finding of Cx30 in the LGCs is intriguing. According to Amir and Devor (1996) cross-depolarization is excitatory and increases neurons' input resistance and spiking for sub-threshold pulses and changes chemical mediated membrane conductance. Excitation was modulated by afferent spike activity and voltage-dependent. It could be induced by the elevation of extracellular potassium (Utzschneider et al., 1992) or the release of chemical mediators, such as excitatory amino acids, eicosanoids, and nitric oxide from neuron soma (Amir and Devor, 1996), whose receptors are also widely expressed in humans.

Cochlear Implantation, Voice Fundamentals, and Phase Locking

Patients with severe sensorineural hearing loss (SNHL) can be treated with CIs to regain substantial hearing and speech comprehension (Michelson, 1971; House and Urban, 1973; Clark et al., 1979; Burian Hochmair-Desoyer and Hochmair, 1981; Hochmair et al., 2015). By placing an electrode array inside the cochlea, plentiful hearing can be regained through electrically generated APs along the NFs. Even congenitally deaf children may achieve speech comprehension and production. This remarkable outcome, despite limited spectral information, suggests that alternate coding principles are involved, such as envelope extraction and temporal cues (Shannon et al., 1995). To improve auditory outcomes with CI, models are created to better understand how external electric stimulation induces neurophysiological responses (Wilhelm-Bade et al., 2009; Bruce et al., 2018). Mapping VGIC and spike generators may reveal new strategies to approach natural hearing (Liu Q, et al., 2014). Today's implants fail to reproduce the traveling wave, spatial resolution from OHCs, and compression of IHC synapse/nerve thresholds through different spontaneous activity. According to Davis and Crozier (2015), ganglion cell bodies are endowed with VGICs that vary along the cochlea, mounting evidence for diverse firing patterns, including thresholds and accommodation. A similar gradient expression may exist in humans. For these variances, potassium channels play an essential role, and in the future, the distribution and molecular diversity along the human cochlear spiral may be examined in more detail. It is notable that Kv1 currents appear only after loosening of the myelin sheath from the axonal membrane, such as the juxta-paranode (Chiu and Ritchie, 1980), a normal situation in human cell soma that could act as a distinguished NR. Un-myelination raises opportunities for wider nerve interaction, cross-excitation, summation, and sub-threshold firing as well as synchronization. In the brain, synchronization depends on spike-frequency adaptations and is essential in auditory perceptual processing (Pantev et al., 1991). In the human ear, several ganglion cell bodies form structural units surrounded by the same SGCs that occasionally allow direct soma-soma interaction. Whether these clusters represent "functional units" representing inputs from one or several IHCs or broader areas is unknown. Acoustic information generated by assemblies of frequency-coded hair cells may be integrated and synchronized to broaden intensity levels and modulate dynamic range. A cell-to-cell communication among similarly tuned cell bodies may coordinate neurite activity and increase tuning sharpness (**Figure 15**). These units are particularly prevalent in the apical cochlea, where voice fundamentals are coded. A large-scale cross-depolarization may combine place and rate coding for low-frequency temporal excitation, which is essential for speech perception and synchronized phase-locking. This could partially explain why patients lacking peripheral dendrites also discriminate speech through external electric stimulation. Several neurons can fire synchronously (Bennett and Zukin, 2004; Shinozaki et al., 2013) in response to sub-threshold electric activity in clustered neurons (Connors and Long, 2004), such as in the inferior olivary nucleus and inhibitory interneurons of the neocortex, hippocampus, and thalamus through Cx36 (Gibson et al., 1999; Connors and Long, 2004). In the visual system, APs are highly synchronized and mediated by many GJs (Meister et al., 1995) shown to consist of Cx36. More studies are needed to characterize the membrane specializations in the human SG, such as hemi-channel purinergic intercellular signaling, HCN channels, and alternate types of connecting proteins.

Apical neurons are commonly preserved in patients with SNHL, such as in the presbyacusis. However, they are acoustically compressed, obstructing selective stimulation of frequency-coded neurons. A more polarized electric CI stimulation might increase spectral resolution and could even induce activity-based dynamic intercellular communication. This could be induced by the production and modulation of cell connecting protein/molecules establishing novel electrical circuits, a property usually dedicated to the CNS. A broader molecular and genetic diversity of such units may be exposed in

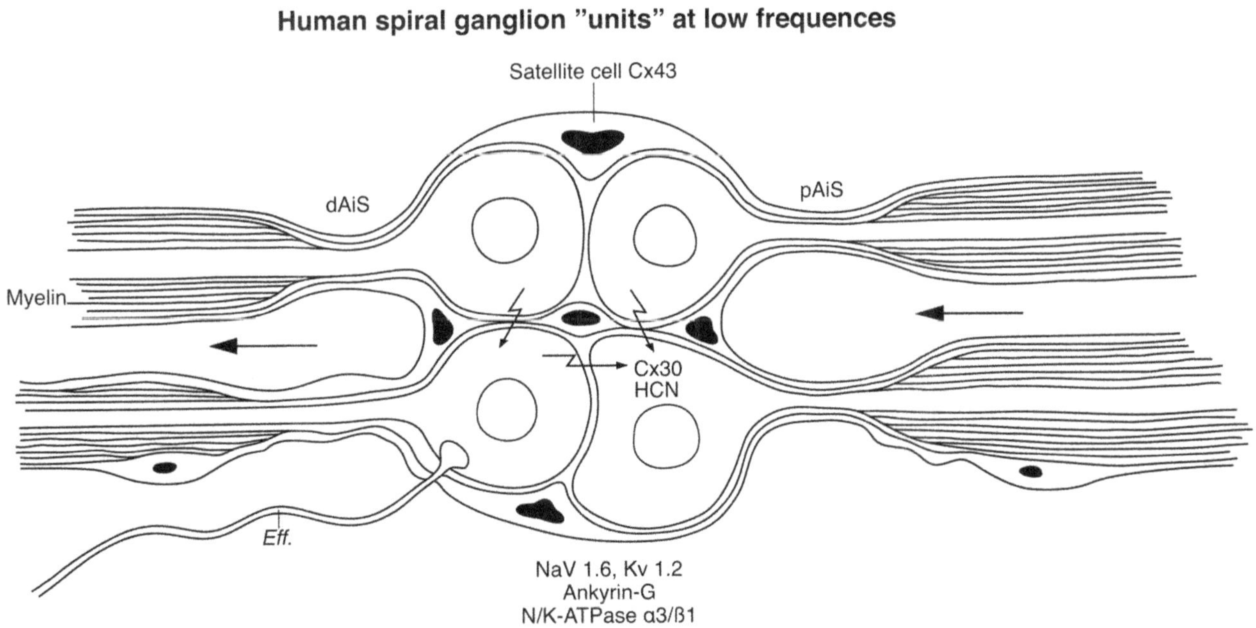

FIGURE 15 | Principal model of large or type I spiral ganglion cell "units" in the human modiolus. Cell bodies and distal (dAIS) and proximal (pAIS) axonal initial segments are unmyelinated in human and surrounded by satellite glial cells. The close proximity between the perikarya may allow inter-cellular communication suggesting an electric filtering at this level. HCN channels were identified in the perikarya with particular intense staining of HCN 1, 2, and 4 at adjoining cell membranes which may boost coupling and synchronize AP firing (Luque et al., 2021). Cx30 was so far not identified in the plasmalemma. Eff., efferent.

future studies, such as those already identified and genetically defined through single-cell RNA sequencing of intensity-coding properties in the murine cochlea (Petitpré et al., 2018; Sun et al., 2018).

CONCLUSION

It is challenging to obtain well-fixed human inner ear tissue since it is surrounded by the hardest bone in the body, and neurosensory tissues undergo rapid degeneration. So far, our knowledge of the molecular of the human auditory pathway is fairly limited, and most studies are based on laboratory animals (Kiang, 1980; Rusznák and Szucs, 2009; Davis and Crozier, 2015; Reijntjes and Pyott, 2016; Reijntjes et al., 2019). Results herein indicate that surgically acquired tissue may provide useful information, but it is limited by the relatively small amount of obtainable tissue. It also influences the practical management of control analyses including positive and negative staining and ab-neutralization tests (Burry, 2011). We used RNA scope technique to further validate our findings. A first attempt to use SR-SIM in *in situ* hybridization for gene localization in human cochlear tissue sections was made. Findings suggest surprisingly that molecular expression and nerve signaling may differ in the human auditory nerve compared with that of laboratory animals. A complete understanding of how it relates to various inner ear disorders and strategies for future CI stimulation has not yet been reached. More knowledge about the heterogeneous signal properties in individual neurons, intensity coding, and inter-neural communication and synchrony may be required.

ETHICS STATEMENT

The studies involving human participants were reviewed and approved by the local ethics committee (Etikprövningsnämnden Uppsala, no. 99398, 22/9 1999, cont, 2003, no. C254/4; no. C45/7 2007, Dnr. 2013/190), and patient consent was obtained. The study adhered to the rules of the Declaration of Helsinki. The surgical specimens were from patients suffering from life-threatening posterior cranial fossa meningioma compressing the brain stem. Human cochleas were harvested at major trans-cochlear skull base surgeries, including facial nerve rerouting. The operations were performed at Uppsala University Hospital by a team of neurosurgeons and otoneurosurgeons. Five cochleae were dissected out using diamond drills of various sizes (**Table 1**). Ethics approval for the microCT project was obtained from the University of Western Australia (UWA, RA/4/1/5210), and the human temporal bones were provided by the Department of Anatomy at UWA. The patients/participants provided their written informed consent to participate in this study. The animal study was reviewed and approved by the local ethics committee (no. C254/4, C209/10).

AUTHOR CONTRIBUTIONS

WL performed immunohistochemistry for super-resolution microscopy and performed RNA-scope. AS-F, RG, and ML performed immunohistochemistry of cadaver temporal bones at the Innsbruck University, Austria. GR performed micro-CT of human cadaver. ST supplied (**Figure 14**) and shared the work related to it. HL performed image processing and 3D visualization of scanned objects provided by SA, HL, and GR. HR-A was the head of laboratory and planned the project, analyzed the images, and wrote the manuscript. All authors contributed to the article and approved the submitted version.

ACKNOWLEDGMENTS

This study was supported by ALF grants from Uppsala University Hospital and Uppsala University, and by the Tysta Skolan Foundation, Sellanders Foundation, and the Swedish Deafness Foundation (HRF). We also acknowledge the kind donations of private funds by Arne Sundström, Sweden. We are grateful to SciLife Laboratories and the Bio-Vis Platform at Uppsala University for providing SR-SIM microscope equipment and personal support throughout the study. We gratefully thank Med-El Austria and the Austrian Science Fund FWF for Project Funding (ion channel project and FWF project I 3154-B27—Gapless Man: Machine Interface). We especially thank Susanne Braun, Carolyn Garnham, and Heval Benav from Med-El Innsbruck. We wish to thank and honor those individuals who donated their bodies and tissues for the advancement of education and research to the Department of Anatomy, Medical University of Innsbruck. The project was supported by Med-El Inc. Austria under an agreement and contract with Uppsala University. X-ray microCT scans were conducted by Jeremy Shaw, and we wish to acknowledge the facilities and the scientific and technical assistance of Microscopy Australia at the Centre for Microscopy, Characterization & Analysis and the University of Western Australia, a facility funded by the university, state, and commonwealth governments. We thank Karin Lodin for her skillful artwork.

SUPPLEMENTARY MATERIAL

Supplementary Figure 1 | (A) CM of Cx30 expression in the human and guinea pig cochlea. Cx30 is richly expressed in the lateral wall, OC, and spiral limbus in both species. Cx30 is expressed in human SGNs [framed area and **(B)**] but not in the guinea pig SGNs [framed area and **(C)**]. TUJ1; Neuron marker. DAPI; Cell nucleus marker (**Supplementary Video 1**). Cx30 is expressed in the human SGNs.

Supplementary Figure 2 | (A) Immune fluorescence and SR-SIM (inset) show expression of Cx26 and Cx30 in the human OC. Cx30 is heavily expressed at the inner and outer hair cell region and among Hensen cells. SR-SIM shows that Cx26 and Cx30 are separately expressed RNAscope and four channel SR-SIM show localization of ATP1A1, ATP1B1 and GJB6 in the OC **(B,C)** and the lateral wall **(D,E)**. Gene transcripts are expressed both in the cytoplasm and cell nuclei (**Supplementary Video 2**). 3D visualization of the CX26 and Cx30 expression shown in **Figure 2A**.

Supplementary Figure 3 | Illustration of the human habenular canal opening into the organ of Corti based on SEM and TEM. Neurons are accompanied by thin glial cells from which they exit surrounded by supporting cells and populate the sub-receptor zone. Synaptic terminals are not surrounded by supporting cells.

REFERENCES

Adamson, C. L., Reid, M. A., Mo, Z. L., Bowne-English, J., and Davis, R. L. (2002). Firing features and potassium channel content of murine spiral ganglion neurons vary with cochlear location. *J. Comp. Neurol.* 447, 331–350. doi: 10.1002/cne.10244

Amir, R., and Devor, M. (1996). Chemically mediated cross-excitation in rat dorsal root ganglia. *J. Neurosci.* 16, 4733–4741. doi: 10.1523/jneurosci.16-15-04733.1996

Ariyasu, L., Galey, F. R., Hilsinger, R., and Byl, F. M. (1989). Computer-generated three-dimensional reconstruction of the cochlea. *Otolaryngol. Neck Surg.* 100, 87–91. doi: 10.1177/019459988910000201

Arnold, W. (1987). Myelination of the human spiral ganglion. *Acta Otolaryngol.* 436, 76–84. doi: 10.3109/00016488709124979

Arnold, W., Wang, J. B., and Linnenkohl, S. (1980). [Anatomical observations in the spiral ganglion of human newborns (author's transl)]. *Arch. Otorhinolaryngol.* 228, 69–84.

Bender, K. J., and Trussell, L. O. (2012). The Physiology of the Axon Initial Segment. *Annu. Rev. Neurosci.* 35, 249–265. doi: 10.1146/annurev-neuro-062111-150339

Bennett, M. V. L. (2009). Gap junctions and electrical synapses. *Encyclopedia Neurosci.* 529–548. doi: 10.1016/B978-008045046-9.01256-0

Bennett, M. V. L., and Zukin, R. S. (2004). Electrical coupling and neuronal synchronization in the mammalian brain. *Neuron* 41, 495–511. doi: 10.1016/S0896-6273(04)00043-1

Bewick, G. S., and Banks, R. W. (2014). Mechanotransduction in the muscle spindle. *Pflugers Arch. Eur. J. Physiol.* 457, 197–209. doi: 10.1007/s00424-014-1536-9

Bishop, D. V. M., Hardiman, M., Uwer, R., and Von Suchodoletz, W. (2007). Atypical long-latency auditory event-related potentials in a subset of children with specific language impairment: REPORT. *Dev. Sci.* 10, 576–587. doi: 10.1111/j.1467-7687.2007.00620.x

Bodian, D. (1978). Synapses involving auditory nerve fibers in primate cochlea. *Proc. Natl. Acad. Sci. U.S.A.* 75, 4582–4586. doi: 10.1073/pnas.75.9.4582

Boulet, J., White, M., and Bruce, I. C. (2016). Temporal Considerations for Stimulating Spiral Ganglion Neurons with Cochlear Implants. *JARO - J. Assoc. Res. Otolaryngol.* 17, 1–17. doi: 10.1007/s10162-015-0545-5

Bramhall, N., Beach, E. F., Epp, B., Le Prell, C. G., Lopez-Poveda, E. A., Plack, C. J., et al. (2019). The search for noise-induced cochlear synaptopathy in humans: mission impossible? *Hear. Res.* 377, 88–103. doi: 10.1016/j.heares.2019.02.016

Bruce, I. C., Erfani, Y., and Zilany, M. S. A. (2018). A phenomenological model of the synapse between the inner hair cell and auditory nerve: implications of limited neurotransmitter release sites. *Hear. Res.* 360, 40–54. doi: 10.1016/j.heares.2017.12.016

Burian Hochmair-Desoyer, I. J., and Hochmair, E. S. K. (1981). Hoeren ueber ein cochlea implantat. *Arch. Onk-heilkd.* 231, 569–570.

Burry, R. W. (2011). Controls for immunocytochemistry: an update. *J. Histochem. Cytochem.* 59, 6–12. doi: 10.1369/jhc.2010.956920

Camilieri-Asch, V., Shaw, J. A., Mehnert, A., Yopak, K. E., Partridge, J. C., and Collin, S. P. (2020). Dicect: a valuable technique to study the nervous system of fish. *eNeuro* 7, 1–23. doi: 10.1523/ENEURO.0076-20.2020

Carrasco, D. I., Vincent, J. A., and Cope, T. C. (2017). Distribution of TTX-sensitive voltage-gated sodium channels in primary sensory endings of mammalian muscle spindles. *J. Neurophysiol.* 117, 1690–1701. doi: 10.1152/jn.00889.2016

Cherkas, P. S., Huang, T.-Y., Pannicke, T., Tal, M., Reichenbach, A., and Hanani, M. (2004). The effects of axotomy on neurons and satellite glial cells in mouse trigeminal ganglion. *Pain* 110, 290–298. doi: 10.1016/j.pain.2004.04.007

Chiu, S. Y., and Ritchie, J. M. (1980). Potassium channels in nodal and internodal axonal membrane of mammalian myelinated fibres. *Nature* 284, 170–171. doi: 10.1038/284170a0

Clark, G. M., Pyman, B. C., and Bailey, Q. R. (1979). The surgery for multiple-electrode cochlear implantations. *J Laryngol Otol* 93, 215–223.

Connors, B. W., and Long, M. A. (2004). Electrical synapses in the mammalian brain. *Annu. Rev. Neurosci.* 27, 393–418. doi: 10.1146/annurev.neuro.26.041002.131128

Culling, C. F. A. (1974). *Handbook of Histopathological and Histochemical Techniques*. Butterworth. doi: 10.1016/c2013-0-04011-x

Damodaram, S., Thalakoti, S., Freeman, S. E., Garrett, F. G., and Durham, P. L. (2009). Tonabersat inhibits trigeminal ganglion neuronal-satellite glial cell signaling. *Headache J. Head Face Pain* 49, 5–20. doi: 10.1111/j.1526-4610.2008.01262.x

Davis, R. L., and Crozier, R. A. (2015). Dynamic firing properties of type I spiral ganglion neurons. *Cell Tissue Res.* 361, 115–127. doi: 10.1007/s00441-014-2071-x

Devor, M., and Wall, P. D. (1990). Cross-excitation in dorsal root ganglia of nerve-injured and intact rats. *J. Neurophysiol.* 64, 1733–1746. doi: 10.1152/jn.1990.64.6.1733

Dublin, P., and Hanani, M. (2007). Satellite glial cells in sensory ganglia: their possible contribution to inflammatory pain. *Brain Behav. Immun.* 21, 592–598. doi: 10.1016/j.bbi.2006.11.011

Dunn, R. A., and Morest, D. K. (1975). Receptor synapses without synaptic ribbons in the cochlea of the cat. *Proc. Natl. Acad. Sci. U.S.A.* 72, 3599–3603. doi: 10.1073/pnas.72.9.3599

Dzhashiashvili, Y., Zhang, Y., Galinska, J., Lam, I., Grumet, M., and Salzer, J. L. (2007). Nodes of Ranvier and axon initial segments are ankyrin G-dependent domains that assemble by distinct mechanisms. *J. Cell Biol.* 177, 857–870. doi: 10.1083/jcb.200612012

Flock, Å., Flock, B., and Ulfendahl, M. (1986). Mechanisms of movement in outer hair cells and a possible structural basis. *Arch. Otorhinolaryngol.* 243, 83–90. doi: 10.1007/BF00453755

Fryatt, A. G., Mulheran, M., Egerton, J., Gunthorpe, M. J., and Grubb, B. D. (2011). Ototrauma induces sodium channel plasticity in auditory afferent neurons. *Mol. Cell. Neurosci.* 48, 51–61. doi: 10.1016/j.mcn.2011.06.005

Fryatt, A. G., Vial, C., Mulheran, M., Gunthorpe, M. J., and Grubb, B. D. (2009). Voltage-gated sodium channel expression in rat spiral ganglion neurons. *Mol. Cell. Neurosci.* 42, 399–407. doi: 10.1016/j.mcn.2009.09.001

Fuchs, P. A. (2005). Time and intensity coding at the hair cell's ribbon synapse. *J. Physiol. (Lond).* 566, 7–12. doi: 10.1113/jphysiol.2004.082214

Gatto, C. L., Walker, B. J., and Lambert, S. (2003). Local ERM activation and dynamic growth cones at schwann cell tips implicated in efficient formation of nodes of Ranvier. *J. Cell Biol.* 162, 489–498. doi: 10.1083/jcb.200303039

Geering, K. (1991). The functional role of the β-subunit in the maturation and intracellular transport of Na,K-ATPase. *FEBS Lett.* 285, 189–193. doi: 10.1016/0014-5793(91)80801-9

Geisler, C. D. (1981). A model for discharge patterns of primary auditory-nerve fibers. *Brain Res.* 212, 198–201. doi: 10.1016/0006-8993(81)90051-2

Gibson, J. R., Beierlein, M., and Connors, B. W. (1999). Two networks of electrically coupled inhibitory neurons in neocortex. *Nature* 402, 75–79. doi: 10.1038/47035

Glowatzki, E., and Fuchs, P. A. (2002). Transmitter release at the hair cell ribbon synapse. *Nat. Neurosci.* 5, 147–154. doi: 10.1038/nn796

Grabinski, T. M., Kneynsberg, A., Manfredsson, F. P., and Kanaan, N. M. (2015). A method for combining rnascope *in situ* hybridization with immunohistochemistry in thick free-floating brain sections and primary neuronal cultures. *PLoS ONE* 10:e0120120. doi: 10.1371/journal.pone.0120120

Grant, L., Yi, E., and Glowatzki, E. (2010). Two modes of release shape the postsynaptic response at the inner hair cell ribbon synapse. *J. Neurosci.* 30, 4210–4220. doi: 10.1523/JNEUROSCI.4439-09.2010

Guild, S. R., Crowe, S. J., Bunch, C. C., and Polvogt, L. M. (1931). Correlations of differences in the density of innervation of the organ of Corti with differences in the acuity of hearing, including evidence as to the location in the human cochlea of the receptors for certain tones. *Acta Otolaryngol.* 15, 269–308. doi: 10.3109/00016483109119096

Gustafsson, M. G., Shao, L., Carlton, P. M., Wang, C. J., Golubovskaya, I. N., Cande, W. Z., et al. (2008). Three-dimensional resolution doubling in wide-field fluorescence microscopy by structured illumination. *Biophys. J.* 94, 4957–4970. doi: 10.1529/biophysj.107.120345

Han, K. S., Guo, C., Chen, C. H., Witter, L., Osorno, T., and Regehr, W. G. (2018). Ephaptic coupling promotes synchronous firing of cerebellar purkinje cells. *Neuron 100*, 564–578.e3. doi: 10.1016/j.neuron.2018.09.018

Hanani, M., Huang, T. Y., Cherkas, P. S., Ledda, M., and Pannese, E. (2002). Glial cell plasticity in sensory ganglia induced by nerve damage. *Neuroscience* 114, 279–283. doi: 10.1016/S0306-4522(02)00279-8

Hochmair, I., Hochmair, E., Nopp, P., Waller, M., and Jolly, C. (2015). Deep electrode insertion and sound coding in cochlear implants. *Hear. Res.* 322, 14–23. doi: 10.1016/j.heares.2014.10.006

Hockett, C. F., Ascher, R., Agogino, G. A., Birdwhistell, R. L., Bryan, A. L., Clark, J. D., et al. (1964). The human revolution [and comments and reply]. *Curr. Anthropol.* 5, 135–168. doi: 10.1086/200477

Hossain, W. A., Antic, S. D., Yang, Y., Rasband, M. N., and Morest, D. K. (2005). Where is the spike generator of the cochlear nerve? Voltage-gated sodium channels in the mouse cochlea. *J. Neurosci.* 25, 6857–6868. doi: 10.1523/JNEUROSCI.0123-05.2005

House, W. F., and Urban, J. (1973). Long term results of electrode implantation and electronic stimulation of the cochlea in man. *Ann. Otol. Rhinol. Laryngol* 82, 504–517. doi: 10.1177/000348947308200408

JoséGarrido, J., Giraud, P., Carlier, E., Fernandes, F., Moussif, A., Fache, M. P., et al. (2003). A targeting motif involved in sodium channel clustering at the axonal initial segment. *Science (80-.).* 300, 2091–2094. doi: 10.1126/science.1085167

Jyothi, V., Li, M., Kilpatrick, L. A., Smythe, N., LaRue, A. C., Zhou, D., et al. (2010). Unmyelinated auditory type i spiral ganglion neurons in congenic Ly5.1 mice. *J. Comp. Neurol.* 518, 3254–3271. doi: 10.1002/cne.22398

Kantardzhieva, A., Liberman, M. C., and Sewell, W. F. (2013). Quantitative analysis of ribbons, vesicles, and cisterns at the cat inner hair cell synapse: correlations with spontaneous rate. *J. Comp. Neurol.* 521, 3260–3271. doi: 10.1002/cne.23345

Keen, E. C., and Hudspeth, A. J. (2006). Transfer characteristics of the hair cell's afferent synapse. *Proc. Natl. Acad. Sci. U.S.A.* 103, 5537–5542. doi: 10.1073/pnas.0601103103

Kemp, D. T. (1979). The evoked cochlear mechanical response and the auditory microstructure - evidence for a new element in cochlear mechanics. *Scand Audiol Suppl.* 8(suppl. 9), 35–47.

Khalifa, S. A. M., Friberg, U., Illing, R. B., and Rask-Andersen, H. (2003). Synaptophysin immunohistochemistry in the human cochlea. *Hear. Res.* 185, 35–42. doi: 10.1016/S0378-5955(03)00228-4

Khanna, S. M., and Teich, M. C. (1989). Spectral characteristics of the responses of primary auditory nerve fibers to frequency-modulated signals. *Hear. Res.* 39, 159–175. doi: 10.1016/0378-5955(89)90088-9

Kiang, N. Y. S. (1980). Processing of speech by the auditory nervous system. *J. Acoust. Soc. Am.* 68, 830–835. doi: 10.1121/1.384822

Kim, K. X., and Rutherford, M. A. (2016). Maturation of NaV and KV channel topographies in the auditory nerve spike initiator before and after developmental onset of hearing function. *J. Neurosci.* 36, 2111–2118. doi: 10.1523/jneurosci.3437-15.2016

Kim, Y. S., Anderson, M., Park, K., Zheng, Q., Agarwal, A., Gong, C., et al. (2016). Coupled activation of primary sensory neurons contributes to chronic pain. *Neuron* 91, 1085–1096. doi: 10.1016/j.neuron.2016.07.044

Kimura, R. S., Ota, C. Y., and Takahashi, T. (1979). Nerve fiber synapses on spiral ganglion cells in the human cochlea. *Ann. Otol. Rhinol. Laryngol. Suppl.* 88, 1–17.

Kimura, R. S., Schuknecht, H. F., Ota, C. Y., and Jones, D. D. (1980). Obliteration of the ductus reuniens. *Acta Otolaryngol.* 89, 295–309. doi: 10.3109/00016488009127141

Kordeli, E., Lambert, S., and Bennett, V. (1995). Ankyrin(G). A new ankyrin gene with neural-specific isoforms localized at the axonal initial segment and node of Ranvier. *J. Biol. Chem.* 270, 2352–2359. doi: 10.1074/jbc.270.5.2352

Kujawa, S. G., and Liberman, M. C. (2015). Synaptopathy in the noise-exposed and aging cochlea: primary neural degeneration in acquired sensorineural hearing loss. *Hear. Res.* 330(Pt B), 191–9. doi: 10.1016/j.heares.2015.02.009

Lacas-Gervais, S., Guo, J., Strenzke, N., Scarfone, E., Kolpe, M., Jahkel, M., et al. (2004). βIVΣ1 spectrin stabilizes the nodes of Ranvier and axon initial segments. *J. Cell Biol.* 166, 983–990. doi: 10.1083/jcb.200408007

Lai, C. S. L., Fisher, S. E., Hurst, J. A., Vargha-Khadem, F., and Monaco, A. P. (2001). A forkhead-domain gene is mutated in a severe speech and language disorder. *Nature* 413, 519–523. doi: 10.1038/35097076

Leterrier, C. (2016). The axon initial segment, 50 years later: a nexus for neuronal organization and function. *Curr. Top. Membr.* 77, 185–233. doi: 10.1016/bs.ctm.2015.10.005

Leterrier, C., Clerc, N., Rueda-Boroni, F., Montersino, A., Dargent, B., and Castets, F. (2017). Ankyrin G membrane partners drive the establishment and maintenance of the axon initial segment. *Front. Cell. Neurosci.* 11:6. doi: 10.3389/fncel.2017.00006

Li, H., Schart-Morén, N., Rohani, S. A., Ladak, H. M., Rask-Andersen, H., and Agrawal, S. (2018). Synchrotron radiation-based reconstruction of the human spiral ganglion: implications for cochlear implantation. *Ear Hear.* 41, 173–181. doi: 10.1097/AUD.0000000000000738

Liu, Q., Lee, E., and Davis, R. L. (2014). Heterogeneous intrinsic excitability of murine spiral ganglion neurons is determined by Kv1 and HCN channels. *Neuroscience* 257, 96–110. doi: 10.1016/j.neuroscience.2013.10.065

Liu, W., Boström, M., Kinnefors, A., and Rask-Andersen, H. (2009). Unique expression of connexins in the human cochlea. *Hear. Res.* 250, 55–62. doi: 10.1016/j.heares.2009.01.010

Liu, W., Edin, F., Atturo, F., Rieger, G., Löwenheim, H., Senn, P., et al. (2015). The pre- and post-somatic segments of the human type I spiral ganglion neurons - Structural and functional considerations related to cochlear implantation. *Neuroscience* 284, 470–482. doi: 10.1016/j.neuroscience.2014.09.059

Liu, W., Glueckert, R., Linthicum, F. H., Rieger, G., Blumer, M., Bitsche, M., et al. (2014). Possible role of gap junction intercellular channels and connexin 43 in satellite glial cells (SGCs) for preservation of human spiral ganglion neurons: a comparative study with clinical implications. *Cell Tissue Res.* 355, 267–278. doi: 10.1007/s00441-013-1735-2

Liu, W., Glueckert, R., Schrott-Fischer, A., and Rask-Andersen, H. (2020). Human cochlear microanatomy–an electron microscopy and super-resolution structured illumination study and review. *Hear. Balanc. Commun.* 18, 1–14. doi: 10.1080/21695717.2020.1807259

Liu, W., Luque, M., Glueckert, R., Danckwardt-Lillieström, N., Nordström, C. K., Schrott-Fischer, A., et al. (2019). Expression of Na/K-ATPase subunits in the human cochlea: a confocal and super-resolution microscopy study with special reference to auditory nerve excitation and cochlear implantation. *Ups. J. Med. Sci.* 124, 168–179. doi: 10.1080/03009734.2019.1653408

Liu, W., Molnar, M., Garnham, C., Benav, H., and Rask-Andersen, H. (2018). Macrophages in the human cochlea: Saviors or predators-A study using super-resolution immunohistochemistry. *Front. Immunol.* 9:223. doi: 10.3389/fimmu.2018.00223

Loewenstein, W. R., and Ishiko, N. (1960). Effects of polarization of the receptor membrane and of the first Ranvier node in a sense organ. *J. Gen. Physiol.* 43, 981–998. doi: 10.1085/jgp.43.5.981

Lopez-Poveda, E. A., and Eustaquio-Martin, A. (2013). On the controversy about the sharpness of human cochlear tuning. *JARO - J. Assoc. Res. Otolaryngol.* 14, 673–686. doi: 10.1007/s10162-013-0397-9

Luque, M., Schrott-Fischer, A., Dudas, J., Pechriggl, E., Brenner, E., Rask-Andersen, H., et al. (2021). HCN channels in the mammalian cochlea: Expression pattern, subcellular location, and age-dependent changes. *J. Neurosci. Res.* 99, 699–728. doi: 10.1002/jnr.24754

Matthews, G., and Fuchs, P. (2010). The diverse roles of ribbon synapses in sensory neurotransmission. *Nat. Rev. Neurosci.* 11, 812–822. doi: 10.1038/nrn2924

McLean, W. J., Smith, K. A., Glowatzki, E., and Pyott, S. J. (2009). Distribution of the Na,K-ATPase α subunit in the rat spiral ganglion and organ of corti. *JARO - J. Assoc. Res. Otolaryngol.* 10:37. doi: 10.1007/s10162-008-0152-9

Mei, X., Glueckert, R., Schrott-Fischer, A., Li, H., Ladak, H. M., Agrawal, S. K., et al. (2020). Vascular supply of the human spiral ganglion: novel three-dimensional analysis using synchrotron phase-contrast imaging and histology. *Sci. Rep.* 10:5877. doi: 10.1038/s41598-020-62653-0

Meister, M., Lagnado, L., and Baylor, D. A. (1995). Concerted signaling by retinal ganglion cells. *Science (80-.).* 270, 1207–1210. doi: 10.1126/science.270.5239.1207

Merchan-Perez, A., and Liberman, M. C. (1996). Ultrastructural differences among afferent synapses on cochlear hair cells: correlations with spontaneous discharge rate. *J. Comp. Neurol.* 371, 208–221. doi: 10.1002/(SICI)1096-9861(19960722)371:2<208::AID-CNE2>3.0.CO;2-6

Michelson, R. P. (1971). The results of electrical stimulation of the cochlea in human sensory deafness. *Ann. Otol. Rhinol. Laryngol.* 80, 914–919. doi: 10.1177/000348947108000618

Mo, Z. L., and Davis, R. L. (1997). Heterogeneous voltage dependence of inward rectifier currents in spiral ganglion neurons. *J. Neurophysiol.* 78, 3019–3027. doi: 10.1152/jn.1997.78.6.3019

Moser, T., and Beutner, D. (2000). Kinetics of exocytosis and endocytosis at the cochlear inner hair cell afferent synapse of the mouse. *Proc. Natl. Acad. Sci. U.S.A.* 97, 883–888. doi: 10.1073/pnas.97.2.883

Nadol, J. B. (1983). Serial section reconstruction of the neural poles of hair cells in the human organ of Corti. I. Inner hair cells. *Laryngoscope* 93, 599–614. doi: 10.1002/lary.1983.93.5.599

Nadol, J. B. (1988). Comparative anatomy of the cochlea and auditory nerve in mammals. *Hear. Res.* 34, 253–266. doi: 10.1016/0378-5955(88)90006-8

Newbury, D. F., Bishop, D. V. M., and Monaco, A. P. (2005). Genetic influences on language impairment and phonological short-term memory. *Trends Cogn. Sci. (Regul. Ed).* 9, 528–534. doi: 10.1016/j.tics.2005.09.002

Nouvian, R., Beutner, D., Parsons, T. D., and Moser, T. (2006). Structure and function of the hair cell ribbon synapse. *J. Membr. Biol.* 209, 153–165. doi: 10.1007/s00232-005-0854-4

Oak, M. H., and Yi, E. (2014). Voltage-gated K^+ channels contributing to temporal precision at the inner hair cell-auditory afferent nerve fiber synapses in the mammalian cochlea. *Arch. Pharm. Res.* 37, 821–833. doi: 10.1007/s12272-014-0411-8

Ota, C. Y., and Kimura, R. S. (1980). Ultrastructural study of the human spiral ganglion. *Acta Otolaryngol.* 32, 161–167. doi: 10.1002/jhet.5570320126

Pan, Z., Kao, T., Horvath, Z., Lemos, J., Sul, J. Y., Cranstoun, S. D., et al. (2006). A common ankyrin-G-based mechanism retains KCNQ and Na V channels at electrically active domains of the axon. *J. Neurosci.* 26, 2599–2613. doi: 10.1523/JNEUROSCI.4314-05.2006

Pannese, E. (2020). The structure of the perineuronal sheath of satellite glial cells (SGCs) in sensory ganglia * ennio pannese. *Neuron Glia Biol.* 6, 3–10. doi: 10.1017/S1740925X10000037

Pantev, C., Makeig, S., Hoke, M., Galambos, R., Hampson, S., and Gallen, C. (1991). Human auditory evoked gamma-band magnetic fields. *PNAS.* 88, 8996–9000. doi: 10.1073/pnas.88.20.8996

Petitpré, C., Wu, H., Sharma, A., Tokarska, A., Fontanet, P., Wang, Y., et al. (2018). Neuronal heterogeneity and stereotyped connectivity in the auditory afferent system. *Nat. Commun.* 9:3692. doi: 10.1038/s41467-018-06033-3

Rasband, M. N. (2010). The axon initial segment and the maintenance of neuronal polarity. *Nat. Rev. Neurosci.* 11, 552–562. doi: 10.1038/nrn2852

Rask-Andersen, H., Liu, W., Erixon, E., Kinnefors, A., Pfaller, K., Schrott-Fischer, A., et al. (2012). Human cochlea: anatomical characteristics and their relevance for cochlear implantation. *Anat. Rec.* 295, 1791–1811. doi: 10.1002/ar.22599

Rask-Andersen, H., Tylstedt, S., Kinnefors, A., and Illing, R. B. (2000). Synapses on human spiral ganglion cells: a transmission electron microscopy and immunohistochemical study. *Hear. Res.* 141, 1–11. doi: 10.1016/S0378-5955(99)00179-3

Rask-Andersen, H., Tylstedt, S., Kinnefors, A., and Schrott-Fischer, A. (1997). Nerve fibre interaction with large ganglion cells in the human spiral ganglion: a TEM study. *Auris Nasus Larynx* 24, 1–11. doi: 10.1016/S0385-8146(96)00039-9

Reijntjes, D. O. J., Lee, J. H., Park, S., Schubert, N. M. A., van Tuinen, M., Vijayakumar, S., et al. (2019). Sodium-activated potassium channels shape peripheral auditory function and activity of the primary auditory neurons in mice. *Sci. Rep.* 9, 1–18. doi: 10.1038/s41598-019-39119-z

Reijntjes, D. O. J., and Pyott, S. J. (2016). The afferent signaling complex: regulation of type I spiral ganglion neuron responses in the auditory periphery. *Hear. Res.* 336, 1–16. doi: 10.1016/j.heares.2016.03.011

Retzius, G. (1884). *Das Gehörorgan der Wirbelthiere: morphologisch-histologische Studien*. Stockholm: Samson and Wallin.
Rhode, W. S. (1971). Observations of the vibration of the basilar membrane in squirrel monkeys using the mössbauer technique. *J. Acoust. Soc. Am.* 49, 1218–1231. doi: 10.1121/1.1912485
Rosbe, K. W., Burgess, B. J., Glynn, R. J., and Nadol, J. B. (1996). Morphologic evidence for three cell types in the human spiral ganglion. *Hear. Res.* 93, 120–127. doi: 10.1016/0378-5955(95)00208-1
Ross, M. D. (1969). The general visceral efferent component of the eighth cranial nerve. *J. Comp. Neurol.* 135, 453–477. doi: 10.1002/cne.901350405
Ross, M. D., and Burkel, W. (1973). Multipolar neurons in the spiral ganglion of the rat. *Acta Otolaryngol.* 76, 381–394. doi: 10.3109/00016487309121526
Roux, I., Safieddine, S., Nouvian, R., Grati, M., Simmler, M.-C., Bahloul, A., et al. (2006). Otoferlin, defective in a human deafness form, is essential for exocytosis at the auditory ribbon synapse. *Cell* 127, 277–289. doi: 10.1016/j.cell.2006.08.040
Ruggero, M. A., and Temchin, A. N. (2005). Unexceptional sharpness of frequency tuning in the human cochlea. *Proc. Natl. Acad. Sci. U.S.A.* 102, 18614–18619. doi: 10.1073/pnas.0509323102
Rusznák, Z., and Szucs, G. (2009). Spiral ganglion neurones: An overview of morphology, firing behaviour, ionic channels and function. *Pflugers Arch. Eur. J. Physiol.* 457, 1303–1325. doi: 10.1007/s00424-008-0586-2
Rutherford, M. A., Chapochnikov, N. M., and Moser, T. (2012). Spike encoding of neurotransmitter release timing by spiral ganglion neurons of the cochlea. *J. Neurosci.* 32, 4773–4789. doi: 10.1523/JNEUROSCI.4511-11.2012
Safieddine, S., El-Amraoui, A., and Petit, C. (2012). The auditory hair cell ribbon synapse: from assembly to function. *Annu. Rev. Neurosci.* 35, 509–528. doi: 10.1146/annurev-neuro-061010-113705
Schaette, R., and McAlpine, D. (2011). Tinnitus with a normal audiogram: physiological evidence for hidden hearing loss and computational model. *J. Neurosci.* 31, 13452–13457. doi: 10.1523/JNEUROSCI.2156-11.2011
Schnee, M. E., Lawton, D. M., Furness, D. N., Benke, T. A., and Ricci, A. J. (2005). Auditory hair cell-afferent fiber synapses are specialized to operate at their best frequencies. *Neuron* 47, 243–254. doi: 10.1016/j.neuron.2005.06.004
Shannon, R. V., Zeng, F. G., Kamath, V., Wygonski, J., and Ekelid, M. (1995). Speech recognition with primarily temporal cues. *Science* 270, 303–304. doi: 10.1126/science.270.5234.303
Sheets, L., He, X. J., Olt, J., Schreck, M., Petralia, R. S., Wang, Y. X., et al. (2017). Enlargement of ribbons in zebrafish hair cells increases calcium currents but disrupts afferent spontaneous activity and timing of stimulus onset. *J. Neurosci.* 37, 6299–6313. doi: 10.1523/JNEUROSCI.2878-16.2017
Shera, C. A., Guinan, J. J., and Oxenham, A. J. (2010). Otoacoustic estimation of cochlear tuning: validation in the chinchilla. *JARO - J. Assoc. Res. Otolaryngol.* 11, 343–365. doi: 10.1007/s10162-010-0217-4
Shinozaki, T., Naruse, Y., and Câteau, H. (2013). Gap junctions facilitate propagation of synchronous firing in the cortical neural population: a numerical simulation study. *Neural Networks* 46, 91–98. doi: 10.1016/j.neunet.2013.04.011
Siegel, J. H. (1992). Spontaneous synaptic potentials from afferent terminals in the guinea pig cochlea. *Hear. Res.* 59, 85–92. doi: 10.1016/0378-5955(92)90105 V
Siegel, J. H., and Dallos, P. (1986). Spike activity recorded from the organ of Corti. *Hear. Res.* 22, 245–248. doi: 10.1016/0378-5955(86)90101-2
Smith, K. E., Browne, L., Selwood, D. L., McAlpine, D., and Jagger, D. J. (2015). Phosphoinositide modulation of heteromeric Kv1 channels adjusts output of spiral ganglion neurons from hearing mice. *J. Neurosci.* 35, 11221–11232. doi: 10.1523/JNEUROSCI.0496-15.2015
Spoendlin, H. (1972). Innervation densities of the cochlea. *Acta Otolaryngol.* 73, 235–248. doi: 10.3109/00016487209138937
Spoendlin, H., and Schrott, A. (1988). The spiral ganglion and the innervation of the human organ of corti. *Acta Otolaryngol.* 105, 403–410. doi: 10.3109/00016488809119493
Spoendlin, H., and Schrott, A. (1989). Analysis of the human auditory nerve. *Hear. Res.* 43, 23–38. doi: 10.1016/0378-5955(89) 90056-7
Stakhovskaya, O., Sridhar, D., Bonham, B. H., and Leake, P. A. (2007). Frequency map for the human cochlear spiral ganglion: implications for cochlear implants. *JARO - J. Assoc. Res. Otolaryngol.* 8:220. doi: 10.1007/s10162-007-0076-9
Sumner, C. J., Wells, T. T., Bergevin, C., Sollini, J., Kreft, H. A., Palmer, A. R., et al. (2018). Mammalian behavior and physiology converge to confirm sharper cochlear tuning in humans. *Proc. Natl. Acad. Sci. U.S.A.* 115, 11322–11326. doi: 10.1073/pnas.1810766115
Sun, S., Babola, T., Pregernig, G., So, K. S., Nguyen, M., Su, S. S. M., et al. (2018). Hair cell mechanotransduction regulates spontaneous activity and spiral ganglion subtype specification in the auditory system. *Cell* 174, 1247–1263.e15. doi: 10.1016/j.cell.2018.07.008
Thalakoti, S., Patil, V. V., Damodaram, S., Vause, C. V., Langford, L. E., Freeman, S. E., et al. (2007). Neuron-glia signaling in trigeminal ganglion: implications for migraine pathology. *Headache* 47, 1008–1023. doi: 10.1111/j.1526-4610.2007.00854.x
Theunissen, F. E., and Elie, J. E. (2014). Neural processing of natural sounds. *Nat. Rev. Neurosci.* 15, 355–366. doi: 10.1038/nrn3731
Tokhtaeva, E., Clifford, R. J., Kaplan, J. H., Sachs, G., and Vagin, O. (2012). Subunit isoform selectivity in assembly of Na,K-ATPase α-β heterodimers. *J. Biol. Chem.* 287, 26115–26125. doi: 10.1074/jbc.M112.370734
Tylstedt, S., Kinnefors, A., and Rask-Andersen, H. (1997). Neural interaction in the human spiral ganglion: a TEM study. *Acta Otolaryngol.* 117, 505–512. doi: 10.3109/00016489709113429
Tylstedt, S., and Rask-Andersen, H. (2001). A 3-D model of membrane specializations between human auditory spiral ganglion cells. *J. Neurocytol.* 30, 465–473. doi: 10.1023/A:1015628831641
Utzschneider, D., Kocsis, J., and Devor, M. (1992). Mutual excitation among dorsal root ganglion neurons in the rat. *Neurosci. Lett.* 146, 53–56. doi: 10.1016/0304-3940(92)90170-C
Viana, L. M., O'Malley, J. T., Burgess, B. J., Jones, D. D., Oliveira, C. A. C. P., Santos, F., et al. (2015). Cochlear neuropathy in human presbycusis: confocal analysis of hidden hearing loss in post-mortem tissue. *Hear. Res.* 327, 78–88. doi: 10.1016/j.heares.2015.04.014
Wahl-Schott, C., and Biel, M. (2009). HCN channels: structure, cellular regulation and physiological function. *Cell. Mol. Life Sci.* 66, 470–494. doi: 10.1007/s00018-008-8525-0
Wiener, L. F. (1984). The evolution of language: a primate perspective. *WORD.* 35, 255–269. doi: 10.1080/00437956.1984.11435760
Wilhelm-Bade, P., Rudnicki, M., and Hemmert, W. (2009). A model of auditory spiral ganglion neurons. *Front. Comput. Neurosci. Conference Abstract: Bernstein Conference on Computational Neuroscience.* doi: 10.3389/conf.neuro.10.2009.14.131
Wright, A., Davis, A., Bredberg, G., Ülehlová, L., and Spencer, H. (1987). Hair cell distributions in the normal human cochlea: a report of a european working group. *Acta Otolaryngol.* 436, 15–24. doi: 10.3109/00016488709124972
Zuo, Y., Zhuang, D. Z., Han, R., Isaac, G., Tobin, J. J., McKee, M., et al. (2008). ABCA12 maintains the epidermal lipid permeability barrier by facilitating formation of ceramide linoleic esters. *J Biol Chem* 283, 36624–36635. doi: 10.1074/jbc.M807377200

6

Navigating Hereditary Hearing Loss: Pathology of the Inner Ear

*Teresa Nicolson**

Department of Otolaryngology, Stanford University, Stanford, CA, United States

***Correspondence:**
Teresa Nicolson
tnicolso@stanford.edu

Inherited forms of deafness account for a sizable portion of hearing loss among children and adult populations. Many patients with sensorineural deficits have pathological manifestations in the peripheral auditory system, the inner ear. Within the hearing organ, the cochlea, most of the genetic forms of hearing loss involve defects in sensory detection and to some extent, signaling to the brain *via* the auditory cranial nerve. This review focuses on peripheral forms of hereditary hearing loss and how these impairments can be studied in diverse animal models or patient-derived cells with the ultimate goal of using the knowledge gained to understand the underlying biology and treat hearing loss.

Keywords: cochlea, organ of corti, hair cells, afferent neurons, stria vascularis, endolymph

INTRODUCTION

Impairment of hearing can be due to several factors including environmental insults, the effects of aging, and hereditary defects. Of these three forms, the most common form is due to aging (Bowl and Dawson, 2019; Keithley, 2020), which can affect the function of the delicate bones and tympanic membrane that mediate the transfer of sound to the hearing organ within the skull, the cochlea. Inside the cochlea, aging typically leads to loss of the sensory receptors for sound known as hair cells owing to a tuft of "hairs" or microvilli-like protrusions at the apical surface. Age-related hearing loss can be greatly exacerbated by a lifelong exposure to damaging levels of sound. If traumatic enough, sound can destroy or weaken the delicate structure of the hair bundle of the sensory cells, leading to permanent damage. In contrast, long term exposure to a less traumatic yet still noisy environment may not adversely affect the hair bundles but may rather cause the disconnection or de-innervation of neurons that receive signals from the hair cells and transmit that information to the brain (Moser and Starr, 2016; Liberman, 2017; Liberman and Kujawa, 2017). Loss of neuronal contacts or synapses with hair cells can eventually result in the death of some of the neurons. Weakened synaptic transmission is usually not apparent in standard hearing tests, but often leads to the inability to hear in noisy environments, also known as the "cocktail party problem." Aside from loud noise, other environmental insults to the ear include exposure to ototoxic drugs such as aminoglycoside antibiotics that are used to treat life threatening infections or platinum-based drugs used for chemotherapy (Guo et al., 2019). The unintended target of these drugs inside the ear are primarily the hair cells, which can die upon accumulation of the drug inside the hair-cell body (O'Sullivan et al., 2017). The third form of hearing loss involves genetic factors (Korver et al., 2017; Sheffield and Smith, 2019). Hereditary hearing loss is less common than impairments caused by aging and environmental insults, but it is among the most prevalent monogenic diseases in humans.

Hereditary hearing loss is one of the most common sensory deficits in humans affecting one out every 500 newborns (Sheffield and Smith, 2019). The level of impairment can vary widely from profound deafness to mild hearing loss, sometimes varying even among family members with the same mutation. Particular forms of hereditary hearing loss may affect the ability to hear particular frequencies of sound. In addition, the onset of hearing loss can be at the time of birth (congenital), or it can occur in a progressive manner much later in life. To date, hundreds of genes are associated with syndromic (more than the auditory system affected) and non-syndromic (auditory system only) deafness (see text footnote 1).[1] Of the non-syndromic forms, more than 120 genes have been implicated in hearing loss and the majority of cases involve recessive mutations in which both copies of the gene are mutated. Approximately a third of the cases are dominant, requiring only one copy to be mutated. As with aging, sometimes the middle ear is affected, leading to a loss of conduction of sound. However, the majority of mutations are sensorineural in nature, mainly affecting the inner ear, with many having developmental or functional consequences for hair cells.

Efforts to understand the etiologies associated with hearing loss have been ongoing for several decades. The purpose of this review is to highlight a few recent studies of non-syndromic hereditary hearing loss that illustrate the different types of pathology found in the inner ear. The following studies focus on three different tissue or cell types of the cochlea, namely the stria vascularis, sensory epithelium and the afferent neurons of the spiral ganglion. These studies were also chosen based on the variety of animal models or the use of human-derived cell lines to determine the function of the genes. Due to the inaccessibility of the inner ear in patients, a basic scientific approach with models is necessary to gain a better understanding of the nature of the defects caused by genetic variants that are associated with human hearing loss.

GENERATION OF THE RIGHT ENVIRONMENT FOR DETECTING SOUNDS: THE STRIA VASCULARIS

An important prerequisite for hair-cell function is the presence of an ionic environment that is conducive to excitation. Unlike other extracellular fluids throughout the body, the fluid inside the scala media of the inner ear is exceedingly rich in potassium ions (**Figure 1**). The high concentration of potassium ions on the apical side of hair-cell neuroepithelium contrasts greatly to the low concentration of potassium that bathes the basolateral surfaces of hair-cell somas. This striking difference between the two concentrations of potassium generates a dramatic electrochemical potential that facilitates excitation of auditory hair cells. The generation of this unique, high potassium fluid, known as "endolymph," is carried out by a specialized structure called the stria vascularis (**Figure 1**, green structure denoted as 1). The tissue of the stria vascularis is comprised of three cell layers. The marginal cells that face the endolymph are positioned on top of a layer of intermediate cells, which are followed by a layer of basal cells. The layers work together to pump and secrete potassium ions from the perilymph to the endolymph [for in-depth reviews, see Wangemann (2006) and Zdebik et al. (2009)].

[1] http://hereditaryhearingloss.org

Accordingly, mutations in ion channels and their regulatory subunits that are expressed in the stria vascularis such as KCNQ1, KCNE1, KCNQ10, and BARTTIN or tight junction molecules such as CLDN11 that are required for the integrity of the cell layers lead to the loss of endocochlear potential and consequently the loss of hearing (Gow et al., 2004; Kitajiri et al., 2004; Rickheit et al., 2008; Chen and Zhao, 2014; Chang et al., 2015; Faridi et al., 2019). In terms of novel gene networks operating in the stria vascularis, recent findings using a single cell RNA-seq approach have revealed expression profiles and further subtypes of cells beyond the marginal, intermediate and basal cells (Gu et al., 2020). In addition, known deafness genes that were thought to act elsewhere such as in the organ of Corti were also found to be expressed in the stria vascularis (Korrapati et al., 2019). The involvement of multiple tissues in causing deafness may mean that robust rescue of hearing using gene therapy will require targeting several cell types.

Although marginal or "dark" cells found in the vestibular inner ear of vertebrates are thought to perform a similar function to the stria vascularis, the electrochemical potential created is substantially lower and defined cell layers are not evident (Wangemann et al., 1995). Furthermore, the structure itself is not present in the hearing end-organs of non-mammalian vertebrates, thus necessitating the study of the pathological consequences of mutations in mammalian model organisms such as the mouse.

A recent example of such a study is illustrated by efforts to understand human hearing loss associated with deletions in the 3′ UTR of hepatocyte growth factor (*HGF*). Despite the name suggesting a specific role in the liver, this extracellular ligand has been implicated in many biological processes involving cell proliferation, survival, and motility. More surprisingly, the only disease in humans associated with mutations in *HGF* is non-syndromic hearing loss. In mice, the knock-out of *Hgf* results in embryonic lethality, whereas a conditional knock-out in the inner ear does indeed result in deafness (Schultz et al., 2009). However, to demonstrate that microdeletions in the non-coding region 3′UTR are causal to the deafness, Morell et al. (2020) engineered a 10 bp deletion in the mouse to mimic the mutation in humans. They found that the stria vascularis was abnormally thin and detached in their mouse model, likely due to a developmental defect wherein neural crest cells fail to migrate and populate the structure. Such a defect is fitting with the role of the HGF protein in cell migration. The failure of cell migration into the stria vascularis was inferred by the reduction of an array of genes expressed by melanocytes, a pigmented neural crest cell that acts as a progenitor source for the intermediate cells. Interestingly, it is this cell type, the intermediate cells, that expresses the receptor for HGF, which is a transmembrane receptor tyrosine kinase known as mesenchymal epithelial transition (MET). Accordingly, a reduction in the endocochlear potential was reported by the authors. Progressive death of hair cells also occurred, presumably due to the changes in the composition of the endolymph.

This example serves as an illustration of the ability to test the causality of specific mutations found in human patients in an animal model such as mice. There is a pressing need for such an

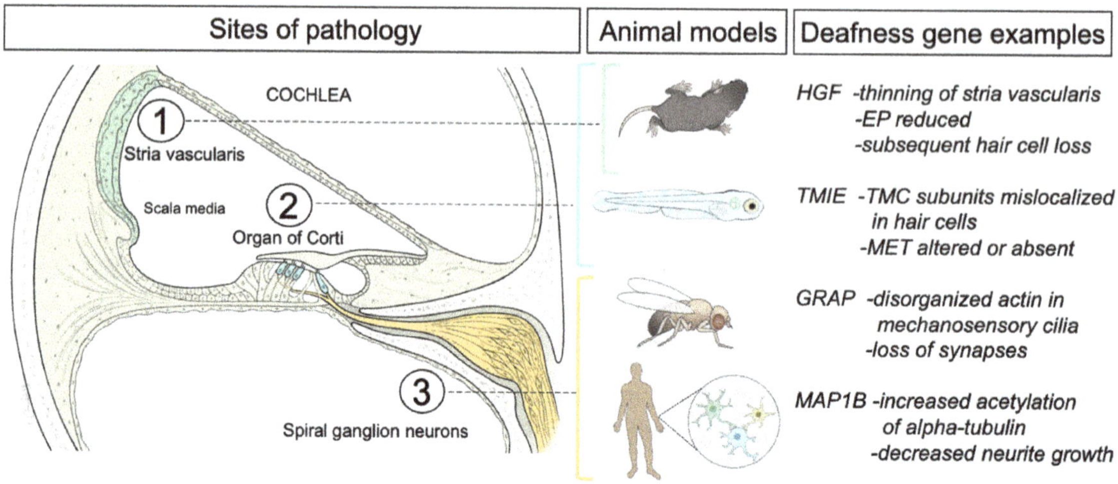

FIGURE 1 | Left panel, schematic of a cross sectional view of the cochlea, the hearing organ of the inner ear. The three regions of interest for this review are indicated. The fluid-filled middle compartment (scala media) contains the stria vascularis, a multilayer of cells (green) that generates the high concentration of potassium ions that are needed for sound detection. The neuroepithelium (organ of Corti) is comprised of sensory hair cells (inner and outer hair cells indicated in blue) embedded in a layer of supporting cells. Auditory hair cells are innervated by afferent or spiral ganglion neurons (yellow) that project to the hindbrain. Middle panel indicates the animal and cell models (*Mus Musculus* mice, *Danio rerio* zebrafish larvae, *Drosophila* flies, and human-derived cells) used for the studies of pathology induced by mutations in the orthologs of four different examples of human deafness genes (right panel). A brief summary of the findings is included. EP, endocochlear potential; TMC, transmembrane channel-like; MET, mechanotransduction.

approach as genome sequencing of many more affected families forges onward and the putative mutations are identified.

DETECTION OF SOUND: SENSORY HAIR CELL RECEPTORS

The generation of the high potassium endolymph is key to the function of auditory hair cells. Hair cells rely on the passive movement of potassium from the endolymph to the perilymph *via* their somas for excitation. The mechanism involves mechanoelectrical transduction in which a mechanical stimulus is converted into an electrical signal (Fettiplace, 2017; Ó Maoiléidigh and Ricci, 2019). Hair cells transduce sounds when the wave energy results in a deflection of the apical hair bundle that is exposed to the endolymph. Deflection along the excitatory axis of the hair bundle is thought to cause tension on fine extracellular filaments known as tip links that open mechanotransduction channels (Richardson and Petit, 2019). The passage of potassium through these channels leads to excitation or the depolarization of the cell body. Voltage changes are registered by voltage-gated channels in the basolateral membrane such as Cav1.3a, ultimately leading to the release of neurotransmitter at specialized contacts called ribbon synapses (Moser et al., 2020). Unlike neurons which have all or nothing responses, the excitation of sensory hair cells is a graded response, which is key to passing along information about the intensity of a sound. Information about frequency is based on the mechanics of the cochlea whereby the position itself of the hair cell in the snail-like structure favors the response to a particular pitch of sound (Fettiplace, 2017). For example, hair cells located at the base of the cochlea respond strongly to higher frequencies (in humans up to 20 kHz), whereas hair cells present at the apex are more responsive to lower frequencies (as low as 20 Hz in humans). In the organ of Corti in mammals, hair cells occur in two distinct types: a row of inner hair cells that responds to sound and three rows of outer hair cells that amplify those sounds when needed (**Figure 1**, structure denoted as 2). Each hair cell is surrounded by supporting cells, which participate in supportive functions such as maintaining structural integrity of the neuroepithelium, clearing potassium and excess neurotransmitter, and generation of extracellular structures that facilitate mechanotransduction [for a comprehensive review see Wan et al. (2013)].

With respect to sensorineural deafness, the vast majority of mutations identified thus far have deleterious effects on hair cells. The list of genes associated with hearing loss affects a wide array of biological processes in hair cells including transcription of genes, organization of the cytoskeleton, mechanotransduction, and synaptic transmission (Hilgert et al., 2009; Müller and Barr-Gillespie, 2015). In mouse models of human deafness, the most common phenotype is the degeneration of hair cells. This outcome is similar to the eventual loss of hair cells induced by defects in the function of the stria vascularis. Thus, examination of earlier stages of development before the onset of degeneration in animal models is often key to understanding the function of particular deafness genes. For example, the architecture of the hair bundle and/or mechanotransduction may be disrupted well before degeneration sets in.

Although many cell types of the cochlea are unique to mammals, the detection of sound by sensory receptors in the inner ear is an ancient sense, and most of the fundamental mechanisms of hair-cell function are highly conserved among vertebrates. For this reason, it is possible to study hair-cell function in a wide range of species. With CRISPR-based gene editing or other genetic methods such as mutagenesis screens, it is also possible to generate animal models of hearing loss outside of rodent models.

As an illustration of (i) using a non-rodent model, the zebrafish, to study human hearing loss, and (ii) the ability to compare the findings with this animal model to that of the mouse model, this review will focus on two recent studies of transmembrane inner ear (*TMIE*). Zebrafish have an inner ear that is anatomically similar to the vestibular portion of human ears. For hearing, they use the saccular end-organ. The sensory hair cells in the zebrafish inner ear rely on many of the same basic components necessary for hearing and balance in humans, and well over a dozen models of human hearing loss have been generated and studied in detail [for comprehensive reviews of studies in zebrafish see Nicolson et al. (1998); Nicolson (2015); Blanco-Sánchez et al. (2017); and Pickett and Raible (2019)].

Previous reports on *TMIE* demonstrated that loss of *TMIE* function resulted in deafness in fish, mice and humans, indicating the importance and conserved function of this gene among vertebrates (Mitchem et al., 2002; Naz et al., 2002; Cho et al., 2006; Shen et al., 2008; Gleason et al., 2009; Zhao et al., 2014). The mechanism, however, was not clear. In zebrafish, the studies of *tmie* were grounded in unbiased forward genetic screens for mutants with balance and hearing defects (Gleason et al., 2009; Pacentine and Nicolson, 2019). In mice, spontaneous mutations in *Tmie* were also identified (Naz et al., 2002; Cho et al., 2006). Initially it was reported that a striking developmental defect in the growth and maturation of hair bundles was observed in *tmie* zebrafish mutants (Shen et al., 2008; Gleason et al., 2009), but this defect was not observed in later studies of hair bundles in either the zebrafish or mouse knock-out mutants (Zhao et al., 2014; Pacentine and Nicolson, 2019; Cunningham et al., 2020). Instead, the main effect of the loss of TMIE protein appeared to be a functional defect resulting in the absence of mechanotransduction (Zhao et al., 2014; Pacentine and Nicolson, 2019; Cunningham et al., 2020). In both fish and mouse mutants, there is a pronounced reduction in the trafficking and localization of a component of the mechanotransduction machinery, the transmembrane channel-like (TMC) TMC1 protein. *TMC1* is a known deafness gene and collective evidence largely supports the idea that the multi-pass transmembrane proteins TMC1 and TMC2 are subunits of the mechanotransduction channel in hair cells [for a review see Corey et al. (2019)]. Mice rely mainly on *Tmc1* at the onset of hearing. In fish where the *tmc2* gene is duplicated, both duplicates (*tmc2a* and *tmc2b*) play a more critical role in hearing (Chen et al., 2020; Smith et al., 2020). Indeed, in *tmie* null mutants, GFP-tagged Tmc2b proteins are not detectable in the hair bundle (Pacentine and Nicolson, 2019). Aside from the role in trafficking of the TMCs to the hair bundles where they are thought to form the pore of the channel, TMIE itself is highly enriched in hair bundles, and is required for the stability of the TMCs at the site of mechanotransduction in both fish and mice (Pacentine and Nicolson, 2019; Cunningham et al., 2020). Therefore, TMIE acts as more than a chaperone for the TMCs, that is, TMIE is also an integral component of the transduction machinery. In *Tmie-/-* mice TMC2 is still present in cochlear hair bundles but inactive without TMIE, however, partial loss-of-function mutations in TMIE can affect TMC2-dependent mechanotransduction channel properties in hair cells (Cunningham et al., 2020). These results suggest that TMIE contributes to the function of the mechanotransduction channel.

The above studies demonstrate that the principal role of TMIE in mechanotransduction is similar among vertebrates. Nevertheless, it also reveals differences that are reflective of having a more flexible array of paralogs or interchangeable components for the mechanotransduction machinery in hair cells. What is common to both animal models is the mislocalization of TMC1, which is essential for hearing in humans. Using a diversity of animal models to explore the basic understanding of how hearing works allows us to identify what is conserved at the core of a biological process such as mechanotransduction and to infer that mutations in the human orthologs will cause similar pathologies in humans.

TRANSMISSION OF AUDITORY INFORMATION TO THE BRAIN: AFFERENT NEURONS

As mentioned above, hair cells release neurotransmitter at their basolateral surface, which is innervated by afferent neurons. The contacts between hair cells and afferent neurons are referred to as the first order synapses of the ascending auditory system. Auditory afferent neurons have a bipolar-type of morphology with their dendrites or peripheral processes forming the synapses with hair cells and their long axons (central process) projecting out of the bone-encased inner ear into the hindbrain. The fibers of the afferent neurons in the cochlea along with the cell bodies comprising the spiral ganglion are shown in yellow in **Figure 1** (denoted as 3). Recent efforts using single cell RNA-seq have identified several subtypes that either belong to the class of spiral ganglion neurons known as Type I that innervate inner hair cells, or a less numerous Type II class that synapses with outer hair cells [for an in depth review see Pavlinkova (2020)]. The tonotopic organization of the cochlea is largely preserved in the projection pattern of the spiral ganglion neurons to their target in the hindbrain, the cochlear nucleus. Thus, information about frequency is also represented spatially at the second order synapse of the auditory system.

As with the stria vascularis and the organ of Corti, hereditary mutations can affect the spiral ganglion neurons and the impairments are known as auditory neuropathies (De Siati et al., 2020). However, there are just a handful of spiral ganglion genes to date that are associated with human hearing loss. These include the deafness genes *DIAPH1*, *TMPRSS3* and *PJVK* (Lynch et al., 1997; Scott et al., 2001; Delmaghani et al., 2006), but as the following examples illustrate, the list is growing.

Using fruit flies to study human deafness genes may seem like a surprising choice but there are remarkable parallels between the mechanisms employed in insect and vertebrate hearing [for reviews see Boekhoff-Falk (2005); Boekhoff-Falk and Eberl (2014); and Hehlert et al. (2020)]. Moreover, similarities exist in the expression patterns of several homologous genes in both the *Drosophila* hearing organ (known as Johnston's organ) and the vertebrate inner ear. Of the genes required for auditory function in fruit flies, 20% have human orthologs implicated in deafness (Senthilan et al., 2012). For example, like vertebrate ears the developmental genes such as *atonal* and *distalless* are expressed in the auditory organ of *Drosophila*, as are the homologs of known deafness genes such as *myosin VIIa*, *diaphanous*, and *prestin*. The expression of shared genes is indicative that an ancestral mechanosensory cell, if not an ancestral hearing organ, existed in a predecessor that lived before the split of the insect and animal lineages.

A recent study of a novel deafness gene serves as an excellent example of the use of flies to study hereditary hearing loss (Li et al., 2019). In this study, a missense mutation predicted to result in a Q104L substitution in the growth factor receptor-bound adaptor protein (GRAP) was identified in two families. This protein couples small GTPase protein signaling with receptor activation and the authors demonstrated that the gene is expressed in mouse afferent fibers and the sensory organs or "scolopidia" of the fly auditory organ. A conditional knockout of the fly homolog of *GRAP* called downstream of receptor kinase (*drk*) in the antenna harboring the Johnston's organ caused deficits in gravity sensing and balance in adult flies. At the cellular level, the sensory scolopidia were disorganized, including abnormalities of internal structures such as actin bundles, and there was a loss of synapses formed by scolopidia neurons in the fly brain. To test the whether the Gln104Leu variant was causative, the authors compared rescue of the behavioral defects in the *drk* fly mutant by expressing the wild type human gene and the human Q104L variant and found that the variant form of GRAP was ineffective at rescuing the fly phenotype. The ability to rescue the deficits of an animal model with the corresponding human gene and test newly identified variants is an important and much needed approach for establishing causality of mutations found in the genome of hearing loss patients.

The study of animal models is invaluable for understanding the potential etiology caused by mutations. Nevertheless, with the recent advances in stem cell biology, it is also possible to take cells from patients such as blood cells and reprogram them into cells that resemble those in the auditory system. Cui et al. (2020) used precisely this approach to study the effects of a progressive form of hearing loss that they identified in three families. They focused on one mutation predicted to cause a substitution, S1400G, in the microtubule associated protein 1B (MAP1B). This protein promotes microtubule assembly and neurite extension primarily during development. To assess the effects of the dominant S1400G mutation in auditory neurons, pluripotent stem cells were generated from blood cells collected from hearing-impaired patients and their unaffected family members. A portion of the stem cells were "corrected" using CRISPR gene editing to eliminate the dominant mutation. The stem cells were then coaxed into differentiating into otic sensory neuron-like cells for *in vitro* experiments. The authors found that sensory neural-like cells heterozygous for the S1400G mutation had defects in later steps of differentiation and physiological responses. These defects were accompanied by a decrease in microtubule dynamics. Most of the heterozygous S1400G cells had shorter neurites in contrast to the CRISPR-corrected cells or sibling-derived cells. To further confirm their findings, the authors engineered a mouse model expressing the same dominant mutation. Heterozygous mutant mice displayed moderate yet progressive hearing loss. In addition, primary cultures of the spiral ganglion neurons exhibited similar decreases in neurite length and altered electrophysiological properties.

The above study highlights the utility of reprogramming patient-derived cells into a desired cell type for *in vitro* studies. This approach is an invaluable method for assessing the pathological consequences of a mutation in human cells. Although the technology is in its infancy, another potentially useful method is to generate human organoids of the inner ear. These 3D structures contain cell types that resemble hair cells and the sensory neurons that innervate them (Koehler et al., 2017; Roccio and Edge, 2019). Inner ear organoids can be generated from either human embryonic stem cells or human pluripotent stem cells. Overall, the process requires several weeks and involves manipulation of four signaling pathways to guide cells to adopt multiple cell fates. Perhaps further improvements in the reproducibility of generating 3D cultures will eventually lead to a more routine use of patient-derived cells to generate inner ear organoids, which would presumably create a more physiological environment in which to study a particular mutation.

CONCLUSION

In summary, hereditary sensorineural forms of hearing loss primarily affect the tissues and cell types of the inner ear that are vital to sensing sound and transmitting signals to the brain. Our knowledge of the genetics of hearing loss is growing as the pace of identifying novel human mutations associated with impairments in hearing is rapidly increasing (Shearer and Smith, 2015; McDermott et al., 2019). This increase is fueled by the accessibility and affordability of genome sequencing. Furthermore, the time for therapeutic interventions for hearing loss such as gene therapy is also rapidly approaching (Müller and Barr-Gillespie, 2015; Omichi et al., 2019; Taiber and Avraham, 2019; Delmaghani and El-Amraoui, 2020). The need to understand the underlying pathology induced by a mutation, and whether an approach such as gene therapy, or even whether a currently available therapy like cochlear implantation is likely to work requires the type of studies highlighted in this review. The ability to test the causality of new variants discovered *via* genomic sequencing and to establish animal models or study patient derived cells is a key step toward selecting the appropriate therapeutic approaches to ameliorate hearing loss.

The choice of animal or cell model is dictated by several factors. Although the genetic methods in *Drosophila* are highly advanced, the existence of an obvious ortholog of a human deafness gene is not always the case. In addition, extrapolating the pathological defects in fly mutants to potential defects in human patients can be challenging due to the very different structures of the hearing organs in flies. With respect to zebrafish, some deafness genes may be duplicated due to the large-scale duplication of approximately 40% of the genome in teleost fish during evolution. Depending on the expression pattern of the gene duplicates, it may be necessary knock out and analyze two genes instead of one. Also, fish do not have a cochlea; questions about the structures or tissues present only in the mammalian cochlea cannot be addressed. In mice, the need for dissection and cochlear explants to study the cellular defects makes the work more challenging. Generally, research with this particular animal model tends to be more costly and time consuming. Branching out to the use of human stem cells and organoids to study hearing loss is certainly exciting and gaining traction. Whether *in vitro* differentiated cells truly resemble desired cell types or how well the organoids recapitulate the environment of the inner ear is, however, not clear. To date, generating auditory hair cells from stem cells has yet to be achieved. Despite the above shortcomings, animal and cell models have been very valuable for studies of human hearing loss and continuing efforts with these models will undoubtedly yield more insights into the defects and pathology at the molecular, cellular and physiological level.

Aside from helping patients navigate hearing loss, research with animal models and patient-derived cells increases our basic understanding of how the inner ear works. These studies also add fascinating insights of how this remarkable sensory organ evolved and they provide clues about strategies that are employed to suit the auditory needs of a particular animal. On the whole, the interplay between basic and translational research is a fruitful one and offers hope to patients with hearing loss.

AUTHOR CONTRIBUTIONS

The author wrote the manuscript and confirms being the sole contributor of this work and has approved it for publication.

REFERENCES

Blanco-Sánchez, B., Clément, A., Phillips, J. B., and Westerfield, M. (2017). Zebrafish models of human eye and inner ear diseases. *Methods Cell Biol.* 138, 415–467. doi: 10.1016/bs.mcb.2016.10.006

Boekhoff-Falk, G. (2005). Hearing in Drosophila: development of Johnston's organ and emerging parallels to vertebrate ear development. *Dev. Dyn.* 232, 550–558. doi: 10.1002/dvdy.20207

Boekhoff-Falk, G., and Eberl, D. F. (2014). The Drosophila auditory system. *Wiley Interdiscip. Rev. Dev. Biol.* 3, 179–191.

Bowl, M. R., and Dawson, S. J. (2019). Age-Related Hearing Loss. *Cold Spring Harb. Perspect. Med.* 9:a033217.

Chang, Q., Wang, J., Li, Q., Kim, Y., Zhou, B., Wang, Y., et al. (2015). Virally mediated *Kcnq1* gene replacement therapy in the immature scala media restores hearing in a mouse model of human Jervell and Lange-Nielsen deafness syndrome. *EMBO Mol. Med.* 7, 1077–1086. doi: 10.15252/emmm.201404929

Chen, J., and Zhao, H.-B. (2014). The role of an inwardly rectifying K(+) channel (Kir4.1) in the inner ear and hearing loss. *Neuroscience* 265, 137–146. doi: 10.1016/j.neuroscience.2014.01.036

Chen, Z., Zhu, S., Kindig, K., Wang, S., Chou, S.-W., Davis, R. W., et al. (2020). Tmc proteins are essential for zebrafish hearing where Tmc1 is not obligatory. *Hum. Mol. Genet.* 29, 2004–2021. doi: 10.1093/hmg/ddaa045

Cho, K. I., Suh, J.-G., Lee, J. W., Hong, S. H., Kang, T.-C., Oh, Y.-S., et al. (2006). The circling mouse (C57BL/6J-cir) has a 40-kilobase genomic deletion that includes the transmembrane inner ear (tmie) gene. *Comp. Med.* 56, 476–481.

Corey, D. P., Akyuz, N., and Holt, J. R. (2019). Function and Dysfunction of TMC Channels in Inner Ear Hair Cells. *Cold Spring Harb. Perspect. Med.* 9:a033506. doi: 10.1101/cshperspect.a033506

Cui, L., Zheng, J., Zhao, Q., Chen, J.-R., Liu, H., Peng, G., et al. (2020). Mutations of MAP1B encoding a microtubule-associated phosphoprotein cause sensorineural hearing loss. *JCI Insight* 5:e136046.

Cunningham, C. L., Qiu, X., Wu, Z., Zhao, B., Peng, G., Kim, Y.-H., et al. (2020). TMIE Defines Pore and Gating Properties of the Mechanotransduction Channel of Mammalian Cochlear Hair Cells. *Neuron* 107, 126–143.e8.

De Siati, R. D., Rosenzweig, F., Gersdorff, G., Gregoire, A., Rombaux, P., and Deggouj, N. (2020). . Auditory Neuropathy Spectrum Disorders: from Diagnosis to Treatment: literature Review and Case Reports. *J. Clin. Med.* 9:1074. doi: 10.3390/jcm9041074

Delmaghani, S., del Castillo, F. J., Michel, V., Leibovici, M., Aghaie, A., Ron, U., et al. (2006). Mutations in the gene encoding pejvakin, a newly identified protein of the afferent auditory pathway, cause DFNB59 auditory neuropathy. *Nat. Genet.* 38, 770–778. doi: 10.1038/ng1829

Delmaghani, S., and El-Amraoui, A. (2020). Inner Ear Gene Therapies Take Off: current Promises and Future Challenges. *J. Clin. Med.* 9:2309. doi: 10.3390/jcm9072309

Faridi, R., Tona, R., Brofferio, A., Hoa, M., Olszewski, R., Schrauwen, I., et al. (2019). Mutational and phenotypic spectra of KCNE1 deficiency in Jervell and Lange-Nielsen Syndrome and Romano-Ward Syndrome. *Hum. Mutat.* 40, 162–176.

Fettiplace, R. (2017). Hair Cell Transduction, Tuning, and Synaptic Transmission in the Mammalian Cochlea. *Compr. Physiol.* 7, 1197–1227. doi: 10.1002/cphy.c160049

Gleason, M. R., Nagiel, A., Jamet, S., Vologodskaia, M., López-Schier, H., and Hudspeth, A. J. (2009). The transmembrane inner ear (Tmie) protein is essential for normal hearing and balance in the zebrafish. *Proc. Natl. Acad. Sci. U. S. A.* 106, 21347–21352. doi: 10.1073/pnas.0911632106

Gow, A., Davies, C., Southwood, C. M., Frolenkov, G., Chrustowski, M., Ng, L., et al. (2004). Deafness in Claudin 11-null mice reveals the critical contribution of basal cell tight junctions to stria vascularis function. *J. Neurosci.* 24, 7051–7062. doi: 10.1523/jneurosci.1640-04.2004

Gu, S., Olszewski, R., Taukulis, I., Wei, Z., Martin, D., Morell, R. J., et al. (2020). Characterization of rare spindle and root cell transcriptional profiles in the stria vascularis of the adult mouse cochlea. *Sci. Rep.* 10:18100.

Guo, J., Chai, R., Li, H., and Sun, S. (2019). Protection of Hair Cells from Ototoxic Drug-Induced Hearing Loss. *Adv. Exp. Med. Biol.* 1130, 17–36. doi: 10.1007/978-981-13-6123-4_2

Hehlert, P., Zhang, W., and Göpfert, M. C. (2020). Drosophila Mechanosensory Transduction. *Trends Neurosci.* 44, 323–335. doi: 10.1016/j.tins.2020.11.001

Hilgert, N., Smith, R. J. H., and Van Camp, G. (2009). Function and expression pattern of nonsyndromic deafness genes. *Curr. Mol. Med.* 9, 546–564. doi: 10.2174/156652409788488775

Keithley, E. M. (2020). Pathology and mechanisms of cochlear aging. *J. Neurosci. Res.* 98, 1674–1684. doi: 10.1002/jnr.24439

Kitajiri, S., Miyamoto, T., Mineharu, A., Sonoda, N., Furuse, K., Hata, M., et al. (2004). Compartmentalization established by claudin-11-based tight junctions in stria vascularis is required for hearing through generation of endocochlear potential. *J. Cell. Sci.* 117, 5087–5096. doi: 10.1242/jcs.01393

Koehler, K. R., Nie, J., Longworth-Mills, E., Liu, X.-P., Lee, J., Holt, J. R., et al. (2017). Generation of inner ear organoids containing functional hair cells from human pluripotent stem cells. *Nat. Biotechnol.* 35, 583–589. doi: 10.1038/nbt.3840

Korrapati, S., Taukulis, I., Olszewski, R., Pyle, M., Gu, S., Singh, R., et al. (2019). Single Cell and Single Nucleus RNA-Seq Reveal Cellular Heterogeneity and Homeostatic Regulatory Networks in Adult Mouse Stria Vascularis. *Front. Mol. Neurosci.* 12:316. doi: 10.3389/fnmol.2019.00316

Korver, A. M. H., Smith, R. J. H., Van Camp, G., Schleiss, M. R., Bitner-Glindzicz, M. A. K., Lustig, L. R., et al. (2017). Congenital hearing loss. *Nat. Rev. Dis. Primer* 3:16094.

Li, C., Bademci, G., Subasioglu, A., Diaz-Horta, O., Zhu, Y., Liu, J., et al. (2019). Dysfunction of GRAP, encoding the GRB2-related adaptor protein, is linked to sensorineural hearing loss. *Proc. Natl. Acad. Sci. U. S. A.* 116, 1347–1352. doi: 10.1073/pnas.1810951116

Liberman, M. C. (2017). Noise-induced and age-related hearing loss: new perspectives and potential therapies. *F1000Res.* 6:927. doi: 10.12688/f1000research.11310.1

Liberman, M. C., and Kujawa, S. G. (2017). Cochlear synaptopathy in acquired sensorineural hearing loss: manifestations and mechanisms. *Hear. Res.* 349, 138–147. doi: 10.1016/j.heares.2017.01.003

Lynch, E. D., Lee, M. K., Morrow, J. E., Welcsh, P. L., León, P. E., and King, M. C. (1997). Nonsyndromic deafness DFNA1 associated with mutation of a human homolog of the Drosophila gene diaphanous. *Science* 278, 1315–1318. doi: 10.1126/science.278.5341.1315

McDermott, J. H., Molina-Ramírez, L. P., Bruce, I. A., Mahaveer, A., Turner, M., Miele, G., et al. (2019). Diagnosing and Preventing Hearing Loss in the Genomic Age. *Trends Hear.* 23:2331216519878983.

Mitchem, K. L., Hibbard, E., Beyer, L. A., Bosom, K., Dootz, G. A., Dolan, D. F., et al. (2002). Mutation of the novel gene Tmie results in sensory cell defects in the inner ear of spinner, a mouse model of human hearing loss DFNB6. *Hum. Mol. Genet.* 11, 1887–1898. doi: 10.1093/hmg/11.16.1887

Morell, R. J., Olszewski, R., Tona, R., Leitess, S., Wafa, T. T., Taukulis, I., et al. (2020). Noncoding Microdeletion in Mouse Hgf Disrupts Neural Crest Migration into the Stria Vascularis, Reduces the Endocochlear Potential, and Suggests the Neuropathology for Human Nonsyndromic Deafness DFNB39. *J. Neurosci.* 40, 2976–2992. doi: 10.1523/jneurosci.2278-19.2020

Moser, T., Grabner, C. P., and Schmitz, F. (2020). Sensory Processing at Ribbon Synapses in the Retina and the Cochlea. *Physiol. Rev.* 100, 103–144. doi: 10.1152/physrev.00026.2018

Moser, T., and Starr, A. (2016). Auditory neuropathy–neural and synaptic mechanisms. *Nat. Rev. Neurol.* 12, 135–149. doi: 10.1038/nrneurol.2016.10

Müller, U., and Barr-Gillespie, P. G. (2015). New treatment options for hearing loss. *Nat. Rev. Drug Discov.* 14, 346–365. doi: 10.1038/nrd4533

Naz, S., Giguere, C. M., Kohrman, D. C., Mitchem, K. L., Riazuddin, S., Morell, R. J., et al. (2002). Mutations in a novel gene, TMIE, are associated with hearing loss linked to the DFNB6 locus. *Am. J. Hum. Genet.* 71, 632–636. doi: 10.1086/342193

Nicolson, T. (2015). Ribbon synapses in zebrafish hair cells. *Hear. Res.* 330, 170–177. doi: 10.1016/j.heares.2015.04.003

Nicolson, T., Rüsch, A., Friedrich, R. W., Granato, M., Ruppersberg, J. P., and Nüsslein-Volhard, C. (1998). Genetic analysis of vertebrate sensory hair cell mechanosensation: the zebrafish circler mutants. *Neuron* 20, 271–283. doi: 10.1016/s0896-6273(00)80455-9

Ó Maoiléidigh, D., and Ricci, A. J. (2019). A Bundle of Mechanisms: inner-Ear Hair-Cell Mechanotransduction. *Trends Neurosci.* 42, 221–236. doi: 10.1016/j.tins.2018.12.006

Omichi, R., Shibata, S. B., Morton, C. C., and Smith, R. J. H. (2019). Gene therapy for hearing loss. *Hum. Mol. Genet.* 28, R65–R79.

O'Sullivan, M. E., Perez, A., Lin, R., Sajjadi, A., Ricci, A. J., and Cheng, A. G. (2017). Towards the Prevention of Aminoglycoside-Related Hearing Loss. *Front. Cell Neurosci.* 11:325. doi: 10.3389/fncel.2017.00325

Pacentine, I. V., and Nicolson, T. (2019). Subunits of the mechano-electrical transduction channel, Tmc1/2b, require Tmie to localize in zebrafish sensory hair cells. *PLoS Genet.* 15:e1007635. doi: 10.1371/journal.pgen.1007635

Pavlinkova, G. (2020). Molecular Aspects of the Development and Function of Auditory Neurons. *Int. J. Mol. Sci.* 22:131. doi: 10.3390/ijms22010131

Pickett, S. B., and Raible, D. W. (2019). Water Waves to Sound Waves: using Zebrafish to Explore Hair Cell Biology. *J. Assoc. Res. Otolaryngol.* 20, 1–19. doi: 10.1007/s10162-018-00711-1

Richardson, G. P., and Petit, C. (2019). Hair-Bundle Links: genetics as the Gateway to Function. *Cold Spring Harb. Perspect. Med.* 9:a033142. doi: 10.1101/cshperspect.a033142

Rickheit, G., Maier, H., Strenzke, N., Andreescu, C. E., De Zeeuw, C. I., Muenscher, A., et al. (2008). Endocochlear potential depends on Cl- channels: mechanism underlying deafness in Bartter syndrome IV. *EMBO J.* 27, 2907–2917. doi: 10.1038/emboj.2008.203

Roccio, M., and Edge, A. S. B. (2019). Inner ear organoids: new tools to understand neurosensory cell development, degeneration and regeneration. *Development* 146:dev177188,

Schultz, J. M., Khan, S. N., Ahmed, Z. M., Riazuddin, S., Waryah, A. M., Chhatre, D., et al. (2009). Noncoding mutations of HGF are associated with nonsyndromic hearing loss, DFNB39. *Am. J. Hum. Genet.* 85, 25–39. doi: 10.1016/j.ajhg.2009.06.003

Scott, H. S., Kudoh, J., Wattenhofer, M., Shibuya, K., Berry, A., Chrast, R., et al. (2001). Insertion of beta-satellite repeats identifies a transmembrane protease causing both congenital and childhood onset autosomal recessive deafness. *Nat. Genet.* 27, 59–63. doi: 10.1038/83768

Senthilan, P. R., Piepenbrock, D., Ovezmyradov, G., Nadrowski, B., Bechstedt, S., Pauls, S., et al. (2012). Drosophila auditory organ genes and genetic hearing defects. *Cell* 150, 1042–1054. doi: 10.1016/j.cell.2012.06.043

Shearer, A. E., and Smith, R. J. H. (2015). Massively Parallel Sequencing for Genetic Diagnosis of Hearing Loss: the New Standard of Care. *Otolaryngol. Head Neck Surg.* 153, 175–182. doi: 10.1177/0194599815591156

Sheffield, A. M., and Smith, R. J. H. (2019). The Epidemiology of Deafness. *Cold Spring Harb. Perspect. Med.* 9:a033258. doi: 10.1101/cshperspect.a033258

Shen, Y.-C., Jeyabalan, A. K., Wu, K. L., Hunker, K. L., Kohrman, D. C., Thompson, D. L., et al. (2008). The transmembrane inner ear (tmie) gene contributes to vestibular and lateral line development and function in the zebrafish (Danio rerio). *Dev. Dyn.* 237, 941–952. doi: 10.1002/dvdy.21486

Smith, E. T., Pacentine, I., Shipman, A., Hill, M., and Nicolson, T. (2020). Disruption of tmc1/2a/2b Genes in Zebrafish Reveals Subunit Requirements in Subtypes of Inner Ear Hair Cells. *J. Neurosci.* 40, 4457–4468. doi: 10.1523/jneurosci.0163-20.2020

Taiber, S., and Avraham, K. B. (2019). Genetic Therapies for Hearing Loss: accomplishments and Remaining Challenges. *Neurosci. Lett.* 713:134527. doi: 10.1016/j.neulet.2019.134527

Wan, G., Corfas, G., and Stone, J. S. (2013). Inner ear supporting cells: rethinking the silent majority. *Semin. Cell. Dev. Biol.* 24, 448–459. doi: 10.1016/j.semcdb.2013.03.009

Wangemann, P. (2006). Supporting sensory transduction: cochlear fluid homeostasis and the endocochlear potential. *J. Physiol.* 576, 11–21. doi: 10.1113/jphysiol.2006.112888

Wangemann, P., Liu, J., and Shiga, N. (1995). The pH-sensitivity of transepithelial K+ transport in vestibular dark cells. *J. Membr. Biol.* 147, 255–262.

Zdebik, A. A., Wangemann, P., and Jentsch, T. J. (2009). Potassium ion movement in the inner ear: insights from genetic disease and mouse models. *Physiology* 24, 307–316. doi: 10.1152/physiol.00018.2009

Zhao, B., Wu, Z., Grillet, N., Yan, L., Xiong, W., Harkins-Perry, S., et al. (2014). TMIE is an essential component of the mechanotransduction machinery of cochlear hair cells. *Neuron* 84, 954–967. doi: 10.1016/j.neuron.2014.10.041

7

Successful Treatment of Noise-Induced Hearing Loss by Mesenchymal Stromal Cells: An RNAseq Analysis of Protective/Repair Pathways

Athanasia Warnecke[1,2†], Jennifer Harre[1,2†], Matthew Shew[3], Adam J. Mellott[4], Igor Majewski[1], Martin Durisin[1] and Hinrich Staecker[5]*

[1] Clinic for Otolaryngology–Head & Neck Surgery, Hanover Medical School, Hanover, Germany, [2] Cluster of Excellence "Hearing4all" of the German Research Foundation (EXC 2177/1), Oldenburg, Germany, [3] Department of Otolaryngology–Head & Neck Surgery, Washington University School of Medicine in St. Louis, St. Louis, MO, United States, [4] Ronawk Inc., Olathe, KS, United States, [5] Department of Otolaryngology–Head & Neck Surgery, University of Kansas School of Medicine, Kansas City, KS, United States

***Correspondence:**
Athanasia Warnecke
warnecke.athanasia@mh-hannover.de

† These authors have contributed equally to this work and share first authorship

Mesenchymal stromal cells (MSCs) are an adult derived stem cell-like population that has been shown to mediate repair in a wide range of degenerative disorders. The protective effects of MSCs are mainly mediated by the release of growth factors and cytokines thereby modulating the diseased environment and the immune system. Within the inner ear, MSCs have been shown protective against tissue damage induced by sound and a variety of ototoxins. To better understand the mechanism of action of MSCs in the inner ear, mice were exposed to narrow band noise. After exposure, MSCs derived from human umbilical cord Wharton's jelly were injected into the perilymph. Controls consisted of mice exposed to sound trauma only. Forty-eight hours post-cell delivery, total RNA was extracted from the cochlea and RNAseq performed to evaluate the gene expression induced by the cell therapy. Changes in gene expression were grouped together based on gene ontology classification. A separate cohort of animals was treated in a similar fashion and allowed to survive for 2 weeks post-cell therapy and hearing outcomes determined. Treatment with MSCs after severe sound trauma induced a moderate hearing protective effect. MSC treatment resulted in an up-regulation of genes related to immune modulation, hypoxia response, mitochondrial function and regulation of apoptosis. There was a down-regulation of genes related to synaptic remodeling, calcium homeostasis and the extracellular matrix. Application of MSCs may provide a novel approach to treating sound trauma induced hearing loss and may aid in the identification of novel strategies to protect hearing.

Keywords: noise trauma, hearing loss, mesenchymal stroma cells, Wharton's jelly, cochlear transcriptome, hearing protection

INTRODUCTION

Sound trauma can lead to hearing loss with protean manifestations. With exposures ranging from acute blast injury to chronic noise exposure, a wide range of pathological effects are induced in the cochlea. The degree of injury that occurs is related to the energy and frequency of the input sound combined with the time of exposure (Le et al., 2017). At higher levels of sound exposure, damage to stereocilia and loss of hair cells in a basal to apical gradient occurs resulting in a permanent threshold shift. Damage to the spiral ganglion can occur through excitotoxicity, inflammation and loss of trophic support (Chen et al., 1997; Puel et al., 1997; Lin et al., 2011). Additionally, severe sound trauma results in degradation of the blood labyrinthine barrier. Sound trauma therefore causes a range of cellular damage that includes both hair cells and spiral ganglion neurons as well as changes in the cochlear blood supply. The molecular mechanisms involved in these processes have been extensively investigated. Initial sound overexposure results in oxidative stress with overproduction of reactive oxygen and nitrogen species leading to hair cell lipid membranes peroxidation and disruption of mitochondrial homeostasis (Yamane et al., 1995). The mitochondrion has also been implicated as a primary generator of free radicals and appears to be intimately involved in the generation sound trauma related pathophysiology (Kurabi et al., 2017). Multiple studies have shown that antioxidant defenses and the ability to buffer free calcium of the cells can prevent noise trauma (Huang et al., 2000; Gonzalez-Gonzalez, 2017). Ultimately, there is an activation of a variety of mitogen-activated protein (MAP) kinase stress pathways including c-Jun N-terminal (JNK) kinase leading to programmed cell death/apoptosis. Apoptosis can also be activated through tumor necrosis factor alpha (TNFα), which is produced during sound trauma (Kurabi et al., 2017). Other pro-inflammatory cytokines are produced in a delayed fashion via an nuclear factor kappa-light-chain-enhancer of activated B-cells (NFκB) signaling cascade (Kurabi et al., 2017). More recent studies have focused on erythroid two related factor 2 (Nrf2) being a key signal mediator at the center of multiple pathways (Fetoni et al., 2019). This molecule acts as a reactive oxygen species (ROS) sensor and normally exists in a bound state in the cytoplasm. It controls a variety of stress responses and events such as oxidative stress and inflammation can cause it to enter the nucleus and activate a variety of signaling cascades (Fetoni et al., 2019). Evaluation of gene expression networks after sound trauma has implicated several key pathways in sound trauma mainly relating to inflammation, heat shock response and detoxification of ROS (Clifford et al., 2016; Yang et al., 2016). Changes in regulation of genes related to cytokine signaling and pathways related to innate immunity appear to play an important role in the early response to sound trauma (Patel et al., 2013; Vethanayagam et al., 2016; Yang et al., 2016). Single cell RNAseq analysis after sound trauma demonstrates that a mix of adaptive and innate immune cells infiltrate the cochlea after sound trauma highlighting the complexity of the damage response (Rai et al., 2020). Antioxidants and anti-inflammatory drugs clearly can protect against noise induced hearing loss although, given the complexity of the induced reactome, it is unlikely that a single pharmaceutical agent would adequately protect against all aspects of damage (Rajguru, 2013; Maeda et al., 2017).

Many of the transcriptome changes seen in sound trauma are also seen in traumatic brain injury (TBI) and stroke, suggesting common mechanisms and potentially common approaches to attenuating these injuries (Meng et al., 2017; Li et al., 2020). An alternate approach to cochlear protection is treatment of inner ear injury with neuronal or mesenchymal stem cells/mesenchymal stromal cells (MSCs). MSCs have been demonstrated to have a wide range of immunomodulatory and protective effects after tissue injury and have been tested in diverse disorders such as stroke, acute kidney injury and myocardial infarction (Squillaro et al., 2016; Fu et al., 2017; Chang et al., 2018; Cunningham et al., 2018; Harrell et al., 2019; Tsintou et al., 2020). Fat derived MSCs have been shown to express growth factors in sound exposed inner ears (Fetoni et al., 2014). Both peripheral and local delivery of MSCs have been shown to have protective effects in a variety of hearing loss models but the molecular consequences of MSC delivery after sound trauma have not been evaluated [Reviewed in Warnecke et al. (2017); Kanzaki et al. (2020)].

Mesenchymal stromal cells have been postulated to work through two distinct mechanisms. When delivered into the peripheral circulation, MSCs can home into areas of damaged tissue and through a range of distinct signaling pathways including TGFβ, CCL2, IL6, IDO, VEGF, and WNT modulate inflammation and induce tissue protection and repair. It has been shown that in this delivery approach, the majority of injected MSCs are trapped in in the pulmonary circulation and are phagocytosed by pulmonary macrophages. This process of efferocytosis results in the release of factors inducing immune tolerance such as IL-10 and TGFβ, which may provide additional beneficial effects (Galipeau and Sensébé, 2018). Local delivery of MSCs also induces immunomodulatory and protective effects through direct delivery of growth factors and extracellular vesicles in their secretome. Some studies suggest that interaction between the MSCs and the damaged tissue is needed for the most complete protective effects (Wakabayashi et al., 2010; Drago et al., 2013; Hsieh et al., 2013). Local delivery of MSCs to the brain after TBI has been shown to partially normalize pathologic gene expression induced by trauma, resulting in a return to normal immune signaling, receptor mediated cell signaling, neuronal plasticity and glycolysis (Darkazalli et al., 2017). This suggests that cell therapy with MSCs has the capacity to provide multi-mechanistic protection and repair. To evaluate the mechanisms underlying the effects of MSCs on the inner ear, we treated adult mice exposed to an acute narrow band sound trauma with Wharton's jelly-derived MSCs (WJCs) directly delivered into the inner ear. Umbilical cord-derived cells like WJCs, were chosen since they have been shown to have a secretome that supports neuronal repair (Hsieh et al., 2013). After treatment, changes in the cochlear transcriptome and in hearing threshold were evaluated. With this investigative approach, we identified up and down regulated genes in mice exposed to noise and treated with WJC when compared to mice exposed to noise trauma only.

MATERIALS AND METHODS

All animal procedures were approved by the Institutional Animal Care and Use Board. A total of 25 4 week old female C57BL/6 mice (Jackson Laboratories) weighing between 18 and 23 grams were utilized for the experiments described below.

Procurement and Expansion of Mesenchymal Stromal Cells

Human MSCs were isolated from Wharton's jelly of umbilical cords according to the protocols approved by the University of Kansas Human Subjects Committee (KU-Lawrence IRB approval #15402) and Stormont-Vail (SMV) Hospital (SMV IRB Approval conferred by IRB Chair, Jo-Ann S. Harris, MD). Informed consent was obtained from the patients before collection of the umbilical cords. Three umbilical cords (n = 3) were obtained from Stormont-Vail (Topeka, KS, United States). All cords were from males that were born at full term and delivered under normal delivery conditions. Human MSCs were isolated and cultured according to previously published protocols (Mellott et al., 2016). Cells were cultured in medium consisting of 1% penicillin-streptomycin (Life Technologies), 10% fetal bovine serum (FBS) mesenchymal stem cell qualified (MSCq) (Life Technologies), and fibroblast basal medium (Lonza Group Ltd., Basel, Switzerland), and expanded to passage 5 for all experiments. For delivery, cells were harvested, washed in phosphate buffered saline (PBS) and resuspended to a concentration of 1×10^6 cells/ml in sterile PBS.

Experimental Design

Three groups were evaluated with five animals in each experimental condition. Group one consisted of animals (n = 5) that underwent assessment of baseline hearing by auditory brainstem response (ABR) followed by MSC delivery into the left ear. The same animals underwent re-evaluation of hearing with ABR 7 days post-MSC delivery. Group two animals were exposed unilaterally to sound followed by treatment with MSC (n = 5) or artificial perilymph (n = 5) at 48 h post-sound trauma. These animals were sacrificed 72 h post-MSC delivery for extraction of RNA from the treated (left-sided) cochlea. Group 3 animals were unilaterally exposed to sound followed by MSC (n = 5) or artificial perilymph (n = 5) at 48 h post-sound trauma. These animals underwent hearing testing with ABR at 14 days post-cell or perilymph therapy to evaluate rescue of hearing and thereafter sacrificed for histological analysis. Group 4 animals were exposed unilaterally to sound followed by treatment with MSC (n = 8) or artificial perilymph (n = 8) at 48 h post-sound trauma. These animals were sacrificed 72 h post-MSC delivery for extraction of RNA from the treated (left-sided) cochlea (n = 5) or perfused for immunohistochemistry (n = 3). An additional set of age matched untreated control animals underwent extraction of RNA from the cochlea (n = 5) or were perfused for immunohistochemistry (n = 3).

Auditory Brainstem Response Measurements

For ABR testing, the mice were anesthetized intraperitoneally using a mixture of ketamine (100 mg/kg) and xylazine (10 mg/kg). Mice were then placed inside a double-walled, sound attenuated chamber. Body temperature was maintained at 37°C using a MediHeat V500Vstat Heated Operating Table Digital Thermostat (PECO Services). ABR measurements were acquired using the Smart EP program from Intelligent Hearing Systems. Needle electrodes were placed on the vertex (+), behind the left ear (−) and behind the opposite ear (ground). Tone bursts were presented at 4, 8, 16, and 32 kHz, with duration of 500 μs using a high frequency transducer. Recording was carried out using a total gain equal to 100 K and using 100 Hz and 15 kHz settings for the high and low-pass filters. A minimum of 128 sweeps was presented at 90 dB sound pressure level (SPL). The SPL was decreased in 10 dB steps. Near the threshold level, 5 dB SPL steps using up to 1024 presentations were carried out at each frequency. Threshold was defined as the SPL at which at least one of the waves could be identified in 2 or more repetitions of the recording.

Sound Exposure

For the noise trauma (sound exposure), the mice were anesthetized as described above. Mice were then exposed to a 16 kHz pure tone presented at 118 dB SPL in the left ear for 4 h. Sound was delivered through a speaker equipped with a ribbon tweeter (Radio Shack 40-1310 Horn Super Tweeter). The speaker was coupled to the left ear via a short plastic tube, 12 mm in inner diameter and 45 mm in length. Prior to exposure, the sound output was calibrated using a Quest Electronics Precision Integrating Sound Level Meter (model 1800). The Sound Level Meter was calibrated using a 1000 Hz Bruel & Kjaer 4230 Sound Level Calibrator. After sound exposure, animals were allowed to recover for 48 h before initiating treatment.

Delivery of Mesenchymal Stromal Cells

Mice were anesthetized as described above. A dorsal post-auricular incision was made, and the left posterior semicircular canal exposed. Using a microdrill, a canalostomy was created, exposing the perilymphatic space. Subsequently 1 μl of MSCs (1×10^6 cells/ml in sterile PBS) were injected using a Hamilton microsyringe with 0.1 μl graduations and a 36-gauge needle). Control animals received 1 μl injection of artificial perilymph into the canal. The canalostomy was sealed with bone wax. The mice showed no signs of vestibular dysfunction or head tilt post-operatively.

RNA Extraction and Analysis

Group 2 animals (noise trauma plus MSC or perilymph treatment) were anesthetized with Beuthanasia 75 mg/kg (Schering-Plough Animal Health Corp., Union, NJ, Canada). The treated (left) cochlea was removed and immediately placed in RNAlater (Qiagen, cat #76104). Total RNA was extracted with Trizol reagent (Thermofisher, cat #15596018) and purified by centrifuging with phase lock heavy gel (Tiagen, cat # WMS-2302830). Concentration and quality of RNA were assessed using an Agilent Bioanalyzer 2100. Analysis of cochlear RNAs was carried out using the NuGen Universal Plus Assay on a NovaSeq sequencer as per manufacturer instructions. Trimming, quality control and alignment was carried out using the A.I.R. software package[1] with noise damage only specimens as a reference and noise damage with MSC treatment as the analyzed data package. There were five replicates for each experimental condition. The C57Bl/6 mouse genome (C57Bl6NJvi/ENSEMBL release) was used as a reference genome. Statistical analysis was carried out by the NOISeq method. Up regulated and down regulated genes were identified and organized according to their gene ontology (GO) classification. A combination of the enrichment score and the false discovery rate (FDR) was then used to develop a gene ontology enrichment analysis (GOEA). Analysis of potential biological significance was carried out using Ingenuity Pathway Analysis (IPA) software (Qiagen Bioinformatics, Redwood City, CA, United States) and the Reactome Knowledgebase[2] (Jassal et al., 2019). Using the IPA software package, results were organized into the most common pathways that were altered in response to MSC treatment and which keys genes were up or down regulated. The most up and down regulated genes were additionally evaluated using Pharos software[3] for identification of molecules in clinical use that can down or up-regulate the identified genes.

Expression of bcl2 and tnf was quantified in group 4 animals. cDNA from the control, noise exposed and noise + MSC samples was synthesized using the miScript II reverse transcription kit (Qiagen, cat#218161). Semi quantitative PCR for bcl-2 and tnf (Origene cat MP201255; NM013693) was then performed on the Bio-Rad CFX using the Quantitect SYBR Green PCR kit (Qiagen, cat# 204141). Tranthyretin expression was measured using the Bio-Rad qMMuCID0006861 primer pairs.

All reactions were performed in triplicate and the Cq value was determined using the threshold calculated by the Bio-Rad software. Fold change was calculated using the $2^{-\Delta\Delta CT}$ method.

Histological Analysis

Group 3 animals were anesthetized with Beuthanasia (Merck Animal Health) 14 days after treatment with MSCs or artificial perilymph and fixed via intracardiac perfusion with 4% paraformaldehyde in PBS. The cochleae were removed and postfixed in 2.5% glutaraldehyde, 1.5% paraformaldehyde in 0.1 M phosphate buffer overnight at 4°C. Cochleae were decalcified in 1% glutaraldehyde in 0.12 M ethylene diamine tetraacetic acid (ETDA) in 0.1 M phosphate buffer for 4 days at 4°C. The specimen were then stained with osmium 1% for 1 h. After washing in distilled water specimens were dehydrated in a graded series of ethanol. After 30 min in propylene oxide (obtained from Electron Microscopy Sciences, Hatfield, PA, United States #20401), cochleae were transferred to araldite/P mix (obtained from Electron Microscopy Sciences, Hatfield, PA, United States #10900) and kept on a rotating shaker overnight. Specimen were then embedded in araldite in a vacuum oven. The blocks were baked in a 60°C oven. Serial sections at 30 μm were performed and stained with toluidine blue. After air drying, sections were mounted on slides with Permount for microscopic analysis.

Fog group 4 animals, the temporal bones were removed, the stapes extracted, and the round window was opened. The temporal bones were postfixed overnight in 4% paraformaldehyde in PBS at 4°C. After rinsing in PBS three times for 30 min, the temporal bones were decalcified in 10% ETDA for 48 h. The temporal bones were rinsed in PBS, dehydrated, and embedded in paraffin. Ten μm sections were cut in parallel to the modiolus, mounted on Fisherbrand® Superfrost®/Plus Microscope Slides (Fisher Scientific, Pittsburgh, PA, United States) and dried overnight. Samples were deparaffinized and rehydrated in PBS two times for 5 min, then three times in 0.2% Triton X-100 in PBS for 5 min and finally in blocking solution 0.2% Triton X-100 in PBS with 10% FBS for 30 min at room temperature. Sections underwent antigen retrieval in a microwave using 1:10 Dako® Target Retrieval Solution (DAKO Corporation, Carpinteria, CA, United States) for 30 s. Immunohistochemistry was carried out with anti-Bcl-2 rabbit polyclonal antibody diluted 1:200 (BD Biosciences, Inc., San Jose, CA, United States). The tissue was incubated overnight at 4°C in a humid chamber. After three rinses in PBS, immunohistochemical detection was carried out with an anti-Rabbit IgG (1:50; Vectastain Elite ABC Kit of Vector Laboratories, Inc., Burlingame, CA, United States). The secondary antibody incubated for 3 h at room temperature in a humid chamber and reactions carried out per manufacturer instructions. For TNFα immunohistochemistry the tissue was incubated for 48 h at 4°C in a humid chamber in TNFα polyclonal antibody (1:500, Thermo Fisher, PA5-19810). After three rinses in 0.2% Triton X-100 in PBS, immunohistochemical detection was carried out with an Alexa Fluor Donkey 555 anti-Rabbit (1:1000; Abcam). The secondary antibody was incubated for 6 h at room temperature in a humid chamber. The slides were rinsed in 0.2% Triton X-100 in PBS three times for 5 min and finally cover slipped with ProLong® Gold antifade reagent (Invitrogen™ Molecular Probes, Eugene, OR, United States). For detection of Bcl-2 expression, sections underwent antigen retrieval in a microwave using 1:10 Dako® Target Retrieval Solution (DAKO Corporation, Carpinteria, CA, United States) for 30 s. Immunohistochemistry was carried out with anti-human Bcl-2 rabbit polyclonal antibody diluted 1:200 (BD Biosciences, Inc., San Jose, CA, United States). The tissue was incubated overnight at 4°C in a humid chamber. After three rinses in PBS, immunohistochemical detection was carried out with an anti-Rabbit IgG (1:50; Vectastain Elite ABC Kit of Vector Laboratories, Inc., Burlingame, CA, United States). The secondary antibody incubated for 3 h at room temperature in a humid chamber.

Statistical Analysis

Statistical analysis of hearing outcomes was performed with ANOVA for repeated measures. RT PCR results were analyzed using ANOVA (Prism V8).

[1] sequentiabiotech.com

[2] reactome.org

[3] Pharos.nih.gov

RESULTS

Delivery of Mesenchymal Stromal Cells to the Mouse Cochlea Does Not Induce Hearing Loss

After documentation of baseline hearing by ABR, 1 month old C57Bl/6 mice ($n = 5$) underwent delivery of 1 μl of human Wharton's Jelly-derived MSCs into their left posterior semicircular canal. One week post-delivery of cells, their hearing was re-evaluated. ABR recording prior to treatment at 4, 8, 16, and 32 kHz showed an average hearing threshold of 28.3 ± 7, 35 ± 5, 30 ± 5, and 30 ± 17, respectively. The average hearing threshold for each frequency did not change significantly after cell therapy (30 ± 0, 35 ± 5, 30 ± 0, and 40 ± 17 for 4, 8, 16, and 32 kHz, respectively) (**Figure 1**).

Delivery of Mesenchymal Stromal Cells to the Mouse Inner Ear Provides Significant Hearing Rescue After Severe Noise Trauma

Pre-treatment ABR measurements showed normal hearing threshold in both groups (**Figure 2**; control ore and MSC treated pre). After noise exposure, animals of the control group (treated with artificial perilymph) demonstrated a severe to profound hearing loss across all frequencies at 14 days post-sound exposure (**Figure 2**; control post). There was a significant rescue effect seen in the MSC treated animals at 4 and 8 kHz ($p < 0.01$) and at 32 kHz ($p < 0.05$) (**Figure 2**; MSC treated post) when compared to the thresholds of the control group after noise exposure and application of artificial perilymph (**Figure 2**; control post). At 16 kHz, treated animals showed better hearing thresholds than sound trauma and artificial perilymph treated animals, but this was not statistically significant. Histological analysis of the organ of Corti performed separately for the basal and mid turn showed loss of hair cells both inner and outer hair cells for both groups after sound trauma (MSCs and artificial perilymph treated) in the basal turn (**Figures 3A,B**). When compared to the artificial perilymph treated animals (**Figure 3C**), the MSC-treated animals did show preservation in the mid turn of the cochlea (**Figure 3D**). DPOAEs were not measurable after sound trauma and were not restored by MSC therapy (data not shown).

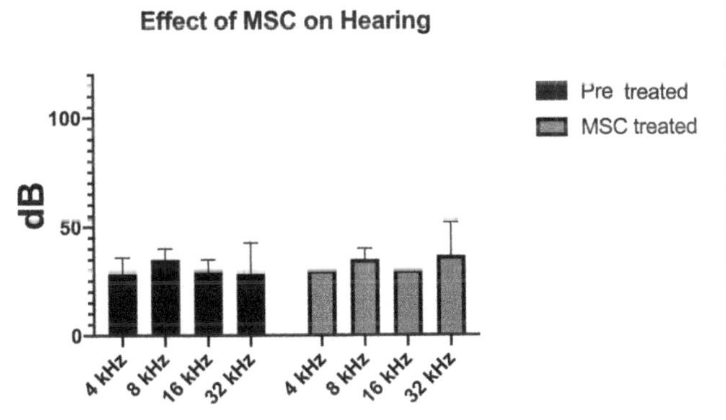

FIGURE 1 | Delivery of MSCs did not have any effect on baseline hearing. Hearing thresholds measured by ABR at four different frequencies prior to (black bars) and 7 days after transplantation of MSC to the inner ear via the posterior semicircular canal (gray bars) are depicted. There is no significant difference between the pre- and post-transplantation thresholds.

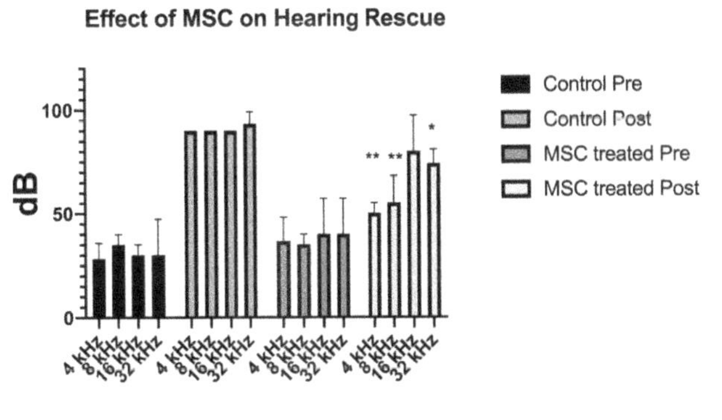

FIGURE 2 | Delivery of MSCs rescue hearing after noise exposure. Exposure to sound for 4 h results in a profound hearing loss across all frequencies (medium gray bars; Control Post). Delivery of MSCs into the posterior semicircular canal of animals after sound exposure resulted in significant rescue of hearing at 4 and 8 kHz ($p < 0.01$**) as well as at 32 kHz ($p < 0.05$*) (light gray bars; MSC treated Post) when compared to the control animals treated with artificial perilymph (Control Post).

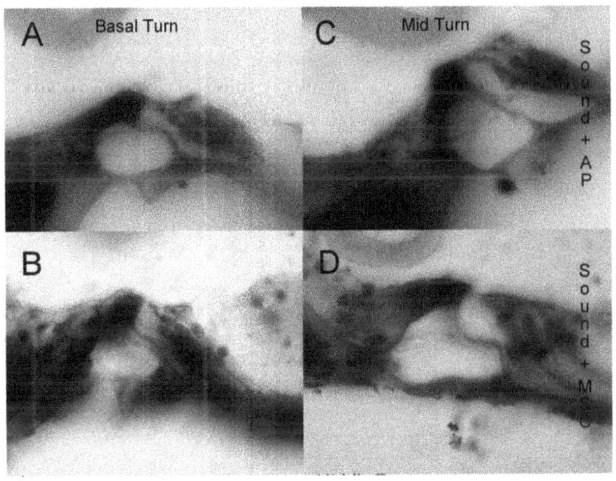

FIGURE 3 | Histological evaluation of organ of Corti integrity in sound trauma **(A,C)** and sound trauma and MSC **(B,D)** treated cochlea. Loss of inner hair cells is consistently seen in the basal turns of both groups **(A,B)**. The MSC treated group showed occasional survival of inner hair cells at the midturn **(D)**.

Delivery of Mesenchymal Stromal Cell Alters Cochlear Gene Expression

For control cochleae, an average of 155 ng/μl of RNA and for MSC treated cochleae 182 ng/μl of RNA were extracted. An average of 13,789,205 and 13,472,844 input reads for control and MSC treated cochleae were performed yielding 15,671 mapped genes. Delivery of MSCs caused a greater down-regulatory than up-regulatory effect on gene expression in sound traumatized animals treated with MSCs. A total of 2742 genes were down-regulated, and 1138 genes were found to be up-regulated. Significantly changed genes were considered to have an FDR of <0.05 and two fold change (up or down). Key down-regulated genes are shown in **Supplementary Table 1** and up-regulated genes are shown in **Supplementary Table 2**.

Analysis of Gene Ontologies and Functional Networks

The effects of MSC delivery after sound trauma were evaluated using GO expression analysis using IPA "Core" and "Bioprofiler" analysis. The GO classification for genes that are regulated by MSC delivery were broken down into the biological processes, molecular functions and cellular components and weighted according to their enrichment (FPKM) and FDR score. These were also visualized as a Voronoi tree plots to facilitate identification of key pathways. Down-regulated genes were enriched for processes related to neuronal function and repair with ion transport, nervous system transport, positive regulation of synapse assembly, modulation of synaptic transmission, regulation of membrane potential, synaptic transmission, regulation of post-synaptic membrane potential and long-term synaptic potentiation GO classifications dominating (**Figure 4**). The GO molecular function classification showed significant changes in genes related to protein binding although these were not highly enriched. Genes related to transmitter-gated ion channel activity, voltage gated ion activity, syntaxin-1 binding, sodium channel activity and calcium channel activity were found. Interestingly, processes relating to dynein light and intermediate chain binding were also seen. The GO terms relating to cellular components concentrated on the excitatory synapse, components of the axon, dendrites, and myelin sheath as well as mitochondrion related annotations (**Figure 5**). Voronoi tree-maps that improved hierarchical representation of the GOEA data were additionally evaluated and groups of genes that appear significantly represented were identified (Bernhardt et al., 2009).

Down-regulated genes included miRNAs such as miR-9, miR-124a, miR-124-2, and miR-133a. Regulation of heat shock proteins has been implicated in sound trauma and in this data set, delivery of MSCs resulted in down-regulation of Hspa1b, Hsp1l, Hsph1, Ahsa1, Hsp9, and Hsp90ab1 (Gratton et al., 2011). Key effectors of cell death were also down-regulated whereas protective genes such as bcl-2 were up-regulated.

Up-regulated genes were enriched for processes involved in adaptive and innate immune responses, extracellular matrix organization, cell adhesion and a wide range of cell repair and developmental processes (**Table 1**). Additional processes included transcription factor function, wound healing, regulation of apoptotic process and response to hypoxia. Molecular function annotations centered on a range of protein receptor signaling processes and processes related to matrix binding. Signaling processes related to insulin like growth factor binding, TGFβ, fibroblast growth factor and Wnt binding were represented.

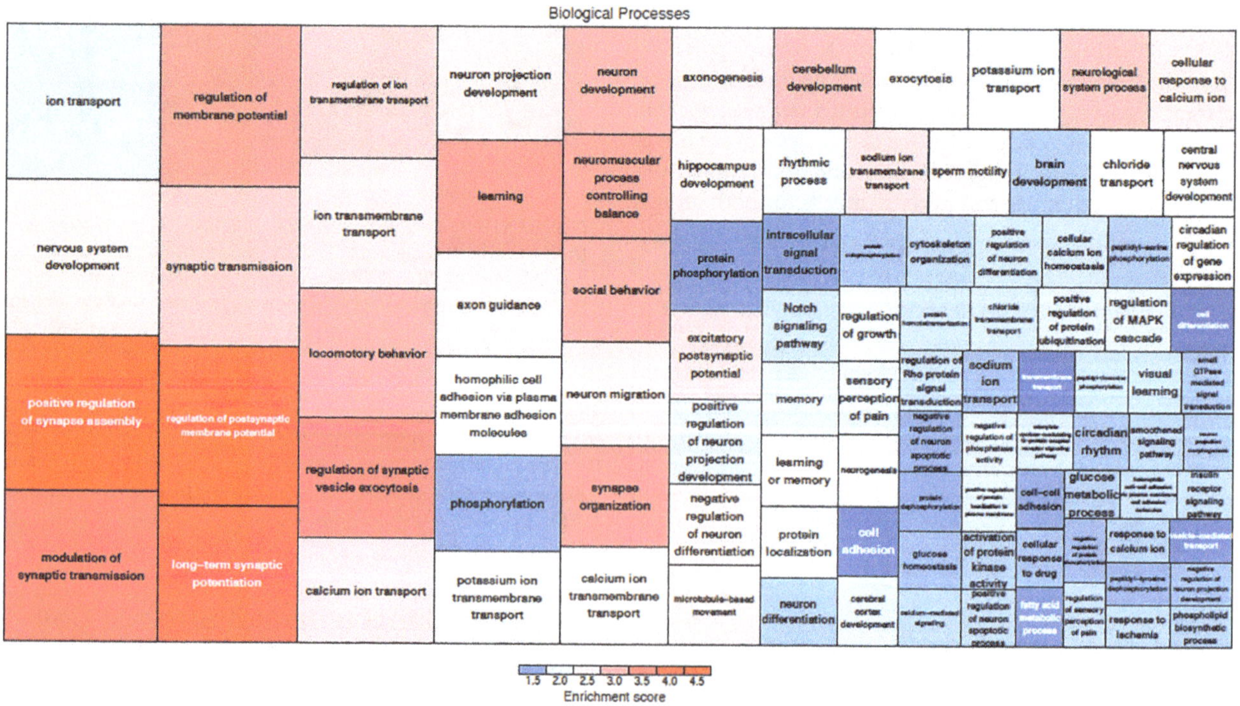

FIGURE 4 | Down-regulated biological processes classified by gene ontology. The size of the category corresponds to a lower FDR with the more deeply red groups representing a higher enrichment score. The graphic representation of gene expression demonstrates that a key element in MSC treatment is modulation of synaptic assembly which is represented in multiple groups of down-regulated genes.

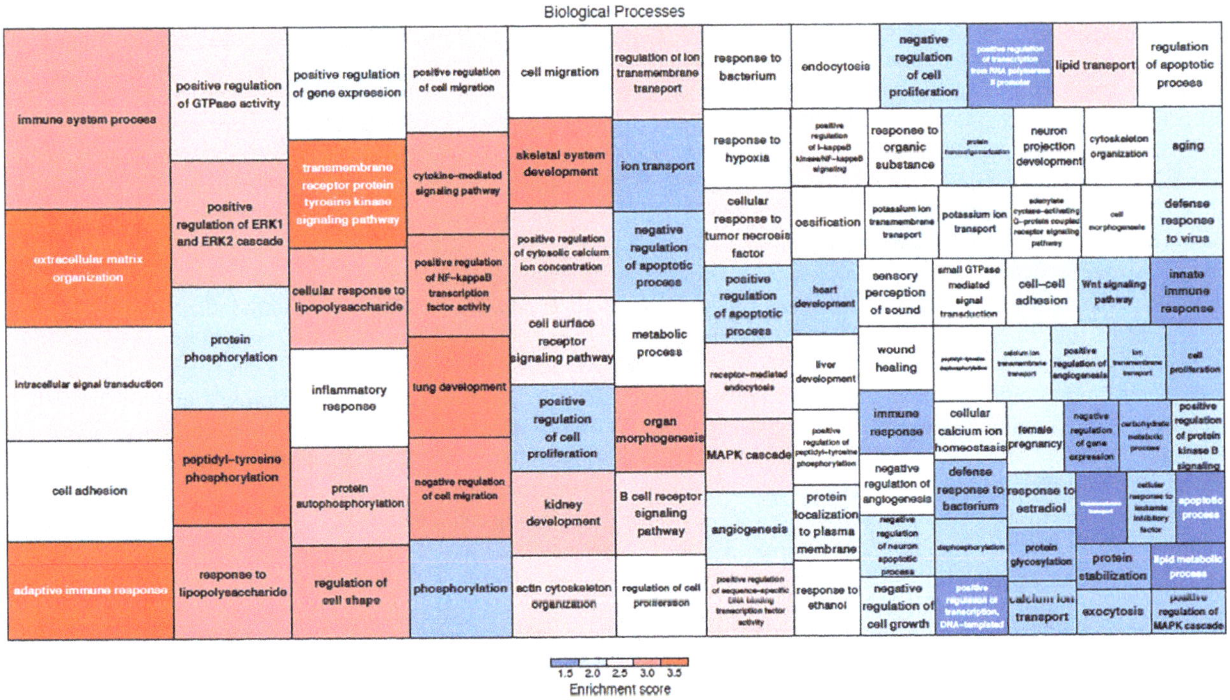

FIGURE 5 | Up-regulated biological processes classified by gene ontology. The size of the category corresponds to a lower FDR with the more deeply red groups representing a higher enrichment score. Up-regulation of genes related to immune function are a key component of MSC treatment.

Annotations showed that these genes were related to the cell surface, the extracellular matrix and the Golgi apparatus. Processes involving membrane repair and transmembrane tyrosine kinase signaling were also represented. Also represented were processes such as negative regulation of neuronal apoptosis, protein stabilization and sensory response to sound, which we would expect to see in a repair process involving the inner ear. Up-regulated genes related to response to sound are specific to the ear, associated with development of the inner ear, associated with syndromes that include hearing loss or when mutated are associated with sensorineural hearing loss (Shearer et al., 1993). We identified 14 up-regulated genes including Myo1A (Kwon et al., 2014), Ripor2 (Diaz-Horta et al., 2018), Nipbl, Ccdc50 (Modamio-Høybjør et al., 2007), Lhfpl5 (Ge et al., 2018), Fgfr1 (Pirvola et al., 2002), Diaph1 (Neuhaus et al., 2017), Pou4f3 (Walters et al., 2017), P2rx2 (Mittal et al., 2016), Otog (Schraders et al., 2012), Otoa (Lukashkin et al., 2012), Cntn5, Icam1 (Schmutzhard et al., 2011), and Hexa. The identified genes ranged from hair cell, spiral ganglion and stria specific to affecting tectorial membrane function, emphasizing that the MSC treatment affects multiple areas of the inner ear. Treatment with MSC resulted in both up and down regulation of genes that have been associated with noise induced hearing loss in other studies. Regulation of complement and toll receptor signaling has been shown to be associated with noise induced hearing loss (Patel et al., 2013; Vethanayagam et al., 2016; Yang et al., 2016). Members of the complement cascade identified included C1qtnf4, C1ql2, and Cfd (down-regulated) and C1rl and C3 (up-regulated). Other members of the innate immune system that showed differential expression were members of the Toll signaling system including Tlr4, Tlr6, and Tiarp, which were up-regulated. To more clearly identify effects of cell

TABLE 1 | Down- and up-regulated canonical pathways.

Down-regulated canonical pathways	Up-regulated canonical pathways
Calcium Signaling	Cardiovascular Disease, Cardiovascular System Development and Function
Synaptogenesis Signaling Pathway	Cancer, Organismal Injury and Abnormalities
GABA Receptor Signaling	Cell-To-Cell Signaling and Interaction, Hematological System Development and Function, Inflammatory Response, Organismal Functions
Endocannabinoid Neuronal Synapse Pathway	Hematological System Development and Function, Immune Cell Trafficking, Inflammatory Response, Tissue Development
Oxidative Phosphorylation	Cancer, Hematological Disease, Immunological Disease, Organismal Injury and Abnormalities
Opioid Signaling Pathway	Connective Tissue Development and Function, Skeletal and Muscular System Development and Function, Tissue Development
Mitochondrial Dysfunction	Cancer, Gastrointestinal Disease, Organismal Injury and Abnormalities
GNRH Signaling	Cellular Function and Maintenance
Synaptic Long Term Depression	Cell-To-Cell Signaling and Interaction, Cellular Function and Maintenance, Inflammatory Response
Corticotropin Releasing Hormone Signaling	Cancer, Gastrointestinal Disease, Organismal Injury and Abnormalities

therapy the IPA software was used to compare only significantly up- and down-regulated genes to evaluate the relationship between expression data and potential pathways involved in injury and protection. Key canonical pathways identified were calcium signaling, synaptogenesis signaling, endocaniboid neuronal synapse pathway, GABA receptor signaling and CREB signaling in neurons. Key predicted upstream regulators include BDNF, which has been shown to be produced by MSCs and has been identified as a mechanism of MSC protection of neurons in stroke models (Gu et al., 2014; Mukai et al., 2018). When graphically represented, TNFα can be seen as playing a central role in the predicted changes in biological function and signaling pathways (**Figure 6**). This was further evaluated using immunohistochemistry and semi quantitative PCR (**Figures 7–9**). Immunofluorescent labeling showed that MSC therapy reduced expression of TNFα protein in the lateral wall (**Figures 7B vs. C**), however expression was higher than controls in the inner hair cells of both sound trauma only (**Figure 7B**) and sound trauma + MSC treated animals (**Figure 7C**). RNAseq analysis demonstrated a 0.8 fold up-regulation of TNFα mRNA in MSC vs. sound trauma treated animals. Evaluation using RT-PCR demonstrated that both sound trauma only and sound trauma + MSC treated animals showed significantly up-regulated mRNA levels compared to controls (p = 0.0021; p = 0.0002) but were not significantly different from each other (p = 0.2517). IPA comparison analysis (**Figure 6**) also identified NeuroD1 as a significantly down-regulated transcription factor that is predicted to modulate multiple pathways related to neuronal growth and survival. Many of the survival effects are mediated through neurotrophin signaling. One of the downstream effects of neuroD signaling are alterations in the balance of bcl-2 and bax modulating apoptosis (Wy, 2013). MSCs have also been shown to modulate bcl-2 expression in a variety of injury models (Xiang et al., 2009; Gu et al., 2014). Our data showed that there was a 0.4 fold up-regulation of bcl-2 in MSC treated animals vs. sound only controls. There were no identifiable changes in bax expression in our data suggesting induction of an anti-apoptotic state. This was confirmed using immunohistochemistry and RT-PCR (**Figure 8**). MSC treated animals showed an increase of bcl-2 immunolabeling in the organ of Corti, particularly in the supporting cells (**Figure 8C**) and demonstrated an up-regulation of bcl-2 mRNA (**Figure 8D**). One of the most down-regulated genes identified in our study was transthyretin (5.377 fold decrease in expression after MSC treatment). Transthyretin plays multiple roles in the nervous system and is a key modulator of metabolism, which was predicted to be altered in the IPA comparison analysis (**Figure 6**). We confirmed down-regulation

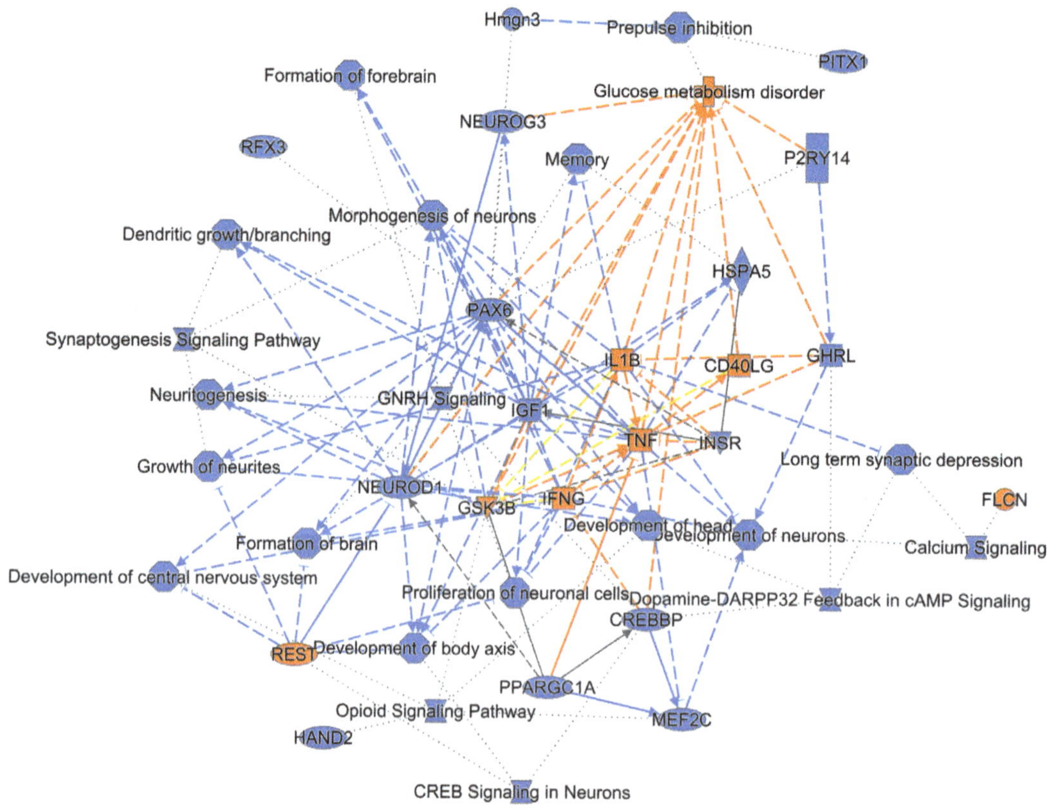

FIGURE 6 | Graphical representation of IPA analysis of up- and down-regulated genes and processes. Using IPA core analysis of down-regulated genes and processes (blue) predicted up-regulation of genes and processes (orange). There is an overall down-regulation of pathways related to synaptogenesis, development of neurons and excitatory signaling. TNFα is a key factor that influences multiple processes and genes.

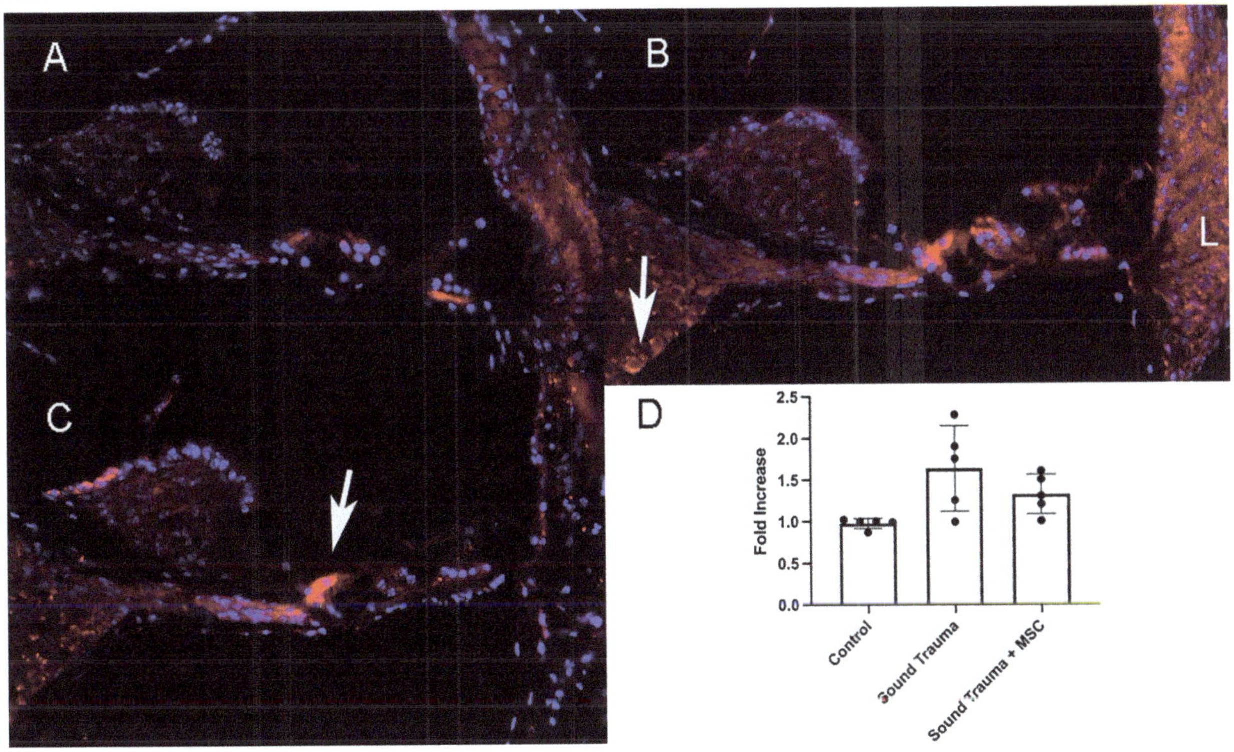

FIGURE 7 | Expression of TNFα protein (Red **A–C**) and semi quantitative RT PCR of TNFα mRNA **(D)**. Control cochlea showed minimal TNF expression in the hair cells and lateral wall **(A)**. After sound trauma there was a clear increase in TFN alpha immunolabeling in hair cells, the spiral ganglion (arrow) and the lateral wall **(B)**. Treatment with MSCs after sound trauma reduced TNFα expression in the lateral wall and outer hair cells but expression remained high in the inner hair cell (arrow **C**). Semi quantitative RT-PCR showed an up-regulation of TNF gene expression after sound trauma. This was slightly reduced after MSC treatment but not to control levels **(D)**.

of transthyretin by semi quantitative RT-PCR (**Figure 9**). Finally, we identified molecules in clinical use that could modulate most significantly regulated genes, identifying 46 drugs that could potentially be used to study some of the effects induced by MSCs (**Table 2**). Transthyretin can be down-regulated using thyroxine hormone (T4). Based on the Pharos analysis, multiple modulators of GABA neurotransmission are available, raising the possibility of using small molecules to modulate this pathway.

Besides neurotrophins, MSCs produce a variety of immunomodulatory molecules and other growth factors. Using the predictive functions of IPA, we analyzed the potential effect of several growth factors and cytokines known to be delivered by MSC on our data set and found that the observed changes in HSP90, complement factor 3 and toll like receptor 4 could potentially be modulated by MSCs (**Figure 10**).

DISCUSSION

Intra-labyrinthine application of WJCs after noise trauma showed significant protection of hearing threshold at the lower frequencies at 4 and 8 kHz and to a lesser degree at 32 kHz in mice. Histological changes related to sound trauma could be identified in the organ of Corti in both groups. There was preservation of some mid turn hair cells in the MSC treated group. The changes underlying the altered threshold could also be the result of damage to other regions, for example of the stria vascularis or the synapses. Since the focus of the present study was the functional restoration and RNA changes induced by cell therapy rather than the histological changes, synapses and the stria vascularis were not investigated. We identified more than 2700 down-regulated and 1138 up-regulated genes after treatment with WJC. To understand the biological effects of the differentially regulated genes, the cellular components, molecular function, and biological process were analyzed by GO annotation. Using IPA, specific analysis of genes related to cell death and survival showed the regulation of 365 molecules related to necrosis and 353 molecules related to apoptosis with a predictive effect of decreasing both death mechanisms and increasing cell survival. We could demonstrate that there are MSC induced reductions of TNFα expression in the cochlear lateral wall (**Figure 7**) and MSC induced increases in bcl-2 expression in the organ of Corti (**Figure 8**). TNFα up-regulation has been associated with sound trauma (Frye et al., 2019). Our data demonstrated an up-regulation in TNFα gene expression which could not be confirmed by PCR (**Figure 7D**). However, distribution of TNFα expression was reduced in the lateral wall of the cochlea (**Figures 7C vs. B**). Increased expression of TNFα in the sound damaged cochlea has been demonstrated for days 1–3 post-sound trauma followed by a

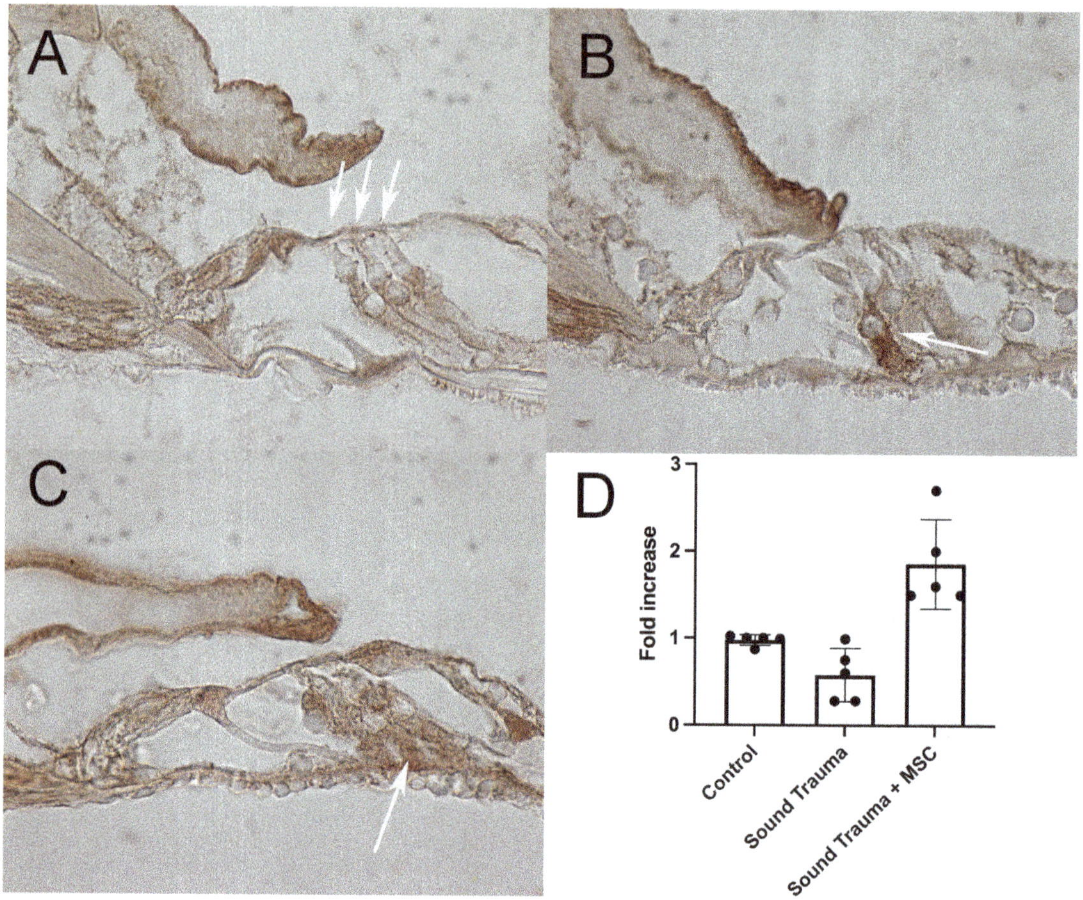

FIGURE 8 | Expression of bcl-2 (brown **A–C**) and semi quantitative RT PCR of bcl-2 mRNA **(D)**. Control cochlea showed bcl-2 expression in the pillar, in the inferior portion of the outer hair cells (arrows) and neurites **(A)**. After sound trauma there was an occasional increase in bcl-2 immunolabeling in isolated supporting cells (arrow) **(B)**. Treatment with MSCs after sound trauma increased expression of bcl-2 in supporting cells (arrow **C**). Semi quantitative RT-PCR showed reduction of bcl-2 mRNA expression after sound trauma. Treatment with MSC after sound trauma showed a significant up-regulation of bcl-2 mRNA compared to both controls and sound trauma only treated animals (p = 0.003) **(D)**.

decrease and then a further expression increase at 28 days post-noise exposure (Fujioka et al., 2006). Additional time points will be needed to evaluate the long term effects of MSC treatment. We additionally evaluated the effect of MSC treatment on bcl-2 expression in the sound damaged inner ear. Our RNAseq data demonstrated a down-regulation of cell death effector genes and an up-regulation of the antiapoptotic bcl-2 (**Figure 8**) consistent with other MSC experiments (Gu et al., 2014). Up-regulation of bcl-2 has been shown to be an underlying mechanism in sound conditioning protection from noise trauma (Niu et al., 2003).

Many of the identified genes and GO annotations have been found in or belong to a similar GO pattern seen in stroke or TBI suggesting that severe sound trauma and TBI (Spaethling et al., 2008; Darkazalli et al., 2017; Meng et al., 2017; Trivedi et al., 2019; Li et al., 2020) involve similar molecular mechanisms. By evaluating the diverse pathways activated in this recovering system, we may be able to select new targets for the pharmacological mitigation of sound trauma. Significant advances have been made in the pharmacologic treatment of brain injury and many of the drugs that are in experimental or clinical trials (Diaz-Arrastia et al., 2014) may also be applicable to the inner ear. Use of the Pharos database identified that 46 of the most up and down regulated genes could potentially be targeted by molecules that are already in use. NMDA receptors in particular have already been targeted in clinical trials for sound induced tinnitus, demonstrating that MSC induced protection in part functions through previously identified mechanisms (Bing et al., 2015; Staecker et al., 2017).

In the cellular component category, the most represented term is "AMPA glutamate receptor complex," followed by "post-synaptic density membrane" and "excitatory and inhibitory synapses" for the down-regulated genes. In the molecular function category, the term "transmitter-gated ion channel activity involved in regulation of post-synaptic membrane potential" and "syntaxin-1 binding was found to be represented. The underlying biological processes in the down-regulated genes were related to synaptic functions. Most striking, synapse-specific processes like excitatory as well as inhibitory

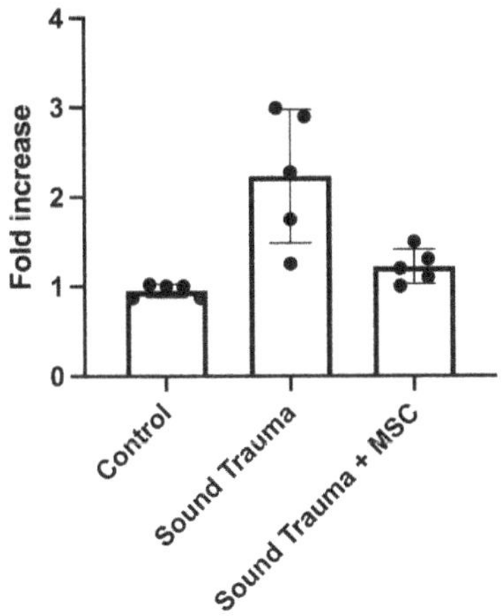

FIGURE 9 | Expression of cochlear transthyretin by semi quantitative RT-PCR. Sound trauma treated animals showed a relative increase in expression of transthyretin mRNA. MSC treatment resulted in a significant reduction in expression of transthyretin mRNA after sound trauma (p = 0.001).

synapse, AMPA glutamate receptor complex synapse assembly, regulation of post-synaptic membrane potential, modulation of synaptic transmission and long-term synaptic potentiation were significantly down-regulated. This suggests that neuronal repair and control of excitotoxicity could be key components of recovery from severe sound trauma. For the up-regulated genes, "*trans*-Golgi network transport vesicles" is the most over-represented term in the cellular component category. Looking at molecular functions, extracellular binding, Wnt-protein and insulin-like growth factor binding were most abundant alongside with cytokine receptor activity. In the biological processes category, the terms extracellular matrix organization, adaptive immune response as well as transmembrane receptor protein tyrosine kinase (Trk) signaling pathway were found to be strongly represented. Immunomodulation and activation of Trk signaling pathways are known to be potent enhancers of survival. For example, systemic transplantation of MSC in a TBI model led to a lower density of microglia, macrophages as well as peripheral infiltrating leukocytes at the injury site, to reduced levels of pro-inflammatory cytokines and increased anti-inflammatory cytokines (Zhang et al., 2013). Even in a model of xenotransplantation of MSC derived from adipose tissue after ventral root avulsion, an increased neuronal survival and partial preservation of synaptophysin-positive nerve terminals as well as a reduction of pro-inflammatory reactions were elicited (Ribeiro et al., 2015). It is assumed that by suppressing lymphocyte, astroglia and microglia effects, MSC can prevent a second delayed neuronal injury (Ribeiro et al., 2015). Furthermore, MSCs can prevent neuronal cell death not only via restoration of the local microenvironment but also by the release of classic inhibitors of apoptosis (Tran and Damaser, 2014).

Looking at the top down-regulated genes, mainly genes coding for transcription factors or for proteins and receptors related to synaptic function are among the most regulated. Down-regulation of oxidative stress pathways might be key

TABLE 2 | Pharos analysis of genes showing greatest up- and down-regulation that can be modulated by small molecules in clinical use.

Symbol	Gene name	Symbol	Gene name
Cacna1a	Voltage-dependent calcium channel subunit alpha-1/alpha	Hrh3	Histamine H3 receptor
Cacna1i	Voltage-dependent T-type calcium channel subunit alpha	Htr2c	5-hydroxytryptamine receptor 2C
Car4	Carbonic anhydrase 4	Irs4	Insulin receptor substrate 4
Cck	Cholecystokinin	Kcnd2	Potassium voltage-gated channel subfamily D member 2
Ccl3	C-C motif chemokine 3	Kcnh6	Potassium voltage-gated channel, subfamily H, member 6
Cnr1	Cannabinoid receptor 1	Kcns2	Potassium voltage-gated channel subfamily S member 2
Gabra1	Gamma-aminobutyric acid receptor subunit alpha-1	Krt1	Keratin, type II cytoskeletal 1
Gabra4	Gamma-aminobutyric acid receptor subunit alpha-4	Lipf	Gastric triacylglycerol lipase
Gabra6	Gamma-aminobutyric acid receptor subunit alpha-6	Muc1	Mucin 1, transmembrane
Gabrb1	Gamma-aminobutyric acid receptor subunit beta-1	Ngf	Beta-nerve growth factor
Gabrb2	Gamma-aminobutyric acid receptor subunit beta-2	Pou1f1	Pituitary-specific positive transcription factor 1
Gabrp	Gamma-aminobutyric acid receptor subunit pi	Prl	Prolactin
Gal	Galanin peptides	Prlr	Prolactin receptor
Gh	Growth hormone	Rnf112	RING finger protein 112
Gnrhr	Gonadotropin releasing hormone receptor	Scn2a1	Sodium channel protein
Gp2	Pancreatic secretory granule membrane major glycoprotein GP2	Slc5a1	SGLT1 protein
Gria1	Glutamate receptor 1	Slc6a1	Sodium- and chloride-dependent GABA transporter 1
Gria2	Glutamate receptor 2	Slc6a5	Sodium-dependent noradrenaline transporter
Grik2	Glutamate receptor ionotropic, kainate 2	Sstr3	Somatostatin receptor type 3
Grin2a	Glutamate receptor ionotropic, NMDA 2A; NMDA 2B; NMDA 2D	Stum	Protein stum homolog
Grin2b	Glutamate receptor ionotropic, NMDA 2B	Tnr	Tenascin-R
Grin2c	Glutamate receptor, ionotropic, NMDA2C	Trpm8	Transient receptor potential cation channel subfamily M member 8
Grm5	Metabotropic glutamate receptor 5	Ttr	Transthyretin

for the mediation of protective effects. According to our RNA sequencing data, transthyretin (Ttr), a neuronal stress marker, is one of the most significantly down-regulated genes by the application of MSC after noise-induced trauma. It has been

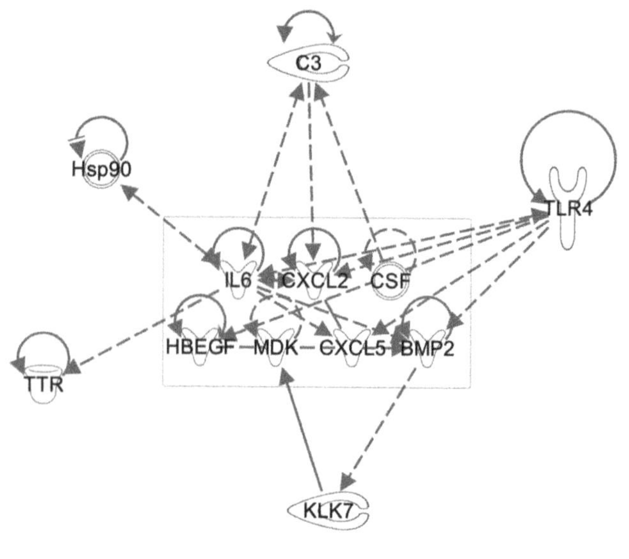

FIGURE 10 | The known WJC secretome regulates multiple genes found to be altered after sound trauma and MSC delivery. Components of the WJC secretome (boxed area) were evaluated for potential interactions with genes that we found to undergo significant change using the IPA knowledgebase. This demonstrates the potential biological basis for the protective effects that WJCs have on noise trauma.

shown that Ttr level correlate with ROS or reactive nitrogen species (RNS) (Saito et al., 2005; Fong and Vieira, 2013). In addition, the expression of the Ttr gene is regulated by glucocorticoids, which are stress hormones (Li et al., 2011; Martinho et al., 2012). On a protein level, Ttr can initiate oxidative stress in the endoplasmic reticulum and is thereby involved in the unfolded protein response (UPR) (Teixeira et al., 2006; Genereux et al., 2015; Chen J. et al., 2016). Thus, down-regulation of ttr might result in inhibition of formation of reactive oxygen and nitrogen species thereby reducing the extent of trauma-associated damage. Recent TBI studies using drop-seq have demonstrated that up-regulation of ttr is one of the major markers of trauma in a wide range of cell types (Arneson et al., 2018). This study also documented functional recovery induced by dosing TBI animals with thyroxine (T4) which down-regulates transthyretin. We demonstrated an MSC induced normalization of ttr gene expression by RNAseq and semiquantitative PCR (**Figure 9**) raising the possibility that thyroxine could be used to limit sound trauma induced damage. Other factors involved in the production of ROS belong to the kallikrein-kinin system. This system includes plasma or tissue related kinins and they mediate vascular permeability, edema formation, inflammation and the release of glutamate in the case of neurodegenerative disease associated with neuroinflammation such as TBI or Alzheimer's disease (Naffah-Mazzacoratti Mda et al., 2014; Hopp and AlbertWeissenberger, 2015). Tissue-derived kallikreins belong to the chymotrypsin- and trypsin-like serine endopeptidases. Especially kallikrein-7, originally identified as an inflammation–induced proteolytic enzyme in the skin, is down regulated by the application of WJS after sound trauma (Kidana et al., 2018). In addition, stress-related heat shock proteins that are involved in the response to stress and metabolic damage to the inner ear such as Hspa1b, Hsp1l, Hsph1, Ahsa1, Hsp9, and Hsp90ab1 are also down-regulated by MSC treatment (Sheehan-Rooney et al., 2013).

Moreover, several transcription factors, e.g., BarHl2, Neurod2, EN2, and Pax6, are down-regulated by application of MSC in noise trauma as demonstrated by our results. The homeobox protein BarH-like 2 (Barhl2) acts as transcription factor and possesses an enhancer that can be activated by the basic helix-loop-helix factor Atoh1 and can drive spinal cord-specific gene expression. Interestingly, this gene is significantly down-regulated when comparing noise-damaged cochlea treated with MSC to the sham-treated. Similar is observed for the neuronal differentiation factor 2, Pax6 and homeobox protein engrailed-2 (EN2). The later may alter the excitation/inhibition balance, and its down-regulation may rescue or regain homeostasis by MSC to reduce damage. NeuroD2 and Pax6 are important regulators of neuronal development in the central nervous system and their down-regulation after treatment with MSC seems quite surprising (Yogarajah et al., 2016). Whether damage leads to dedifferentiation and induction of neurogenesis thereby making the inner ear more susceptible to secondary damage mediated by oxidative stress and therewith associated metabolites remains speculative and needs further investigation. In addition to neuronal development, NeuroD2 balances synaptic neurotransmission and intrinsic excitability in the adult system, thereby decreasing neuronal excitability of cortical pyramidal neurons both *in vitro* and *in vivo* (Chen F. et al., 2016). After trauma, as has been shown for example in models of TBI, there is an excitation/inhibition imbalance as also reflected by the GABA/glutamate imbalance. Excitatory pathways in the brain are regulated by GABA and loss of GABA releasing cells after trauma further enhances cell injury and apoptosis (Guerriero et al., 2015). Although glutamate is the excitatory transmitter in the brain required for proper function, post-traumatic burst release of glutamate leads to excitotoxicity and subsequent cellular injury as has been also shown after noise-induced damage of the inner ear. By down-regulation of both, glutamate and GABA receptor subunits, MSC might down regulate the neuronal activity thereby possibly preventing further damage and transforming the cochlea to a state for protection and regeneration. The availability of multiple small molecules modulating this pathway (**Table 2**) raises the possibility of novel treatments of sound trauma.

Several miRNAs (miR-9, miR-124a, miR-124-2, and miR-133a) are also down-regulated after treatment with MSCs. These miRNAs play a variety of important developmental roles; miRNA-9 is the most significantly up-regulated miRNA in the developing brain, targeting the transcription factors FoxG1, Hes1, or Tlx, thereby playing an important role in the regulation of neuronal progenitors (Coolen et al., 2013). MicroRNA-9 has also been shown to regulate Schwann cell migration in neuronal injury, and is thought to play an important role in peripheral neuronal repair (Zhou et al., 2014). Similarly, miRNA-124a is an important developmental regulator and is involved in neurogenesis of the hippocampus and retinal cones (Sanuki et al., 2011). This miRNA has also been shown to be up-regulated in repetitive brain injury (Huang et al., 2018). Therefore, the down-regulation of miR-124 observed in this study may represent a positive effect of MSC treatment. Both miR-9 and -124 have been identified as biomarkers of TBI (Ji et al., 2016). Thus, MSCs regulate not only transcription factors involved in neurogenesis, but also miRNAs involved in the regulation of transcription factors. Another miRNA that we found to be down-regulated (miR-133) is involved in organogenesis, regulating the hedgehog pathway in myogenesis (Mok et al., 2018; Yu et al., 2019). This miRNA has been found to protect neurons when up-regulated but is also involved in the remodeling of connective tissue after injury (Xin et al., 2012; Li et al., 2018). To fully understand the relevance of the changes induced by MSC in the inner ear, investigation of further time points after damage and treatment or even transcriptomics at single cell resolution will be needed.

The biological effects of MSCs have been widely studied. MSCs produce a wide range of growth factors, extracellular vesicles and miRNAs that taken as a whole have a wide range of potential effects on a tissue. The secretome of umbilical cord MSCs has been shown to contain Ntf3, Egf, Mdk, Hbegf, Cxcl5, Cxcl2, and Fgf9 (Hsieh et al., 2013). Interestingly, many of these factors are involved in neurogenesis and *in vitro*, they up-regulate a variety of transcription factors that enhance local release of some of the same growth factors, thereby amplifying the repair process. Many of the regulated genes we also identified in this study. Immunomodulation is also a well characterized feature of MSCs (Hsieh et al., 2013). We evaluated the potential effect of some of these reported growth factors by modeling their regulation of genes we saw change using IPA software. As depicted in **Figure 10**, the IPA knowledge base predicts that growth factors produced by WJCs can regulate factors such as C3, Tlr4, bcl2, and Ttr that we identified. Fully characterizing the links between MSC signaling and our findings is difficult since interactions of MSCs with their target tissue may actually alter their secretome (Drago et al., 2013). Evaluation of extracellular vesicles produced by WJCs for the mitigation of sound trauma has demonstrated that similar protective effects can be achieved using only the secretome alone (Warnecke et al., 2020).

Several limitations are associated with the present study. The study was focused on identifying the effects of MSC cell therapy on the cochlear transcriptome after noise exposure. Further insights could be gained by including analysis of the transcriptome from a group of mice not exposed to noise with and without treatment with MSC. Sound trauma-induced changes in gene expression have been evaluated in numerous publications (Cai et al., 2012; Patel et al., 2013). We chose a severe form of sound trauma to test the ability of WJC type MSCs to rescue an inner ear function. The identified pathways are similar to the ones seen in other MSC-based rescue of models and in analysis of TBI induced neuronal injury. To further characterize these effects, a more moderate sound trauma paradigm with multiple sample time points after MSC delivery and verification of the effects using PCR and immunohistochemistry will be needed. Despite these limitations, main cell signaling pathways involved in MSC-mediated inner ear protection after noise trauma have been identified by applying pathway enrichment analysis. In future studies, we could mimic the effects of MSCs or inhibit potential protective pathways with small molecules to better characterize regulatory pathways by using large-scale transcriptome analysis in well-defined sets of experiments (Islam et al., 2019).

CONCLUSION

Delivery of WJC type MSCs after sound trauma has a significant rescue effect on hearing. RNAseq analysis demonstrates regulatory changes in multiple genes including genes related to excitatory neurotransmission and the innate immune system. Further studies using different sound trauma paradigms and different timing of cell delivery as well as additional replicates are needed to better characterize the effects mediated by MSCs in the present study.

AUTHOR CONTRIBUTIONS

AW and HS research design, data analysis, and writing of the manuscript. JH and MD data analysis and writing of the manuscript. MS electrophysiology and manuscript approval. AM preparation and delivery of MSC and manuscript approval. IM bioinformatics and manuscript approval. All authors contributed to the article and approved the submitted version.

Support grant P30 CA168524 and NIGMS P20GM103418. AW and JH are funded by the German Research Foundation, Cluster of Excellence Hearing4all (EXC 2177/1).

ACKNOWLEDGMENTS

We would like to thank Clark Bloomer and the University of Kansas Medical Center Genomics Core for advice and technical support.

SUPPLEMENTARY MATERIAL

Supplementary Table 1 | Genes down-regulated in response to sound trauma followed by MSC treatment.

Supplementary Table 2 | Genes up-regulated in response to sound trauma followed by MSC treatment.

REFERENCES

Arneson, D., Zhang, G., Ying, Z., Zhuang, Y., Byun, H. R., Ahn, I. S., et al. (2018). Single cell molecular alterations reveal target cells and pathways of concussive brain injury. *Nat. Commun.* 9, 1–18.

Bernhardt, J., Funke, S., Hecker, M., and Siebourg, J. (2009). "Visualizing gene expression data via voronoi treemaps," in *6th International Symposium on Voronoi Diagrams in Science and Engineering* (Copenhagen, Denmark: IEEE), 233–241.

Bing, D., Lee, S. C., Campanelli, D., Xiong, H., Matsumoto, M., Panford-Walsh, R., et al. (2015). Cochlear NMDA Receptors as a Therapeutic Target of Noise-Induced Tinnitus. *Cell. Physiol. Biochem.* 35, 1905–1923. doi: 10.1159/000374000

Cai, Q., Patel, M., Coling, D., and Hu, B. H. (2012). Transcriptional changes in adhesion-related genes are site-specific during noise-induced cochlear pathogenesis. *Neurobiol. Dis.* 45, 723–732. doi: 10.1016/j.nbd.2011.10.018

Chang, Y. H., Wu, K. C., Harn, H. J., Lin, S. Z., and Ding, D. C. (2018). Exosomes and Stem Cells in Degenerative Disease Diagnosis and Therapy. *Cell Transplant.* 27, 349–363. doi: 10.1177/0963689717723636

Chen, F., Moran, J. T., Zhang, Y., Ates, K. M., Yu, D., Schrader, L. A., et al. (2016). The transcription factor NeuroD2 coordinates synaptic innervation and cell intrinsic properties to control excitability of cortical pyramidal neurons. *J. Physiol.* 594, 3729–3744. doi: 10.1113/jp271953

Chen, J., Genereux, J., Suh, E., and Vartabedian, V. (2016). Endoplasmic reticulum proteostasis influences the oligomeric state of an amyloidogenic protein secreted from mammalian cells. *Cell Chem.* 23, 1282–1293. doi: 10.1016/j.chembiol.2016.09.001

Chen, L., Trautwein, P. G., Powers, N., and Salvi, R. J. (1997). Two-tone rate suppression boundaries of cochlear ganglion neurons in chickens following acoustic trauma. *J. Acoust. Soc. Am.* 102, 2245–2254. doi: 10.1121/1.419598

Clifford, R. E., Hoffer, M., and Rogers, R. (2016). The Genomic Basis of Noise-induced Hearing Loss: a Literature Review Organized by Cellular Pathways. *Otol. Neurotol.* 37, e309–16. doi: 10.1097/mao.0000000000001073

Coolen, M., Katz, S., and Bally-Cuif, L. (2013). miR-9: a versatile regulator of neurogenesis. *Front. Cell. Neurosci.* 7:220. doi: 10.3389/fncel.2013.00220

Cunningham, C. J., Redondo-Castro, E., and Allan, S. M. (2018). The therapeutic potential of the mesenchymal stem cell secretome in ischaemic stroke. *J. Cereb. Blood Flow Metab.* 38, 1276–1292. doi: 10.1177/0271678x18776802

Darkazalli, A., Vied, C., Badger, C.-D., and Levenson, C. W. (2017). Human Mesenchymal Stem Cell Treatment Normalizes Cortical Gene Expression after Traumatic Brain Injury. *J. Neurotrauma* 34, 204–212. doi: 10.1089/neu.2015.4322

Diaz-Arrastia, R., Kochanek, P. M., Bergold, P., Kenney, K., Marx, C. E., Grimes, C. J. B., et al. (2014). Pharmacotherapy of traumatic brain injury: state of the science and the road forward: report of the department of defense neurotrauma pharmacology workgroup. *J. Neurotrauma* 31, 135–158. doi: 10.1089/neu.2013.3019

Diaz-Horta, O., Abad, C., Cengiz, F. B., Bademci, G., Blackwelder, P., Walz, K., et al. (2018). Ripor2 is involved in auditory hair cell stereociliary bundle structure and orientation. *J. Mol. Med.* 96, 1227–1238. doi: 10.1007/s00109-018-1694-x

Drago, D., Cossetti, C., Iraci, N., Gaude, E., Musco, G., Bachi, A., et al. (2013). The stem cell secretome and its role in brain repair. *Biochimie* 95, 2271–2285. doi: 10.1016/j.biochi.2013.06.020

Fetoni, A. R., Lattanzi, W., Eramo, S. L. M., Barba, M., Paciello, F., Moriconi, C., et al. (2014). Grafting and Early Expression of Growth Factors from Adipose-Derived Stem Cells Transplanted into the Cochlea, in a Guinea Pig Model of Acoustic Trauma. *Front. Cell. Neurosci.* 8:334. doi: 10.3389/fncel.2014.00334

Fetoni, A. R., Paciello, F., Rolesi, R., Paludetti, G., and Troiani, D. (2019). Targeting dysregulation of redox homeostasis in noise-induced hearing loss: oxidative stress and ROS signaling. *Free Radic. Biol. Med.* 135, 46–59. doi: 10.1016/j.freeradbiomed.2019.02.022

Fong, V., and Vieira, A. (2013). Transthyretin aggregates induce production of reactive nitrogen species. *Neurodegener. Dis.* 11, 42–48. doi: 10.1159/000338153

Frye, M. D., Ryan, A. F., and Kurabi, A. (2019). Inflammation associated with noise-induced hearing loss. *J. Acoust. Soc. Am.* 146, 4020–4032.

Fu, Y., Karbaat, L., Wu, L., Leijten, J., Both, S. K., and Karperien, M. (2017). Trophic Effects of Mesenchymal Stem Cells in Tissue Regeneration. *Tissue Eng. Part B Rev.* 23, 515–528.

Fujioka, M., Kanzaki, S., Okano, H. J., Masuda, M., Ogawa, K., and Okano, H. (2006). Proinflammatory cytokines expression in noise-induced damaged cochlea. *J. Neurosci. Res.* 83, 575–583. doi: 10.1002/jnr.20764

Galipeau, J., and Sensébé, L. (2018). Mesenchymal Stromal Cells: clinical Challenges and Therapeutic Opportunities. *Cell Stem Cell* 22, 824–833. doi: 10.1016/j.stem.2018.05.004

Ge, J., Elferich, J., Goehring, A., Zhao, H., Schuck, P., and Gouaux, E. (2018). Structure of mouse protocadherin 15 of the stereocilia tip link in complex with LHFPL5. *Elife* 7:e38770.

Genereux, J. C., Qu, S., Zhou, M., Ryno, L. M., Wang, S., Shoulders, M. D., et al. (2015). Unfolded protein response-induced ER dj3 secretion links ER stress to extracellular proteostasis. *EMBO J.* 34, 4–19.

Gonzalez-Gonzalez, S. (2017). The role of mitochondrial oxidative stress in hearing loss. *Neurol. Disord. Ther.* 1, 1–5. doi: 10.1097/01.aud.0000191942.36672.f3

Gratton, M. A., Eleftheriadou, A., Garcia, J., Verduzco, E., Martin, G. K., and Lonsbury–Martin, B. L. (2011). Noise-induced changes in gene expression in the cochleae of mice differing in their susceptibility to noise damage. *Hear. Res.* 277, 211–226. doi: 10.1016/j.heares.2010.12.014

Gu, N., Rao, C., Tian, Y., Di, Z., Liu, Z., Chang, M., et al. (2014). Anti-inflammatory and Antiapoptotic Effects of Mesenchymal Stem Cells Transplantation in Rat Brain with Cerebral Ischemia. *J. Stroke Cerebrovasc. Dis.* 23, 2598–2606. doi: 10.1016/j.jstrokecerebrovasdis.2014.05.032

Guerriero, R. M., Giza, C. C., and Rotenberg, A. (2015). Glutamate and GABA Imbalance Following Traumatic Brain Injury. *Curr. Neurol. Neurosci. Rep.* 15:27.

Harrell, C. R., Fellabaum, C., Jovicic, N., Djonov, V., Arsenijevic, N., and Volarevic, V. (2019). Molecular Mechanisms Responsible for Therapeutic Potential of Mesenchymal Stem Cell-Derived Secretome. *Cells* 8:467. doi: 10.3390/cells8050467

Hopp, S., and AlbertWeissenberger, C. (2015). The kallikrein-kinin system: a promising therapeutic target for traumatic brain injury. *Neural Regen. Res.* 10, 885–886. doi: 10.4103/1673-5374.158339

Hsieh, J.-Y., Wang, H.-W., Chang, S.-J., Liao, K.-H., Lee, I.-H., Lin, W.-S., et al. (2013). Mesenchymal stem cells from human umbilical cord express preferentially secreted factors related to neuroprotection, neurogenesis, and angiogenesis. *PLoS One* 8:e72604. doi: 10.1371/journal.pone.0072604

Huang, S., Ge, X., Yu, J., Han, Z., Yin, Z., Li, Y., et al. (2018). Increased miR-124-3p in microglial exosomes following traumatic brain injury inhibits neuronal inflammation and contributes to neurite outgrowth *via* their transfer into neurons. *FASEB J.* 32, 512–528.

Huang, T., Cheng, A. G., Stupak, H., Liu, W., Kim, A., Staecker, H., et al. (2000). Oxidative stress-induced apoptosis of cochlear sensory cells: otoprotective strategies. *Int. J. Dev. Neurosci.* 18, 259–270. doi: 10.1016/s0736-5748(99)00094-5

Islam, A., Urbarova, I., Bruun, J. A., and Martinez-Zubiaurre, I. (2019). Large-scale secretome analyses unveil the superior immunosuppressive phenotype of umbilical cord stromal cells as compared to other adult mesenchymal stromal cells. *Eur. Cell Mater.* 37, 153–174. doi: 10.22203/ecm.v037a10

Jassal, B., Matthews, L., Viteri, G., Gong, C., Lorente, P., Fabregat, A., et al. (2019). The reactome pathway knowledgebase. *Nucleic Acids Res.* 44, D481–D487.

Ji, Q., Ji, Y., Peng, J., Zhou, X., Chen, X., Zhao, H., et al. (2016). Increased brain-specific MiR-9 and MiR-124 in the serum exosomes of acute ischemic stroke patients. *PLoS One* 11:e0163645. doi: 10.1371/journal.pone.0163645

Kanzaki, S., Toyoda, M., Umezawa, A., and Ogawa, K. (2020). Application of Mesenchymal Stem Cell Therapy and Inner Ear Regeneration for Hearing Loss: a Review. *Int. J. Mol. Sci.* 21:5764. doi: 10.3390/ijms21165764

Kidana, K., Tatebe, T., Ito, K., Hara, N., Kakita, A., Saito, T., et al. (2018). Loss of kallikrein-related peptidase 7 exacerbates amyloid pathology in Alzheimer's disease model mice. *EMBO Mol. Med.* 10:e8184.

Kurabi, A., Keithley, E. M., Housley, G. D., Ryan, A. F., and Wong, A. C. Y. (2017). Cellular mechanisms of noise-induced hearing loss. *Hear. Res.* 349, 129–137. doi: 10.1016/j.heares.2016.11.013

Kwon, T. J., Oh, S. K., Park, H. J., Sato, O., Venselaar, H., Choi, S. Y., et al. (2014). The effect of novel mutations on the structure and enzymatic activity of unconventional myosins associated with autosomal dominant non-syndromic hearing loss. *Open Biol.* 4:140107. doi: 10.1098/rsob.140107

Le, T. N., Straatman, L. V., Lea, J., and Westerberg, B. (2017). Current insights in noise-induced hearing loss: a literature review of the underlying mechanism, pathophysiology, asymmetry, and management options. *J. Otolaryngol. Head Neck Surg.* 46:41.

Li, L., Dong, L., Xiao, Z., He, W., Zhao, J., Pan, H., et al. (2020). Integrated analysis of the proteome and transcriptome in a MCAO mouse model revealed the molecular landscape during stroke progression. *J. Adv. Res.* 24, 13–27. doi: 10.1016/j.jare.2020.01.005

Li, N., Zhou, H., and Tang, Q. (2018). miR-133: a suppressor of cardiac remodeling? *Front. Pharmacol.* 9:903. doi: 10.3389/fphar.2018.00903

Li, X., Masliah, E., Reixach, N., and Buxbaum, J. N. (2011). Neurobiology of Disease Neuronal Production of Transthyretin in Human and Murine Alzheimer's Disease: is It Protective? *J. Neurosci.* 31, 12483–12490. doi: 10.1523/jneurosci. 2417-11.2011

Lin, H. W., Furman, A. C., Kujawa, S. G., and Liberman, M. C. (2011). Primary neural degeneration in the Guinea pig cochlea after reversible noise-induced threshold shift. *J. Assoc. Res. Otolaryngol.* 12, 605–616. doi: 10.1007/s10162-011-0277-0

Lukashkin, A. N., Legan, P. K., Weddell, T. D., Lukashkina, V. A., Goodyear, R. J., Welstead, L. J., et al. (2012). A mouse model for human deafness DFNB22 reveals that hearing impairment is due to a loss of inner hair cell stimulation. *Proc. Natl. Acad. Sci. U. S. A.* 109, 19351–19356. doi: 10.1073/pnas.1210159109

Maeda, Y., Omichi, R., Sugaya, A., Kariya, S., and Nishizaki, K. (2017). Cochlear Transcriptome Following Acoustic Trauma and Dexamethasone Administration Identified by a Combination of RNA-seq and DNA Microarray. *Otol. Neurotol.* 38, 1032–1042. doi: 10.1097/mao.0000000000001373

Martinho, A., Gonçalves, I., Costa, M., and Santos, C. R. (2012). Stress and glucocorticoids increase transthyretin expression in rat choroid plexus via mineralocorticoid and glucocorticoid receptors. *J. Mol. Neurosci.* 48, 1–13. doi: 10.1007/s12031-012-9715-7

Mellott, A. J., Detamore, M. S., and Staecker, H. (2016). The use of human Wharton's jelly cells for cochlear tissue engineering. *Methods Mol. Biol.* 1427, 319–345. doi: 10.1007/978-1-4939-3615-1_19

Meng, Q., Zhuang, Y., Ying, Z., Agrawal, R., Yang, X., and Gomez-Pinilla, F. (2017). Traumatic Brain Injury Induces Genome-Wide Transcriptomic, Methylomic, and Network Perturbations in Brain and Blood Predicting Neurological Disorders. *EBioMedicine* 16, 184–194. doi: 10.1016/j.ebiom.2017.01.046

Mittal, R., Grati, M., Sedlacek, M., Yuan, F., Chang, Q., Yan, D., et al. (2016). Characterization of ATPase Activity of P2RX2 Cation Channel. *Front. Physiol.* 7:186. doi: 10.3389/fphys.2016.00186

Modamio-Høybjør, S., Mencía, Á, Goodyear, R., Del Castillo, I., Richardson, G., and Moreno, F. (2007). A mutation in CCDC50, a gene encoding an effector of epidermal growth factor-mediated cell signaling, causes progressive hearing loss. *Am. J. Hum. Genet.* 80, 1076–1089. doi: 10.1086/518311

Mok, G. F., Lozano-Velasco, E., Maniou, E., Viaut, C., Moxon, S., Wheeler, G., et al. (2018). miR-133-mediated regulation of the Hedgehog pathway orchestrates embryo myogenesis. *Development* 145:dev159657.

Mukai, T., Tojo, A., and Nagamura-Inoue, T. (2018). Umbilical Cord-Derived Mesenchymal Stromal Cells Contribute to Neuroprotection in Neonatal Cortical Neurons Damaged by Oxygen-Glucose Deprivation. *Front. Neurol.* 9:466. doi: 10.3389/fneur.2018.00466

Naffah-Mazzacoratti Mda, G., Gouveia, T. L. F., Simões, P. S. R., and Perosa, S. R. (2014). What have we learned about the kallikrein-kinin and renin-angiotensin systems in neurological disorders? *World J. Biol. Chem.* 5, 130–140.

Neuhaus, C., Lang-Roth, R., Zimmermann, U., Heller, R., Eisenberger, T., Weikert, M., et al. (2017). Extension of the clinical and molecular phenotype of *DIAPH1*-associated autosomal dominant hearing loss (*DFNA1*). *Clin. Genet.* 91, 892–901. doi: 10.1111/cge.12915

Niu, X., Shao, R., and Canlon, B. (2003). Suppression of apoptosis occurs in the cochlea by sound conditioning. *Neuroreport* 14, 1025–1029.

Patel, M., Hu, Z., Bard, J., Jamison, J., Cai, Q., and Hu, B. H. (2013). Transcriptome characterization by RNA-Seq reveals the involvement of the complement components in noise-traumatized rat cochleae. *Neuroscience* 248, 1–16. doi: 10.1016/j.neuroscience.2013.05.038

Pirvola, U., Ylikoski, J., Trokovic, R., Hébert, J. M., McConnell, S. K., and Partanen, J. (2002). FGFR1 is required for the development of the auditory sensory epithelium. *Neuron* 35, 671–680. doi: 10.1016/s0896-6273(02)00824-3

Puel, J. L., d'Aldin, C., Ruel, J., Ladrech, S., and Pujol, R. (1997). Synaptic repair mechanisms responsible for functional recovery in various cochlear pathologies. *Acta Otolaryngol.* 117, 214–218. doi: 10.3109/0001648970911 7773

Rai, V., Wood, M. B., Feng, H., Schabla, N. M., Tu, S., and Zuo, J. (2020). The immune response after noise damage in the cochlea is characterized by a heterogeneous mix of adaptive and innate immune cells. *Sci. Rep.* 10:15167.

Rajguru, R. (2013). Military aircrew and noise-induced hearing loss: prevention and management. *Aviat .Space Env. Med.* 84, 1268–1276. doi: 10.3357/asem. 3503.2013

Ribeiro, T. B., Duarte, A. S. S., Longhini, A. L. F., Pradella, F., Farias, A. S., Luzo, A. C. M., et al. (2015). Neuroprotection and immunomodulation by xenografted human mesenchymal stem cells following spinal cord ventral root avulsion. *Sci. Rep.* 5:16167.

Saito, S., Ando, Y., Nakamura, M., Ueda, M., Kim, J., Ishima, Y., et al. (2005). Effect of nitric oxide in amyloid fibril formation on transthyretin-related amyloidosis. *Biochemistry* 44, 11122–11129. doi: 10.1021/bi050327i

Sanuki, R., Onishi, A., Koike, C., Muramatsu, R., Watanabe, S., Muranishi, Y., et al. (2011). miR-124a is required for hippocampal axogenesis and retinal cone survival through Lhx2 suppression. *Nat. Neurosci.* 14, 1125–1134.

Schmutzhard, J., Kositz, C. H., Lackner, P., Pritz, C., Glueckert, R., Fischer, M., et al. (2011). Murine cerebral malaria: histopathology and ICAM 1 immunohistochemistry of the inner ear. *Trop. Med. Int. Health* 16, 914–922. doi: 10.1111/j.1365-3156.2011.02801.x

Schraders, M., Ruiz-Palmero, L., Kalay, E., Oostrik, J., Del Castillo, F. J., Sezgin, O., et al. (2012). Mutations of the gene encoding otogelin are a cause of autosomal-recessive nonsyndromic moderate hearing impairment. *Am. J. Hum. Genet.* 91, 883–889. doi: 10.1016/j.ajhg.2012.09.012

Shearer, A. E., Hildebrand, M. S., and Smith, R. J. (1993). *Hereditary Hearing Loss and Deafness Overview . GeneReviews®* . Seattle: University of Washington.

Sheehan-Rooney, K., Swartz, M. E., Zhao, F., Liu, D., and Eberhart, J. K. (2013). Ahsa1 and Hsp90 activity confers more severe craniofacial phenotypes in a zebrafish model of hypoparathyroidism, sensorineural deafness and renal dysplasia (HDR). *Dis. Model. Mech.* 6, 1285–1291.

Spaethling, J. M., Klein, D. M., Singh, P., and Meaney, D. F. (2008). Calcium-permeable AMPA receptors appear in cortical neurons after traumatic mechanical injury and contribute to neuronal fate. *J. Neurotrauma* 25, 1207–1216. doi: 10.1089/neu.2008.0532

Squillaro, T., Peluso, G., and Galderisi, U. (2016). Clinical trials with mesenchymal stem cells: an update. *Cell Transplant.* 25, 829–848. doi: 10.3727/096368915x689622

Staecker, H., Morelock, M., Kramer, T., Chrbolka, P., Ho Ahn, J., and Meyer, T. (2017). Safety of Repeated-Dose Intratympanic Injections with AM-101 in Acute Inner Ear Tinnitus. *Otolaryngol. Head Neck Surg.* 157, 478–487.

Teixeira, P. F., Cerca, F., Santos, S. D., and Saraiva, M. J. (2006). Endoplasmic reticulum stress associated with extracellular aggregates evidence from transthyretin deposition in familial amyloid polyneuropathy. *J. Biol. Chem.* 281, 21998–22003.

Tran, C., and Damaser, M. S. (2014). Stem cells as drug delivery methods: application of stem cell secretome for regeneration. *Adv. Drug Deliv. Rev.* 8, 1–11. doi: 10.1016/j.addr.2014.10.007

Trivedi, A., Noble-Haeusslein, L. J., Levine, J. M., Santucci, A. D., Reeves, T. M., and Phillips, L. L. (2019). Matrix metalloproteinase signals following neurotrauma are right on cue. *Cell. Mol. Life Sci.* 76, 3141–3156. doi: 10.1007/s00018-019-03176-4

Tsintou, M., Dalamagkas, K., and Makris, N. (2020). Taking central nervous system regenerative therapies to the clinic: curing rodents versus nonhuman primates versus humans. *Neural Regen. Res.* 15, 425–437. doi: 10.4103/1673-5374.266048

Vethanayagam, R. R., Yang, W., Dong, Y., and Hu, B. H. (2016). Toll-like receptor 4 modulates the cochlear immune response to acoustic injury. *Cell Death Dis.* 7:e2245. doi: 10.1038/cddis.2016.156

Wakabayashi, K., Nagai, A., Sheikh, A. M., Shiota, Y., Narantuya, D., Watanabe, T., et al. (2010). Transplantation of human mesenchymal stem cells promotes functional improvement and increased expression of neurotrophic factors in a rat focal cerebral ischemia model. *J. Neurosci. Res.* 88, 1017–1025.

Walters, B. J., Coak, E., Dearman, J., Bailey, G., Yamashita, T., Kuo, B., et al. (2017). In Vivo Interplay between p27Kip1, GATA3, ATOH1, and POU4F3 Converts Non-sensory Cells to Hair Cells in Adult Mice. *Cell Rep.* 19, 307–320.

Warnecke, A., Harre, J., Staecker, H., Prenzler, N., Strunk, D., Couillard-Despres, S., et al. (2020). Extracellular vesicles from human multipotent stromal cells protect against hearing loss after noise trauma in vivo. *Clin. Transl. Med.* 10:e262.

Warnecke, A., Mellott, A. J., Römer, A., Lenarz, T., and Staecker, H. (2017). Advances in translational inner ear stem cell research. *Hear. Res.* 353, 76–86. doi: 10.1016/j.heares.2017.05.011

Wy, K. (2013). NeuroD regulates neuronal migration. *Mol. Cells* 35, 444–449. doi: 10.1007/s10059-013-0065-2

Xiang, M., He, A., Wang, J., and Gui, C. (2009). Protective paracrine effect of mesenchymal stem cells on cardiomyocytes. *J. Zhejiang Univ. Sci. B* 10, 619–624. doi: 10.1631/jzus.b0920153

Xin, H., Li, Y., Buller, B., Katakowski, M., Zhang, Y., Wang, X., et al. (2012). Exosome-Mediated Transfer of miR-133b from Multipotent Mesenchymal Stromal Cells to Neural Cells Contributes to Neurite Outgrowth. *Stem Cells* 30, 1556–1564. doi: 10.1002/stem.1129

Yamane, H., Nakai, Y., Takayama, M., Iguchi, H., Nakagawa, T., and Kojima, A. (1995). Appearance of free radicals in the guinea pig inner ear after noise-induced acoustic trauma. *Eur. Arch. Otorhinolaryngol.* 252, 504–508. doi: 10.1007/bf02114761

Yang, S., Cai, Q., Vethanayagam, R. R., Wang, J., Yang, W., and Hu, B. H. (2016). Immune defense is the primary function associated with the differentially expressed genes in the cochlea following acoustic trauma. *Hear. Res.* 333, 283–294. doi: 10.1016/j.heares.2015.10.010

Yogarajah, M., Matarin, M., Vollmar, C., Thompson, P. J., Duncan, J. S., Symms, M., et al. (2016). PAX6, brain structure and function in human adults: advanced MRI in aniridia. *Ann. Clin. Transl. Neurol.* 3, 314–330. doi: 10.1002/acn3.297

Yu, X., Wang, D., Wang, X., Sun, S., Zhang, Y., Wang, S., et al. (2019). CXCL12/CXCR4 promotes inflammation-driven colorectal cancer progression through activation of RhoA signaling by sponging miR-133a-3p. *J. Exp. Clin. Cancer Res.* 38:32.

Zhang, R., Liu, Y., Yan, K., Chen, L., Chen, X.-R., Li, P., et al. (2013). Anti-inflammatory and immunomodulatory mechanisms of mesenchymal stem cell transplantation in experimental traumatic brain injury. *J. Neuroinflammation* 10:106.

Zhou, S., Gao, R., Hu, W., Qian, T., Wang, N., Ding, G., et al. (2014). miR-9 inhibits Schwann cell migration by targeting Cthrc1 following sciatic nerve injury. *J. Cell Sci.* 127, 967–976.

8

Regenerative Effect of a ROCK Inhibitor, Y-27632, on Excitotoxic Trauma in an Organotypic Culture of the Cochlea

Yutaka Koizumi[1], Tsukasa Ito[1], Kunio Mizutari[2]* and Seiji Kakehata[1]*

[1] Department of Otolaryngology-Head and Neck Surgery, Faculty of Medicine, Yamagata University, Yamagata, Japan,
[2] Department of Otolaryngology-Head and Neck Surgery, National Defense Medical College, Saitama, Japan

***Correspondence:**
Kunio Mizutari
tari@mbf.ocn.ne.jp
Seiji Kakehata
kakehata@med.id.yamagata-u.ac.jp;
seijik06@gmail.com

In the past, most inner ear diseases were thought to start with the impairment of the sensory epithelium of the cochlea before subsequently progressing to secondary neural degeneration. However, recent studies show that loss of primary synapses accompanied by excitotoxic degeneration of peripheral axons is likely to be the underlying pathology in sensorineural hearing loss. Rho-associated coiled-coil containing protein kinase (ROCK) inhibition has been reported to have neuroprotective and regenerative effects on synaptic pathways. Therefore, we analyzed the effect of ROCK inhibition using Y-27632 in a model of peripheral axonal damage in the spiral ganglion neurons created using the glutamate agonists, *N*-methyl-D-aspartate (NMDA) and kainic acid, to induce excitotoxic trauma in the explanted cochlea. The number of axons projecting to hair cells in the cochlea treated with Y-27632 was significantly greater than those in the cochlea treated only with NMDA + kainic acid. Furthermore, there was a significant increase in synapses between the spiral ganglion and the inner hair cells in the cochlea treated with Y-27632. The findings of this study suggest that ROCK inhibition could be a potential strategy for the regeneration of peripheral axons in the spiral ganglion and synapse formation in the inner hair cells of a cochlea that has sustained excitotoxic injury, which is one of the primary etiologies of inner ear disease.

Keywords: cochlea, spiral ganglion, Y-27632, hearing loss, inner ear, synapse, regeneration, Rho-associated coiled-coil containing protein kinase

INTRODUCTION

The etiology of sensorineural hearing loss (SNHL) involves two main mechanisms, the loss of sensory epithelium and/or the loss of sensory neurons (Wang et al., 2002; Sugawara et al., 2005; Liberman and Kujawa, 2017). The sensory epithelium, which includes hair cells and supporting cells, is the primary receptor of sound. Spiral ganglion neurons (SGNs) form synaptic connections with hair cells, which receive sound signals, convert them into action potentials, and convey them to the auditory center via SGNs. The conventional thinking has been that inner ear disease begins with impairment of the sensory epithelium of the cochlea and is followed by secondary neural degeneration (Johnsson, 1974; Bohne and Harding, 2000). Therefore, primary neural degeneration of the cochlea without loss of hair cells is considered to be a rare cause of SNHL. However, recent studies have shown that primary synapse degeneration, known as cochlear neuropathy, which causes a reduction in the amplitude of wave I in the auditory brainstem response (ABR) without elevation of the ABR threshold caused by loss of the synaptic ribbon (Kujawa and Liberman, 2009, 2015), is a common underlying pathology in SNHL. This type of hearing dysfunction has recently been described as hidden hearing loss, the pathology of which is strongly associated with the pathogenesis of tinnitus (Schaette and McAlpine, 2011; Schaette et al., 2012) and hyperacusis (Hickox and Liberman, 2014). The above-mentioned lesions are now recognized as a potential therapeutic target for SNHL.

Rho-associated coiled-coil containing protein kinase (ROCK) is a serine-threonine protein kinase that has been identified as a target protein of small molecular weight GTP-binding protein Ras homologous (Rho) (Madaule and Axel, 1985). Similar to the Rho family, low molecular weight G protein Ras-related C3 botulinum toxin substrate (Rac), and cell division cycle 42 (Cdc42) (Didsbury et al., 1989; Munemitsu et al., 1990), Rho has a specific action in the remodeling of actin (Hall, 1998). ROCK inhibitors inhibit the Rho/ROCK pathway and have multiple effects, including increased blood flow, neuroprotective actions, and neurosynaptic regeneration, and are used clinically as therapeutic agents for glaucoma and cerebral vasospasm. Several clinical trials have been conducted in cardiovascular disease (Shimokawa et al., 2002; Fukumoto et al., 2005; Vicari et al., 2005). Furthermore, ROCK inhibitors have been reported to have a beneficial effect on axonal regeneration in the central nervous system (Sarner et al., 2000; Yamaguchi et al., 2001). There have also been reports on the effect of promoting nerve fiber elongation by using a ROCK inhibitor in the cochlear nerve and in the central nervous system (Lie et al., 2010; Defourny et al., 2013). Therefore, we hypothesized that ROCK inhibitors would affect remodeling of the synapses between hair cells and axons in the SGN even after the cochlea has been damaged by an inner ear disorder.

To validate this hypothesis, we examined the effects of ROCK inhibition on damaged auditory nerve fibers in an organotypic culture of the cochlea. The most straightforward method to test the effectiveness of candidate compounds would be to perform *in vitro* research using the cultured organ. However, there is no established cochlear synaptopathy *in vitro* model. Therefore, we used a *N*-methyl-D-aspartate (NMDA) and kainite-induced auditory nerve damage culture model in our study. Brief exposure to NMDA and kainite (NK) was used to induce the auditory nerve damage. The exposure led to the loss of the synapses between the inner hair cells (IHCs) and synapses in the SGN as well as degeneration of the distal type 1 peripheral axons in the SGN, thus mimicking, *in vivo*, the damage caused by excitotoxicity or noise (Wang and Green, 2011). In addition, this excitotoxicity model has been hypothesized to represent critical aspects of neuropathy or synaptopathy (Han et al., 2019).

MATERIALS AND METHODS

C57BL/6J mice were sourced from Japan SLC, Inc. (Hamamatsu, Japan) on postnatal day 4, 5, or 6. A total of 29 mice, and 58 cochleae were employed in this study. The mice were placed on ice to induce hypothermic anesthesia and euthanized by decapitation. The inner ear was harvested from the mouse temporal bone and the cochlear tissue was isolated in phosphate-buffered saline (PBS) under a stereomicroscope.

The study was approved by the Yamagata University Animal Experiment Committee (approval number, 28156) and carried out in accordance with the rules for animal experimentation at Yamagata University.

Organotypic Culture of the Cochlea

The dissected cochlear tissue isolated from mice of either sex was cultured in Hanks solution. To obtain a flat cochlear surface preparation, the spiral ganglia, Reissner's membrane, and most of the basal cochlear segment were removed. The explants were plated onto 4-well plates coated with 0.01% poly-L-ornithine (Sigma, St. Louis, MO, United States) and 50 μg/ml laminin (BD Biosciences, Franklin Lakes, NJ, United States). All cultures were maintained in a 5% CO_2/20% O_2-humidified incubator. The composition of the culture medium was as follows: Dulbecco's modified Eagle's medium/Ham's F12 medium (Gibco Life Technologies, Paisley, United Kingdom), 10% heat-inactivated fetal bovine serum, 25 mM HEPES (Gibco), N-2 Supplement (Gibco), B-27 Supplement (Gibco), and 100 U/l penicillin G (Wako, Osaka, Japan). The organotypic culture was maintained for up to 72 or 96 h at 37°C.

Excitotoxic Injury of Cochlear Tissue in Organotypic Culture and Treatment With a ROCK Inhibitor

Damaged cochlear tissue were created as described elsewhere (Wang and Green, 2011). Following the original method, *N*-methyl-D-aspartic acid 0.5 mM (NMDA; Tocris Bioscience, Ellisville, MO, United States) 0.5 mM and kainic acid (Tocris Bioscience; NK treatment) were reacted in a culture solution for 2 h.

The following three groups were compared to investigate the effects of a ROCK inhibitor, Y-27632 (257-00511, Wako) in a model of excitotoxic injury of cochlear tissue: a control group; an NK group (NMDA 0.5 mM + kainic acid 0.5 mM for 2 h, followed by washing and culture in normal culture medium); and a ROCK inhibition group (washed after treatment with NK with addition of 10 μM Y-27632 in normal culture medium). Immunohistochemical evaluations were performed at 24 and 72 h after culture.

Quantitative RT-PCR

Before and after NK treatment, harvested cochleae tissues were collected and stored in RNAlater (Ambion, Austin, TX, United States) (n = 6 per group). Total RNAs were extracted with an RNeasy Mini Kit (QIAGEN, Valencia, CA, United States) according to the manufacturer's instructions. Quantitative RT-PCR was performed on a Thermal Cycler Dice Real Time System using the One Step SYBR PrimeScript PLUS RT-PCR Kit (RR096A; TaKaRa Bio, Shiga, Japan). Forward (F) and reverse (R) primer sequences were RhoA-F, 5′-AGCTTGTGGTAAGACATGCTTG-3′ and RhoA-R,

5′-GTGTCCCATAAAGCCAACTCTAC-3′, ROCK1-F, 5′-GACTGGGGACAGTTTTGAGAC-3′ and ROCK1-R, 5′-GGGCATCCAATCCATCCAGC-3′ and ROCK2-F, 5′-TTGGTTCGTCATAAGGCATCAC-3′ and ROCK2-R, 5′-TGTTGGCAAAGGCCATAATATCT-3′. PCR cycling conditions included 40 cycles of 95°C for 5 s and 60°C for 30 s. Expression was determined using the ΔΔCt method with glyceraldehyde 3-phosphate dehydrogenase (GAPDH) as internal control. All reactions were performed in duplicate. mRNA expression was reported as n-fold GAPDH mRNA. For assessment of relative mRNA expression, levels were standardized to cochlear samples extracted before NK treatment.

Immunohistochemistry

The whole-mounted cochlear tissues were reacted with 4% paraformaldehyde/PBS at room temperature for 1-h for fixation. After washing with PBS, 0.3% Triton X, and 5% BSA/PBS, the specimens were reacted at room temperature for 1-h for blocking and permeabilization. The following primary antibodies were reacted at 4°C for 16 h: Rabbit anti-ROCK1 (1:100 Abcam, Cambridge, United Kingdom: ab134181); Rabbit anti-ROCK2 (1:100 Abcam, Cambridge, United Kingdom: ab125025); Rabbit anti-NF200 (1:1000 Sigma: N4142), Chicken anti-NF 200 (1:1000 Chemicon, Temecula, CA, United States: MAB5262), Rabbit anti-NF200 as an auditory nerve marker, Rabbit anti-Myo7a (1:500, Proteus Biosciences Inc., Ramona, CA, United States: 25-6790) as a hair cell marker, Mouse (IgG1) anti-CtBP2 (1:1000 BD Biosciences, San Jose, CA, United States: 612044) as a presynaptic marker, Mouse (IgG2a) anti-PSD95 (1: 5000 Abcam: ab 2723) as a postsynaptic marker. After washing with PBS, the following secondary antibodies, diluted 500-fold, were reacted at 4°C for 16 h: Alexa 405 Goat anti-Rabbit IgG (Invitrogen, Carlsbad, CA, United States: A31556), Alexa 488 Donkey anti-Rabbit IgG (Invitrogen: A21206), Alexa 488 Goat anti-Chicken IgG (Invitrogen: A11039), Alexa 488 Goat anti-Mouse IgG2a (Invitrogen: A 2131), and Alexa 568 Goat anti-Mouse IgG1 (Invitrogen: A-21124). After washing with PBS, the samples were mounted with glycerol and observed.

Quantitative Analysis of Peripheral Axons in the SGN and Synapses

The fluorescently labeled samples, including SGN somata and axons, IHCs, synapses, and other structures, were observed using an LSM-700 confocal laser microscope (Carl Zeiss Microscopy GmbH, Jena, Germany). Optical sections in the x–y plane (z-sections) were recorded at 0.5-μm intervals in the z-axis. The resulting confocal image series (z-stack) contained a three-dimensional image in the entire volume of the explant. The z-stack was reconstructed (to view a plane perpendicular to the x–y plane) as necessary using ImageJ[1] or Photoshop CC (Adobe, San Jose, CA, United States).

We analyzed the number of peripheral axons in the SGN projecting into the IHCs using z-stack images. The methods used to quantify the peripheral neurons, hair cells, presynaptic ribbons, and postsynaptic density in the SGN were mostly consistent with a previous report (Wang and Green, 2011). Every IHC, outer hair cell (OHC), NF200-labeled axon, CtBP2 punctum, and PSD-95 punctum was counted within three randomly chosen volumes in the organ of Corti in the middle turn of the cochlea. Given that the number of afferent synapses on each IHC varies according to location, with a greater number in the middle than in the apex or base (Meyer et al., 2009), we restricted our study to the middle of the cochlea to minimize any location-dependent effects as found in previous research (Wang and Green, 2011).

Axonal growth was quantified as the average number of NF200-labeled fibers in contact with an IHC and was obtained by counting contacts in multiple confocal series, each of which contains 10–12 hair cells. This number was graphed as fibers/IHCs (**Figures 1C, 2G**). Presynaptic ribbons and postsynaptic densities were visualized as CtBP2 and PSD-95 immunoreactive puncta, respectively. Innervation was quantified by counting the number of postsynaptic densities on each IHC in z-stacks containing the bases of the IHCs. Individual postsynaptic densities in the stacks can be resolved and counted using an unbiased stereological method as previously reported (Wang and Green, 2011). The number of synapses made by each IHC was quantified by counting CtBP2 and PSD-95 puncta in contact with the IHC. This number was graphed (see **Figure 3D**) as CtBP2/IHC, or PSD-95 puncta/IHC. The survival rates of IHCs and OHCs, stained by myosin 7a, per field of view were also calculated in the same field by measuring the ratio of the total number of inner or outer hair cells and the number of inner or outer hair cells lost. Hair cells missing from the alignment were defined as lost. Observations were made within the range where the mean number of IHCs was 10–12.

Statistical Analysis

The hair cell and synaptic count data were compared by one-way analysis of variance ($n = 6$ each group). Mean values were compared by one-way analysis of variance, followed by a *post hoc* multiple comparison procedure (Kruskal–Wallis and Dann-Bonferroni tests). The two-tailed Mann–Whitney *U* test was employed to compare differences in mRNA expression. Error bars represent the standard deviation of the mean. All statistical analyses were performed using Prism 7 (GraphPad Software Inc., La Jolla, CA, United States). P-values <0.05 were considered statistically significant.

RESULTS

Excitotoxic Injury and ROCK1, ROCK2 Expression in the SGN and Peripheral Axons After Treatment With NK in an Organotypic Culture of the Cochlea

We first confirmed that the hair cells and peripheral axons in the SGN were morphologically damaged after 2 h of treatment with NK. The number of NF200-positive fibers/IHCs was significantly decreased immediately after treatment with NK (**Figures 1A–C**). The mean number of NF200-positive fibers/IHCs was 1.18 ± 0.77

[1] https://imagej.nih.gov/ij/

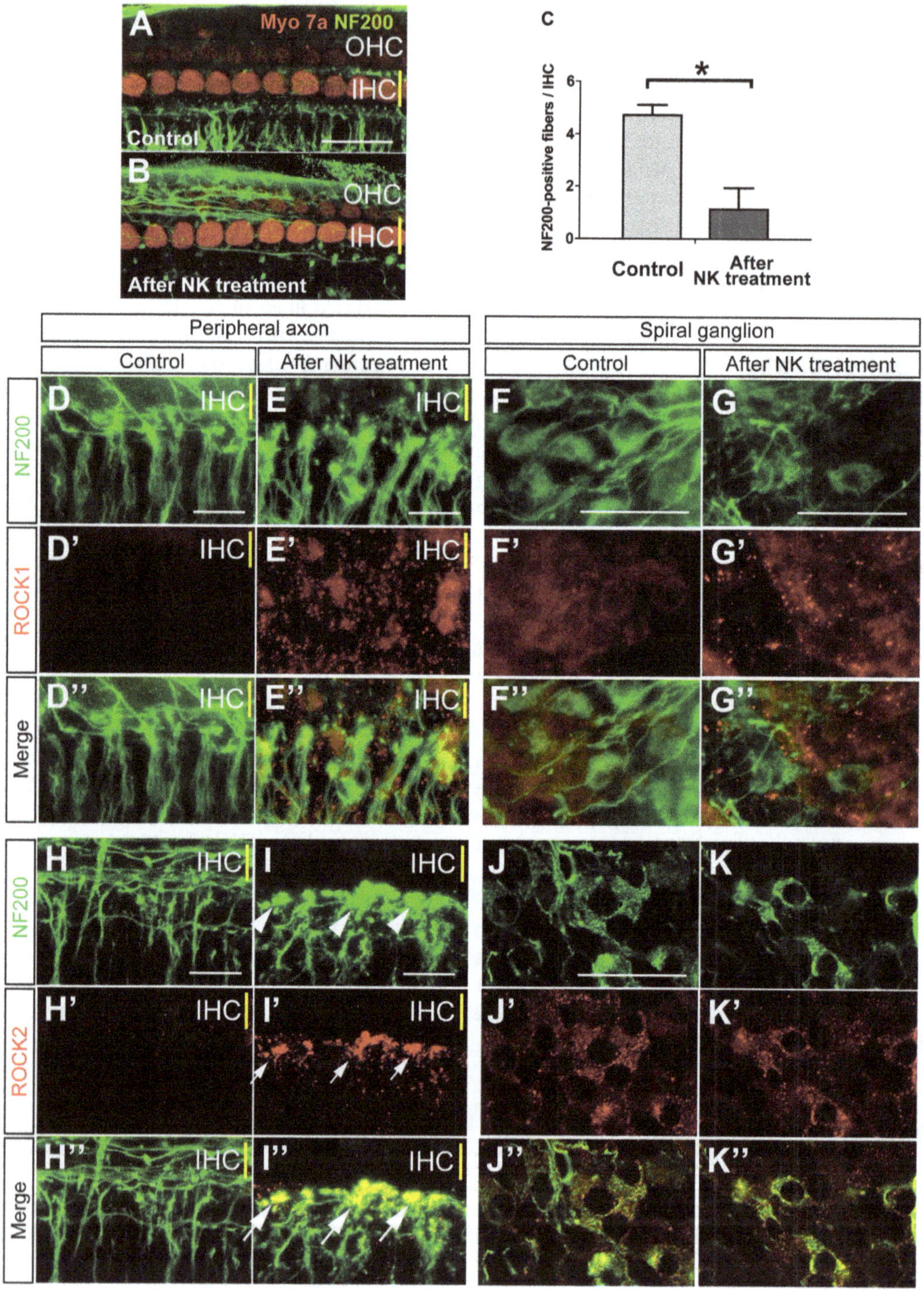

FIGURE 1 | Morphological changes and ROCK1, ROCK2 expression with and without excitotoxic damage caused by NMDA/kainate (NK) treatment in an organotypic culture of the organ of Corti. **(A,B)** Organotypic cochlear explants prepared from the middle turn of the neonatal mouse and cultured hair cells are labeled with anti-myosin 7a (red) and spiral ganglion peripheral axons with anti-NF200 (green). **(A)** A projection image of a confocal series through an explant, including the inner hair cell (IHC) row (yellow line) and the three outer hair cell (OHC) rows, showing the characteristic innervation pattern. **(B)** The peripheral axons of the spiral ganglion showed significant degeneration after 2 h of treatment with NK. **(C)** Peripheral axon counts immediately after 2 h of treatment with NK or no NK (controls) ($n = 6$). *Indicates a significant difference ($p < 0.05$). The data are shown as the mean ± standard deviation. The projection images of a confocal series of cultured explants stained by anti-NF200 antibody [green, **(D–K)**], anti-ROCK1 antibody [red, **(D′–G′)**] and merge images **(D″–G″)**, anti-ROCK2 antibody [red, **(H′–K′)**], and merge images **(H″–K″)**. **(H,I)** SGN peripheral processes, which are the radial fibers that innervate the IHC row, were markedly degenerated and formed debris (white arrowheads) at the ending of the processes **(E,I)**. After excitotoxic damage by NK, ROCK1 expression was slightly elevated around the fibers **(E′,E″)** and the spiral ganglions **(G′,G″)**. At the sites of debris formation, ROCK2 expression was significantly elevated consistent with the debris [white arrows in panel **(I′,I″)**]. However, there were no changes in the ROCK2 expression pattern in the spiral ganglion cell body **(J′,K′)**. Scale bar: 20 μm.

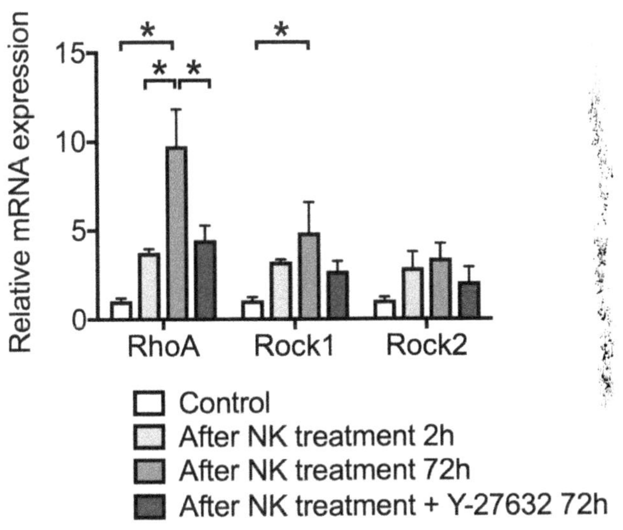

FIGURE 2 | The effect of Y-27632 on relative mRNA expression levels of RhoA, ROCK1 and ROCK2, after cochlear excitotoxic injury. The relative mRNA expression levels were standardized by the expression levels before NK treatment in each mRNA ($n = 6$). *Indicates a significant difference ($p < 0.05$). The data are shown as the mean ± standard errors of mean.

after treatment with NK and 4.77 ± 0.34 in the control group at the same time point (**Figures 1A–C**). Meanwhile, the number of IHCs/OHCs did not change regardless of whether or not NK was administered (data not shown).

Local expression of ROCK1 and ROCK2 were confirmed by immunohistochemistry. Slight ROCK1 expression was identified in the cytoplasm of the somata in the SGN (**Figures 1F–F″**) but was not clearly identified in the peripheral axons (**Figures 1D–D″**). After excitotoxic damage by NK, debris-like expression of ROCK1 was observed around the peripheral ends of the SGN axons (**Figures 1E–E″**). These debris-like expression of ROCK1 was also observed around the somata of the SGN (**Figures 1G–G″**). NF200 allowed the identification of the constant expression of ROCK2 in the cytoplasm of the somata in the SGN (**Figures 1J–J″**) but the expression was not clearly identified in the peripheral axons (**Figures 1H–H″**). However, after excitotoxic damage by NK, the peripheral ends of the SGN axons showed marked degeneration and aggregation that had the appearance of debris formation (**Figure 1I**, white arrowhead). Expression of ROCK2 was significantly increased at the site of the debris (**Figures 1I′,I″**). In contrast, the morphology and ROCK2 expression pattern in the somata of the SGN did not change regardless of treatment with NK (**Figures 1K–K″**).

Effect of Y-27632 on the mRNA Expression Level of RhoA, ROCK1, and ROCK2 in the Cochlear Tissue With Excitotoxic Injury

We confirmed the expression patterns of RhoA, ROCK1, and ROCK2 in the cultured cochlea before and after the excitotoxic damage caused by NK. In the intact cochlea, qPCR analysis revealed that mRNA expression levels of RhoA, ROCK1, and ROCK2 were increased (**Figure 2**). The mRNA expression levels of RhoA and ROCK1 were further increased even after 72-h culture ($p < 0.0001$, RhoA control vs 72 h after NK treatment; $p = 0.0002$, RhoA at 2 vs 72 h after NK treatment; $p = 0.0284$, ROCK1 control vs 72 h after NK treatment). Conversely, the mRNA expression level of RhoA significantly decreased in the Y-27632-treated group compared to the 72-h treatment of the NK group. The expression levels of ROCK1 and ROCK2 in the Y-27632-treated group decreased to near the expression level of the control group, whereas the differences in the 72-h treatment NK group were not significant.

Effect of the ROCK Inhibitor Y-27632 on Neurite Growth in the Cochlea With Excitotoxic Injury

After we confirmed excitotoxic auditory nerve injury in the cultured cochlea, we applied Y-27632 to detect the regenerative effect in the damaged peripheral axon. Twenty-four hours after the excitotoxic injury induced by NK, the peripheral axons in the SGN were degenerated and the peripheral ends of the axons were still aggregated in the same way they had been in the same location immediately after treatment with NK (**Figure 3B**). The mean number of peripheral axons/IHCs in the SGN was 0.49 ± 0.34 in the NK group and 4.69 ± 0.33 in the control group (without NK; **Figure 3A**) with significant difference compared to the NK group (**Figure 3H**). At the same time point, explants with excitotoxic injury treated with Y-27632 also showed degeneration of the ends of the peripheral axons in the SGN; the mean number present was 1.05 ± 0.45/IHC, which was not significantly different from that in the NK group (**Figures 3C,D**).

Seventy-two hours after excitotoxic injury, degenerative changes and aggregation were still observed at the ends of the peripheral axons in the SGN (**Figure 3E′**, white arrowheads) in the group that was not treated with the ROCK inhibitor (**Figure 3E**), although the morphological structure in the same region remained in the control group (**Figures 3D,D′**). However, in the group treated with Y-27632 after excitotoxic injury at the same time point, the peripheral ends of the axons in the SGN were elongated and some had connections with the edge of the IHC (**Figure 3F′**, white dotted line); the number of peripheral axons/IHCs in the SGN was 2.96 ± 0.30, which was significantly greater than that at 24 h after treatment with Y-27632 (**Figure 2H**). This increase was also significant in comparison with the value in the NK treatment group at the same time point. However, the number of peripheral axons in the SGN 72 h after administration of the ROCK inhibitor following treatment with NK remained significantly decreased in comparison with the number in the intact explant at the same time point (**Figure 3H**). We also confirmed whether the elongation of axons was observed by treatment of Y-27632 even at 24 h after excitotoxic injury. The peripheral ends of the axons in the SGN were elongated and some had connections with the IHC edge in some samples (**Figures 3G,G′**), and there were many axonal spheroids at the end of the axons in the NK treatment

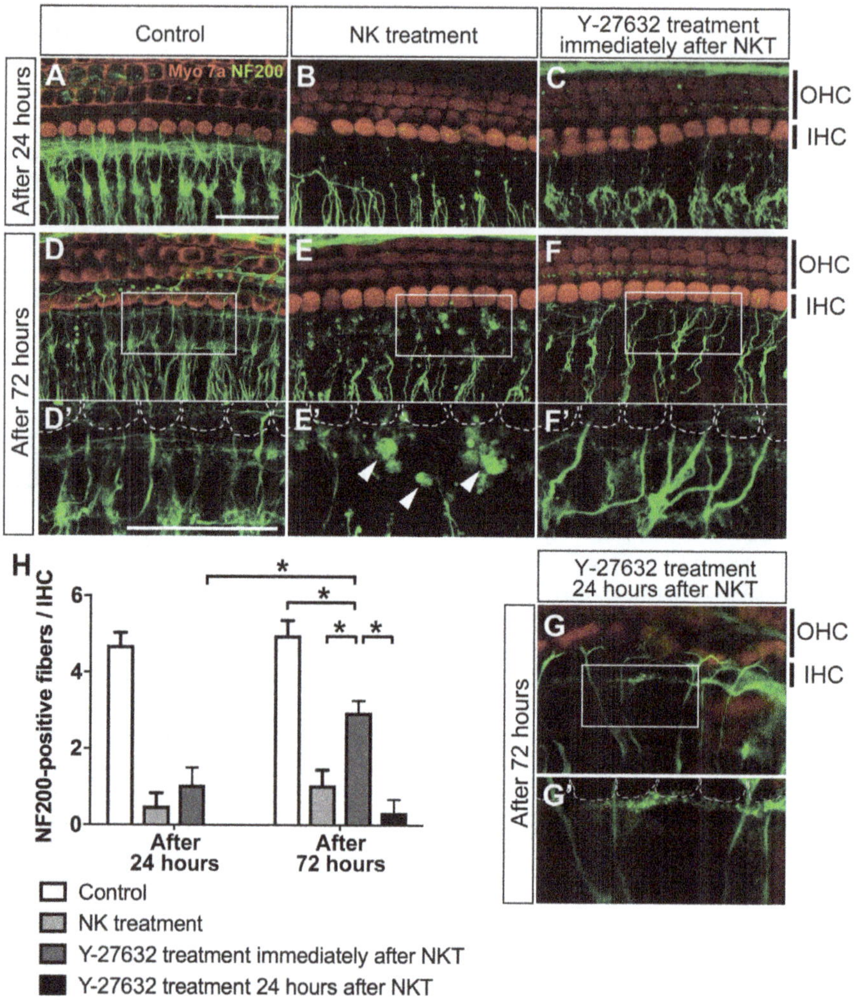

FIGURE 3 | The effect of Y-27632 on the degenerated peripheral axons of the spiral ganglion after cochlear excitotoxic injury. In panels **(A–G)**, hair cells are labeled with anti-myosin 7a (red) and spiral ganglion peripheral processes with anti-NF200 (green). **(A–C)** z-Projections of confocal image stacks of the organ of Corti in explants fixed at 24 h after the end of NK exposure: without NK treatment (control) **(A)**, after NK treatment **(B)**, and with Y-27632 treatment **(C)**. **(D–F)** z-Projections of confocal image stacks of the organ of Corti in explants fixed at 24 h after the end of NK exposure: without NK treatment (control) **(D)**, after NK treatment **(E)**, and with Y-27632 treatment **(F)**. **(D′–F′)** Enlarged images of the white inlets in panels **(D,E)** focusing on the inner hair cells and the end of the peripheral axons of the spiral ganglion. White dotted lines show the contour of the inner hair cells. Arrowheads **(E′)** show the debris formed at the end of a peripheral axon. **(G,G′)** The peripheral ends of the axons in the SGN were elongated and some had connections with the IHC edge after Y-27632 treatment even at 24 h after NK treatment. Scale bar: 20 μm. **(H)** Counts of peripheral axons at two time points after NK treatment (24 and 72 h) with and without Y-27632, and 72-h treatment of Y-27632 even at 24 h after NK treatment (n = 6). *Indicates a significant difference ($p < 0.05$). The data are shown as the mean ± standard deviation.

group (**Figure 3E**) while axonal spheroids were mostly absent in the Y-27632 treatment 24 h after NKT group (**Figure 3G**); however, the mean number of peripheral axons/IHCs in the SGN was 0.40 ± 0.89, which was not significantly different from that in the NK group (**Figure 3H**).

Next, we examined the IHC and OHC survival rates at the same time points by counting the axons in all the study groups. There was no significant change in the IHC and OHC survival rates at any time point regardless of whether or not NK was administered. Furthermore, there was no significant change in the IHC and OHC survival rates after administration of Y-27632 in the group that was treated with NK (data not shown).

Effect of Y-27632 on Acceleration of Synapse Formation in Cochlear Tissue With Excitotoxic Injury

Finally, we quantified the number of synaptic markers in the IHCs, including presynaptic ribbons stained by CtBP2 and postsynaptic densities stained by PSD-95, to explore the functional connection between IHCs and the peripheral axons in the SGN at 72 h after administration of Y-27632. PSD-95 puncta in the NK-treated group were markedly decreased in comparison with the control group (**Figures 4A,A′,B,B′**). The mean number of PSD-95 puncta was 16.49 ± 1.10 in the control group and 1.30 ± 0.36 in the NK group (**Figure 4E**).

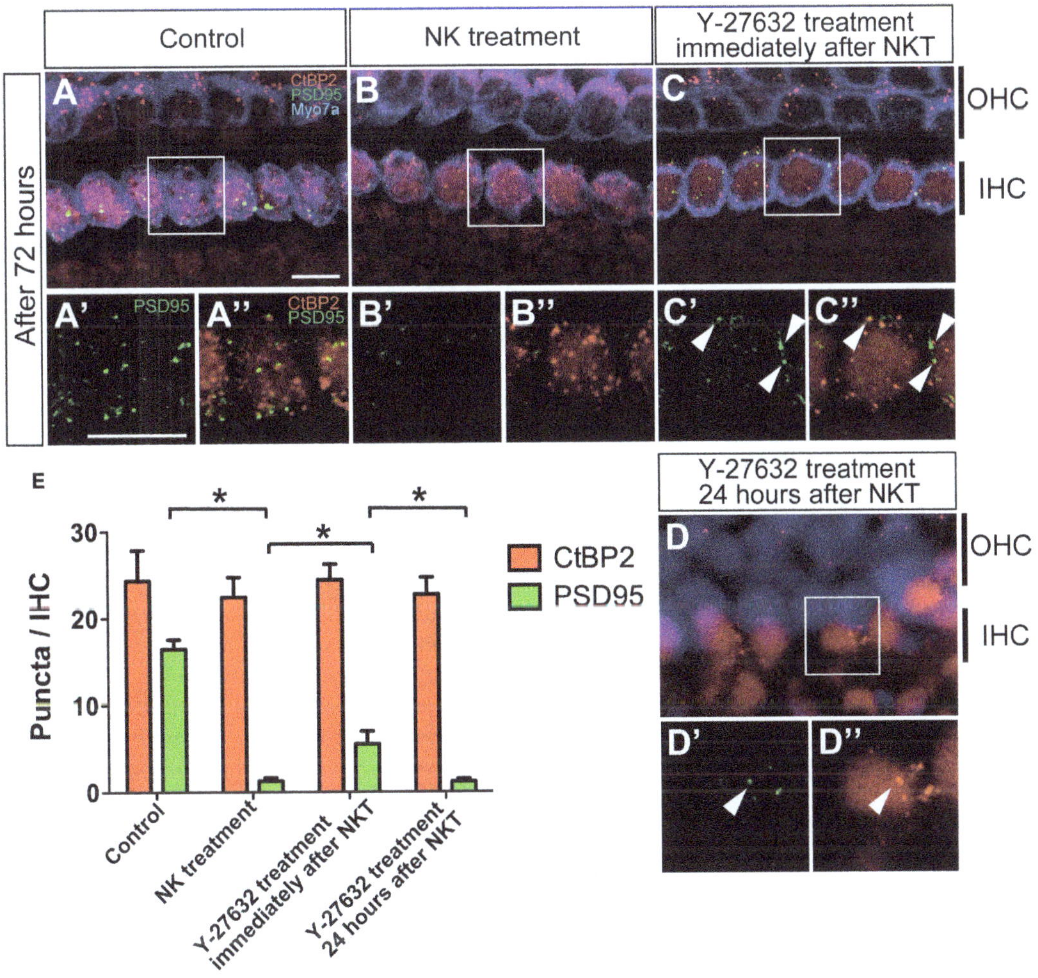

FIGURE 4 | The effect of Y-27632 on the degenerated synapses of the inner hair cells 72 h after cochlear excitotoxic injury. In **(A–D),** presynaptic ribbons (CTBP2-immunoreactive puncta, red) and postsynaptic densities (PSD-95 immunoreactive puncta, green), and hair cells labeled with myosin 7a (blue) are shown. **(A′–D′,A″–D″)** Enlarged images of the white inlets in panels **(A–D)** focusing on the inner hair cells area. Panels **(A′–D′)** Show postsynaptic densities and double-labeled images with presynaptic ribbons are shown in panels **(A″–D″)**. White arrowheads in panel **(C″)** show typical overlapping synaptic density with CtBP2 and PSD-95 after Y-27632 treatment. **(A′–D′,A″–D″)** Scale bar: 20 μm. **(E)** Counts of puncta of presynaptic ribbons and postsynaptic densities 72 h after NK treatment with and without Y-27632, and 72-h Y-27632 treatment even at 24 h after NK treatment ($n = 6$). *Indicates a significant difference ($p < 0.05$). The data are shown as the mean ± standard deviation.

However, the mean number of CtBP2 puncta was 24.53 ± 3.12 in the control group and 22.15 ± 2.28 in the NK group; the difference was not statistically significant and there were no morphological changes (**Figures 4A,A″,B,B″**). However, there was a significant increase in the mean number of PSD-95 puncta after administration of Y-27632 (5.52 ± 1.50) in comparison with the group that was not treated with Y-27632 (**Figure 4E**). Despite the significant increase in PSD-95 puncta in the Y-27632-treated group, the number in this group was still significantly lower than that in the control group (**Figure 4E**). The regenerated PSD-95 puncta were located beside the CtPB2 puncta around the IHC outline, which was considered to be the same region as the regenerated synapse (**Figures 4C′,C″**, arrowheads). Even in the Y-27632-treated group, there were no significant changes in the mean CtBP2 puncta count (24.45 ± 1.77; **Figure 3E**). Conversely, PSD-95 puncta in the treatment of Y-27632 even at 24 h after, decreased in the NKT group compared with the Y-27632-treated group (**Figures 4D,D′**) and CtBP2 puncta did not change (**Figures 4D,D″**). PSD-95 and CtBP2 puncta were 1.18 ± 0.38 and 20.15 ± 1.87, respectively (**Figure 4E**). There were not significantly different from PSD95 and CtBP2 puncta in the NK group.

DISCUSSION

In this study, we observed the regenerative effects of a ROCK inhibitor on NK-treated cochlear tissue, which represents excitotoxic damage, in terms of elongation of axons in the SGN and formation of synapses. We also found that mRNA expression levels of RhoA, ROCK1, and ROCK2 were increased in NK-treated cochlea. While expression of ROCK1 was higher in the whole cochlea, ROCK2 was expressed by the degenerated peripheral axons in the SGN of the NK-treated cochlea. The increased mRNA expression levels of the Rho-ROCK pathway may be suppressed by administration of Y-27632. The changes in the expression levels of RhoA, ROCK1, and ROCK2 and the localized expression of ROCK2 clearly show that the Rho/ROCK pathway is involved in the etiology of degeneration of the spiral ganglion and synapses and their regeneration. This is the first study to confirm that treatment with a ROCK inhibitor can regenerate SGN axons and synapses between IHCs and the auditory nerve in the cochlea after excitotoxic injury.

The mechanism by which of ROCK inhibitors cause regeneration of axons in the central nervous system has been investigated in detail. Axonal elongation requires reorganization of the actin cytoskeletons at the growth cone followed by orientation and stabilization of the microtubules. Activation of RhoA suppresses elongation of axons, and activation of Rac and Cdc42 has been shown to promote their elongation (Sarner et al., 2000; Yamaguchi et al., 2001). ROCK plays an important role in the suppression of axonal outgrowth downstream of RhoA (Govek et al., 2005), and it has been suggested that LIM kinase suppresses depolymerization of actin downstream of ROCK (Bito et al., 2000). Axonal regeneration after injury is due to physical damage from glial scars and myelin/oligodendrocyte-derived axon extension inhibitors, myelin-associated glycoproteins, Nogo-A, chondroitin sulfate proteoglycans (CSPGs), and oligodendrocyte myelin glycoprotein (Schwab, 2004). The effects of these inhibitors are suppressed by inactivation of RhoA and ROCK inhibitors (Alabed et al., 2006; Gopalakrishnan et al., 2008). ROCK2-deficient mice have been reported to recover after axonal injury (Duffy et al., 2009).

In contrast, peripheral axons are known to regenerate spontaneously, but functional reinnervation of the injured axon is often difficult (Navarro et al., 1997). Sensory, motor, and autonomic neurons, Schwann cells, other glial cells, and immune system cells were contained in the peripheral nervous system (Menorca et al., 2013). When peripheral nerves are injured, a process called Wallerian degeneration is initiated, which facilitates the removal of cell debris and enhances conditions favorable for axon regeneration (Rotshenker, 2011). At this time, Schwann cells form a structure called Büngner's band. The Büngner's band secures a scaffold for regenerating axons and supplies neurotrophic factors to help in the growth of regenerating axons (Webber and Zochodne, 2010). Schwann cells also have a phagocytic effect on myelin debris (Lyons et al., 2005), in contrast to glial cells, which suppress nerve regeneration by glial scar formation and persistence of myelin/oligodendrocyte-derived axon extension inhibitors in the central nervous system. However, it has been elucidated that the peripheral nervous system also contains inhibitory components of axon regeneration, such as CSPGs (Zuo et al., 1998a,b,c). Joshi et al. reported on the involvement of CSPGs in the peripheral motor neuron and the regenerative effect of ROCK inhibitors (Joshi et al., 2015). Although the peripheral sensory nerves did not regenerate in their study, they explained that the ability to regenerate depends on their responsiveness to CSPGs and ROCK inhibitors. In this study, we focused on the auditory nerve, which is one of the sensory nerves; however, the suppression of the mRNA expression levels of the Rho-ROCK pathway by Y-27632 administration was observed, as in the aforementioned study. These molecular biological changes suggested the possibility of regeneration of the sensory nerves when they present reactivity to CSPGs or ROCK inhibitors.

Studies on regeneration of the trigeminal nerve of zebrafish larvae indicate that NgR, its coreceptor leucine-rich repeat, immunoglobulin-like domain-containing protein 1 (LINGO-1), RhoA, ROCK, and their intracellular CRMP2 partners work as local inhibitor factors, while the ability of injured axons to reinnervate was improved by antagonizing these factors (O'Brien et al., 2009).

It is known that the tropomyosin receptor kinase (Trk) receptor has a high affinity for neurotrophin-3 (NT-3) and that p75 is a low affinity receptor (Kaplan and Miller, 2000; Reichardt, 2006). Trk C is expressed in the cochlea, and Wang and Green (2011) reported that inhibition of Trk C attenuated the nerve fiber regenerating effect of NT-3. Therefore, it is thought that the Trk C receptor pathway is involved in NT-3 activity in the inner ear. Furthermore, NT-3 has been reported to have a regenerating effect on auditory nerve fibers *in vivo* (Suzuki et al., 2016). In contrast, p75 has been implicated in the formation of dendrites downstream of brain-derived neurotrophic growth factor in the inner ear (Inoue et al., 2014) and is known to control axonal outgrowth in the central nervous system (Lee et al., 1994). p75 binds to and activates RhoA whereas binding of nerve growth factor to p75 has been shown to suppress RhoA activity and promote neurite outgrowth (Yamashita et al., 1999). p75 and Trk receptors are known to interact with each other (Numakawa et al., 2010; Gomes et al., 2012). The ROCK pathway is the downstream protein kinase of these neurotrophins, which include NT-3, nerve growth factor, and brain-derived neurotrophic growth factor (Yamashita et al., 1999; Kaplan and Miller, 2000). Therefore, ROCK inhibition is thought to be a relatively direct mechanism of axonal regeneration. Moreover, it would be easier to apply a ROCK inhibitor for neuronal regeneration in the clinical setting because such agents are already in clinical use. Our present findings point to the possibility of a breakthrough therapeutic strategy for hearing impairment accompanied by primary neural/synaptic degeneration.

In this study, morphological damage of hair cells was not observed in the cultured cochlear tissue. Therefore, we speculated that the ROCK inhibitor at the concentration used in this study had no or very limited toxicity to hair cells. There are few reports on the Rho/ROCK pathway in the cochlear region of the inner ear. With regard to hair cell damage, there are reports on activation of the ROCK pathway in OHCs that have been subjected to acoustic trauma (Chen et al., 2012) and on the protective effect of a Rac inhibitor against drug injury in OHCs (Bodmer et al., 2002). Those studies investigated the activity of the Rho/ROCK and Rac/Cdc42 pathways in OHC disorders. It has been shown that the activity of Rho decreases and conversely that the activity of Rac increases in OHCs that have sustained acoustic trauma or have been damaged by exposure to aminoglycoside antibiotic preparations. Chen et al. (2012) reported that inhibition of the activity of Rho strongly impaired

OHCs while Bodmer et al. (2002) reported that inhibition of the activity of Rac had a protective effect on OHCs. These reports indicate that the balance between the Rho/ROCK and Rac /Cdc42 pathways determines the impairment of OHCs. An increase in the activity of the Rho/ROCK pathway or a decrease in the activity of the Rac/Cdc42 pathway is presumed to promote the survival of OHCs.

The main limitation of this research is that the results were obtained over a short observation period and a limited drug concentration. When Y-27632 was administered at 24 h after NK treatment, there was no significant change as a whole; however, some cases of axonal elongation could be confirmed. This result suggested that the reactivity may decrease depending on the time until drug administration. In addition, as the mRNA expression levels of RhoA were further increased at 72 h after NK treatment, it was suggested that the reactivity may have decreased due to insufficient drug concentration. Therefore, the implication of Y-27632 in the clinical situation would be at an earlier timepoint after hearing loss onset, similar to other preventive drugs. Future studies should include a wide range of observation periods and drug concentrations. Another limitation is that the results of this study only confirmed the effects on morphology but not the effects on hearing. Further research should include an analysis of the effect of ROCK inhibition on nerve elongation and formation of synapse in an *in vivo* model to elucidate the role of the Rho/ROCK and Rac/Cdc42 pathways in the cochlea.

In summary, this study has demonstrated that the Rho/ROCK pathway is involved in axon elongation in the cochlear spiral ganglion even after excitotoxic injury. The Rho/ROCK pathway was involved downstream of neurotrophins and their receptors in nerve regeneration in the cochlea. An advantage of the ROCK inhibitor used in this study is that it is already in clinical use. Further analysis of the RhoA/ROCK pathway in the process of regeneration of the cochlear spiral ganglion and the effect of a ROCK inhibitor in this etiology *in vivo* are expected in the future.

AUTHOR CONTRIBUTIONS

SK organized the whole study. YK, TI, KM, and SK were involved in conceptualization and design of the study. YK and TI conducted the research and analyzed the data. YK wrote early drafts of the manuscript. KM and SK prepared the manuscript. All authors reviewed the final version of the present manuscript.

REFERENCES

Alabed, Y. Z., Grados-Munro, E., Ferraro, G. B., Hsieh, S. H., and Fournier, A. E. (2006). Neuronal responses to myelin are mediated by rho kinase. *J. Neurochem.* 96, 1616–1625. doi: 10.1111/j.1471-4159.2006.03670.x

Bito, H., Furuyashiki, T., Ishihara, H., Shibasaki, Y., Ohashi, K., Mizuno, K., et al. (2000). A critical role for a Rho-associated kinase, p160ROCK, in determining axon outgrowth in mammalian CNS neurons. *Neuron* 26, 431–441. doi: 10.1016/s0896-6273(00)81175-7

Bodmer, D., Brors, D., Pak, K., Gloddek, B., and Ryan, A. (2002). Rescue of auditory hair cells from aminoglycoside toxicity by Clostridium difficile toxin B, an inhibitor of the small GTPases Rho/Rac/Cdc42. *Hear. Res.* 172, 81–86. doi: 10.1016/s0378-5955(02)00514-2

Bohne, B. A., and Harding, G. W. (2000). Degeneration in the cochlea after noise damage: primary versus secondary events. *Am. J. Otol.* 21, 505–509.

Chen, F. Q., Zheng, H. W., Hill, K., and Sha, S. H. (2012). Traumatic noise activates Rho-family GTPases through transient cellular energy depletion. *J. Neurosci.* 32, 12421–12430. doi: 10.1523/JNEUROSCI.6381-11.2012

Defourny, J., Poirrier, A. L., Lallemend, F., Mateo Sanchez, S., Neef, J., Vanderhaeghen, P., et al. (2013). Ephrin-A5/EphA4 signalling controls specific afferent targeting to cochlear hair cells. *Nat. Commun.* 4:1438. doi: 10.1038/ncomms2445

Didsbury, J., Weber, R. F., Bokoch, G. M., Evans, T., and Snyderman, R. (1989). rac, a novel ras-related family of proteins that are botulinum toxin substrates. *J. Biol. Chem.* 264, 16378–16382.

Duffy, P., Schmandke, A., Schmandke, A., Sigworth, J., Narumiya, S., Cafferty, W. B., et al. (2009). Rho-associated kinase II (ROCKII) limits axonal growth after trauma within the adult mouse spinal cord. *J. Neurosci.* 29, 15266–15276. doi: 10.1523/JNEUROSCI.4650-09.2009

Fukumoto, Y., Matoba, T., Ito, A., Tanaka, H., Kishi, T., Hayashidani, S., et al. (2005). Acute vasodilator effects of a Rho-kinase inhibitor, fasudil, in patients with severe pulmonary hypertension. *Heart* 91, 391–392. doi: 10.1136/hrt.2003.029470

Gomes, J. R., Costa, J. T., Melo, C. V., Felizzi, F., Monteiro, P., Pinto, M. J., et al. (2012). Excitotoxicity downregulates TrkB.FL signaling and upregulates the neuroprotective truncated TrkB receptors in cultured hippocampal and striatal neurons. *J. Neurosci.* 32, 4610–4622. doi: 10.1523/JNEUROSCI.0374-12.2012

Gopalakrishnan, S. M., Teusch, N., Imhof, C., Bakker, M. H., Schurdak, M., Burns, D. J., et al. (2008). Role of Rho kinase pathway in chondroitin sulfate proteoglycan-mediated inhibition of neurite outgrowth in PC12 cells. *J. Neurosci. Res.* 86, 2214–2226. doi: 10.1002/jnr.21671

Govek, E. E., Newey, S. E., and Van Aelst, L. (2005). The role of the Rho GTPases in neuronal development. *Genes Dev.* 19, 1–49. doi: 10.1101/gad.1256405

Hall, A. (1998). Rho GTPases and the actin cytoskeleton. *Science* 279, 509–514. doi: 10.1126/science.279.5350.509

Han, B. R., Lin, S. C., Espinosa, K., Thorne, P. R., and Vlajkovic, S. M. (2019). Inhibition of the adenosine A2A receptor mitigates excitotoxic injury in organotypic tissue cultures of the rat cochlea. *Cells* 8:877. doi: 10.3390/cells8080877

Hickox, A. E., and Liberman, M. C. (2014). Is noise-induced cochlear neuropathy key to the generation of hyperacusis or tinnitus? *J. Neurophysiol.* 111, 552–564. doi: 10.1152/jn.00184.2013

Inoue, A., Iwasaki, S., Fujimoto, C., Nakajima, T., and Yamasoba, T. (2014). Developmental changes in the protective effect of exogenous brain-derived neurotrophic factor and neurotrophin-3 against ototoxic drugs in cultured rat vestibular ganglion neurons. *Cell Tissue Res.* 356, 299–308. doi: 10.1007/s00441-014-1813-0

Johnsson, L. G. (1974). Sequence of degeneration of Corti's organ and its first-order neurons. *Ann. Otol. Rhinol. Laryngol.* 83, 294–303. doi: 10.1177/000348947408300303

Joshi, A. R., Bobylev, I., Zhang, G., Sheikh, K. A., and Lehmann, H. C. (2015). Inhibition of Rho-kinase differentially affects axon regeneration of peripheral motor and sensory nerves. *Exp. Neurol.* 263, 28–38. doi: 10.1016/j.expneurol.2014.09.012

Kaplan, D. R., and Miller, F. D. (2000). Neurotrophin signal transduction in the nervous system. *Curr. Opin. Neurobiol.* 10, 381–391. doi: 10.1016/s0959-4388(00)00092-1

Kujawa, S. G., and Liberman, M. C. (2009). Adding insult to injury: cochlear nerve degeneration after "temporary" noise-induced hearing loss. *J. Neurosci.* 29, 14077–14085. doi: 10.1523/JNEUROSCI.2845-09.2009

Kujawa, S. G., and Liberman, M. C. (2015). Synaptopathy in the noise-exposed and aging cochlea: primary neural degeneration in acquired sensorineural hearing loss. *Hear. Res.* 330, 191–199. doi: 10.1016/j.heares.2015.02.009

Lee, K. F., Bachman, K., Landis, S., and Jaenisch, R. (1994). Dependence on p75 for innervation of some sympathetic targets. *Science* 263, 1447–1449. doi: 10.1126/science.8128229

Liberman, M. C., and Kujawa, S. G. (2017). Cochlear synaptopathy in acquired sensorineural hearing loss: manifestations and mechanisms. *Hear. Res.* 349, 138–147. doi: 10.1016/j.heares.2017.01.003

Lie, M., Grover, M., and Whitlon, D. S. (2010). Accelerated neurite growth from spiral ganglion neurons exposed to the Rho kinase inhibitor H-1152. *Neuroscience* 169, 855–862. doi: 10.1016/j.neuroscience.2010.05.020

Lyons, D. A., Pogoda, H. M., Voas, M. G., Woods, I. G., Diamond, B., Nix, R., et al. (2005). erbb3 and erbb2 are essential for schwann cell migration and myelination in zebrafish. *Curr. Biol.* 15, 513–524. doi: 10.1016/j.cub.2005.02.030

Madaule, P., and Axel, R. (1985). A novel ras-related gene family. *Cell* 41, 31–40. doi: 10.1016/0092-8674(85)90058-3

Menorca, R. M., Fussell, T. S., and Elfar, J. C. (2013). Nerve physiology: mechanisms of injury and recovery. *Hand Clin.* 29, 317–330. doi: 10.1016/j.hcl.2013.04.002

Meyer, A. C., Frank, T., Khimich, D., Hoch, G., Riedel, D., Chapochnikov, N. M., et al. (2009). Tuning of synapse number, structure and function in the cochlea. *Nat. Neurosci.* 12, 444–453. doi: 10.1038/nn.2293

Munemitsu, S., Innis, M. A., Clark, R., Mccormick, F., Ullrich, A., and Polakis, P. (1990). Molecular cloning and expression of a G25K cDNA, the human homolog of the yeast cell cycle gene CDC42. *Mol. Cell. Biol.* 10, 5977–5982. doi: 10.1128/mcb.10.11.5977

Navarro, X., Verdu, E., Wendelschafer-Crabb, G., and Kennedy, W. R. (1997). Immunohistochemical study of skin reinnervation by regenerative axons. *J. Comp. Neurol.* 380, 164–174. doi: 10.1002/(sici)1096-9861(19970407)380:2<164::aid-cne2>3.0.co;2-1

Numakawa, T., Suzuki, S., Kumamaru, E., Adachi, N., Richards, M., and Kunugi, H. (2010). BDNF function and intracellular signaling in neurons. *Histol. Histopathol.* 25, 237–258. doi: 10.14670/HH-25.237

O'Brien, G. S., Martin, S. M., Sollner, C., Wright, G. J., Becker, C. G., Portera-Cailliau, C., et al. (2009). Developmentally regulated impediments to skin reinnervation by injured peripheral sensory axon terminals. *Curr. Biol.* 19, 2086–2090. doi: 10.1016/j.cub.2009.10.051

Reichardt, L. F. (2006). Neurotrophin-regulated signalling pathways. *Philos. Trans. R. Soc. Lond. B Biol. Sci.* 361, 1545–1564. doi: 10.1098/rstb.2006.1894

Rotshenker, S. (2011). Wallerian degeneration: the innate-immune response to traumatic nerve injury. *J. Neuroinflammation* 8:109. doi: 10.1186/1742-2094-8-109

Sarner, S., Kozma, R., Ahmed, S., and Lim, L. (2000). Phosphatidylinositol 3-kinase, Cdc42, and Rac1 act downstream of Ras in integrin-dependent neurite outgrowth in N1E-115 neuroblastoma cells. *Mol. Cell. Biol.* 20, 158–172. doi: 10.1128/mcb.20.1.158-172.2000

Schaette, R., and McAlpine, D. (2011). Tinnitus with a normal audiogram: physiological evidence for hidden hearing loss and computational model. *J. Neurosci.* 31, 13452–13457. doi: 10.1523/JNEUROSCI.2156-11.2011

Schaette, R., Turtle, C., and Munro, K. J. (2012). Reversible induction of phantom auditory sensations through simulated unilateral hearing loss. *PLoS One* 7:e35238. doi: 10.1371/journal.pone.0035238

Schwab, M. E. (2004). Nogo and axon regeneration. *Curr. Opin. Neurobiol.* 14, 118–124. doi: 10.1016/j.conb.2004.01.004

Shimokawa, H., Hiramori, K., Iinuma, H., Hosoda, S., Kishida, H., Osada, H., et al. (2002). Anti-anginal effect of fasudil, a Rho-kinase inhibitor, in patients with stable effort angina: a multicenter study. *J. Cardiovasc. Pharmacol.* 40, 751–761. doi: 10.1097/00005344-200211000-00013

Sugawara, M., Corfas, G., and Liberman, M. C. (2005). Influence of supporting cells on neuronal degeneration after hair cell loss. *J. Assoc. Res. Otolaryngol.* 6, 136–147. doi: 10.1007/s10162-004-5050-1

Suzuki, J., Corfas, G., and Liberman, M. C. (2016). Round-window delivery of neurotrophin 3 regenerates cochlear synapses after acoustic overexposure. *Sci. Rep.* 6:24907. doi: 10.1038/srep24907

Vicari, R. M., Chaitman, B., Keefe, D., Smith, W. B., Chrysant, S. G., Tonkon, M. J., et al. (2005). Efficacy and safety of fasudil in patients with stable angina: a double-blind, placebo-controlled, phase 2 trial. *J. Am. Coll. Cardiol.* 46, 1803–1811. doi: 10.1016/j.jacc.2005.07.047

Wang, Q., and Green, S. H. (2011). Functional role of neurotrophin-3 in synapse regeneration by spiral ganglion neurons on inner hair cells after excitotoxic trauma in vitro. *J. Neurosci.* 31, 7938–7949. doi: 10.1523/JNEUROSCI.1434-10.2011

Wang, Y., Hirose, K., and Liberman, M. C. (2002). Dynamics of noise-induced cellular injury and repair in the mouse cochlea. *J. Assoc. Res. Otolaryngol.* 3, 248–268. doi: 10.1007/s101620020028

Webber, C., and Zochodne, D. (2010). The nerve regenerative microenvironment: early behavior and partnership of axons and Schwann cells. *Exp. Neurol.* 223, 51–59. doi: 10.1016/j.expneurol.2009.05.037

Yamaguchi, Y., Katoh, H., Yasui, H., Mori, K., and Negishi, M. (2001). RhoA inhibits the nerve growth factor-induced Rac1 activation through Rho-associated kinase-dependent pathway. *J. Biol. Chem.* 276, 18977–18983. doi: 10.1074/jbc.M100254200

Yamashita, T., Tucker, K. L., and Barde, Y. A. (1999). Neurotrophin binding to the p75 receptor modulates Rho activity and axonal outgrowth. *Neuron* 24, 585–593. doi: 10.1016/s0896-6273(00)81114-9

Zuo, J., Ferguson, T. A., Hernandez, Y. J., Stetler-Stevenson, W. G., and Muir, D. (1998a). Neuronal matrix metalloproteinase-2 degrades and inactivates a neurite-inhibiting chondroitin sulfate proteoglycan. *J. Neurosci.* 18, 5203–5211. doi: 10.1523/jneurosci.18-14-05203.1998

Zuo, J., Hernandez, Y. J., and Muir, D. (1998b). Chondroitin sulfate proteoglycan with neurite-inhibiting activity is up-regulated following peripheral nerve injury. *J. Neurobiol.* 34, 41–54. doi: 10.1002/(sici)1097-4695(199801)34:1<41::aid-neu4>3.0.co;2-c

Zuo, J., Neubauer, D., Dyess, K., Ferguson, T. A., and Muir, D. (1998c). Degradation of chondroitin sulfate proteoglycan enhances the neurite-promoting potential of spinal cord tissue. *Exp. Neurol.* 154, 654–662. doi: 10.1006/exnr.1998.6951

9

Insulin-Like Growth Factor 1 on the Maintenance of Ribbon Synapses in Mouse Cochlear Explant Cultures

*Li Gao, Tomoko Kita, Tatsuya Katsuno, Norio Yamamoto, Koichi Omori and Takayuki Nakagawa**

Department of Otolaryngology, Head and Neck Surgery, Graduate School of Medicine, Kyoto University, Kyoto, Japan

Correspondence:
Takayuki Nakagawa
tnakagawa@ent.kuhp.kyoto-u.ac.jp

Hearing loss has become one of the most common disabilities worldwide. The synaptic connections between inner hair cells (IHCs) and spiral ganglion neurons have specialized synaptic constructions, termed ribbon synapses, which are important for auditory function. The ribbon synapses in the cochlea are quite vulnerable to various insults. As such, the maintenance of ribbon synapses is important for ensuring hearing function. Insulin-like growth factor 1 (IGF1) plays a critical role in the development and maintenance of the cochlea and has the potential to protect cochlear hair cells from various insults. In this study, we examined the role of IGF1 in the maintenance of ribbon synapses in cochlear explants of postnatal day four mice. We cultured cochlear explants with an IGF1 receptor antagonist, JB1, which is an IGF1 peptide analog. Results showed that exposure to JB1 for 24 h resulted in the loss of ribbon synapses. After an additional 24-h culture without JB1, the number of ribbon synapses spontaneously recovered. The application of exogenous IGF1 showed two different aspects of ribbon synapses. Low doses of exogenous IGF1 promoted the recovery of ribbon synapses, while it compromised the spontaneous recovery of ribbon synapses at high doses. Altogether, these results indicate that the paracrine or autocrine release of IGF1 in the cochlea plays a crucial role in the maintenance of cochlear ribbon synapses.

Keywords: cochlea, insulin-like growth factor 1, inner hair cell, ribbon synapse, maintenance

INTRODUCTION

Hearing loss has become one of the most common disabilities worldwide. The World Health Organization (2018) estimates that hearing loss affects over 6.1% (around 466 million people) of the world's population. The cochlea is the sensory organ responsible for auditory function. Hearing is a series of events in which sound vibrations travel into the cochlea and are then converted into electrochemical signals that are perceived by the auditory cortex. In the mammalian cochlea, the conversion is processed by mechanosensory hair cells (HCs) consisting

---

Abbreviations: BDNF, brain-derived neurotrophic factor; CtBP2, C-terminal-binding protein 2; HC, hair cell; IGF1, Insulin-like growth factor 1; IGF1R, Insulin-like growth factor 1 receptor; IHC, Inner hair cell; NT-3, Neurotrophin-3; OHC, Outer hair cell; P, Postnatal day; PBS, phosphate-buffered saline; rhIGF1, Recombinant human insulin-like growth factor 1; RT, Room temperature; SGN, Spiral ganglion neuron.

of outer and inner hair cells (IHCs). Outer hair cells (OHCs) act as motor units that amplify the sound stimuli and contact type II spiral ganglion neurons (SGNs). IHCs play a key role in the process of auditory transduction. IHCs contact type I SGNs and convey electrochemical signals to the central auditory system (Hudspeth, 1997). Synaptic connections between IHCs and type I SGNs have specialized synaptic constructions, termed ribbon synapses, and are important for auditory function (Safieddine et al., 2012; Coate et al., 2019).

The ribbon synapse is an electron-dense structure associated with neurotransmitter-filled vesicles at sensory synapses in the retina, lateral line, and inner ear organs (Becker et al., 2018). Unlike conventional synapses, the ribbon synapse is specialized for the transmission of sensory information. The rapid and sustained neurotransmitter release from ribbon synapses allows for the proper transfer of sensory information to the postsynaptic receptors (Safieddine et al., 2012). The ribbon synapses in the cochlea are highly vulnerable to various insults such as ototoxic agents (Liu et al., 2013) and noise-induced injury (Kujawa and Liberman, 2009). Recent studies have demonstrated the associations between the loss of ribbon synapses and difficulties in understanding speech in noisy environments (Bharadwaj et al., 2014) and age-related hearing impairment (Viana et al., 2015). Therefore, the maintenance of ribbon synapses is crucial for ensuring normal hearing function. This encourages investigation into the protection and regeneration of cochlear ribbon synapses. Both a TrkB agonist (Meltser et al., 2014) and an AMPA receptor blocker (Hu et al., 2020) have demonstrated the protection of cochlear ribbon synapses against noise trauma. In an aminoglycoside-induced degeneration model, the protection of cochlear ribbon synapses by the local application of fibroblast growth factor 22 has also been reported (Li et al., 2016). Although still controversial (Wagner and Shin, 2019), the capacity to regenerate ribbon synapses in the mammalian cochlea was demonstrated *in vitro* (Wang and Green, 2011; Yamahara et al., 2019) and *in vivo* (Wan et al., 2014; Suzuki et al., 2016).

Insulin-like growth factor 1 (IGF1), once known as somatomedin C, is a hormone similar in molecular structure to insulin. IGF1 is essential for controlling cell proliferation, differentiation, and apoptosis in various tissues and organs, including the inner ears (Varela-Nieto et al., 2007; Okano et al., 2011; Allahdadi et al., 2019). IGF1 has the potential to protect HCs from excessive noise (Iwai et al., 2006; Lee et al., 2007), aminoglycoside antibiotics (Hayashi et al., 2017), ischemic trauma (Fujiwara et al., 2008), and surgical invasion (Yamahara et al., 2018). Also, the therapeutic effects of recombinant human IGF1 (rhIGF1) on sudden sensorineural hearing loss refractory to systemic corticosteroids have been confirmed in clinical studies (Nakagawa et al., 2010, 2014, 2016). IGF1 performs its functions by binding to its tyrosine kinase receptor (IGF1R). In the cochlea, IGF1R is expressed on the surface of OHCs, IHCs, and all supporting cells, including pillar cells, Hensen's and Claudius' cells, inner sulcus cells, and Deiters' cells (Okano et al., 2011; Hayashi et al., 2013), as well as SGNs (Sanchez-Calderon et al., 2010). Our previous study confirmed that IGF1 induced the regeneration of ribbon synapses in cochlear explant cultures of postnatal day (P) two mice (Yamahara et al., 2019). In this study, we examined the roles of IGF1 signaling in the maintenance of cochlear ribbon synapses using explant cultures. For the pharmacological inhibition of IGF1Rs, we used a competitive IGF1R antagonist, JB1, which is an IGF1 peptide analog. JB1 is a 12-amino acid cyclic peptide that inhibits the binding of IGF1 to its receptor (Pietrzkowski et al., 1992). We further confirmed the potential for spontaneous recovery of ribbon synapses and the additional effect of exogenous IGF1 in cochlear explants that had previously been damaged by JB1.

MATERIALS AND METHODS

Animals

Institute of Cancer Research (ICR) mice aged postnatal day 4 were purchased from Japan SLC (Hamamatsu, Japan). All animal procedures were performed following the NIH Guide for the Care and Use of Laboratory Animals (NIH Publications No. 8023, revised 1978) and were approved by the Animal Research Committee of Kyoto University Graduate School of Medicine (Med Kyo 17,114, 18,117, 19,536).

Explant Cultures

Cochlear explant cultures were performed as previously described (Yamahara et al., 2019). Briefly, P4 mice were killed with carbon dioxide (CO_2), after which they were decapitated. The cochleae were removed from the temporal bones and dissected in ice-cold sterile 0.1 M phosphate-buffered saline (PBS). The surrounding bony capsules were removed, and cochlear sensory epithelia were carefully dissected to preserve afferent connections with SGNs. To minimize any differences related to the region of cochlea under study, we only used the middle portion (40–60% from the apex) of the cochlear sensory epithelia. The samples were placed on cell culture inserts (Becton Dickinson, Franklin Lake, NJ, USA) and incubated in Dulbecco's modified Eagle's medium (DMEM; Sigma–Aldrich Inc., St. Louis, MO, USA) supplemented with 6 g/l D-glucose (Wako Pure Chemicals, Osaka, Japan) and 0.15 g/l penicillin G (Wako Pure Chemicals, Osaka, Japan) at 37°C in a humidified atmosphere with 5% CO_2. To prevent any effects caused by serum growth factors or hormones, serum-free medium was used in all experiments. Overnight pre-cultures were established to stabilize the cochlear explants.

Pharmacological Inhibition by JB1

After the overnight pre-cultures, cochlear explants were exposed to JB1 (Cat. No. J3705; Sigma–Aldrich Inc., St. Louis, MO, USA) at a concentration of 25, 50, 100, or 150 μg/ml for 24 h ($n = 5$ for each). Cochlear explants that were cultured without exposure to JB1 were used as controls. Cultured samples were histologically assessed for the number of IHCs, density of SGNs, as well as number of density of SGNs, as well as number of presynaptic ribbons, and postsynaptic receptor patches per IHC.

Spontaneous Recovery of Ribbon Synapses

To assess the capacity for spontaneous recovery of ribbon synapses, we used cochlear explants that were pre-treated with

50 μg/ml JB1 for 24 h. After rinsing for 5 min thrice with culture media, cochlear explants ($n = 9$) were incubated in the culture media for another 24 h without being exposed to JB1. The cochlear explants exposed to JB1 for 24 h were used as controls ($n = 9$). The number of presynaptic ribbons and postsynaptic receptor patches per IHC was compared between the two groups.

Effects of Exogenous IGF1 on Ribbon Synapses

To determine the effect of exogenous IGF1 on the recovery of presynaptic ribbons and postsynaptic receptor patches, cochlear explants that had been exposed to 50 μg/ml JB1 for 24 h were incubated with culture media supplemented with rhIGF1 (Orphan Pacific Pharma, Tokyo, Japan) at a concentration of 0, 0.1, 0.15, 0.2, 0.5, 1.0, or 5.0 μg/ml (n = 5–10) for 24 h. The specimens were then histologically examined.

Immunohistochemistry

Specimens were fixed in 4% paraformaldehyde in phosphate buffer (0.1 M; pH 7.4) for 15 min at room temperature (RT) and then rinsed with PBS. We analyzed ribbon synapses by immunohistochemical staining for C-terminal-binding protein 2 (CtBP2) and ionotropic glutamate receptor-2 (GluA2), as previously described (Liberman and Liberman, 2016; Suzuki et al., 2016). After blocking with 10% goat serum in 0.2% Triton™ X-100 for 30 min at RT, we incubated the specimens at 37°C overnight with the primary antibodies shown in **Table 1** diluted in 10% goat serum in PBS. We incubated samples with primary antibody species-specific secondary antibodies with Alexa Fluor® conjugates (**Table 1**) for 1 h at RT.

Presynaptic Ribbon and Postsynaptic Receptor Patch Counting

Cochlear specimens were imaged with a Leica TCS-SPE confocal microscope (Leica Microsystems, Wetzlar, Germany) equipped with 405, 488, 532, and 635 nm solid-state lasers. Scanning was sequential with a 2.5 μs dwell time. Images were sampled at a resolution of 512 by 512 pixels with a 63× oil immersion (NA 1.3) objective, a 1.5× software zoom, and a z-step size of 0.17 μm. A series of images contained at least 10 IHCs from the cuticular plate to the base. For SGN density analysis, a z-step size of 0.5 μm was applied to include the soma and SGN afferent dendrites. Imaris 7.4.2 software (BitPlane AG, Zurich, Switzerland) was used to perform three-dimensional reconstructions and spot analyses to count the number of presynaptic ribbons and postsynaptic receptor, as previously described (Fogarty et al., 2013). Puncta in each IHC with immunoreactivity for CtBP2 were counted as presynaptic ribbons. Puncta in each IHC with immunoreactivity for both CtBP2 and GluA2 were defined as postsynaptic receptor patches. For the spot analysis, the minimum diameter of a punctum was defined as 0.7 μm. For each sample, the number of presynaptic ribbons and postsynaptic receptor patches was manually counted in 10 IHCs.

Statistical Analysis

Student's t-test or one-way analysis of variance (ANOVA) with Tukey *post hoc* test was used. Statistical analysis was performed using GraphPad Prism v6.0 for Mac (GraphPad, San Diego, CA, USA) and SPSS 25 version for Mac (SPSS Inc., Chicago, IL, USA). The data are expressed as the mean ± standard deviation. Differences with p-values <0.05 were considered statistically significant.

RESULTS

An IGF1R Antagonist Induced Loss of Ribbon Synapses in Cochlear Explant Cultures

To assess the effect of pharmacological inhibition of IGF1R on the maintenance of cochlear ribbon synapses, we exposed cochlear explant cultures of P4 mice to an IGF1R antagonist, JB1, at different concentrations, ranging from 0 to 150 μg/ml, for 24 h (**Figure 1A**). All assays were performed using the middle portion (40–60% from the apex) of the cochlea because the numbers of ribbon synapses per IHC varied according to the location in the cochlear turns (Meyer et al., 2009). Immunohistochemistry for CtBP2 for labeling presynaptic ribbons and GluA2 for labeling postsynaptic receptor patches was used to assess the ribbon synapses histologically. The location of IHCs was determined by immunostaining for myosin VIIa. Immunohistochemical analyses for CtBP2 and GluA2 demonstrated ribbon synapses in control specimens that were cultured without JB1 (**Figures 1B–D**). A decrease in the number of ribbon synapses was observed in specimens cultured with JB1 at concentrations of 50 (**Figures 1E–G**) and 150 μg/ml (**Figures 1H–J**). We quantified the number of CtBP2-positive puncta (as presynaptic ribbons) and CtBP2 and GluA2 co-stained puncta (as postsynaptic receptor patches) per IHC, respectively. JB1 had significant effects on both presynaptic ribbons ($p < 0.001$ by one-way ANOVA) and postsynaptic

TABLE 1 | The information of antibodies.

Antibody	Working dilution	Cat. No.	Company
Rabbit polyclonal anti-myosin 7a	1:500	25-6790	Proteus BioScience, Ramona, CA, USA
Mouse monoclonal immunoglobulin G (IgG)1 anti-CtBP2	1:250	612044	BD Biosciences, Franklin Lakes, NJ, USA
Mouse monoclonal IgG2a anti-GluA2	1:2,000	MAB397	Merck Millipore, Burlington, MA, USA
Chicken polyclonal anti-neurofilament-H	1:1,000	AB5539	Merck Millipore, Burlington, MA, USA
Alexa Fluor 405 Goat anti-rabbit IgG (H+L)	1:1,000	A-31556	Thermo Fisher Scientific, Waltham, MA, USA
Alexa Fluor 568 Goat anti-mouse IgG1	1:1,000	A-21124	Thermo Fisher Scientific, Waltham, MA, USA
Alexa Fluor 488 Goat anti-mouse IgG2a	1:1,000	A-21131	Thermo Fisher Scientific, Waltham, MA, USA
Alexa Fluor 647 Goat anti-chicken IgG (H+L)	1:1,000	A-21449	Thermo Fisher Scientific, Waltham, MA, USA

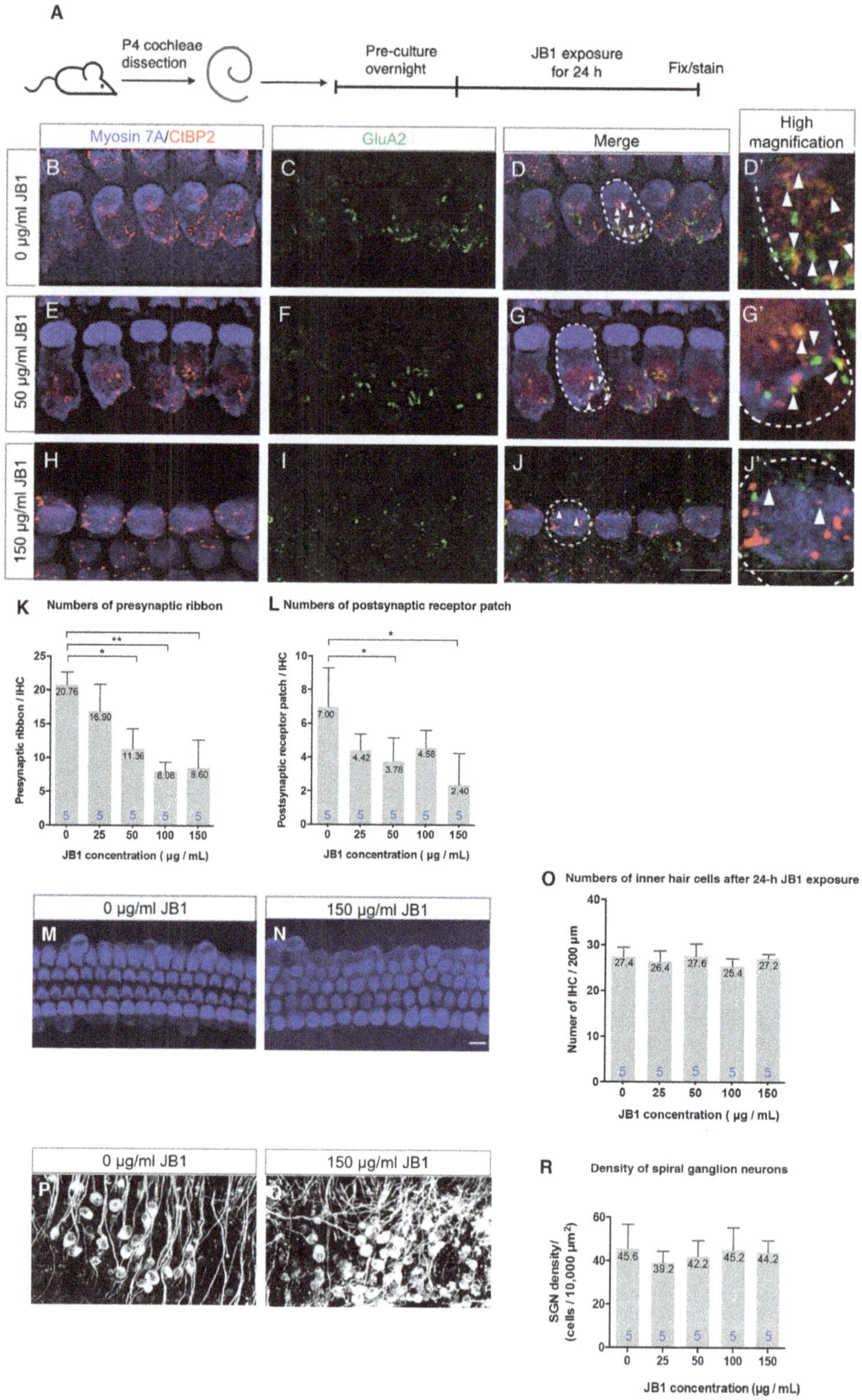

FIGURE 1 | An insulin-like growth factor 1 receptor (IGF1R) antagonist JB1 induced the loss of ribbon synapses in cochlear explant cultures. Cochlear explants of P4 mice were exposed to JB1 at a concentration of 25, 50, 100, or 150 μg/ml for 24 h **(A)**. **(B–D)** Maximal-intensity projection images with *z*-stack of ribbon synapses in control specimens that were cultured without JB1. Panels **(E–J)** are maximal-intensity projection images of the degeneration of ribbon synapses in specimens cultured with JB1 at concentrations of 50 and 150 μg/ml, respectively. Arrows show the postsynaptic receptor patches and dotted lines indicate the location of an IHC. **(K)** JB1 showed significant effects

(Continued)

FIGURE 1 | Continued
on both presynaptic ribbons ($p < 0.001$ by one-way ANOVA) and postsynaptic receptor patches (**L**; $p = 0.004$ by one-way ANOVA). Tukey's *post hoc* test revealed significant losses at concentrations of 50 ($p = 0.001$), 100 ($p < 0.001$), and 150 μg/ml ($p < 0.001$) in the number of presynaptic ribbons, and at concentrations of 50 ($p = 0.032$) and 150 μg/ml ($p = 0.002$) in the number of postsynaptic receptor patches, in comparison with controls which were cultured without JB1. **(M–R)** No inner hair cell (IHC) or spiral ganglion neuron (SGN) loss was found at any JB1 concentrations ($p = 0.428$ by one-way ANOVA for IHC, $p = 0.730$ by one-way ANOVA for SGN). Scale bars: 10 μm. Data are expressed as mean (digits at the top of each bar) ± SD. The digits at the bottom of each bar represent the sample number. $^{*}p < 0.05$; $^{**}p < 0.01$ with Tukey's *post hoc* test. P4, postnatal day 4; IHC, inner hair cell; SGN, spiral ganglion neuron; SD, standard deviation; ANOVA, analysis of variance.

receptor patches ($p = 0.004$ by one-way ANOVA), respectively (**Figures 1K,L**). Tukey's *post hoc* test revealed significant losses at concentrations of 50 ($p = 0.001$), 100 ($p < 0.001$) and 150 μg/ml ($p < 0.001$) in the number of presynaptic ribbons, and at concentrations of 50 ($p = 0.032$) and 150 μg/ml ($p = 0.002$) in the number of postsynaptic receptor patches, in comparison with controls which were cultured without JB1 (**Figures 1K,L**). No significant loss of IHC (**Figures 1M–R**) or SGN (**Figures 1P–R**) was found at any JB1 concentration ($p = 0.428$ by one-way ANOVA for IHC, $p = 0.730$ by one-way ANOVA for SGN). These findings demonstrate that the pharmacological inhibition of IGF1R caused a decrease in both presynaptic ribbons and postsynaptic receptor patches, suggesting that IGF1 is necessary for the maintenance of ribbon synapses in cochlear explant cultures.

Spontaneous Recovery of Ribbon Synapses

To test the spontaneous recovery capacity of ribbon synapses, we performed an additional 24-h culture without the presence of JB1 following a 24-h exposure period to JB1 at a concentration of 50 μg/ml (**Figure 2A**). Compared with cochlear explants exposed to JB1 for 24 h (**Figures 2B–D**), cochlear explants incubated for an additional 24 h without being exposed to JB1 tended to recover their ribbon synapses (**Figures 2E–G**). Statistical analyses using unpaired t-test demonstrated a significant increase in the numbers of both presynaptic ribbons (**Figure 2H**, $p < 0.001$, student's t-test) and postsynaptic receptor patches (**Figure 2I**, $p = 0.046$, student's t-test) in specimens following an additional 24-h culture. These findings indicate that cochlear explants of P4 mice have the capacity for spontaneous recovery of both presynaptic ribbons and postsynaptic receptor patches following their loss because of the pharmacological inhibition of IGF1R.

Effects of Exogenous IGF1 on the Recovery of Cochlear Ribbon Synapses

To assess the additional effects of exogenous IGF1 on the recovery of ribbon synapses, cochlear explants that had been damaged by 24-h exposure to 50 μg/ml JB1 were incubated with culture media supplemented with rhIGF1 for 24 h (**Figure 3A**). Compared with the specimens following an additional 24-h culture without supplementation of rhIGF1 (**Figures 3B–D**), further increase in the number of ribbon synapses was observed in the specimens following an additional 24-h culture with 0.2 μg/ml rhIGF1 (**Figures 3E–G**). However, in those following an additional 24-h culture with 5 μg/ml rhIGF1 (**Figures 3H–J**), a decrease in the number of ribbon synapses was observed. Quantitative analyses showed significant effects of exogenous rhIGF1 on the numbers of both presynaptic ribbons ($p < 0.001$, one-way ANOVA, **Figure 3K**) and postsynaptic receptor patches ($p < 0.001$, one-way ANOVA, **Figure 3L**). Significant differences were identified in the number of presynaptic ribbons between 0 and 0.2 ($p = 0.034$, Tukey *post hoc* test), 1 ($p = 0.017$, Tukey *post hoc* test) or 5 μg/ml ($p = 0.010$, Tukey *post hoc* test), and in the number of postsynaptic receptor patches between 0 and 0.2 ($p = 0.020$, Tukey *post hoc* test) or 5 μg/ml ($p = 0.012$, Tukey *post hoc* test). In summary, exogenous IGF1 at concentrations <0.5 μg/ml exerted positive effects on the recovery of ribbon synapses, but high concentrations diminished spontaneous recovery. We tested the effect of rhIGF1 at a concentration of 5 μg/ml on the survival of IHCs or SGNs. The results demonstrated no significant IHC or SGN loss in specimens treated with 5 μg/ml rhIGF1 compared with those cultured without rhIGF1 (**Supplementary Figure S1**). These findings indicate that the precise regulation of IGF1 levels may be required for the maintenance of ribbon synapses in cochlear explant cultures.

DISCUSSION

In this study, we used the IGF1R antagonist JB1 to pharmacologically inhibit IGF1 signaling. JB1 is a highly selective IGF-IR antagonist, which interferes with the efficacy of IGF1 by competitively inhibiting the binding of IGF1 to IGF1R (Pietrzkowski et al., 1992). Our previous study demonstrated the efficacy of JB1 in attenuating IGF1-mediated regeneration of ribbon synapses in P2 cochlear explants that had been damaged by excitatory amino acids (Yamahara et al., 2019). JB1 has also been used to antagonize IGF1 effects in various organs including the hippocampus (Nelson et al., 2014) and retina (Landi et al., 2009). The present results demonstrated that JB1 decreased the number of both presynaptic ribbons and postsynaptic receptor patches in a dose-dependent manner, indicating that IGF1 is an inevitable factor for the maintenance of ribbon synapses in cochlear explants. Our previous study (Yamahara et al., 2019) used explant cultures of P2 mouse cochleae, while in the present study, we used P4 mouse cochleae for a couple of reasons. One is the maturation process of ribbon synapses. The period from P0 to P12 is an active phase for the maturation of ribbon synapses (Michanski et al., 2019), indicating that ribbon synapses in P4 mice are more mature than those in P2 mice. On the other hand, there is a technical limitation in the preparation of cochlear explant culture. It is difficult to dissect out cochlear sensory epithelia from P5 or older mouse cochleae. Based on these issues, P4 mice were chosen for this study. Ribbon synapses in P4 mouse cochleae are still immature, which can be a limitation of the present study.

Previous studies have revealed the importance of IGF1 for the maturation of cochleae after birth (Camarero et al., 2001, 2002). In homozygous mutants, $IGF1^{-/-}$ mice, no significant

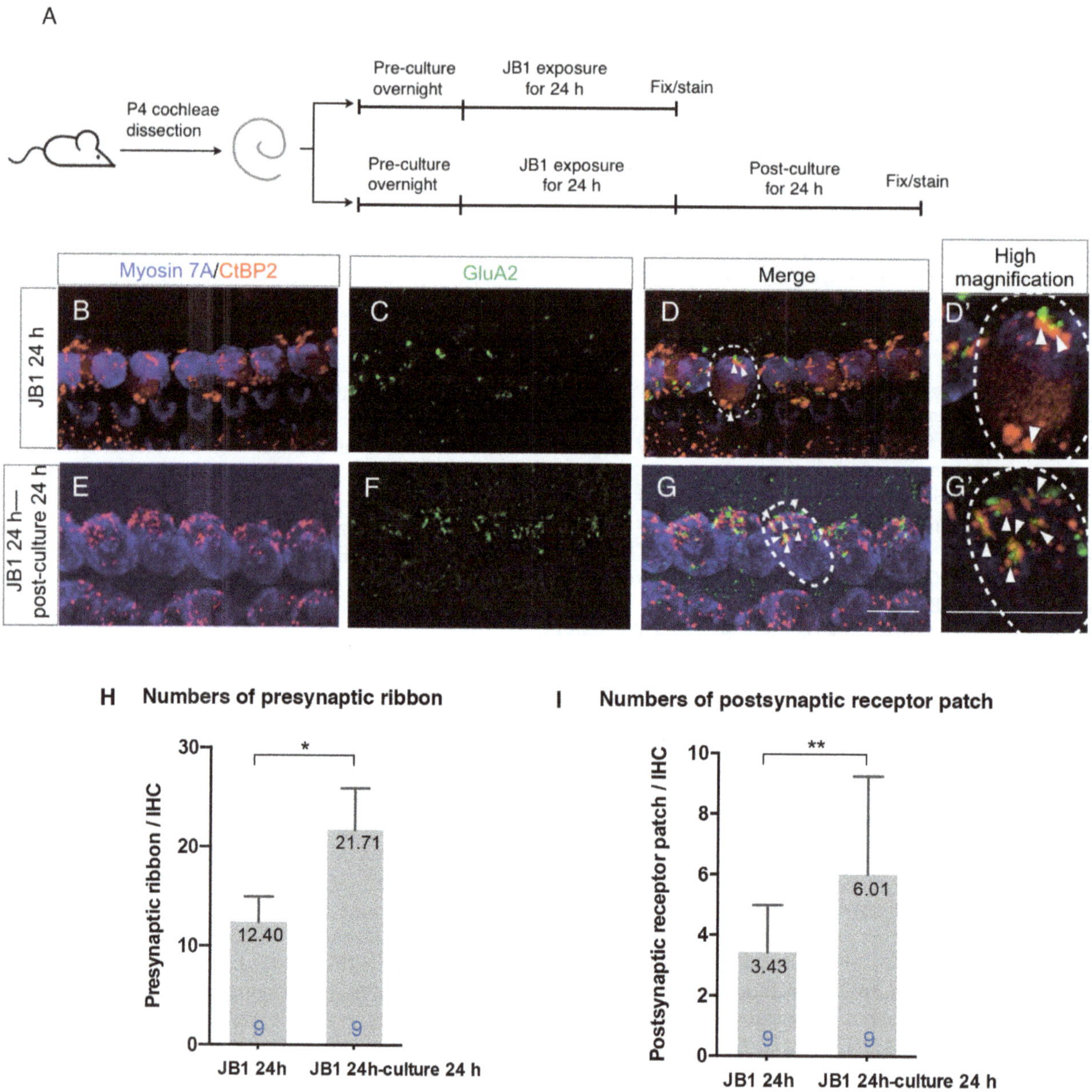

FIGURE 2 | Spontaneous recovery of ribbon synapses. Cochlear explants from P4 mice were exposed to 50 μg/ml JB1 for 24 h, with or without an additional 24 h of culture **(A)**. **(B–D)** Maximal-intensity projection images with *z*-stack of the immunostaining results of specimens immediately after 24-h JB1 exposure. **(E–G)** Maximal-intensity projection images of the specimens following an additional 24-h culture. Arrows show the postsynaptic receptor patches and dotted lines indicate the location of an IHC. **(H)** The number of presynaptic ribbons ($p < 0.001$ by unpaired *t*-test) and postsynaptic receptor patches (**I**; $p = 0.046$ by unpaired *t*-test) in the specimens were significantly increased after an additional 24-h culture. Scale bars: 10 μm. Data are expressed as mean (digits at the top of each bar) ± SD. The digits at the bottom of each bar represent the sample number. $^*p < 0.01$; $^{**}p < 0.05$ by an unpaired *t*-test. P4, postnatal day 4; IHC, inner hair cell; SD, standard deviation.

loss of SGNs was identified at P5, while SGN numbers and sizes were statistically significantly decreased at P20. Moreover, cochlear volumes were also revealed to have the same trend (Camarero et al., 2001). Abnormal innervation of SGN afferent dendrites was observed at P20, but not at P5 (Camarero et al., 2002). Also, IGF1-deficient mice presented profound deafness from 1 month of age onwards, without any obvious worsening of hearing parameters with aging (Riquelme et al., 2010). These findings suggest the importance of IGF1 for the maintenance and maturation of the synaptic contacts between IHCs and SGNs.

IGF1 is mainly produced in the liver and exerts its function through endocrine, autocrine, and paracrine mechanisms (Jenkins and Bustin, 2004). IGF1 is also synthesized in the developing and neonatal cochleae

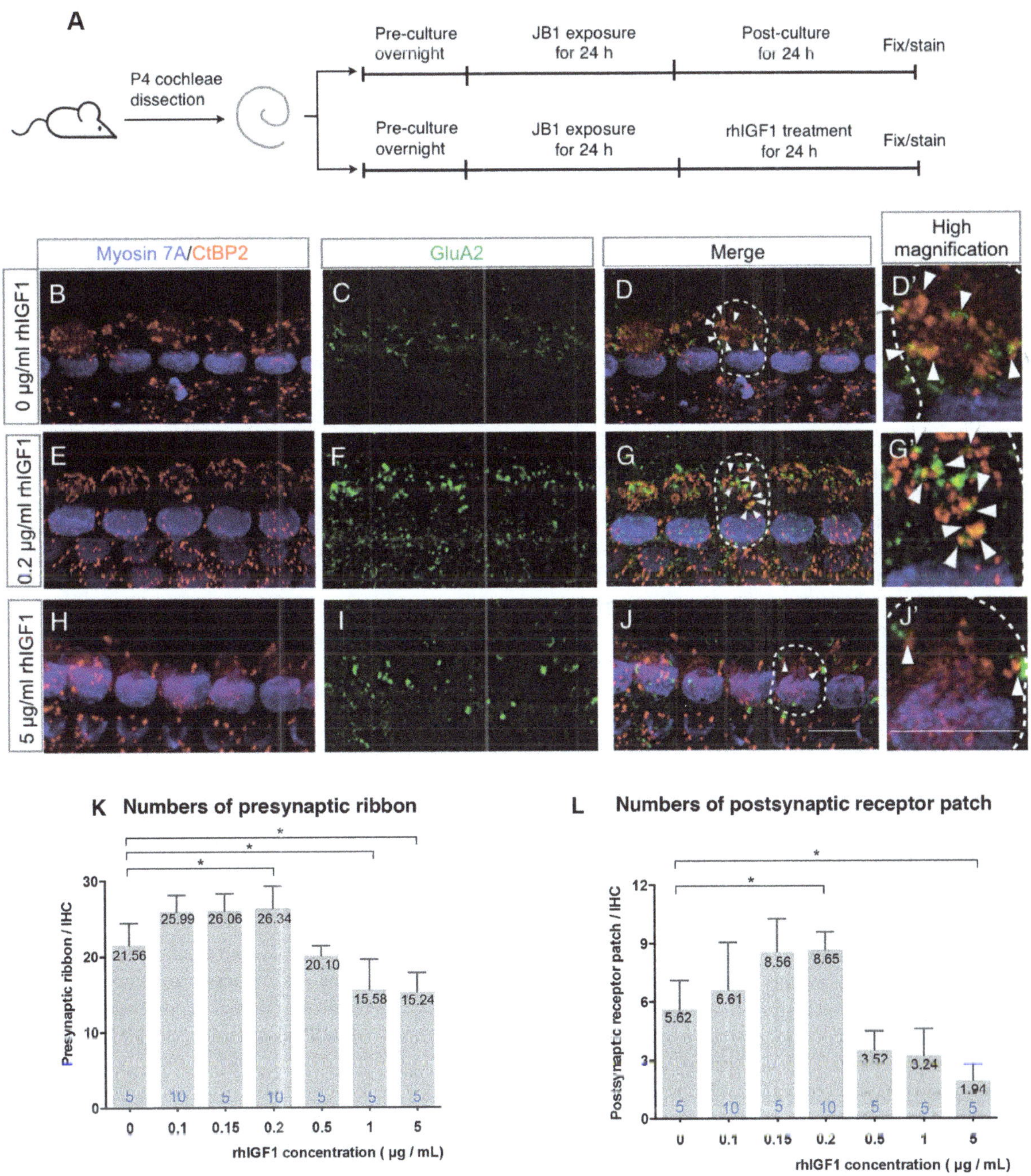

FIGURE 3 | Effect of exogenous IGF1 on the recovery of ribbon synapses. Cochlear explants from P4 mice were exposed to 50 μg/ml JB1 for 24 h, after which they were incubated with culture media supplemented with rhIGF1 at a concentration of 0.1, 0.15, 0.2, 0.5, or 1, 5 μg/ml for 24 h **(A)**. **(B–D)** Maximal-intensity projection images with *z*-stack of the immunostaining images of specimens cultured without rhIGF1. Panels **(E–J)** are maximal-intensity projection images of the recovery of ribbon synapses in specimens cultured with 50 μg/ml JB1 for 24 h, followed by rhIGF1 treatment for 24 h at concentrations of 0.2 and 5 μg/ml, respectively. Arrows show the postsynaptic receptor patches and dotted lines indicate the location of an IHC. Exogenous rhIGF1 showed significant effects on the number of both presynaptic ribbons (**K**; $p < 0.001$ by one-way ANOVA) and postsynaptic receptor patches (**L**; $p < 0.001$ by one-way ANOVA). Tukey's *post hoc* test revealed significant difference at concentrations of 0.2 ($p = 0.034$), 1 ($p = 0.017$), and 5 μg/ml ($p = 0.010$) in the number of presynaptic ribbons, and at concentrations of 0.2 ($p = 0.020$) and 5 μg/ml ($p = 0.012$) in the number of postsynaptic receptor patches, in comparison with controls which were cultured in 0 μg/ml rhIGF1. Scale bars: 10 μm. Data are expressed as mean (digits at the top of each bar) ± SD. The digits at the bottom of each bar represent the sample number. *$p < 0.05$ by one-way ANOVA, followed by Tukey's *post hoc* test. P4, postnatal day 4; IHC, inner hair cell; SD, standard deviation; rhIGF1, recombinant human insulin-like growth factor-1; ANOVA, analysis of variance.

(Sanchez-Calderon et al., 2010; Okano et al., 2011), indicating the existence of paracrine or autocrine systems for IGF1 in the cochlea. In this study, we observed the spontaneous recovery of both presynaptic ribbons and postsynaptic patches after their loss because of the pharmacological inhibition of IGF1R. Therefore, we presume that the paracrine or autocrine systems in the cochlea may contribute to the spontaneous recovery of ribbon synapses in cochlear explants that had been damaged by JB1.

Neurotrophin-3 (NT-3) is a potent factor for the maintenance and regeneration of cochlear ribbon synapses (Wang and Green, 2011; Wan et al., 2014). The selective blockade of endogenous NT-3 signaling reduced the regeneration of axons and postsynaptic densities *in vitro* (Wang and Green, 2011). Endogenous NT-3 promoted the recovery of cochlear ribbon synapses after acoustic trauma *in vivo* (Wan et al., 2014). Brain-derived neurotrophic factor (BDNF) also plays a role in the development and maintenance of ribbon synapses (Zuccotti et al., 2012; Meltser et al., 2014; Wan et al., 2014). In this study, the selective blockade of IGF1R induced the significant loss of cochlear ribbon synapses, suggesting that endogenous NT-3 or BDNF in P4 cochlear explants could not compensate for the loss of IGF1 signaling. In contrast, other factors, including NT-3 and BDNF, may be involved in the process of spontaneous recovery of ribbon synapses that were observed in this study.

In our previous studies using cochlear explants of neonatal mice, exogenous rhIGF1 had protective effects against aminoglycoside ototoxicity on IHCs at concentrations ranging from 0.1 to 1 μg/ml, and on OHCs at concentrations ranging from 10^{-4} to 1 μg/ml (Hayashi et al., 2013; Yamahara et al., 2017). For the regeneration of ribbon synapses after excitotoxic insults, 1 μg/ml exogenous rhIGF1 showed significant effects, but 5 μg/ml did not (Yamahara et al., 2019). Based on these findings, we used exogenous rhIGF1 at concentrations ranging from 0.1 to 5 μg/ml in this study. These results demonstrated the positive effects on the recovery of both presynaptic ribbons and postsynaptic receptor patches at concentrations of rhIGF1 ranging from 0.1 to 0.2 μg/ml, and negative effects at a concentration of 1 and 5 μg/ml. Compared with our previous study using cochlear explants that were damaged by excitatory amino acids (Yamahara et al., 2019), the concentration of rhIGF1 required to promote recovery is lower, which could be due to differences in the method used to induce damage. In contrast to the present results, after the exposure to excitatory amino acids, no spontaneous recovery of ribbon synapses was observed, indicating the lack of endogenous IGF1 production. In the present study, exogenous rhIGF1 exhibited bell-shaped dose-response curves in the numbers of presynaptic ribbons and postsynaptic receptor patches. This type of dose-response curve is common with endocrine disruption (Vandenberg et al., 2012). Some hormones, including androgen and estradiol, show agonist effects at low concentrations and antagonist effects at high concentrations. There are several mechanisms for a bell-shaped dose-response curve, including actions at multiple targets, cytotoxicity, receptor selectivity, receptor down-regulation and desensitization, receptor competition, and endocrine negative feedback loops (Vandenberg et al., 2012). IGF1 is similar in molecular structure to insulin and has a low affinity to insulin receptors. At high concentrations, IGF1 activates insulin receptor-mediated signaling. Altogether, the precise regulation of IGF1 levels may be necessary for the maintenance of cochlear ribbon synapses.

In conclusion, in the current study, we demonstrated that the pharmacological inhibition of IGF1R reduced the number of ribbon synapses in cochlear explant cultures of P4 mice, pointing to the importance of IGF1 for the maintenance of ribbon synapses. Surprisingly, the number of ribbon synapses recovered spontaneously following an additional 24 h of culture, pointing to the contribution of endogenous IGF1 to the maintenance of cochlear ribbon synapses. This confirmation of the effects of exogenous rhIGF1 points to the precise regulation of IGF1 levels for the maintenance of cochlear ribbon synapses. However, ribbon synapses in P4 cochleae are still in their maturation process (Michanski et al., 2019), which is a limitation of this study. We will investigate the role of IGF1 in the maintenance of cochlear ribbon synapses in mature animals *in vivo* shortly.

AUTHOR CONTRIBUTIONS

TN designed the study. LG, TKi and TKa performed the experiments. LG and TN analyzed the data and wrote the manuscript. NY and KO performed a critical review.

ACKNOWLEDGMENTS

We would like to thank Kohei Yamahara (Kyoto University) for valuable suggestions on the design of experiments, Jun Suzuki (Tohoku University) for technical advice for immunostaining, and Editage (www.editage.com) for English language editing.

SUPPLEMENTARY MATERIAL

FIGURE S1 | Effects of exogenous IGF1 on the survival of inner hair cells (IHCs) and spiral ganglion neurons (SGNs). Cochlear explants from P4 mice were exposed to 50 μg/ml JB1 for 24 h, after which they were incubated with culture media supplemented with rhIGF1 at a concentration of 5 μg/ml or without rhIGF1 for 24 h. **(A–D)** Maximal-intensity projection images with *z*-stack of the immunostaining images of specimens cultured with rhIGF1 at concentrations of 0 and 5 μg/ml. **(E,F)** No significant loss of inner hair cell (IHC) or spiral ganglion neuron (SGN) was found with student's *t*-test ($p = 0.578$ for IHC and $p = 0.133$ for SGN). Scale bars: 10 μm. Data are expressed as mean (digits at the top of each bar) ± SD. The digits at the bottom of each bar represent the sample number.

REFERENCES

Allahdadi, K. J., de Santana, T. A., Santos, G. C., Azevedo, C. M., Mota, R. A., Nonaka, C. K., et al. (2019). IGF-1 overexpression improves mesenchymal stem cell survival and promotes neurological recovery after spinal cord injury. *Stem Cell Res. Ther.* 10:146. doi: 10.1186/s13287-019-1223-z

Becker, L., Schnee, M. E., Niwa, M., Sun, W., Maxeiner, S., Talaei, S., et al. (2018). The presynaptic ribbon maintains vesicle populations at the hair cell afferent fiber synapse. *eLife* 12:e30241. doi: 10.7554/eLife.30241

Bharadwaj, H. M., Verhulst, S., Shaheen, L., Liberman, M. C., and Shinn-Cunningham, B. G. (2014). Cochlear neuropathy and the coding of supra-threshold sound. *Front. Syst. Neurosci.* 8:26. doi: 10.3389/fnsys.2014.00026

Camarero, G., Avendano, C., Fernandez-Moreno, C., Villar, A., Contreras, J., de Pablo, F., et al. (2001). Delayed inner ear maturation and neuronal loss in postnatal IGF-1-deficient mice. *J. Neurosci.* 21, 7630–7641. doi: 10.1523/JNEUROSCI.21-19-07630.2001

Camarero, G., Villar, M. A., Contreras, J., Fernández-Moreno, C., Pichel, J. G., Avendaño, C., et al. (2002). Cochlear abnormalities in insulin-like growth factor-1 mouse mutants. *Hear. Res.* 170, 2–11. doi: 10.1016/S0378-5955(02)00447-1

Coate, T. M., Scott, M. K., and Gurjar, M. (2019). Current concepts in cochlear ribbon synapse formation. *Synapse* 73:e22087. doi: 10.1002/syn.22087

Fogarty, M. J., Hammond, L. A., Kanjhan, R., Bellingham, M. C., and Noakes, P. G. (2013). A method for the three-dimensional reconstruction of Neurobiotin™-filled neurons and the location of their synaptic inputs. *Front. Neural. Circuits* 7:153. doi: 10.3389/fncir.2013.00153

Fujiwara, T., Hato, N., Nakagawa, T., Tabata, Y., Yoshida, T., Komobuchi, H., et al. (2008). Insulin-like growth factor 1 treatment *via* hydrogels rescues cochlear hair cells from ischemic injury. *Neuroreport* 19, 1585–1588. doi: 10.1097/WNR.0b013e328311ca4b

Hayashi, Y., Yamamoto, N., Nakagawa, T., and Ito, J. (2013). Insulin-like growth factor 1 inhibits hair cell apoptosis and promotes the cell cycle of supporting cells by activating different downstream cascades after pharmacological hair cell injury in neonatal mice. *Mol. Cell. Neurosci.* 56, 29–38. doi: 10.1016/j.mcn.2013.03.003

Hayashi, Y., Yamamoto, N., Nakagawa, T., Omori, K., and Ito, J. (2017). Activation of IGF1 signaling in the cochlea induces the transcription of its mediators during the protection of cochlear hair cells against aminoglycoside. *Otol. Neurotol.* 38, 278–282. doi: 10.1097/mao.0000000000001276

Hu, N., Rutherford, M. A., and Green, S. H. (2020). Protection of cochlear synapses from noise-induced excitotoxic trauma by blockade of Ca^{2+}-permeable AMPA receptors. *Proc. Natl. Acad. Sci. U S A* 117, 3828–3838. doi: 10.1073/pnas.1914247117

Hudspeth, A. J. (1997). How hearing happens. *Neuron* 19, 947–950. doi: 10.1016/s0896-6273(00)80385-2

Iwai, K., Nakagawa, T., Endo, T., Matsuoka, Y., Kita, T., Kim, T.-S., et al. (2006). Cochlear protection by local insulin-like growth factor-1 application using biodegradable hydrogel. *Laryngoscope* 116, 529–533. doi: 10.1097/01.mlg.0000200791.77819.eb

Jenkins, P. J., and Bustin, S. A. (2004). Evidence for a link between IGF-I and cancer. *Eur. J. Endocrinol.* 151, S17–S22. doi: 10.1530/eje.0.151s017

Kujawa, S. G., and Liberman, M. C. (2009). Adding insult to injury: cochlear nerve degeneration after "temporary" noise-induced hearing loss. *J. Neurosci.* 29, 14077–14085. doi: 10.1523/jneurosci.2845-09.2009

Landi, S., Ciucci, F., Maffei, L., Berardi, N., and Cenni, M. C. (2009). Setting the pace for retinal development: environmental enrichment acts through insulin-like growth factor 1 and brain-derived neurotrophic factor. *J. Neurosci.* 29, 10809–10819. doi: 10.1523/JNEUROSCI.1857-09.2009

Lee, K. Y., Nakagawa, T., Okano, T., Hori, R., Ono, K., Tabata, Y., et al. (2007). Novel therapy for hearing loss: delivery of insulin-like growth factor 1 to the cochlea using gelatin hydrogel. *Otol. Neurotol.* 28, 976–981. doi: 10.1097/MAO.0b013e31811f40db

Li, S., Hang, L., and Ma, Y. (2016). FGF22 protects hearing function from gentamycin ototoxicity by maintaining ribbon synapse number. *Hear. Res.* 332, 39–45. doi: 10.1016/j.heares.2015.11.011

Liberman, L. D., and Liberman, M. C. (2016). Postnatal maturation of auditory-nerve heterogeneity, as seen in spatial gradients of synapse morphology in the inner hair cell area. *Hear. Res.* 339, 12–22. doi: 10.1016/j.heares.2016.06.002

Liu, K., Jiang, X., Shi, C., Shi, L., Yang, B., Shi, L., et al. (2013). Cochlear inner hair cell ribbon synapse is the primary target of ototoxic aminoglycoside stimuli. *Mol. Neurobiol.* 48, 647–654. doi: 10.1007/s12035-013-8454-2

Meltser, I., Cederroth, C. R., Basinou, V., Savelyev, S., Lundkvist, G. S., and Canlon, B. (2014). TrkB-mediated protection against circadian sensitivity to noise trauma in the murine cochlea. *Curr. Biol.* 24, 658–663. doi: 10.1016/j.cub.2014.01.047

Meyer, A. C., Frank, T., Khimich, D., Hoch, G., Riedel, D., Chapochnikov, N. M., et al. (2009). Tuning of synapse number, structure and function in the cochlea. *Nat. Neurosci.* 12, 444–453. doi: 10.1038/nn.2293

Michanski, S., Smaluch, K., Steyer, A. M., Chakrabarti, R., Setz, C., Oestreicher, D., et al. (2019). Mapping developmental maturation of inner hair cell ribbon synapses in the apical mouse cochlea. *Proc. Natl. Acad. Sci. U S A* 116, 6415–6424. doi: 10.1073/pnas.1812029116

Nakagawa, T., Kumakawa, K., Usami, S.-I., Hato, N., Tabuchi, K., Takahashi, M., et al. (2014). A randomized controlled clinical trial of topical insulin-like growth factor-1 therapy for sudden deafness refractory to systemic corticosteroid treatment. *BMC Med.* 12:219. doi: 10.1186/s12916-014-0219-x

Nakagawa, T., Sakamoto, T., Hiraumi, H., Kikkawa, Y. S., Yamamoto, N., Hamaguchi, K., et al. (2010). Topical insulin-like growth factor 1 treatment using gelatin hydrogels for glucocorticoid-resistant sudden sensorineural hearing loss: a prospective clinical trial. *BMC Med.* 8:76. doi: 10.1186/1741-7015-8-76

Nakagawa, T., Yamamoto, M., Kumakawa, K., Usami, S., Hato, N., Tabuchi, K., et al. (2016). Prognostic impact of salvage treatment on hearing recovery in patients with sudden sensorineural hearing loss refractory to systemic corticosteroids: a retrospective observational study. *Auris Nasus Larynx* 43, 489–494. doi: 10.1016/j.anl.2015.12.004

Nelson, B. S., Springer, R. C., and Daniel, J. M. (2014). Antagonism of brain insulin-like growth factor-1 receptors blocks estradiol effects on memory and levels of hippocampal synaptic proteins in ovariectomized rats. *Psychopharmacology* 231, 899–907. doi: 10.1007/s00213-013-3310-7

Okano, T., Xuan, S., and Kelley, M. W. (2011). Insulin-like growth factor signaling regulates the timing of sensory cell differentiation in the mouse cochlea. *J. Neurosci.* 31, 18104–18118. doi: 10.1523/JNEUROSCI.3619-11.2011

Pietrzkowski, Z., Wernicke, D., Porcu, P., Jameson, B. A., and Baserga, R. (1992). Inhibition of cellular proliferation by peptide analogues of insulin-like growth factor 1. *Cancer Res.* 52, 6447–6451.

Riquelme, R., Cediel, R., Contreras, J., Rodriguez-de la Rosa, L., Murillo-Cuesta, S., Hernandez-Sanchez, C., et al. (2010). A comparative study of age-related hearing loss in wild type and insulin-like growth factor I deficient mice. *Front. Neuroanat.* 4:27. doi: 10.3389/fnana.2010.00027

Safieddine, S., El-Amraoui, A., and Petit, C. (2012). The auditory hair cell ribbon synapse: from assembly to function. *Annu. Rev. Neurosci.* 35, 509–528. doi: 10.1146/annurev-neuro-061010-113705

Sanchez-Calderon, H., Rodriguez-de la Rosa, L., Milo, M., Pichel, J. G., Holley, M., and Varela-Nieto, I. (2010). RNA microarray analysis in prenatal mouse cochlea reveals novel IGF-I target genes: implication of MEF2 and FOXM1 transcription factors. *PLoS One* 5:e8699. doi: 10.1371/journal.pone.0008699

Suzuki, J., Corfas, G., and Liberman, M. C. (2016). Round-window delivery of neurotrophin 3 regenerates cochlear synapses after acoustic overexposure. *Sci. Rep.* 6:24907. doi: 10.1038/srep24907

Vandenberg, L. N., Colborn, T., Hayes, T. B., Heindel, J. J., Jacobs, D. R. Jr., Lee, D.-H., et al. (2012). Hormones and endocrine-disrupting chemicals: low-dose effects and nonmonotonic dose responses. *Endocr. Rev.* 33, 378–455. doi: 10.1210/er.2011-1050

Varela-Nieto, I., Hartl, M., Gorospe, I., and Leon, Y. (2007). Anti-apoptotic actions of insulin-like growth factors: lessons from development and implications in neoplastic cell transformation. *Curr. Pharm. Des.* 13, 687–703. doi: 10.2174/138161207780249164

Viana, L. M., O'Malley, J. T., Burgess, B. J., Jones, D. D., Oliveira, C. A., Santos, F., et al. (2015). Cochlear neuropathy in human presbycusis: confocal analysis of hidden hearing loss in post-mortem tissue. *Hear. Res.* 327, 78–88. doi: 10.1016/j.heares.2015.04.014

Wagner, E. L., and Shin, J.-B. (2019). Mechanisms of hair cell damage and repair. *Trends Neurosci.* 42, 414–424. doi: 10.1016/j.tins.2019.03.006

Wan, G., Gómez-Casati, M. E., Gigliello, A. R., Liberman, M. C., and Corfas, G. (2014). Neurotrophin-3 regulates ribbon synapse density in the cochlea and induces synapse regeneration after acoustic trauma. *eLife* 3:e03564. doi: 10.7554/eLife.03564

Wang, Q., and Green, S. H. (2011). Functional role of neurotrophin-3 in synapse regeneration by spiral ganglion neurons on inner hair cells after excitotoxic trauma *in vitro*. *J. Neurosci.* 31, 7938–7949. doi: 10.1523/jneurosci.1434-10.2011

World Health Organization (2018). *Deafness and Hearing Loss.* World Health Organization Fact Sheets. Available online at: https://www.who.int/en/news-room/fact-sheets/detail/deafness-and-hearing-loss

Yamahara, K., Nakagawa, T., Ito, J., Kinoshita, K., Omori, K., and Yamamoto, N. (2017). Netrin 1 mediates protective effects exerted by insulin-like growth factor 1 on cochlear hair cells. *Neuropharmacology* 119, 26–39. doi: 10.1016/j.neuropharm.2017.03.032

Yamahara, K., Asaka, N., Kita, T., Kishimoto, I., Matsunaga, M., Yamamoto, N., et al. (2019). Insulin-like growth factor 1 promotes cochlear synapse regeneration after excitotoxic trauma *in vitro*. *Hear. Res.* 374, 5–12. doi: 10.1016/j.heares.2019.01.008

Yamahara, K., Nishimura, K., Ogita, H., Ito, J., Nakagawa, T., Furuta, I., et al. (2018). Hearing preservation at low frequencies by insulin-like growth factor 1 in a guinea pig model of cochlear implantation. *Hear. Res.* 368, 92–108. doi: 10.1016/j.heares.2018.07.004

Zuccotti, A., Kuhn, S., Johnson, S. L., Franz, C., Singer, W., Hecker, D., et al. (2012). Lack of brain-derived neurotrophic factor hampers inner hair cell synapse physiology, but protects against noise-induced hearing loss. *J. Neurosci.* 32, 8545–8553. doi: 10.1523/JNEUROSCI.1247-12.2012

10

A Novel Small Molecule Neurotrophin-3 Analogue Promotes Inner Ear Neurite Outgrowth and Synaptogenesis *In vitro*

Judith S. Kempfle [1,2†], ***Marlon V. Duro*** [3†], ***Andrea Zhang*** [1†], ***Carolina D. Amador*** [3], ***Richard Kuang*** [1], ***Ryan Lu*** [1], ***Boris A. Kashemirov*** [3], ***Albert S. Edge*** [1], ***Charles E. McKenna*** [3*] ***and David H. Jung*** [1*]

[1]*Department of Otolaryngology, Massachusetts Eye and Ear Infirmary, Harvard Medical School, Boston, MA, United States,* [2]*Department of Otolaryngology, University Medical Center Tübingen, Tübingen, Germany,* [3]*Department of Chemistry, University of Southern California, Los Angeles, CA, United States*

Correspondence:
Charles E. McKenna
mckenna@usc.edu
David H. Jung
david_jung@meei.harvard.edu

Sensorineural hearing loss is irreversible and is associated with the loss of spiral ganglion neurons (SGNs) and sensory hair cells within the inner ear. Improving spiral ganglion neuron (SGN) survival, neurite outgrowth, and synaptogenesis could lead to significant gains for hearing-impaired patients. There has therefore been intense interest in the use of neurotrophic factors in the inner ear to promote both survival of SGNs and re-wiring of sensory hair cells by surviving SGNs. Neurotrophin-3 (NT-3) and brain-derived neurotrophic factor (BDNF) represent the primary neurotrophins in the inner ear during development and throughout adulthood, and have demonstrated potential for SGN survival and neurite outgrowth. We have pioneered a hybrid molecule approach to maximize SGN stimulation *in vivo*, in which small molecule analogues of neurotrophins are linked to bisphosphonates, which in turn bind to cochlear bone. We have previously shown that a small molecule BDNF analogue coupled to risedronate binds to bone matrix and promotes SGN neurite outgrowth and synaptogenesis *in vitro*. Because NT-3 has been shown in a variety of contexts to have a greater regenerative capacity in the cochlea than BDNF, we sought to develop a similar approach for NT-3. 1Aa is a small molecule analogue of NT-3 that has been shown to activate cells through TrkC, the NT-3 receptor, although its activity on SGNs has not previously been described. Herein we describe the design and synthesis of 1Aa and a covalent conjugate of 1Aa with risedronate, Ris-1Aa. We demonstrate that both 1Aa and Ris-1Aa stimulate neurite outgrowth in SGN cultures at a significantly higher level compared to controls. Ris-1Aa maintained its neurotrophic activity when bound to hydroxyapatite, the primary mineral component of bone. Both 1Aa and Ris-1Aa promote significant synaptic regeneration in cochlear explant cultures, and both 1Aa and Ris-1Aa appear to act at least partly through TrkC. Our results provide the first evidence that a small molecule analogue of NT-3 can stimulate SGNs and promote regeneration of synapses between SGNs and inner hair cells. Our findings support the promise of hydroxyapatite-targeting bisphosphonate conjugation as a novel strategy to deliver neurotrophic agents to SGNs encased within cochlear bone.

Keywords: inner ear, regeneration, synaptopathy, neurotrophin-3, bisphosphonate, small molecule, hidden hearing loss, sensorineural hearing loss

INTRODUCTION

Sensorineural hearing loss (SNHL), is associated with loss of cochlear outer hair cells (OHCs), inner hair cells (IHCs), and spiral ganglion neurons (SGNs; Schuknecht and Gacek, 1993; Wu et al., 2019, 2020). The afferent ribbon synapse between IHCs and SGNs appears to be the element most sensitive to noise in rodents and non-human primates (Kujawa and Liberman, 2006, 2009; Valero et al., 2017). In rodents, such loss is associated with an over-compensation in central gain (Chambers et al., 2016). Although the clinical consequences of ribbon synapse loss in human patients remain under investigation (Bramhall et al., 2014), it is therefore reasonable to suspect that such loss could be linked with other symptoms, including tinnitus, hyperacusis, and difficulty hearing in background noise (Auerbach et al., 2014; Bharadwaj et al., 2015; Chambers et al., 2016; Liberman and Kujawa, 2017).

After a synaptic loss, the cell bodies of IHCs and SGNs remain present for months in mice and, potentially, for decades in humans (Sergeyenko et al., 2013; Viana et al., 2015; Wu et al., 2019). The prolonged survival of these cell bodies suggests a therapeutic window for exogenous neurotrophic treatment to promote synapse regeneration. Two major inner ear neurotrophins, neurotrophin-3 (NT-3) and brain-derived neurotrophic factor (BDNF) are essential for wiring during SGN development and for SGN survival postnatally (Ernfors et al., 1995; Bianchi et al., 1996; Silos-Santiago et al., 1997; Stankovic et al., 2004; Green et al., 2012). Postnatally, BDNF and NT-3 are mainly expressed in supporting cells and hair cells and interact with their respective tropomyosin receptor kinase receptors (Trks), TrkB for BDNF, and TrkC for NT-3, which are expressed by SGNs. While BDNF and NT-3 are expressed in the adult cochlea (Bailey and Green, 2014), their endogenous levels do not appear to be sufficient to induce synaptic regeneration following noise damage (Kujawa and Liberman, 2006; Valero et al., 2017) or to preserve synapses during aging (Sergeyenko et al., 2013).

An intense investigation has therefore focused on delivering exogenous neurotrophic activities to the inner ear as a treatment for hearing loss due to ribbon synapse or SGN deficiency. Experiments using genetically modified mice suggest that overexpression of NT-3, but not BDNF, improves cochlear responses and regenerates ribbon synapses after noise damage (Wan et al., 2014). As with any inner ear therapy, however, neurotrophin entry into the labyrinth presents a barrier. A variety of methods have therefore been utilized to directly introduce neurotrophin protein into the cochlea (Noushi et al., 2005; Evans et al., 2009). Expression of neurotrophin protein within the cochlea *via* a viral vector, which similarly requires a labyrinthotomy, has also been reported (Ramekers et al., 2015; Chen et al., 2018; Akil et al., 2019; Hashimoto et al., 2019). However, intracochlear viral overexpression of neurotrophin has also been found to be ototoxic, potentially limiting this approach (Fukui and Raphael, 2013; Akil et al., 2019; Hashimoto et al., 2019). With respect to a non-cochleoinvasive approach, direct application of NT-3 protein on the round window membrane has been reported, with variable results (Sly et al., 2016; Suzuki et al., 2016). In this regard, transport across the RWM is highly variable, and transit of proteins in particular across the RWM is thought to be inefficient (Goycoolea, 2001).

Small molecules that mimic neurotrophin function and act on Trk receptors have therefore been recognized for their potential in preventing neural cell death and supporting neural survival (Lewis et al., 2006; Jang et al., 2007; Lin et al., 2007; Price et al., 2007). With respect to local cochlear delivery, such compounds could offer a promising alternative by promoting diffusion across the RWM, resulting in higher concentration within the perilymph and eliminating the hearing and balance risk associated with a labyrinthotomy (Hao and Li, 2019; Nyberg et al., 2019). Agonists of TrkB and TrkC have been identified, including 7,8-dihydroxyflavone (DHF) for TrkB (Bai et al., 2010; Jang et al., 2010), and 1Aa for TrkC (Zaccaro et al., 2005; Peleshok and Saragovi, 2006). The neurotrophic effect of DHF has been extensively studied in other contexts. DHF treatment protects against neural degeneration in various disease models and promotes neurogenesis in the hippocampus (He et al., 2016; Garcia-Diaz Barriga et al., 2017; Stagni et al., 2017; Aytan et al., 2018). With respect to SGNs, we and others have demonstrated that DHF has neurotrophic effects on SGNs leading to improved neuron survival, axon outgrowth, and synaptic regeneration *in vitro* (Jang et al., 2010; Kramer et al., 2017; Kempfle et al., 2018) and *in vivo* (Fernandez et al., 2021). 1Aa was first identified in a screen of small molecule TrkC agonist peptidomimetics (Zaccaro et al., 2005). However, the neurotrophic activity of a small molecule NT-3 analogue on SGNs has not previously been described.

To promote cochlear drug delivery, we have developed a platform aimed at the exploitation of cochlear bone as a depot for prolonged neurotrophic stimulation of SGNs. In this regard, we have previously demonstrated that a fluorescently-labeled bisphosphonate can cross the RWM in a non-ototoxic manner and bind cochlear bone (Kang et al., 2015). We then described the synthesis of a hybrid small molecule, Ris-DHF, that linked DHF to risedronate (Ris), a bisphosphonate with high bone mineral affinity. Ris-DHF demonstrated strong neurotrophic activity on SGNs, both when free and when bound to hydroxyapatite bone matrix (Kempfle et al., 2018). Here, we utilize similar synthetic chemistry to conjugate a bisphosphonate to a small molecule NT-3 analogue. We synthesized the small molecule TrkC agonist 1Aa (Pattarawarapan et al., 2002; Lee et al., 2004; Zaccaro et al., 2005) and a conjugate of Ris and 1Aa (Ris-1Aa) to study their ability to promote neurite outgrowth and ribbon synapse regeneration *in vitro*.

MATERIALS AND METHODS

General Chemistry

Dry dichloromethane (DCM) was prepared by distillation over CaH_2. Anh. methanol (MeOH) and *N,N*-dimethylformamide (DMF) were purchased from Merck. 2,6-Lutidine and *N,N*-diisopropylethylamine (DIEA) were distilled over KOH. 2-Fluoro-5-nitrobenzoyl chloride (Jackman et al., 1990), 4-({[(9*H*-fluoren-9-yl)methoxy]carbonylamino})butanoic acid (Fmoc-GABA-OH; Aronov et al., 2004), and 1-(3-amino-2-hydroxypropyl)-3-(2-hydroxy-2, 2-diphosphonoethyl)pyridin-1-ium (RIS-linker; Kempfle et al., 2018) were prepared following literature procedures. All other reagents and solvents were obtained from commercial sources and used without further purification. Reactions on solid support were performed in a fritted polypropylene syringe (5 ml, Torviq) at room temperature using a manual control shaking apparatus (VWR OS-500) and standard Fmoc chemistry on Rink amide resin [(4-(2′,4′-dimethoxyphenyl-Fmoc-aminomethyl)phenoxy resin, Advanced ChemTech, SA5030, 100–200 mesh, 0.5 mmol/g)]. Removal of the Fmoc group was monitored by UV spectroscopy (288 and 299 nm) and capping of primary NH_2 groups was monitored by the Kaiser test (ninhydrin). General purification and characterization procedures were done as described previously (Kempfle et al., 2018).

Preparation of Template Compound

4-(Azidomethyl)-2-nitrobenzoic Acid (1)

To a solution of 4-(bromomethyl)-3-nitrobenzoic acid (502 mg, 1.93 mmol) in anh. DMF (9.6 ml) was slowly added sodium azide (1 equiv, 125 mg) and reacted at room temperature overnight, under nitrogen atmosphere. The crude reaction mixture was then extracted with ethyl acetate (2 × 20 ml) and 0.1 M aq. HCl (2 × 20 ml). The organic solvent was dried over anh. $MgSO_4$ and evaporated under reduced pressure. The desired azide **1**, an orange oil, was obtained, with a quantitative yield, and used immediately in the next step without further purification (**Supplementary Figures 2–5**). ^{1}H NMR (400 MHz, methanol-d_4) δ 8.55 (s, ^{1}H), 8.25 (d, J = 8.1 Hz, ^{1}H), 7.78 (d, J = 8.0 Hz, ^{1}H), 4.89 (s, 2H). ^{13}C NMR (101 MHz, Methanol-d_4) δ 165.40, 147.69, 135.86, 134.05, 131.83, 130.43, 125.59, 51.36. MS (ESI) *m/z*: $[M-H]^-$ calcd for $C_8H_5N_4O_4^-$ 221.0; found: 221.2.

4-(Aminomethyl)-3-nitrobenzoic Acid (2)

The azide **1** (1.93 mmol) was dissolved in 1.6 ml of water and 5.1 ml of THF and triphenylphosphine (1.4 equiv, 709 mg) was slowly added to the reaction mixture and reacted at room temperature overnight (Marinzi et al., 2004; Xu et al., 2011). The solvent was evaporated to dryness, and the residue was re-dissolved in basic water (pH adjusted to 11 with aq. NH_4OH) and the solution was centrifuged. The solution was evaporated to dryness yielding 192 mg (50% yield) of the desired benzylamine **2** (**Supplementary Figures 6, 7**), which was used in the next step without further purification. ^{1}H NMR (600 MHz, D_2O) δ 8.34 (s, ^{1}H), 7.99 (d, J = 8.0 Hz, ^{1}H), 7.51 (d, J = 8.0 Hz, ^{1}H), 3.91 (s, 2H). MS (ESI) *m/z*: $[M-H]^-$ calcd for $C_8H_7N_2O_4^-$ 195.1; found: 195.1

This method is a significant improvement from the one described in the literature (Lee et al., 2004) due to the absence of side products. When 4-(bromomethyl)-3-nitrobenzoic acid reacts with liquid ammonia in ethanol, yielding amine **2**, the alcohol counterpart is formed as a byproduct. This side product is believed to be carried out over the course of the synthetic route, since it is very difficult to separate it from the desired amine, and it could potentially be carried out into the solid phase reactions. Therefore, the method described here *via* an intermediate azide **1** confers a much cleaner method.

4-({[(4-Methylphenyl)diphenylmethyl]amino}methyl)-3-nitrobenzoic Acid (3)

A reported procedure (Lee et al., 2004) was adapted as follows: in a round bottom flask, 4-methyltrityl chloride (2.9 g, 10.2 mmol) was dissolved in a mixture of anh. chloroform (20 ml) and anh. DMF (10 ml) and the mixture was stirred vigorously. The benzylamine **2** (2.0 g, 10.2 mmol) was added to the reaction mixture at room temperature and the reaction mixture was stirred for 30 min. Distilled and anh. triethylamine (2 equiv, 2.8 ml) was added dropwise. The reaction progress was monitored by TLC. After a total of 130 min the reaction mixture was evaporated to dryness. After automated flash chromatography (40 g silica, hexane to ethyl acetate, then to methanol, **Supplementary Figure 8**), the pure desired protected amine **3** was obtained (1.4 g of 31% yield, **Supplementary Figures 9, 10**). ^{1}H NMR (500 MHz, acetone-d_6) δ 8.49 (s, ^{1}H), 8.40–8.34 (m, 2H), 7.56 (d, J = 9.2 Hz, 4H), 7.43 (d, J = 8.3 Hz, 2H), 7.31 (t, J = 7.2 Hz, 4H), 7.21 (t, J = 7.3 Hz, 2H), 7.13 (d, J = 8.5 Hz, 2H), 3.69 (s, 2H), 2.29 (s, 3H). MS (ESI) *m/z*: $[M-H]^-$ calcd for $C_{28}H_{23}N_2O_4^-$ 451.2; found: 451.2

3-Amino-4-({[(4-methylphenyl)diphenylmethyl]amino}methyl)benzoic Acid (4)

Following a procedure reported in the literature (Lee et al., 2004): in a Schlenk flask, the protected amine **3** (700 mg, 1.55 mmol), ethyl acetate (18 ml), and platinum dioxide (70 mg, 20 mol%) were combined and, under nitrogen atmosphere, the reaction mixture was degassed by using the freeze-pump-thaw method (3×). The atmosphere in the flask was changed to hydrogen by placing an H_2-filled balloon, connected to a needle which was inserted directly into the solution. The hydrogenation reaction was left stirring for 24 h at 25°C. The reaction progress was monitored by mass spectrometry. The crude material was then filtered with kieselguhr and the filtrate was evaporated under reduced pressure. The desired product **4** was obtained with a quantitative yield (655 mg, **Supplementary Figures 11, 12**) and was used in the next step without further purification. Spectral data agree with those previously reported. ^{1}H NMR (600 MHz, methanol-d_4) δ 7.48 (d, J = 8.2 Hz, 4H), 7.36–7.33 (m, 3H), 7.29–7.25 (m, 5H), 7.20–7.15 (m, 3H), 7.10 (d, J = 8.1 Hz, 2H),

3.35 (s, 2H), 2.29 (s, 3H). MS (ESI) m/z: $[M-H]^-$ calcd for $C_{28}H_{25}N_2O_2^-$ 421.1 found: 421.3.

Assembly of 1Aa on Solid Phase

Coupling of Template Compound to the Rink Amide Resin

The steps leading up to the macrocyclization were adapted from procedures in the literature (Pattarawarapan et al., 2002; Lee et al., 2004; Zaccaro et al., 2005). The Rink amide resin (0.09 mmol, 0.5 mmol/g, 180 mg) was swollen overnight in dry DCM (1.8 ml) in a plastic fritted syringe. To remove the Fmoc protective group, the resin was treated with a solution of 20% (v/v) piperidine in anh. DMF (1.5 ml) for 1.5 h, and then a fresh portion of the same solution (1.5 ml) was added for another h. The resin was washed with solvent following this sequence (1.5 ml each): DMF, MeOH, DMF, MeOH, DCM (2×), MeOH (2×), and DCM (3×). The beads were then drained and carried over to the next step. A solution of template compound **4** (3 equiv); HBTU (3 equiv, 102 mg); HOBt (3 equiv, 36 mg) and DIEA (5 equiv, 79 μl) in anh. DMF (1.5 ml) was added to the fritted syringe carrying the rink resin, and the syringe was gently shaken for 2 h. The solvents were drained, and the resin (**5**) washed.

Incorporation of Fmoc-Lys (Boc)-OH

The reaction mixture with **5** was treated with a solution of Fmoc-Lys-(Boc)-OH (4 equiv, 169 mg), PyBrOP (6 equiv, 252 mg) and distilled and anh. 2, 6-lutidine (15 equiv, 157 μl) in dry DCM (1.5 ml) and it was left shaking gently overnight. Then, the solvents of the original crude material were drained, the beads were washed and the Fmoc group cleaved (2 × 1.5 ml, 1 h each turn). The resin (**6**) was then washed as described above.

Incorporation of Fmoc-Ile-OH

Resin **6** was treated with a solution of Fmoc-Ile-OH (3 equiv, 95 mg), DIC (3 equiv, 42 μl); HOBt (3 equiv, 36 mg) and anh. DIEA (5 equiv, 79 μl) in 4:1 (v/v) anh. DCM/DMF (1.5 ml) and the vessel was gently shaken for 4 h. The solvents were drained, the beads were washed and the Fmoc group was cleaved with 20% (v/v) piperidine in anh. DMF (2 × 1.5 ml, 10 min first, then 15 min). The resin (**7**) was then washed as described above.

Incorporation of 2-fluoro-5-nitrobenzoyl Chloride

Resin **7** was treated with a solution of 2-fluoro-5-nitrobenzoyl chloride (3 equiv, 55 mg) and anh. and distilled DIEA (3 equiv, 47 μl) in dry DCM (1.5 ml) for 50 min. The reaction was monitored by checking the color of the solution after using the ninhydrin test. The solvents were drained, and the beads were washed. The Mtt protecting group was removed by treatment with a solution of 1% TFA and 5% TIS in DCM (2 ml portions, eight times, or until the yellow color disappeared completely). Lastly, the resin (**8**) was washed as described above.

Macrocyclization to 1Aa-NO₂

Intermediate **8** was treated with a suspension of K_2CO_3 (10 equiv, 124 mg) in anh. DMF (2 ml) at 25°C, with gentle shaking, for 2 d. To monitor the cyclization, a small portion of beads were isolated, washed with water, dried under vacuum for 1 h, and then cleaved from the resin with 1 ml of 18:1:1 TFA/TIS/H_2O for 2 h. The solvent was then evaporated under reduced pressure. LC-MS analysis was then performed on the residue [column: Waters Xterra analytical column, 4.6 × 150 mm; solvent system: A—1% formic acid in water, B—0.1% formic acid in MeCN; program: gradient of 0–100%B over 15 min; flow rate: 1.0 ml/min; UV detection at 254 and 280 nm; t_r = 8.1 min, **Supplementary Figure 13**]. After completion of the cyclization, the resin (**9**) was washed as described above and carried over to the next step. MS (ESI) *m/z*: $[M + H]^+$ calcd for $C_{27}H_{36}N_7O_6^+$ 554.3, found 554.4.

Nitro Group Reduction

9, 13 was treated with 1.5 ml of 2 M $SnCl_2{\bullet}2H_2O$ in anh. DMF for 22 h with gentle shaking. The resin (**10**) was washed with water (3 × 1.5 ml) before washing as above, then dried under vacuum for 1 h and carried over to the next step.

(12S,15S)-20-Amino-12-(4-aminobutyl)-15-(butan-2-yl)-11,14,17-trioxo-2,10,13,16-tetraazatricyclo[16.4.0.0^{4,9}] docosa-1(18),4(9), 5,7,19,21-hexaene-7-carboxamide (1Aa, 11)

A solution of 18:1:1 TFA/TIS/H_2O was added to the syringe containing **10** and the mixture was gently shaken for 2 h. The solvent was drained, and the resin was rinsed with water (3×) and ethyl ether (3×). The solution was evaporated to dryness. The final product (1Aa, **11**) was purified by semi-preparative reversed-phase HPLC (column: Hamilton PRP-1, 10 × 250 mm, 7 μm; solvent system: A—5% MeCN with 0.1% formic acid, B—10% MeCN with 0.1% formic acid; program: 0%B for 20 min, 100%B for 15 min; flow rate: 3.5 ml/min; UV detection at 280 nm; t_r = 25.9 min, **Supplementary Figure 14**) to obtain the title compound (7.4 mg, 16% overall yield, **Supplementary Figure 16**), with an estimated purity of 90%. The purity was confirmed by LC–MS analysis (column: Waters Xterra analytical column, 4.6 × 150 mm; solvent system: A—2% MeCN with 0.1% formic acid, B—10% MeCN with 0.1% formic acid; program: 0%B for 10 min, 100%B for 15 min; flow rate: 1.0 ml/min; UV detection at 254 and 280 nm; t_r = 25.9 min, **Supplementary Figure 15**). ^1H NMR (400 MHz, D_2O) δ 7.95 (s, ^1H), 7.79–7.73 (m, 2H), 7.28 (s, ^1H), 7.21 (d, *J* = 8.6 Hz, ^1H), 7.10 (d, *J* = 8.8 Hz, ^1H), 4.36–4.29 (m, 2H), 4.21–4.14 (m, ^1H), 4.02–3.94 (m, ^1H), 3.64–3.56 (m, ^1H), 3.03 (t, *J* = 7.6 Hz, 2H), 2.05–1.91 (m, 2H), 1.85–1.64 (m, 6H), 1.04 (d, *J* = 6.7 Hz, 3H), 1.03–0.93 (m, 3H). MS (ESI) *m/z*: $[M + H]^+$ calcd for $C_{27}H_{38}N_7O_4^-$ 524.3; found: 524.3.

Synthesis of Boc-1Aa-linker

Incorporation of Fmoc-GABA-OH

The synthesis of resin-immobilized 1Aa (**10**) was scaled up using 320 mg (0.16 mmol) of starting resin. **10** was then treated with a mixture of Fmoc-GABA-OH (156.1 mg, 3 equiv), HBTU (182.0 mg, 3 equiv), and DIEA (110 μl, 5 equiv) in anh. DMF (2.5 ml) for 15 h. After washing the resin following the above sequence, the Fmoc group was removed with 1:4 (v/v) piperidine/DMF (2 × 1.5 ml, 1 h each). The resin (**12**) was then washed as above.

Reaction With Succinic Anhydride

Resin **12** was treated with succinic anhydride (480.3 mg, 36 equiv) in anh. DMF (2.5 ml) for 21 h. The resin (**13**) was then washed as described above.

3-[(3-{[(12S,15S)-15-[(2S)-Butan-2-yl]-12-(4-{[(tert-butoxy)carbonyl]amino}butyl)-7-carbamoyl-11,14,17-trioxo-2,10,13,16-tetraazatricyclo [16.4.0.0^{4,9}]docosa-1(22),4(9),5,7,18,20-hexaen-20-yl]carbamoyl}propyl)carbamoyl]propanoic acid (Boc-1Aa-linker, 14)

13 was treated with 18:1:1 (v/v) TFA/TIS/H_2O (3 ml) for 3 h. The resin beads were removed by filtration and the yellow filtrate was evaporated under reduced pressure, leaving an oily residue which was treated with cold diethyl ether (5 ml), causing precipitation of a yellow solid. After centrifugation, the precipitate was washed with cold diethyl ether (2 × 5 ml), then dried under vacuum. The crude cleavage product was obtained as a yellow solid (39.5 mg) and used in the following step without further purification. MS (ESI) *m/z* [M-H]$^-$: calcd for $C_{35}H_{47}N_8O_8^-$ 707.4; found 707.5.

The product was dissolved in 1:2 (v/v) anh. DMF/MeOH (9.0 ml) and to the solution was added di(*tert*-butyl) dicarbonate (74 μl, 2 equiv) and TEA (22 μl, 1.1 equiv) with stirring. After stirring overnight at room temperature, the solution was then evaporated under reduced pressure. The residue was taken up in 2:1 DMF/water (2 ml), then centrifugated. The solution of crude product was purified by semi-preparative reversed-phase HPLC [column: Hamilton PRP-1, 21.2 × 250 mm, 7 μm; solvent system: A—20% MeCN, 50 mM TEAB (pH 7.8), B—75% MeCN, 50 mM TEAB (pH 7.8); program: 0%B for 5 min, gradient of 0–34%B over 30 min, then an isocratic hold at 100%B for 10 min; flow rate: 8 ml/min; UV detection at 260 nm; t_r = 27.4 min] to afford **14** as a light-yellow powder (26.8 mg, 20% from starting resin, **Supplementary Figures 17, 18**). ^{1}H NMR (400 MHz, DMSO-d_6) δ 9.70 (s, ^{1}H), 9.64 (s, ^{1}H), 8.33 (s, ^{1}H), 8.16 (d, *J* = 8.7 Hz, ^{1}H), 7.91 (s, ^{1}H), 7.85 (t, *J* = 5.5 Hz, ^{1}H), 7.68 (d, *J* = 7.4 Hz, ^{1}H), 7.56 (s, 2H), 7.48 (d, *J* = 2.5 Hz, ^{1}H), 7.41 (dd, *J* = 8.8, 2.5 Hz, ^{1}H), 7.30 (s, ^{1}H), 6.76 (d, *J* = 5.8 Hz, ^{1}H), 6.69 (d, *J* = 8.9 Hz, ^{1}H), 6.00 (br. s, ^{1}H), 4.64 (dd, *J* = 14.7, 6.4 Hz, ^{1}H), 4.35 (q, *J* = 6.8 Hz, ^{1}H), 4.20 (dd, *J* = 15.2, 3.3 Hz, ^{1}H), 3.95 (t, *J* = 9.2 Hz, ^{1}H), 3.04 (q, *J* = 6.7 Hz, 2H), 2.89 (q, *J* = 6.6 Hz, 2H), 2.39 (t, *J* = 6.9 Hz, 2H), 2.28 (t, *J* = 6.9 Hz, 2H), 2.23 (t, *J* = 7.4 Hz, 2H), 1.85–1.56 (m, 7H), 1.43–1.34 (m, 1^{1}H), 1.30–1.22 (m, 2H), 0.93–0.86 (m, 6H). MS (ESI) *m/z*: [M–H]$^-$ calcd for $C_{40}H_{55}N_8O_{10}^-$ 807.4; found 807.6.

Coupling to Ris-linker

Activation and Reaction With Ris-linker

To a solution of **14** (27.8 mg, 34 μmol) in anh. DMF (0.8 ml) was added TEA (4.2 μl, 2 equiv), followed by a freshly prepared 0.05 M solution of TSTU in anh. DMF (300 μl, 1 equiv). After stirring for 2 h at room temperature, the solution of the crude NHS ester intermediate **15**, MS (ESI) *m/z*: [M + Na]$^+$ calcd for $C_{44}H_{59}N_9O_{12}Na^+$ 928.4; found 928.6 was used directly in the next step.

The "magic-linker" procedure (Sun et al., 2016) was adapted to that step as follows: Ris-linker (**16**) (2× TEA salt, 14.0 mg, 2.5 equiv) was dissolved in water (1.2 ml) and the pH was set to 7.5 using Na_2CO_3. The DMF solution of the crude intermediate (**15**) was added to the aqueous Ris-linker solution dropwise with stirring and the pH of the solution was readjusted to 8.4 with Na_2CO_3. Stirring was continued for 3 h, then the mixture was centrifugated. The pellet was then taken up in 0.05 M TEAB (1:4 (v/v) MeCN/water, pH 7.6, 500 μl) and the mixture was centrifuged. The supernatants containing the crude product were filtered through a 0.45 μm syringe filter, then purified on a semi-preparative reversed-phase HPLC [column: Hamilton PRP-1, 10 × 250 mm, 7 μm; solvent system: A—20% MeCN, 50 mM TEAB (pH 7.8), B—75% MeCN, 50 mM TEAB (pH 7.8); program: 0%B for 5 min, gradient of 0–25%B over 20 min, then an isocratic hold at 60%B for 10 min; flow rate: 2.5 ml/min; UV detection at 260 nm; t_r = 24.8 min, **Supplementary Figure 19**] to yield the TEA salt (1.5×) of the conjugate (**17**) as a white powder (10.1 mg, 52% over 2 steps, **Supplementary Figures 20–22**). ^{1}H NMR (400 MHz, D_2O, pD 6.71) δ 8.76 (s, ^{1}H), 8.55 (d, *J* = 6.4 Hz, ^{1}H), 8.44 (d, *J* = 7.4 Hz, ^{1}H), 7.97 (s, ^{1}H), 7.85 (t, *J* = 6.9 Hz, ^{1}H), 7.73–7.63 (m, 2H), 7.45 (s, ^{1}H), 7.28 (d, *J* = 8.6 Hz, ^{1}H), 6.94 (d, *J* = 8.9 Hz, ^{1}H), 4.36–4.11 (m, 6H), 3.48–3.32 (m, 5H), 3.29–3.23 (m, 2H), 3.08 (t, *J* = 6.4 Hz, 2H), 2.59–2.48 (m, 4H), 2.41 (t, *J* = 6.9 Hz, 2H), 1.99–1.65 (m, 7H), 1.61–1.48 (m, 4H), 1.39 (s, 9H), 1.03 (d, *J* = 6.6 Hz, 3H), 0.97 (t, *J* = 7.3 Hz, 3H). ^{31}P NMR (162 MHz, D_2O) δ 16.25 (d, *J* = 25.9 Hz), 16.02 (d, *J* = 26.3 Hz). MS (ESI) *m/z*: [M–2H]$^-$ calcd for $C_{50}H_{71}N_{10}O_{17}P_2^{2-}$ 1145.5; found 1145.3.

1-(3-{3-[(3-{[(12S,15S)-15-[(2S)-Butan-2-yl]-12-(4-amino butyl)-7-carbamoyl-11,14,17-trioxo-2,10,13,16-tetraa zatricyclo[16.4.0.0^{4,9}]docosa-1(22),4(9),5,7,18,20-hexaen-20-yl]carbamoyl}propyl)carbamoyl]propanamido}-2-hydroxypropyl)-3-(2-hydroxy-2,2-diphosphonoethyl) pyridin-1-ium (Ris-1Aa, 18)

To a solution of **17** in water (600 μl) was added TFA (300 μl). After 3 h, the solution was evaporated under reduced pressure, then the residue was taken up in 10% MeCN in water (0.05 M TEAB, pH 9.0). The mixture was then centrifugated, and the supernatant was purified by semi-preparative reversed-phase HPLC [column: Hamilton PRP-1, 10 × 250 mm, 7 μm; solvent system: A—10% MeCN, 50 mM TEAB (pH 9.0), B—75% MeCN, 50 mM TEAB (pH 9.0); program: 0%B for 5 min, gradient of 0–25%B over 20 min, then an isocratic hold at 60%B for 10 min; flow rate: 3 ml/min; UV detection at 260 nm; t_r = 18.0 min, **Supplementary Figure 23**] to yield the final product (Ris-1Aa, **18**) as an off-white powder (4.8 mg, 57%, **Supplementary Figures 24, 25**); the amount of total bisphosphonate was quantified by ^{31}P NMR using pamidronate as the external standard and H_3PO_4 in D_2O (capillary) as the internal standard. Purity was confirmed by LC–MS [column: Hamilton PRP-C18, 4.6 × 150 mm, 7 μm; solvent system: A—10% MeCN, 50 mM TEAB (pH 9.0), B—50% MeCN, 50 mM TEAB (pH 9.0); program: gradient of 0–100%B over 20 min; flow rate: 0.8 ml/min; UV detection at 266 nm; t_r = 6.3 min, **Supplementary Figure 26**]. ^{1}H NMR (400 MHz, D_2O, pD 8.9) δ 8.76 (s, ^{1}H), 8.51 (d, *J* = 7.7 Hz, ^{1}H), 8.33 (d, *J* = 9.2 Hz, ^{1}H), 7.98 (s, ^{1}H), 7.80 (t, *J* = 8.0 Hz, ^{1}H), 7.72–7.63 (m, 2H), 7.44 (s, ^{1}H), 7.25 (d, *J* = 8.6 Hz, ^{1}H), 6.92 (d, *J* = 9.2 Hz, ^{1}H), 4.36–4.22 (m, 3H), 4.21–4.10 (m, 2H), 3.48–3.39 (m, 2H), 3.34–3.22 (m, 6H), 2.96 (t, *J* = 6.6 Hz, 2H), 2.60–2.47 (m, 4H), 2.44–2.33 (m, 2H), 2.02–1.92 (m, 2H), 1.92–1.79 (m, 3H), 1.77–1.64 (m, 3H), 1.55–1.38 (m, 3H), 1.02 (d, *J* = 6.3 Hz,

3H), 0.96 (t, J = 6.8 Hz, 3H). ^{31}P NMR (162 MHz, D_2O, pD 8.9) δ 16.50 (d, J = 20.3 Hz), 16.30 (d, J = 20.3 Hz). MS (ESI) m/z: $[M{-}2H]^-$ calcd for $C_{45}H_{63}N_{10}O_{15}P_2^{2-}$ 1045.4; found 1045.5.

In vitro Spiral Ganglion Neurite Outgrowth Model

The animal portion of this study was conducted according to the NIH Guide for the Care and Use of Laboratory Animals and approved by the Institutional Animal Care and Use Committee (IACUC) at Mass Eye and Ear.

CBA/CaJ pups at postnatal day (p4) were decapitated, and cochleae were extracted from temporal bones and otic capsules in Hank's Balanced Salt Solution (HBSS, Life Technologies). The stria vascularis and sensory epithelium were removed, leaving the modiolus containing SGNs, which were then horizontally and vertically dissected into six pieces.

Sterilized round glass coverslips were added to 4-well dish plates (CellStar). Coverslips were then covered with 1:10 dilution of Matrigel (Corning) in culture medium [DMEM/F12 (GIBCO), N2 (ThermoFisher), B27 (Thermofisher), 50 μl/ml Ampicillin (Sigma-Aldrich), 1:300 Fungizone (250 μg/ml, GIBCO), and 1:100 Hepes (1 M, GIBCO)] and placed in the incubator at 37°C for 10 min. Plates were washed with HBSS. The divided modiolus pieces containing SGNs were allowed to attach to glass coverslips overnight in 50 μl of culture medium at 37°C, 5% CO_2. All drugs were stored as stock solutions in DMSO at 400 μM at −20°C. After tissue attachment was confirmed under the microscope, SGNs were treated with Risedronate, 1Aa, Ris-1Aa, or DMSO medium alone (control) at final concentrations of 400 nM in darkness due to light sensitivity of compounds. DMSO was used for drug dilution at a ratio of 1: 5 - DMSO : water, final DMSO concentration in culture was < 1:1,000. Cultures were kept at 37°C for an additional 48 h after drug applications.

For analysis of phosphorylated TrkC expression, we included treatment with TrkC antibody (Santa Cruz, #sc517245) to block the receptor. SGNs were plated as described above, and additional conditions included pretreatment of SGNs with TrkC antibody at 4 μg/ml for 24 h, followed by 24 h of 1Aa 400 nM treatment, or simultaneous treatment of SGNs with 1Aa at 400 nM and TrkC antibody at 4μg/ml.

For comparison of neurite outgrowth between 1Aa and DHF, n = 4. In cases of outgrowth with Ris-1Aa compared to Ris and 1Aa n = 7, and for HA nanoparticle bound outgrowth, n = 4. The outgrowth study for phosphorylated TrkC was performed n = 3 times. Neurite outgrowth varied in degree based on the compound. In control samples, on average 10–30 neurites were traceable per picture. In treated samples, generally more neurites were found to grow out of the tissue sample, between 20–60 neurons.

Samples were fixed with 4% paraformaldehyde in phosphate-buffered saline (PBS) for 10 min, washed with PBS, then permeabilized and blocked with blocking solution (15% goat serum and 0.3% Triton X-100 in PBS) for 1 h at room temperature. Primary antibody for mouse anti-TUJ1 (1:300, Biolegend, #801201) to detect neurons, or phosphorylated TrkC, pTrkC (1:50, Sigma, #SAB4504648) were diluted in antibody solution (10% goat serum and 0.1% Triton X-100 in PBS) was applied to cultures overnight at 4°C. Samples were washed three times, then incubated with secondary antibody, goat anti-mouse Alexa Fluor 568 (1:500, Invitrogen, #A-11004) diluted in antibody solution for 1 h at room temperature. The tissues were washed three times with PBS. Nuclei were labeled with DAPI (1:1,000, BD Biosciences) diluted in PBS. After washing again as above, coverslips were mounted on glass slides using Fluoromount-G Medium (Invitrogen) and sealed with clear nail polish (Electron Microscopy Sciences). The tissues were then visualized with Leica Sp8 confocal microscopy at 10 × .

In vitro Hydroxyapatite Outgrowth Assays

Hydroxyapatite (HA) nanopowder (10 mg, Sigma-Aldrich) was suspended in 1 ml of culture medium and filtered through a 40 μm sterile filter to remove agglutinated nanoparticles. Four 1 ml suspensions of HA, each containing ~500 μg of nanopowder, in culture medium were prepared in the dark. 6-Fam-Ris (8 nM, 1:50 relative to other compounds added, BioVinc) was added to each suspension. Risedronate, 1Aa, Ris-1Aa, and DMSO alone at final concentrations of 400 nM were added to each dilution, briefly vortexed, then incubated at 37°C for 1 h.

Particles were centrifuged at 2,000 rpm for 2 min and the supernatant was removed. Residues were washed four times with a fresh culture medium. HA pellets were then resuspended in 40 μl of 1:5 Matrigel in the culture medium. The Matrigel-HA solution was spread onto sterilized round glass coverslips and placed in the incubator at 37°C for 15 min.

CBA/CaJ pups (p4) were euthanized and modiolus containing SGNs were extracted as described above. Tissues were plated onto solidified Matrigel-HA suspension for 48 h. Outgrowth was analyzed using immunocytochemistry and confocal imaging as described above.

Neurite Tracing Analysis

Neurite tracing for soluble and HA SGN outgrowth assays was performed blinded to treatment identities. z-stacks were imported to ImageJ and the Simple Neurite Tracer plug-in was used to trace neurite paths through the z-stack. Only neurites with visible start and endpoints were traced. Paths were then compiled into a skeleton, and average neurite lengths were compared between treatments.

In vitro Cochlear Synaptopathy Model

CBA/CaJ pups (p4) were euthanized and cochleae were extracted from temporal bones and otic capsules as described above. The stria vascularis was removed leaving the organ of Corti attached to the modiolus. The middle turn was isolated and cut into two pieces using breakable scalpel blades and a blade holder (Fine Science Tools).

Explants were plated on 1:10 Matrigel pretreated 4-well dish plates with sterilized round glass coverslips as described above. Explants attached onto coverslips overnight in culture medium. After confirming attachment under the microscope, explants were treated in darkness with 0.5 mM kainic acid (KA, Abcam) diluted in the culture medium in the incubator at 37°C for 2 h. An untreated explant was kept as a negative control. KA was removed and explants were washed with culture medium. KA treated cultures were treated in darkness with either the 1st group (1Aa, DHF, DHF, and 1Aa, or DMSO alone) or the 2nd group of drugs (Ris, 1Aa, Ris-1Aa, or, DMSO alone). All drugs were diluted to a final concentration of 400 nM. Synapse experiments for comparison of 1Aa and DHF were performed $n = 4$ times, and synapse experiments with Ris, 1Aa, and Ris-1Aa were performed $n = 10$ times.

Samples were fixed and blocked with blocking solution (5% goat serum, 0.3% Triton X-100 in PBS) in preparation for immunocytochemical analysis as described above. Mouse (IgG1) anti-CtBP2 (1:200, BD Biosciences, #612044) for presynaptic ribbons, mouse (IgG2a) anti-PSD95 (1:1,000, Neuromab, #75-028) for postsynaptic neural densities, and rabbit anti-myosin VIIa (1:500, Proteus, #25-6790) for hair cells, diluted in antibody solution (1% goat serum, 0.3% Triton X-100 in PBS) were applied to samples overnight at room temperature. After washing in PBS three times, Alexa Fluor antibodies (1:500 in antibody solution), goat anti-mouse IgG2a 488 (Invitrogen, #A-21131), goat anti-mouse IgG1 568 (Invitrogen, #A-21124), goat anti-rabbit 647 (Invitrogen, #A-21244), were applied for 1 h at room temperature. After another washing step, coverslips were mounted on glass slides as described above. Explants were visualized with Leica SP8 confocal microscope at 63× with an additional 3.17× zoom.

Synaptic Ribbon Quantification and Colocalization Analysis

Image analysis was performed blinded to treatment identities. z-stacks were imported to Amira imaging software (Visage Imaging, version 6.4). Isosurface functions and connected components were used to create 3D renderings of the images and synaptic colocalizations were analyzed as previously described (Suzuki et al., 2016; Kempfle et al., 2018).

Statistics

This work was conducted with support from the Biostatistics Program at Harvard Catalyst | The Harvard Clinical and Translational Science Center (National Center for Advancing Translational Sciences, National Institutes of Health Award UL 1TR002541) and financial contributions from Harvard University and its affiliated academic healthcare centers. The content is solely the responsibility of the authors and does not necessarily represent the official views of Harvard Catalyst, Harvard University and its affiliated academic healthcare centers, or the National Institutes of Health. Statistical analysis was performed using Student's *t*-test, one-way and two-way ANOVA with Tukey's multiple comparisons test in PRISM software (Version 9.0). A *p*-value less than 0.05 was considered statistically significant.

RESULTS

We synthesized a TrkC agonist, 1Aa, to assess its neurotrophic activity. In a second step, we utilized synthetic chemistry to create a novel small molecule, Ris-1Aa, that linked 1Aa to risedronate (Ris), a bisphosphonate with high bone mineral affinity. We studied both molecules for their ability to promote neurite outgrowth and ribbon synapse regeneration *in vitro*.

Synthesis of the Small Molecule TrkC Agonist, 1Aa

For our investigations of the biochemical activity of 1Aa, we first prepared the compound by solid-phase synthesis (**Figure 1**; **Supplementary Figure 1**). Starting from 4-(bromomethyl)-3-nitrobenzoic acid (**1**), we prepared the corresponding 4-(4-methyltritylaminomethyl-3-aminobenzoic acid (**4**) in four steps by a modification of the literature procedure (Lee et al.,

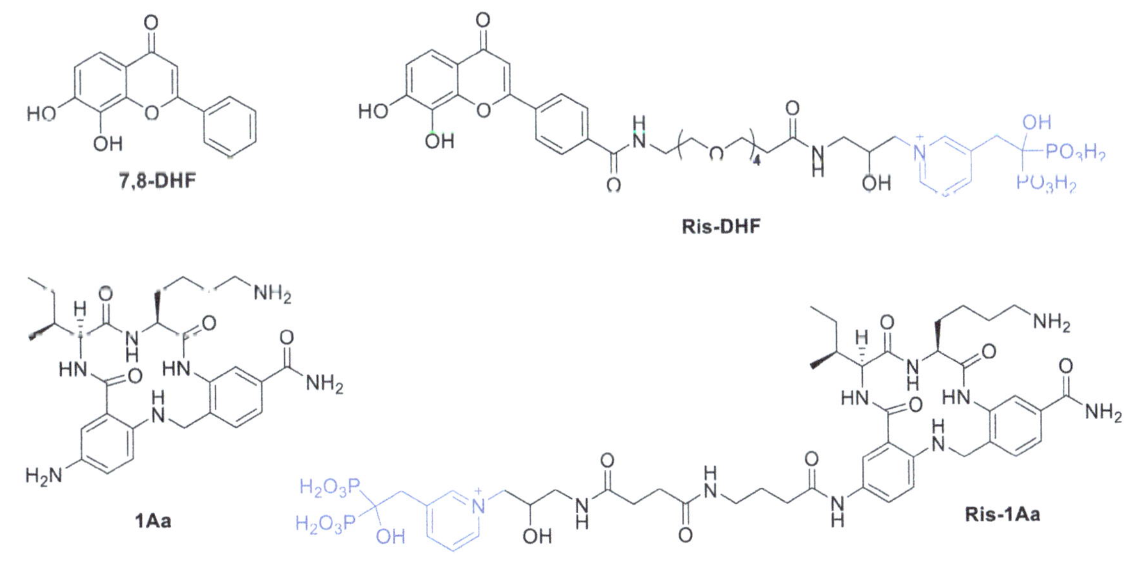

FIGURE 1 | Structures of 7,8-DHF, 1Aa, and their conjugates with risedronate (Ris).

2004). Assembly of 1Aa was initiated by coupling **4** to Rink amide resin, giving the resin-attached intermediate (**5**, **Supplementary Figure 1**, Step e). This was reacted with ϵ-Boc-α-Fmoc protected lysine, giving **6** which after removal of the Fmoc with piperidine, was condensed with Fmoc-protected isoleucine, providing after deprotection at the Ile α-amino group the dipeptide derivative (**7**). After reaction with 2-fluoro-5-nitrobenzoyl chloride and macrocyclization, the nitro group on the resulting intermediate (**9**) was reduced to an amino group by $SnCl_2$ in DMF, yielding resin-bound 1Aa (**10**). Reactions involving resin-bound compounds were monitored by cleavage of a portion of the sample with TFA, then analysis by LC-MS. Treatment of **10** with 1:1:18 H_2O/TIS/TFA followed by removal of the resin beads and evaporation of the filtrate afforded crude 1Aa (**11**) which was isolated as its formate salt after semi-preparative reverse-phase HPLC and characterized by ^{1}H NMR and LC-MS.

Design and Synthesis of the Ris-1Aa Conjugate

The synthetic route is outlined in **Figure 2**. Boc-protected 1Aa immobilized on the resin (**10**) was first decorated with a Fmoc-protected γ-aminobutanoic acid (GABA) linker, which was then deprotected with piperidine to give **12** and further modified by reaction with succinic anhydride to give **13**. After cleavage from the resin, Boc protection was reinstalled on the lysine ε-amine in the 1Aa moiety and the terminal carboxyl function of the resulting intermediate **14** was activated as an unisolated *N*-hydroxy succinimidyl ester **15**, which was reacted *in situ* with risedronate equipped at the pyridyl nitrogen with a 3-(2-hydroxy)-1-aminopropyl (**16**) to form **17**. After deprotection of **17** with aqueous TFA, the final product (**18**, Ris-1Aa) was purified by reversed-phase HPLC and characterized by ^{1}H NMR ^{31}P NMR and LC-MS.

1Aa Stimulates Neurite Outgrowth *In vitro*

In order to compare the effect of 1Aa on neurite outgrowth to our previously published results on DHF, we treated postnatal SGNs in culture with 400 nM of 1Aa, DHF, a combination of equal amounts of DHF and 1Aa, or control with DMSO for 48 h. Immunohistochemistry for neural marker TuJ was performed and TuJ positive neurites were quantified. The average neurite outgrowth ranged between 100 nm and 600 nm. Compared to control, outgrowth significantly increased by 2- to 2.5-fold for DHF and 1Aa and DHF + 1Aa treated samples (**Figure 3**). There was no significant increase in neurite outgrowth upon treatment with both DHF and 1Aa. In summary, these results suggest that 1Aa can promote spiral ganglion neurite outgrowth *in vitro* to a level comparable to DHF.

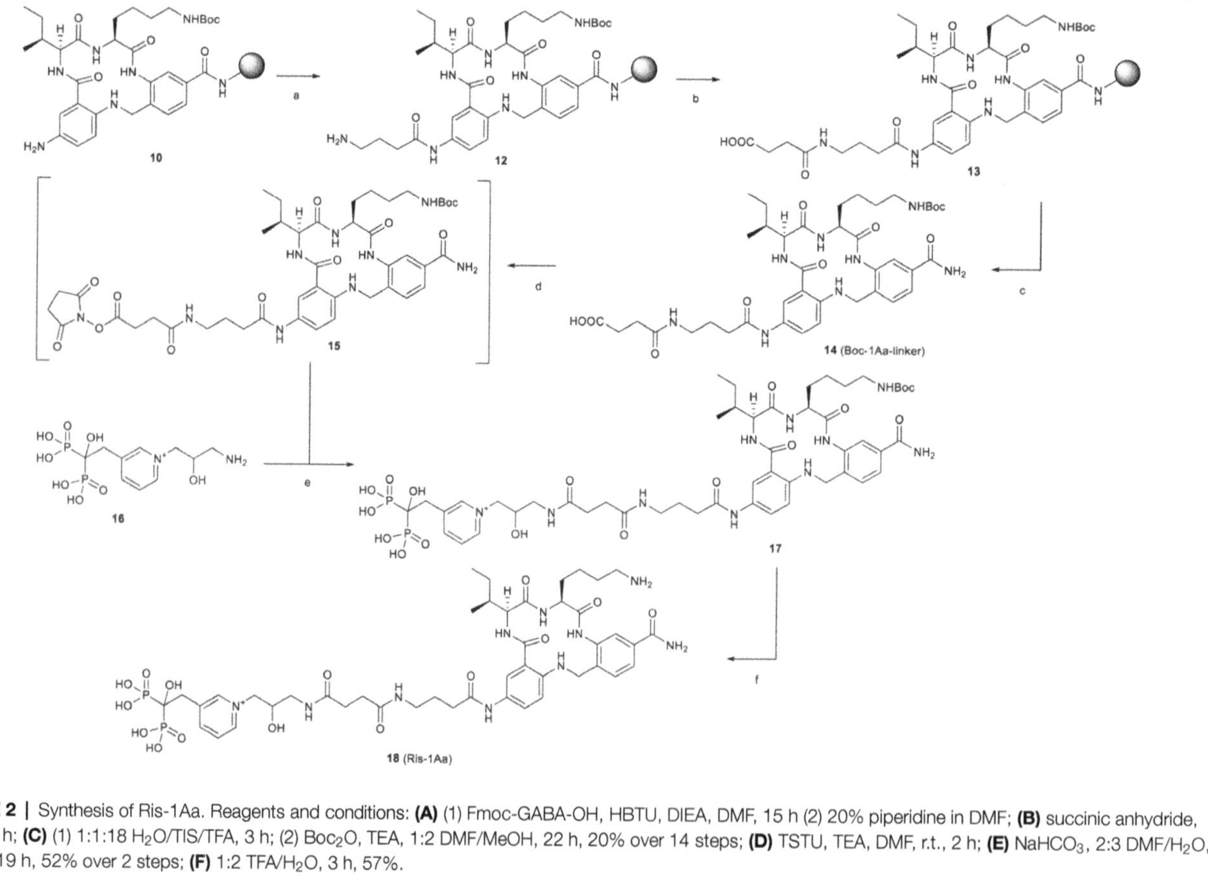

FIGURE 2 | Synthesis of Ris-1Aa. Reagents and conditions: **(A)** (1) Fmoc-GABA-OH, HBTU, DIEA, DMF, 15 h (2) 20% piperidine in DMF; **(B)** succinic anhydride, DMF, 25 h; **(C)** (1) 1:1:18 H_2O/TIS/TFA, 3 h; (2) Boc_2O, TEA, 1:2 DMF/MeOH, 22 h, 20% over 14 steps; **(D)** TSTU, TEA, DMF, r.t., 2 h; **(E)** $NaHCO_3$, 2:3 DMF/H_2O, pH 8.3, 19 h, 52% over 2 steps; **(F)** 1:2 TFA/H_2O, 3 h, 57%.

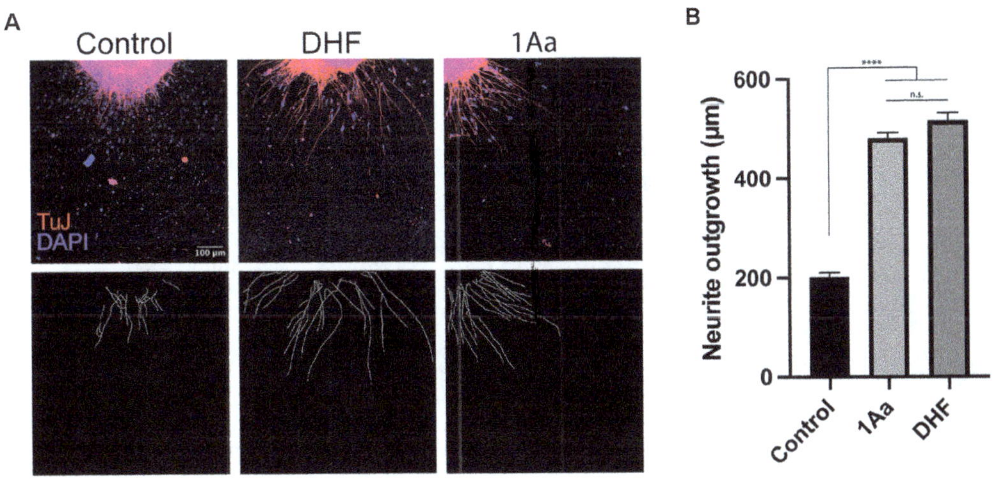

FIGURE 3 | 1Aa promotes neurite outgrowth *in vitro*. **(A)** SGN neurite outgrowth *in vitro*. Neurites were stained with neuronal marker TuJ (red), and nuclei were labeled with DAPI (blue). Scale bar represents 100 μm. Images are representative of four independent experiments. **(B)** Quantification of neurite outgrowth in μm compared to DMSO control and DHF (n.s., not significant; **** represents $p \leq 0.0001$).

Ris-1Aa Promotes Neurite Growth *In vitro*

We next analyzed the ability of Ris-1Aa to promote neurite outgrowth. We treated postnatal SGNs in culture with 400 nM of Ris, 1Aa, and Ris-1Aa, or control with DMSO for 48 h, and quantified the lengths of axons staining positive for TuJ (**Figure 4A**). Average neurite outgrowth ranged between 100 nm to 600 nm. Relative outgrowth for Ris-1Aa was comparable to our prior experiments with 1Aa (**Figure 4B**). This finding suggests that the neurotrophic activity of 1Aa *in vitro* is not abrogated by conjugation with Ris.

Ris-1Aa Promotes Neurite Outgrowth After Pre-binding to Hydroxyapatite

We have previously established an assay to assess the activity of novel hybrid compounds containing bisphosphonates conjugated with neurotrophic small molecules, following binding to hydroxyapatite bone matrix (Kempfle et al., 2018). Ris-1Aa or control molecules were pre-bound to hydroxyapatite nanoparticles and assessed for their ability to promote SGN neurite outgrowth (**Figure 5A**). Ris-1Aa demonstrated the strongest outgrowth compared to control, Ris, or 1Aa (**Figure 5B**). A small positive effect on outgrowth was seen by Ris alone, which is consistent with our prior data. The modest outgrowth demonstrated in response to 1Aa may be from trapping within the hydroxyapatite particles after rinsing.

1Aa Acts at Least in Part Through TrkC *In vitro*

To provide mechanistic insight into whether 1Aa acts *via* TrkC in primary auditory neurons, we treated SGNs in our organotypic culture model with either 1Aa alone, in combination with a blocking antibody specific to the extracellular portion of TrkC, or following pretreatment with the blocking antibody. To assess for activation of TrkC receptors in SGNs, we stained for phosphorylated TrkC after treatment and quantified the number of phosphorylated receptors found on each neurite (**Figures 6A,A′,B**). We compared the number of phosphorylated receptors to untreated SGNs, or SGNs treated with Ris or Ris-1Aa (**Figures 6A′,B**). We demonstrated that, in the presence of 1Aa, the number of phosphorylated receptors increased significantly compared to control or samples treated with the blocking anti-TrkC antibody. Pretreatment with the anti-TrkC antibody resulted in the lowest number of phosphorylated receptors on the neurites across all treatment conditions. Ris-1Aa also demonstrated activity through TrkC, although the amount of phosphorylated TrkC appeared to be lower than after treatment with 1Aa. Interestingly, the number of phosphorylated TrkC receptors on neurites treated with Ris alone was not significantly different compared to control, suggesting that Ris does not act through TrkC (**Figure 6B**).

1Aa Stimulates Regeneration of Cochlear Ribbon Synapses *In vitro*

To assess synaptic regeneration after 1Aa treatment, we isolated organ of Corti (OC) explants with intact ribbon synapses and SGNs for *in vitro* culture (**Figure 7A**). After treatment with kainic acid (KA), which induces excitotoxic damage to ribbon synapses, OC explants were treated with 400 nM of 1Aa, DHF, 1Aa + DHF, or DMSO (control). Quantification of intact synapses per IHC (**Figure 7B**), as measured by the proximity of pre- and post-synaptic markers, revealed an average synapse count of 11–12 synapses for the untreated control OC explants (KA-). KA-treated OC explants without any regenerative treatment (KA+) averaged around two synapses. Treatment with DHF, 1Aa or 1Aa + DHF demonstrated a significant and statistically similar increase in synaptic counts after KA treatment, with an average number of 8–10 synapses per IHC. These data suggest that the small molecule TrkC agonist 1Aa has the ability to regenerate ribbon synapses following KA damage *in vitro*, comparable to the previously described effect of DHF. Furthermore, there

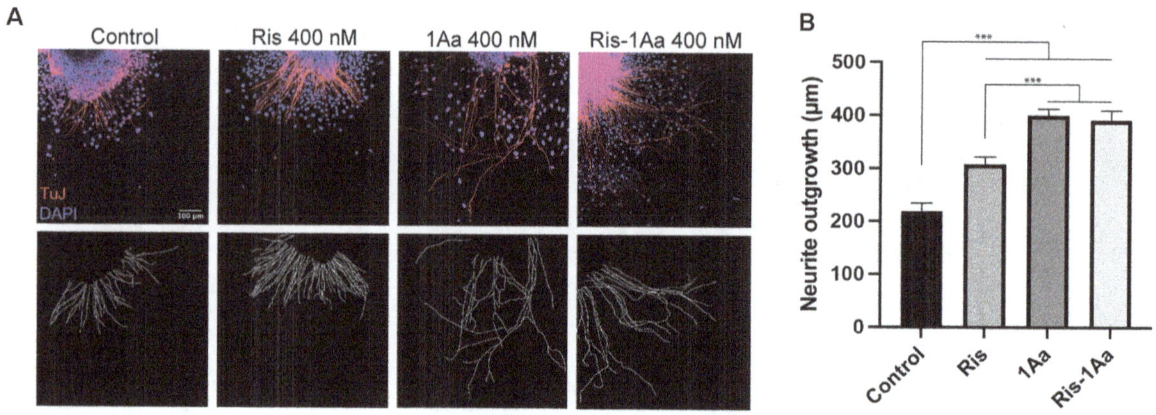

FIGURE 4 | Ris-1Aa supports neurite outgrowth *in vitro* in a manner comparable to 1Aa. **(A)** SGN neurite outgrowth *in vitro*. Neurites were stained with neuronal marker TuJ (red), and nuclei were labeled with DAPI (blue). Scale bar represents 100 μm. Images are representative of seven independent experiments. **(B)** Quantification of neurite outgrowth compared to DMSO control (*** represents $p \leq 0.001$).

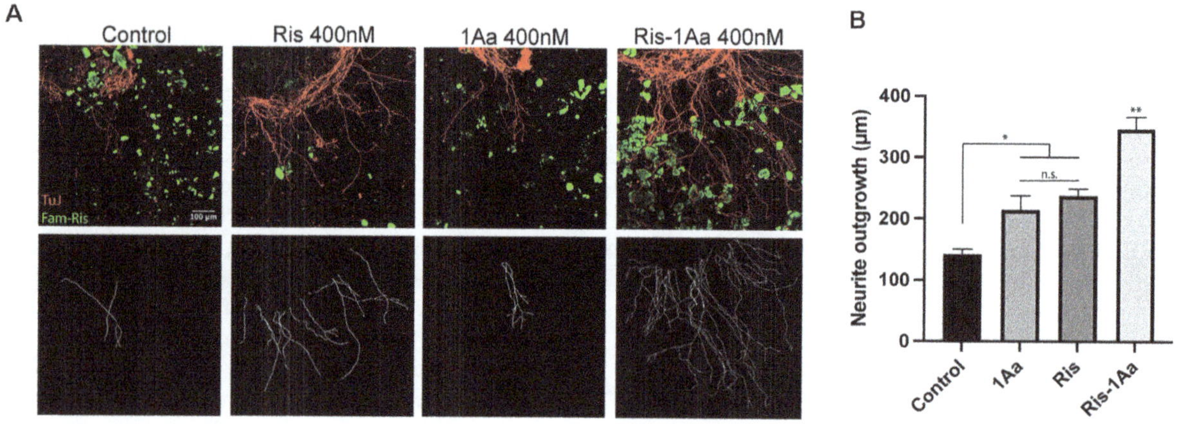

FIGURE 5 | Ris-1Aa retains neurotrophic activity following binding to the bone matrix *in vitro*. **(A)** SGN neurite outgrowth after preincubation of drugs with hydroxyapatite nanoparticles (HA). Neurites were stained with neuronal marker TuJ (red), HA was visualized with Fam-Ris (green), and nuclei were labeled with DAPI (blue). Scale bar represents 100 μm. Images are representative of four independent experiments. **(B)** Quantification of neurite outgrowth compared to DMSO control (* represents $p \leq 0.05$, ** represents $p \leq 0.01$; n.s., not significant).

does not appear to be an additive effect of both TrkB and TrkC stimulation for increasing synaptic counts under these experimental conditions.

Ris-1Aa Promotes Synaptic Regeneration *In vitro*

Finally, we evaluated the ability of the bisphosphonate conjugate Ris-1Aa to promote synaptic regeneration. As above, we treated OC explants *in vitro* with KA to destroy synapses to inner hair cells (**Figure 8A**). OC explants were then treated with 400 nM of 1Aa, Ris, Ris-1Aa, or DMSO (control). Pre- and postsynaptic portions were quantified and demonstrated a significant increase in synaptic regeneration after treatment with Ris-1Aa (**Figure 8B**). This was comparable to numbers of synapses obtained after treatment with 1Aa. These data suggest that Ris-1Aa maintains the ability of 1Aa to increase synaptic counts following KA treatment.

DISCUSSION

We report that neurotrophin-3 small molecule analogue 1Aa promotes SGN outgrowth and regeneration of inner ear ribbon synapses *in vitro*. These effects were similar to those of DHF, a small molecule analogue of BDNF. Bone-binding hybrid molecule Ris-1Aa retained most of native 1Aa's neurotrophic ability *in vitro*, both when freely available in culture and when pre-bound to hydroxyapatite. Our results suggest that 1Aa and Ris-1Aa may be attractive candidates to promote the regeneration of cochlear ribbon synapses *in vivo*.

These data are the first to establish the activity of an NT-3 small molecule analogue, 1Aa, upon SGNs. Previous work identified 1Aa in a screen of small molecule peptidomimetics capable of activating TrkA and/or TrkC. This report defined 1Aa as a TrkC agonist as it bound TrkC, induced TrkC phosphorylation, and promoted differentiation of a cell line

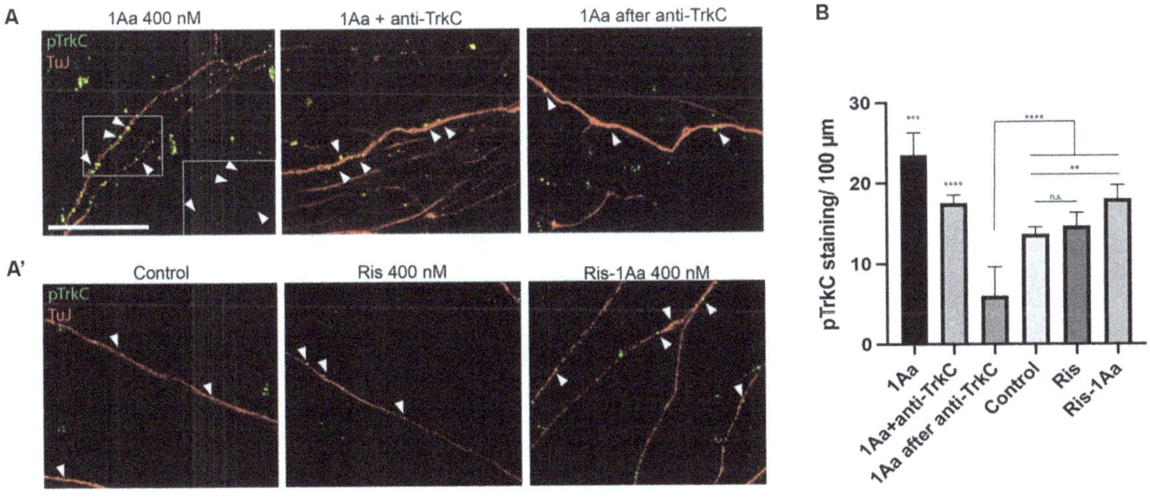

FIGURE 6 | 1Aa and Ris-1Aa activate TrkC *in vitro*. **(A)** and **(A')** Expression of phosphorylated TrkC (pTrkC) on SGN neurites *in vitro*. Neurites were stained with neuronal marker TuJ (red), and phosphorylated TrkC (green), and nuclei were labeled with DAPI (blue). Scale bar represents 10 µm. The outgrowth of 1Aa was compared to pre-treatment with a blocking anti TrkC antibody (1Aa after anti-TrkC) or simultaneous treatment with 1Aa and anti-TrkC (1Aa + TrkC). **(A')** pTrkC staining for control, Ris or Ris-1Aa of the same experiment. Images are one representative experiment of three independently performed experiments. Inlay and arrowheads in **(A)** and **(B)** mark examples of pTrkC staining. **(B)** Quantification of pTrkC per 100 µm. 1Aa and 1Aa+anti-TrkC were each significant compared to all other conditions (**represents $p \leq 0.01$, *** represents $p \leq 0.001$, **** represents $p \leq 0.0001$; n.s., not significant).

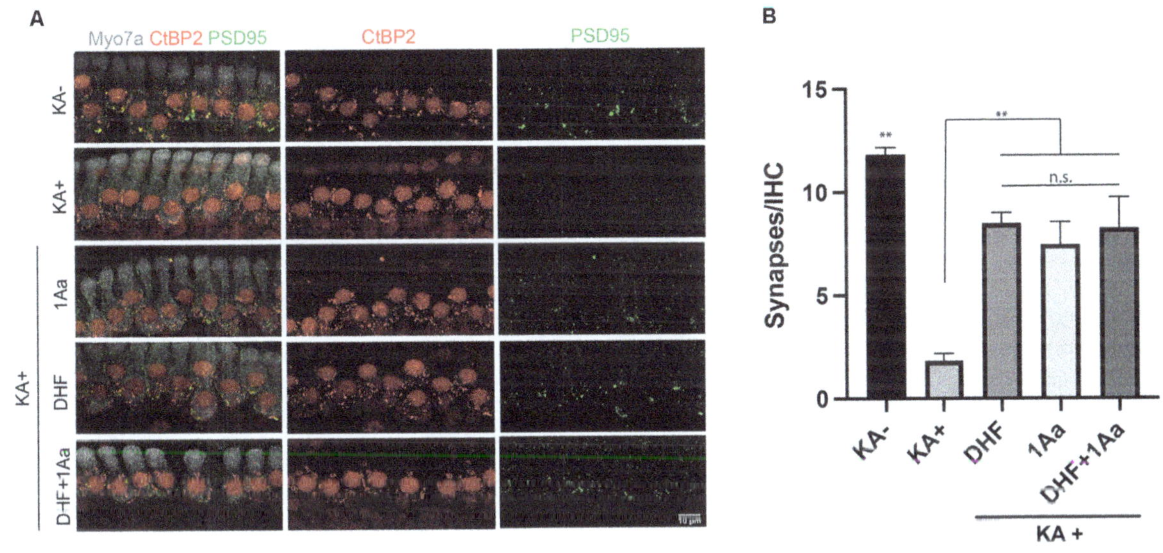

FIGURE 7 | 1Aa promotes synapse regeneration *in vitro*. **(A)** Immunohistochemistry of untreated control (KA-), control treated with KA (KA+), explant treated with KA+DHF (DHF), explant treated with KA+1Aa (1Aa), and explant treated with KA and 1Aa+DHF (1Aa+DHF). Hair cells were labeled with Myo7A (white), presynaptic ribbon synapse was labeled with CtBP2 (red), and postsynaptic ribbon synapse was stained with PSD95 (green). Images are representative of four independent experiments. Scale bar represents 10 µm. **(B)** Quantification of number of synapses per inner hair cell (** represents $p \leq 0.01$, n.s., not significant).

expressing TrkC. 1Aa also potentiated the activity of NT-3 (Zaccaro et al., 2005). Here, we extend these findings to demonstrate that 1Aa and Ris-1Aa have neurotrophic activity on mature SGNs *in vitro* to induce neurite elongation and regeneration of synapses between IHCs and SGNs. Moreover, treatment of SGNs with 1Aa and Ris-1Aa induced TrkC phosphorylation, which is the first step in TrkC signaling following ligand binding. Therefore, it is reasonable to conclude that the effects on SGNs we observe are, at least in part, due to activity through TrkC. Our present data do not, however, rule out that 1Aa and Ris-1Aa also activate TrkB. Critically, stimulation *via* TrkC has been shown in various systems to be superior to TrkB stimulation with respect to cochlear synaptic regeneration (Wang and Green, 2011; Wan et al., 2014). In this regard, DHF,

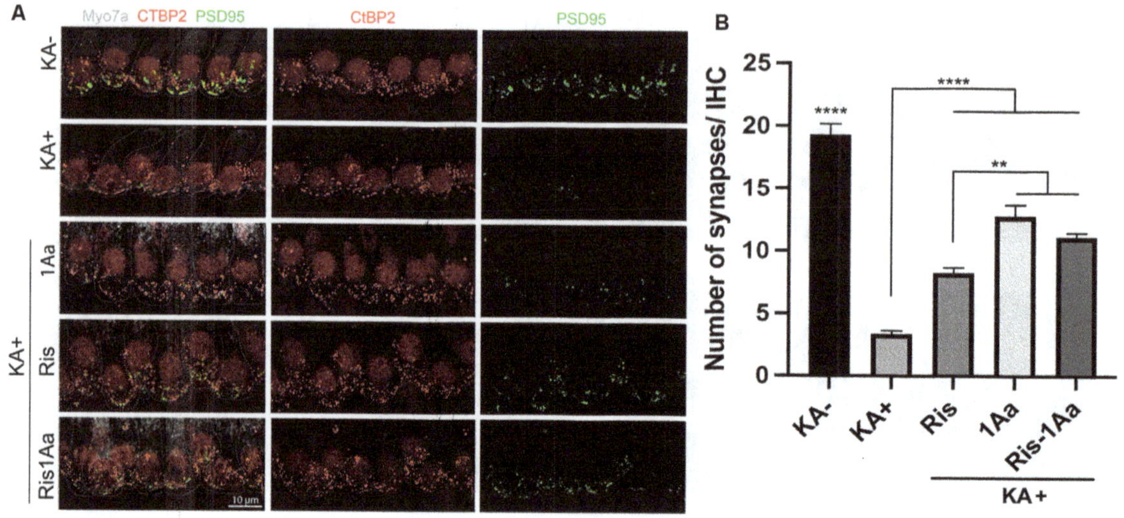

FIGURE 8 | Ris-1Aa promotes synapse regeneration *in vitro*. **(A)** Immunohistochemistry of untreated control (KA-), control treated with KA (KA+), explant treated with KA+ 1Aa, explant treated with KA+ Ris, and explant treated with KA and Ris-1Aa. Hair cells were labeled with Myo7A (white), presynaptic ribbon synapse was labeled with CtBP2 (red), and postsynaptic ribbon synapse was stained with PSD95 (green). Images are representative of 10 independent experiments. Scale bar represents 10 µm. **(B)** Quantification of synapses per inner hair cell for various treatment conditions (****$p \leq 0.0001$, denotes that counted synapses in both KA- and KA+ were statistically significant relative to all other samples; **$p \leq 0.01$).

a small molecule TrkB agonist, can partially restore cochlear ribbon synapses *in vivo* following noise damage, although this effect requires a high concentration of DHF directly injected into perilymph *via* a labyrinthotomy (Fernandez et al., 2021). 1Aa, by acting at least in part through TrkC, may exhibit a more powerful regenerative effect *in vivo*.

Two of the primary challenges of inner ear drug delivery are the complex anatomy of the labyrinth and the labyrinth's existence as a closed, bone-encased system that restricts access *via* the round (RW) and oval (OW) windows and the blood-labyrinth barrier (Swan et al., 2008). Prior approaches have focused on systemic or local delivery to the inner ear. While systemic administration may be relatively straightforward, it has the potential for greater side effects and insufficient drug levels delivered to the inner ear. In cases where hearing loss is not a concern, a local direct approach *via* a cochleostomy affords the potential to maximize drug delivery in a highly controlled manner. However, opening the cochlea presents a risk in patients with residual hearing, as the disturbance of inner ear fluid homeostasis can lead to significant hearing and balance loss. Therefore, local intratympanic delivery to the RW and OW may be a preferred procedure in patients with at least some preserved hearing. In this regard, intratympanic injection, including steroids for sudden hearing loss and gentamicin for Meniere's disease, is commonly performed in human patients. Previous studies have suggested, however, that the percentage of drug that ultimately enters the inner ear *via* these approaches may be low, ranging between 0.1–2%, and bioavailability depends on multiple factors such as size, hydrophobicity, and distribution processes (Salt and Plontke, 2009).

To address these limitations, we have developed a drug delivery platform for the inner ear that relies on bisphosphonate conjugation to maximize co-localization of neurotrophic activity with SGNs. Bisphosphonates have a high affinity for hydroxyapatite, and drug-bisphosphonate conjugates exploit this chemical property to specifically target bone (Sedghizadeh et al., 2017; Farrell et al., 2018; McKenna et al., 2020). We have previously shown that a fluorescently-labeled bisphosphonate can cross the RWM and avidly label the osseous spiral lamina, which is in close proximity to SGNs (Kang et al., 2015). The use of bisphosphonate conjugates to target the cochlea may also have the advantage of prolonged binding to the bony labyrinth and enable long-term stimulation of SGNs (Kempfle et al., 2018). As we have now described novel small conjugated molecules with neurotrophic activity *in vitro*, we anticipate that other small molecules with desired activities within the cochlea could potentially be delivered *via* this platform. Additional work, perhaps utilizing modified hybrid molecules with the ability to release the neurotrophin analogues from the bisphosphonate, may be needed to optimize neurotrophic delivery and activity.

In this regard, our data describe a general synthetic chemistry approach to conjugate a variety of small molecules with a range of bisphosphonates. This approach allows for fine-tuning of delivery. These novel applications derive from our previously reported procedures for the conjugation of fluorescent dyes to bisphosphonates (Kashemirov et al., 2008; Sun et al., 2016). The design for Ris-1Aa includes a long-chain linker between the 1Aa moiety and risedronate, and the attachment point we used to add the linker and conjugate to Ris ensured that the 1Aa moiety retained its TrkC agonism its neurotrophic activity. We successfully incorporated the linker during solid-phase synthesis of 1Aa, then adapted our established "magic linker" method procedure to conjugate 1Aa to Ris.

Interestingly, in our experimental system Ris itself has the intrinsic ability to drive the regeneration of ribbon synapses *in vitro*. We were the first to show that some bisphosphonates have intrinsic activity and can support ribbon synapse regeneration *in vitro* (Kempfle et al., 2018), a finding that we recapitulate with the present results. This result was unexpected, although recent work replicates these findings and further suggests that some bisphosphonates can promote ribbon synapse regeneration *in vivo* following noise damage (Seist et al., 2020). The mechanisms by which bisphosphonates exert this activity remain unclear. Indeed, the broad spectrum of bisphosphonate activity outside the skeletal system is an active area of investigation (Panagiotakou et al., 2020). Our present data and our previous work (Kempfle et al., 2018), however, strongly suggest that this effect occurs independently of TrkB or TrkC signaling as Ris does not appear to induce either TrkB or TrkC phosphorylation *in vitro*.

We present here the first demonstration that an NT-3 small molecule analogue and its bisphosphonate-linked derivative have neurotrophic activity on SGNs *in vitro*. Our findings may hold important implications for the regeneration of cochlear ribbon synapses, as well as for intralabyrinthine drug delivery more generally.

AUTHOR CONTRIBUTIONS

JK: biological study design, acquisition of biological data, data analysis, and manuscript preparation. CA: compound synthesis and manuscript preparation. AZ: acquisition of biological data, data analysis, and manuscript preparation. MD: compound synthesis and manuscript preparation. RK: data analysis and preparation of manuscript. RL: data analysis. BK: synthesis design, and manuscript preparation. AE: manuscript preparation. CM: project concept, synthesis design, data analysis, and manuscript preparation. DJ: project concept, biological study design, data analysis, and manuscript preparation. All authors contributed to the article and approved the submitted version.

ACKNOWLEDGMENTS

We thank Ms. Inah Kang for her invaluable assistance in the preparation of this manuscript.

REFERENCES

Akil, O., Blits, B., Lustig, L. R., and Leake, P. A. (2019). Virally mediated overexpression of glial-derived neurotrophic factor elicits age- and dose-dependent neuronal toxicity and hearing loss. *Hum. Gene. Ther.* 30, 88–105. doi: 10.1089/hum.2018.028

Aronov, O., Horowitz, A. T., Gabizon, A., Fuertes, M. A., Perez, J. M., and Gibson, D. (2004). Nuclear localization signal-targeted poly(ethylene glycol) conjugates as potential carriers and nuclear localizing agents for carboplatin analogues. *Bioconjug. Chem.* 15, 814–823. doi: 10.1021/bc049 9331

Auerbach, B. D., Rodrigues, P. V., and Salvi, R. J. (2014). Central gain control in tinnitus and hyperacusis. *Front. Neurol.* 5:206. doi: 10.3389/fneur.2014.00206

Aytan, N., Choi, J. K., Carreras, I., Crabtree, L., Nguyen, B., Lehar, M., et al. (2018). Protective effects of 7,8-dihydroxyflavone on neuropathological and neurochemical changes in a mouse model of Alzheimer's disease. *Eur. J. Pharmacol.* 828, 9–17. doi: 10.1016/j.ejphar.2018.02.045

Bai, Y., Xu, J., Brahimi, F., Zhuo, Y., Sarunic, M. V., and Saragovi, H. U. (2010). An agonistic TrkB mAb causes sustained TrkB activation, delays RGC death and protects the retinal structure in optic nerve axotomy and in glaucoma. *Invest. Ophthalmol. Vis. Sci.* 51, 4722–4731. doi: 10.1167/iovs.09-5032

Bailey, E. M., and Green, S. H. (2014). Postnatal expression of neurotrophic factors accessible to spiral ganglion neurons in the auditory system of adult hearing and deafened rats. *J. Neurosci.* 34, 13110–13126. doi: 10.1523/JNEUROSCI. 1014-14.2014

Bharadwaj, H. M., Masud, S., Mehraei, G., Verhulst, S., and Shinn-Cunningham, B. G. (2015). Individual differences reveal correlates of hidden hearing deficits. *J. Neurosci.* 35, 2161–2172. doi: 10.1523/JNEUROSCI. 3915-14.2015

Bianchi, L. M., Conover, J. C., Fritzsch, B., DeChiara, T., Lindsay, R. M., and Yancopoulos, G. D. (1996). Degeneration of vestibular neurons in late embryogenesis of both heterozygous and homozygous BDNF null mutant mice. *Development* 122, 1965–1973.

Bramhall, N. F., Shi, F., Arnold, K., Hochedlinger, K., and Edge, A. S. (2014). Lgr5-positive supporting cells generate new hair cells in the postnatal cochlea. *Stem Cell Rep.* 2, 311–322. doi: 10.1016/j.stemcr.2014.01.008

Chambers, A. R., Resnik, J., Yuan, Y., Whitton, J. P., Edge, A. S., Liberman, M. C., et al. (2016). Central gain restores auditory processing following near-complete cochlear denervation. *Neuron* 89, 867–879. doi: 10.1016/j.neuron.2015.12.041

Chen, H., Xing, Y., Xia, L., Chen, Z., Yin, S., and Wang, J. (2018). AAV-mediated NT-3 overexpression protects cochleae against noise-induced synaptopathy. *Gene. Ther.* 25, 251–259. doi: 10.1038/s41434-018 -0012-0

Ernfors, P., Kucera, J., Lee, K. F., Loring, J., and Jaenisch, R. (1995). Studies on the physiological role of brain-derived neurotrophic factor and neurotrophin-3 in knockout mice. *Int. J. Dev. Biol.* 39, 799–807.

Evans, A. J., Thompson, B. C., Wallace, G. G., Millard, R., O'Leary, S. J., Clark, G. M., et al. (2009). Promoting neurite outgrowth from spiral ganglion neuron explants using polypyrrole/BDNF-coated electrodes. *J. Biomed. Mater. Res.* 91, 241–250. doi: 10.1002/jbm.a.32228

Farrell, K. B., Karpeisky, A., Thamm, D. H., and Zinnen, S. (2018). Bisphosphonate conjugation for bone specific drug targeting. *Bone Rep.* 9, 47–60. doi: 10.1016/j. bonr.2018.06.007

Fernandez, K. A., Watabe, T., Tong, M., Meng, X., Tani, K., Kujawa, S. G., et al. (2021). Trk agonist drugs rescue noise-induced hidden hearing loss. *JCI Insight* 6:e142572. doi: 10.1172/jci.insight.142572

Fukui, H., and Raphael, Y. (2013). Gene therapy for the inner ear. *Hear Res.* 297, 99–105. doi: 10.1016/j.heares.2012.11.017

Garcia-Diaz Barriga, G., Giralt, A., Anglada-Huguet, M., Gaja-Capdevila, N., Orlandi, J. G., Soriano, J., et al. (2017). 7,8-dihydroxyflavone ameliorates cognitive and motor deficits in a Huntington's disease mouse model through specific activation of the PLCgamma1 pathway. *Hum. Mol. Genet.* 26, 3144–3160. doi: 10.1093/hmg/ddx198

Goycoolea, M. V. (2001). Clinical aspects of round window membrane permeability under normal and pathological conditions. *Acta Otolaryngol.* 121, 437–447. doi: 10.1080/000164801300366552

Green, S. H., Bailey, E., Wang, Q., and Davis, R. L. (2012). The Trk A, B, C' s of neurotrophins in the cochlea. *Anat. Rec. (Hoboken)* 295, 1877–1895. doi: 10.1002/ar.22587

Hao, J., and Li, S. K. (2019). Inner ear drug delivery: Recent advances, challenges and perspective. *Eur. J. Pharm. Sci.* 126, 82–92. doi: 10.1016/j.ejps.2018.05.020

Hashimoto, K., Hickman, T. T., Suzuki, J., Ji, L., Kohrman, D. C., Corfas, G., et al. (2019). Protection from noise-induced cochlear synaptopathy by virally mediated overexpression of NT3. *Sci. Rep.* 9: 15362. doi: 10.1038/s41598-019-51724-6

He, J., Xiang, Z., Zhu, X., Ai, Z., Shen, J., Huang, T., et al. (2016). Neuroprotective effects of 7, 8-dihydroxyflavone on midbrain dopaminergic neurons in MPP(+)-treated monkeys. *Sci. Rep.* 6:34339. doi: 10.1038/srep34339

Jackman, A. L., Marsham, P. R., Thornton, T. J., Bishop, J. A., O' Connor, B. M., Hughes, L. R., et al. (1990). Quinazoline antifolate thymidylate synthase inhibitors: 2′-fluoro-N10-propargyl-5,8-dideazafolic acid and derivatives with modifications in the C2 position. *J. Med. Chem.* 33, 3067–3071. doi: 10.1021/jm00173a025

Jang, S. W., Liu, X., Yepes, M., Shepherd, K. R., Miller, G. W., Liu, Y., et al. (2010). A selective TrkB agonist with potent neurotrophic activities by 7,8-dihydroxyflavone. *Proc. Natl. Acad. Sci. U S A* 107, 2687–2692. doi: 10.1073/pnas.0913572107

Jang, S. W., Okada, M., Sayeed, I., Xiao, G., Stein, D., Jin, P., et al. (2007). Gambogic amide, a selective agonist for TrkA receptor that possesses robust neurotrophic activity, prevents neuronal cell death. *Proc. Natl. Acad. Sci. U S A* 104, 16329–16334. doi: 10.1073/pnas.0706662104

Kang, W. S., Sun, S., Nguyen, K., Kashemirov, B., McKenna, C. E., Hacking, S. A., et al. (2015). Non-ototoxic local delivery of bisphosphonate to the mammalian cochlea. *Otol. Neurotol.* 36, 953–960. doi: 10.1097/MAO.0000000000000786

Kashemirov, B. A., Bala, J. L., Chen, X., Ebetino, F. H., Xia, Z., Russell, R. G., et al. (2008). Fluorescently labeled risedronate and related analogues: "magic linker" synthesis. *Bioconjug. Chem.* 19, 2308–2310. doi: 10.1021/bc800369c

Kempfle, J. S., Nguyen, K., Hamadani, C., Koen, N., Edge, A. S., Kashemirov, B. A., et al. (2018). Bisphosphonate-linked TrkB agonist: cochlea-targeted delivery of a neurotrophic agent as a strategy for the treatment of hearing loss. *Bioconjug. Chem.* 29, 1240–1250. doi: 10.1021/acs.bioconjchem.8b00022

Kramer, B., Tropitzsch, A., Muller, M., and Lowenheim, H. (2017). Myelin-induced inhibition in a spiral ganglion organ culture - approaching a natural environment in vitro. *Neuroscience* 357, 75–83. doi: 10.1016/j.neuroscience.2017.05.053

Kujawa, S. G., and Liberman, M. C. (2006). Acceleration of age-related hearing loss by early noise exposure: evidence of a misspent youth. *J. Neurosci.* 26, 2115–2123. doi: 10.1523/JNEUROSCI.4985-05.2006

Kujawa, S. G., and Liberman, M. C. (2009). Adding insult to injury: cochlear nerve degeneration after "temporary" noise-induced hearing loss. *J. Neurosci.* 29, 14077–14085. doi: 10.1523/JNEUROSCI.2845-09.2009

Lee, H. B., Zaccaro, M. C., Pattarawarapan, M., Roy, S., Saragovi, H. U., and Burgess, K. (2004). Syntheses and activities of new C10 β-turn peptidomimetics. *J. Org. Chem.* 69, 701–713. doi: 10.1021/jo034167x

Lewis, M. A., Hunihan, L., Franco, D., Robertson, B., Palmer, J., Laurent, D. R., et al. (2006). Identification and characterization of compounds that potentiate NT-3-mediated Trk receptor activity. *Mol. Pharmacol.* 69, 1396–1404. doi: 10.1124/mol.105.020255

Liberman, M. C., and Kujawa, S. G. (2017). Cochlear synaptopathy in acquired sensorineural hearing loss: manifestations and mechanisms. *Hear Res.* 349, 138–147. doi: 10.1016/j.heares.2017.01.003

Lin, B., Pirrung, M. C., Deng, L., Li, Z., Liu, Y., and Webster, N. J. (2007). Neuroprotection by small molecule activators of the nerve growth factor receptor. *J. Pharmacol. Exp. Ther.* 322, 59–69. doi: 10.1124/jpet.106.118034

Marinzi, C., Offer, J., Longhi, R., and Dawson, P. E. (2004). An o-nitrobenzyl scaffold for peptide ligation: synthesis and applications. *Bioorg. Med. Chem.* 12, 2749–2757. doi: 10.1016/j.bmc.2004.02.039

McKenna, C., Haratipour, P., Duro, M. V. V., and Ebetino, F. H. (2020). "Chemistry of bisphosphonates," in *Encyclopedia of Bone Biology*, ed M. Zaidi (Netherlands: Elsevier), 551–564.

Noushi, F., Richardson, R. T., Hardman, J., Clark, G., and O' Leary, S. (2005). Delivery of neurotrophin-3 to the cochlea using alginate beads. *Otol. Neurotol.* 26, 528–533. doi: 10.1097/01.mao.0000169780.84588.a5

Nyberg, S., Abbott, N. J., Shi, X., Steyger, P. S., and Dabdoub, A. (2019). Delivery of therapeutics to the inner ear: the challenge of the blood-labyrinth barrier. *Sci. Transl. Med.* 11:eaao0935. doi: 10.1126/scitranslmed.aao0935

Panagiotakou, A., Yavropoulou, M., Nasiri-Ansari, N., Makras, P., Basdra, E. K., Papavassiliou, A. G., et al. (2020). Extra-skeletal effects of bisphosphonates. *Metabolism* 110:154264. doi: 10.1016/j.metabol.2020.154264

Pattarawarapan, M., Zaccaro, M. C., Saragovi, U. H., and Burgess, K. (2002). New templates for syntheses of ring-fused, C10 β-turn peptidomimetics leading to the first reported small-molecule mimic of neurotrophin-3. *J. Med. Chem.* 45, 4387–4390. doi: 10.1021/jm0255421

Peleshok, J., and Saragovi, H. U. (2006). Functional mimetics of neurotrophins and their receptors. *Biochem. Soc. Trans.* 34, 612–617. doi: 10.1042/BST0340612

Price, R. D., Milne, S. A., Sharkey, J., and Matsuoka, N. (2007). Advances in small molecules promoting neurotrophic function. *Pharmacol. Ther.* 115, 292–306. doi: 10.1016/j.pharmthera.2007.03.005

Ramekers, D., Versnel, H., Strahl, S. B., Klis, S. F., and Grolman, W. (2015). Temporary neurotrophin treatment prevents deafness-induced auditory nerve degeneration and preserves function. *J. Neurosci.* 35, 12331–12345. doi: 10.1523/JNEUROSCI.0096-15.2015

Salt, A. N., and Plontke, S. K. (2009). Principles of local drug delivery to the inner ear. *Audiol. Neurootol.* 14, 350–360. doi: 10.1159/000241892

Schuknecht, H. F., and Gacek, M. R. (1993). Cochlear pathology in presbycusis. *Ann. Otol. Rhinol. Laryngol.* 102, 1–16. doi: 10.1177/00034894931020S101

Sedghizadeh, P. P., Sun, S., Junka, A. F., Richard, E., Sadrerafi, K., Mahabady, S., et al. (2017). Design, synthesis and antimicrobial evaluation of a novel bone-targeting bisphosphonate-ciprofloxacin conjugate for the treatment of osteomyelitis biofilms. *J. Med. Chem.* 60, 2326–2343. doi: 10.1021/acs.jmedchem.6b01615

Seist, R., Tong, M., Landegger, L. D., Vasilijic, S., Hyakusoku, H., Katsumi, S., et al. (2020). Regeneration of cochlear synapses by systemic administration of a bisphosphonate. *Front. Mol. Neurosci.* 13:87. doi: 10.3389/fnmol.2020.00087

Sergeyenko, Y., Lall, K., Liberman, M. C., and Kujawa, S. G. (2013). Age-related cochlear synaptopathy: an early-onset contributor to auditory functional decline. *J. Neurosci.* 33, 13686–13694. doi: 10.1523/JNEUROSCI.1783-13.2013

Silos-Santiago, I., Fagan, A. M., Garber, M., Fritzsch, B., and Barbacid, M. (1997). Severe sensory deficits but normal CNS development in newborn mice lacking TrkB and TrkC tyrosine protein kinase receptors. *Eur. J. Neurosci.* 9, 2045–2056. doi: 10.1111/j.1460-9568.1997.tb01372.x

Sly, D. J., Campbell, L., Uschakov, A., Saief, S. T., Lam, M., and O' Leary, S. J. (2016). Applying neurotrophins to the round window rescues auditory function and reduces inner hair cell synaptopathy after noise-induced hearing loss. *Otol. Neurotol.* 37, 1223–1230. doi: 10.1097/MAO.0000000000001191

Stagni, F., Giacomini, A., Guidi, S., Emili, M., Uguagliati, B., Salvalai, M. E., et al. (2017). A flavonoid agonist of the TrkB receptor for BDNF improves hippocampal neurogenesis and hippocampus-dependent memory in the Ts65Dn mouse model of DS. *Exp. Neurol.* 298, 79–96. doi: 10.1016/j.expneurol.2017.08.018

Stankovic, K., Rio, C., Xia, A., Sugawara, M., Adams, J. C., Liberman, M. C., et al. (2004). Survival of adult spiral ganglion neurons requires erbB receptor signaling in the inner ear. *J. Neurosci.* 24, 8651–8661. doi: 10.1523/JNEUROSCI.0733-04.2004

Sun, S. T., Blazewska, K. M., Kadina, A. P., Kashemirov, B. A., Duan, X. C., Triffitt, J. T., et al. (2016). Fluorescent bisphosphonate and carboxyphosphonate probes: a versatile imaging toolkit for applications in bone biology and biomedicine. *Bioconjug. Chem.* 27, 329–340. doi: 10.1021/acs.bioconjchem.5b00369

Suzuki, J., Corfas, G., and Liberman, M. C. (2016). Round-window delivery of neurotrophin 3 regenerates cochlear synapses after acoustic overexposure. *Sci. Rep.* 6:24907. doi: 10.1038/srep24907

Swan, E. E. L., Mescher, M. J., Sewell, W. F., Tao, S. L., and Borenstein, J. I. (2008). Inner ear drug delivery for auditory applications. *Adv. Drug. Deliv. Rev.* 60, 1583–1599. doi: 10.1016/j.addr.2008.08.001

Valero, M. D., Burton, J. A., Hauser, S. N., Hackett, T. A., Ramachandran, R., and Liberman, M. C. (2017). Noise-induced cochlear synaptopathy in rhesus monkeys *(Macaca mulatta)*. *Hear Res.* 353, 213–223. doi: 10.1016/j.heares.2017.07.003

Viana, L. M., O' Malley, J. T., Burgess, B. J., Jones, D. D., Oliveira, C. A., Santos, F., et al. (2015). Cochlear neuropathy in human presbycusis: confocal analysis of hidden hearing loss in post-mortem tissue. *Hear Res.* 327, 78–88. doi: 10.1016/j.heares.2015.04.014

Wan, G., Gomez-Casati, M. E., Gigliello, A. R., Liberman, M. C., and Corfas, G. (2014). Neurotrophin-3 regulates ribbon synapse density in the cochlea and induces synapse regeneration after acoustic trauma. *eLife* 3:e03564. doi: 10.7554/eLife.03564

Wang, Q., and Green, S. H. (2011). Functional role of neurotrophin-3 in synapse regeneration by spiral ganglion neurons on inner hair cells after excitotoxic trauma *in vitro*. *J. Neurosci.* 31, 7938–7949. doi: 10.1523/JNEUROSCI.1434-10.2011

Wu, P. Z., Liberman, L. D., Bennett, K., de Gruttola, V., O' Malley, J. T., and Liberman, M. C. (2019). Primary neural degeneration in the human cochlea: evidence for hidden hearing loss in the aging ear. *Neuroscience* 407, 8–20. doi: 10.1016/j.neuroscience.2018.07.053

Wu, P. Z., O' Malley, J. T., de Gruttola, V., and Liberman, M. C. (2020). Age-related hearing loss is dominated by damage to inner ear sensory cells, not the cellular battery that powers them. *J. Neurosci.* 40, 6357–6366. doi: 10.1523/JNEUROSCI.0937-20.2020

Xu, L., Cohen, A. E., and Boxer, S. G. (2011). Electrostatic fields near the active site of human aldose reductase: 2. new inhibitors and complications caused by hydrogen bonds. *Biochemistry* 50, 8311–8322. doi: 10.1021/bi200930f

Zaccaro, M. C., Lee, H. B., Pattarawarapan, M., Xia, Z., Caron, A., L' Heureux, P. J., et al. (2005). Selective small molecule peptidomimetic ligands of TrkC and TrkA receptors afford discrete or complete neurotrophic activities. *Chem. Biol.* 12, 1015–1028. doi: 10.1111/jnc.14599

11

A Novel Variant in the TBC1D24 Lipid-Binding Pocket Causes Autosomal Dominant Hearing Loss: Evidence for a Genotype-Phenotype Correlation

Thomas Parzefall[1], Alexandra Frohne[1,2], Martin Koenighofer[1], Juergen Neesen[3], Franco Laccone[3], Julia Eckl-Dorna[1], Jonathan J. Waters[4], Markus Schreiner[5], Sami Samir Amr[6,7], Emma Ashton[4], Christian Schoefer[2], Wolfgang Gstœttner[1], Klemens Frei[1] and Trevor Lucas[2]*

[1]Department of Otorhinolaryngology, Head and Neck Surgery, Medical University of Vienna, Vienna, Austria, [2]Department for Cell and Developmental Biology, Orphan Disease Genetics Group, Center for Anatomy and Cell Biology, Medical University of Vienna, Vienna, Austria, [3]Institute of Medical Genetics, Center for Pathobiochemistry and Genetics, Medical University of Vienna, Vienna, Austria, [4]Rare and Inherited Disease Laboratory, London North Genomic Laboratory Hub, Great Ormond Street Hospital for Children NHS Foundation Trust, London, United Kingdom, [5]Department of Biomedical Imaging and Image-Guided Therapy, Medical University of Vienna, Vienna, Austria, [6]Laboratory for Molecular Medicine, Partners Healthcare Personalized Medicine, Cambridge, MA, United States, [7]Department of Pathology, Brigham and Women's Hospital and Harvard Medical School, Boston, MA, United States

***Correspondence:**
Klemens Frei
klemens.frei@meduniwien.ac.at

Background: Hereditary hearing loss is a disorder with high genetic and allelic heterogeneity. Diagnostic screening of candidate genes commonly yields novel variants of unknown clinical significance. *TBC1D24* is a pleiotropic gene associated with recessive DOORS syndrome, epileptic encephalopathy, myoclonic epilepsy, and both recessive and dominant hearing impairment. Genotype-phenotype correlations have not been established to date but could facilitate diagnostic variant assessment and elucidation of pathomechanisms.

Methods and Results: Whole-exome and gene panel screening identified a novel (c.919A>C; p.Asn307His) causative variant in *TBC1D24* in two unrelated Caucasian families with Autosomal dominant (AD) nonsyndromic late-onset hearing loss. Protein modeling on the *Drosophila* TBC1D24 ortholog Skywalker crystal structure showed close interhelix proximity (6.8Å) between the highly conserved residue p.Asn307 in α18 and the position of the single known pathogenic dominant variation (p.Ser178Leu) in α11 that causes a form of deafness with similar clinical characteristics.

Conclusion: Genetic variants affecting two polar hydrophilic residues in neighboring helices of TBC1D24 cause AD nonsyndromic late-onset hearing loss. The spatial proximity of the affected residues suggests the first genotype-phenotype association in *TBC1D24*-related disorders. Three conserved residues in α18 contribute to the formation of a functionally relevant cationic phosphoinositide binding pocket that regulates synaptic vesicle trafficking which may be involved in the molecular mechanism of disease.

Keywords: TBC1D24, DFNA65, genotype-phenotype association, exome sequencing, autosomal dominant, nonsyndromic, hearing loss

INTRODUCTION

Autosomal dominant (AD) nonsyndromic hearing loss (HL) is a heterogeneous condition regarding the age of onset, frequencies affected, progression, and severity. In total, 49 genes have been identified as causative to date (hereditaryhearingloss.org) that have a wide range of pleiotropy and function. The high genetic and allelic heterogeneity of HL poses a challenge to the clinical assessment of novel variants routinely encountered during the diagnostic screening. Identification of novel genes and variants not only expands diagnosis and genetic counseling but increases understanding of human hearing and deafness and can lead to personalized medicine approaches. Whole-exome sequencing (WES) and targeted next-generation sequencing of HL genetic panels have greatly facilitated the analysis of genetic HL in recent years. *TBC1D24*, coding for TBC1 Domain Family Member 24, is a pleiotropic gene that has been associated with autosomal recessive (AR) HL (DFNB86), ADHL (DFNA65), and a range of epilepsy syndromes (Mucha et al., 2017). Attempts to establish TBC1D24 genotype-phenotype correlations with AR variants have been unsuccessful, complicating the evaluation of variant pathogenicity. Here, we report a novel (c.919A>C; p.Asn307His) mutation in *TBC1D24* identified during WES and diagnostic panel screening of two unrelated ADHL families from Austria and the UK implying an association between AD HL disease phenotype and genetic variation affecting structural elements involved in phospholipid binding (Fischer et al., 2016).

SUBJECTS AND METHODS

Patient Recruitment and Clinical Testing

Study participants were recruited at the Department of Otorhinolaryngology at the Medical University of Vienna, Austria, as part of an ongoing screening project for genetic HL and for diagnostic testing at the Great Ormond Street Hospital for Children, London, UK. Selected probands underwent speech audiometry, brainstem evoked response audiometry (BERA), otoacoustic emission (OAE) testing, video head thrust tests, vestibular caloric assessments, and neurocranial magnetic resonance imaging (MRI). Degrees of HL were defined as mild (20–40), moderate (41–70), and severe (71–95) in threshold dB values. The study met the WMA Helsinki Declaration criteria and was approved by the local Ethics Committee of the Medical University of Vienna (ECS 198/2004, with annual extensions to date). Informed consent was obtained from all participants.

DNA Sequence Analysis and Variant Assessment

Chromosomal DNA was extracted from venous blood using a commercial extraction kit (Invisorb blood universal kit 1000, STRATEC Molecular, Berlin, Germany) or the Chemagic STAR system (Perkin Elmer, Waltham, MA, USA) for British family members. Patients IV.3, IV.5, IV.6, and IV.8, and the normal-hearing father (III.10) in the Austrian family (**Figure 1A**) were selected for WES. Libraries were prepared with a commercial (SureSelectXT All Exon, V5) and a custom capture kit of 95 genes[1] for the screening of the Austrian family and the UK proband (SureSelectXT Agilent Technologies, Santa Clara, CA, USA) respectively, followed by sequencing on an Illumina HiSeq 2000 (Austrian family) or MiSeq (UK proband) device (Illumina Biotechnology, San Diego, CA, USA). The UK sample was processed with an in-house bioinformatics pipeline, involving alignment with Burrows-Wheeler read aligner (BWA), variant calling with Freebayes, annotation with VEP95, re-annotation using Alamut batch, and variant analysis on an in-house system "GOSHG2P." Reads from the Austrian family were mapped to the human genome reference build hg19 with the BWA (Li and Durbin, 2009) and variants were called with the Genome Analysis Tool Kit (Mckenna et al., 2010). All missense, deletion, and insertion variants in coding regions and splice sites were analyzed on an online massive parallel sequencing analysis platform (Genomatix GeneGrid, Genomatix GmbH, Munich, Germany) and visualized by interrogation of bam/bai files with the Integrative Genomics Viewer (IGV; Broad Institute, Cambridge, MA, USA). Variants were filtered at a maximum non-Finnish GnomAD European allele frequency of 0.00075 (Lek et al., 2016). A single common artifact in PPIAL4G (Gln24Leu; rs6604516) was removed by reference to a local WES database. All genomic positions listed refer to hg19. Candidate validation and segregation analysis were performed by PCR and standard Sanger sequencing. Primers were designed with Primer-BLAST interface[2]. All PCR reactions were performed in 2.5 mM $MgCl_2$, 200 mM of dNTPs, 100 ng of chromosomal DNA, and 20 pmol of primers to amplify the segments of interest in *TBC1D24* (5′-CTTCCTGGCCTTTGAGTCGT-3′/5′-AGGATAGGACCCGATGTCCC-3′), *SYNE4* (5′-CGGGATGGGAAATGGGTTGA-3′/5′-CGAACACCTGGGTCAAAGGA-3′) and *CCNF* (5′-CCCTTCCTGCCTGTCATGTG-3′/5′-TGTGCTAGGAGACAGCAGTAGG-3′) in 35 cycles of denaturation (95°C, 30 s), annealing (60°C, 30 s), and elongation (72°C, 90 s). To exclude genes not expressed in the cochlea as

[1] www.labs.gosh.nhs.uk/media/529754/nsd_and_usher_v6.pdf
[2] www.ncbi.nlm.nih.gov/tools/primer-blast

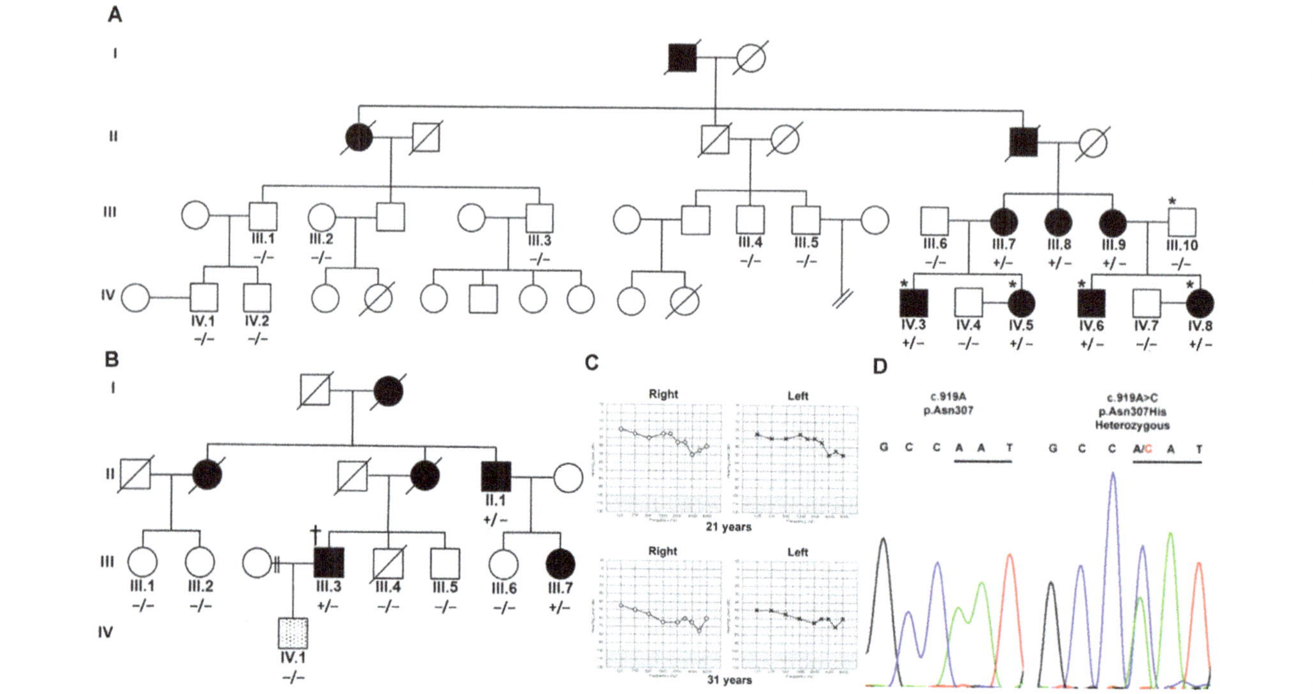

FIGURE 1 | Segregation of TBC1D24 p.Asn307His with autosomal dominant (AD) nonsyndromic hearing loss (HL). **(A)** Four affected (shaded) family members and a normal-hearing (open) father in an Austrian family were analyzed by whole-exome sequencing (*). **(B)** In a UK family, one affected family member (†) was analyzed with panel sequencing. Segregation of heterozygous (+/–) c.919A>C in *TBC1D24* was tested in all available members of both families by Sanger sequencing. A single member of the UK family (lined; IV.1) developed a very-late-onset, predominantly mild high-frequency HL and did not segregate p.Asn307His. **(C)** Unaided, masked pure-tone audiograms in dB hearing levels of patient IV.8 at the ages of 21 and 31 years show progression to moderately severe pantonal HL. **(D)** Representative chromatograms show the A>C variation in IV.8 and the wildtype sequence in control subject IV.4. Codon 307 is underlined.

HL candidates, expression data for adult mouse inner (IHC) and outer hair cells (OHC; Liu et al., 2014) cochlear HC, supporting cells (SC; Scheffer et al., 2015) and spiral ganglion neurons (Lu et al., 2011) at different developmental stages and overall inner ear soft tissue of 9-week-old mice (Geo GSE13421) were retrieved from the SHIELD[3] and mouse cochlea gene[4] databases. For FACS-sorted HC and SC data, the baseline for expression was set at a total of 15 reads from RNA-Seq across all samples (Scheffer et al., 2015) and at intensity levels of 10.9 for adult IHC and OHC microarray data (Liu et al., 2014). The isolated candidate variant was analyzed with SIFT[5] and PolyPhen-2[6].

Protein Modeling and Cross-Species Alignment

The TBC domain was modeled on the Skywalker (human TBC1D24 equivalent residues 21–310; PDB 5HJN) and zebrafish TLDc domain-oxidation resistance protein 22 (residues 333–548; 4ACJ) crystal structures with the Protein Homology/analogY Recognition Engine V 2.0 (Phyre2[7]; Kelley et al., 2015). The PDB file of the generated model was analyzed in JMOL[8] to illustrate bulkiness with Corey-Pauling-Koltun sphere representations and calculate atomic distances. TBC1D24 ortholog sequences from *Homo sapiens* (NP_001186036), *Pan troglodytes* (XP_016784129), *Rattus norvegicus* (NP_001099239), *Mus musculus* (NP_001157319), *Canis lupus familiaris* (XP_013970162), *Gallus gallus* (NP_001244200), *Xenopus laevis* (NP_001090574), *Danio rerio* (XP_009295920), and *Drosophila melanogaster* Skywalker (NP_610073.1) were aligned at Clustal Omega[9] and visualized in AliView (University of Uppsala) with SeaView residue annotation.

RESULTS

Clinical Phenotype in the Patients

Austrian (**Figure 1A**) and British Caucasian families (**Figure 1B**) were identified suffering from recurrent cases of nonsyndromic progressive ADHL. Onset was observed at an average age of 19 years 4 months ± 15 months for three members (IV.5, IV.6, and IV.8) of the Austrian family and 27 years ± 7.5 years in the British family (II.1, III.3, and III.7). HL developed from an initial mainly mild (below 2,000 Hz) to moderate (above

[3] www.shield.hms.harvard.edu
[4] research.meei.harvard.edu/Otopathology/tbimages/mouse.html
[5] https://sift.bii.a-star.edu.sg/
[6] https://genetics.bwh.harvard.edu/pph2/
[7] www.sbg.bio.ic.ac.uk/phyre2
[8] www.jmol.org
[9] www.ebi.ac.uk/Tools/msa/clustalo

5,000 Hz) accentuated high-frequency HL slowly progressing to moderate-to-severe pantonal HL after 10 years (**Figure 1C**). Bone conduction results were not significantly different in the probands analyzed and no air-bone gap was observed (data not shown) consistent with sensorineural HL and excluding a conductive or mixed type of hearing loss. All affected family members use hearing aids for daily communication. Caloric reflex testing and video head thrust testing showed bilateral vestibular normoreflexia in all Austrian study patients. There was no history of syndromic neurologic disease, and brain MRI and neurological examinations showed no abnormalities in a member of the Austrian family (IV.8). One member (IV.1) of the UK family had grommets fitted as a child because of perceived hearing difficulties which were attributed to "glue ear." At 35 years of age, he had normal hearing up to 4,000 Hz but began to develop a bilateral, predominantly mild, high-frequency HL. Due to the different clinical presentation compared to the other family members, a different cause of HL was considered likely.

Genetic Screening Results

Patients IV.3, IV.5, IV.6, and IV.8 and the normal hearing father (III.10) in the Austrian family were selected for WES. Without utilizing coverage or quality filters, potential heterozygous pathogenic variants with a cutoff non-Finnish gnomAD European allele frequency (Lek et al., 2016) for a single heterozygous alteration at 0.00075 were identified in the genes *TPSG1* (16:1,272,028; NM_012467; c.726G>C; p.Trp242Cys; rs551902061), *TBC1D24* (16:2,547,068; NM_001199107.2; c.919A>C; p.Asn307His; submitted as rs1555501320) and *CCNF* (16:2,481,223; NM_001761.3; c.109G>A; p.Glu37Lys) at 16p13.3 and *SYNE4* (19:36,497,711; NM_001039876.3; c.559C>T; p.Arg187Ter; rs750797779). *TPSG1*, *TBC1D24*, *CCNF*, and *SYNE4* variants are all segregated by Sanger sequencing in the family as potential causes of HL (**Figure 1D**). *TPSG1* cochlear expression was below the threshold levels set for cochlear expression and was therefore not further considered as an HL candidate. In the UK family, a *TBC1D24* c.919A>C variant was identified as a sole candidate in targeted HL screening with a panel of 95 genes. The variant segregated in three affected members of the family by Sanger sequencing (**Figure 1B**). The c.109G>A *CCNF* and c.559C>T *SYNE4* variants identified in the Austrian family were not present in the affected UK family members shown by Sanger sequencing. The hearing-impaired family member IV.1 with a different clinical presentation carried the c.919A *TBC1D24* wildtype allele (**Figure 1B**). In contrast to p.Ser178Leu (non-Finnish European allele frequency 2/112,984; 0.000018), p.Asn307His is not listed in the gnomAD database. A single variant at p.307 (p.Asn307Ser; 1/111,448; 0.000009) is listed. The p.Asn307His variant was predicted to be probably damaging with Polyphen-2 (score 1.000, sensitivity 0.00, specificity 1.00) and tolerated (score 0.21) with SIFT. Concerning the American College of Medical Genetics and Genomics/Association for Molecular Pathology guidelines applied to ADHL (Oza et al., 2018), p.Asn307His would be classified as likely pathogenic based on the criteria PM2 (absent or ≤0.00002 in population databases), PS4_supporting (two unrelated probands with the variant) and PP1_strong (segregation in five affected relatives).

TABLE 1 | Homology model predictions of TBC domain alpha helical elements in TBC1D24.

TBC alpha helix	Amino acid coordinates (p.)
1	12–21
2	32–40
3	48–59
4	62–67
5	73–81
6	90–95
7	103–105
8	108–124
9	134–144
10	148–160
11	173–190
12	192–200
13	206–219
14	222–234
15	238–253
16	254–259
17	265–274
18	282–315

Protein Model and Cross-Species Alignment

The TBC domain of TBC1D24 based on the homology model is predicted to contain the alpha-helical elements α1–18 (**Table 1**). Residue p. Asn307 in α18 is conserved in vertebrates (**Figure 2A**). Seven residues in helical elements α2 (p.Gln33 and p.Arg40), α15 (p.Lys238 and p.Arg242), and α18 (p.Arg293, p.Leu294, and p.Arg297) are human equivalent positions involved in the formation of a lipid-binding pocket recently identified in the *Drosophila* orthologue Skywalker. Cross-species alignments reveal full conservation of the residues p.Arg40, p.Lys238, p.Arg242 (data not shown), and p.Arg293 between human TBC1D24 and Skywalker. A single TBC1D24 variation (p.Ser178Leu) exchanging a highly conserved polar uncharged residue for a hydrophobic residue has been described previously in a European and a Chinese family by independent groups that cause AD HL with a similar age of onset and clinical course as the families under study (Azaiez et al., 2014; Zhang et al., 2014). The model predicts an interaction between p.Ser178 (α11) and p.Asn307 (α18) at an interhelix proximity of 6.8Å (**Figure 2B**). Cross-species alignments for α11 are shown in **Figure 2C**.

DISCUSSION

Genetic testing revealed a novel rare missense (c.919A>C; p.Asn307His) variant in *TBC1D24* as the cause of disease in two unrelated families from Austria and the UK with late-onset, progressive, nonsyndromic ADHL. Whereas this variant was the sole candidate identified in the UK proband during diagnostic panel screening that segregated in all tested affected family members by Sanger sequencing, two further variations in *SYNE4*

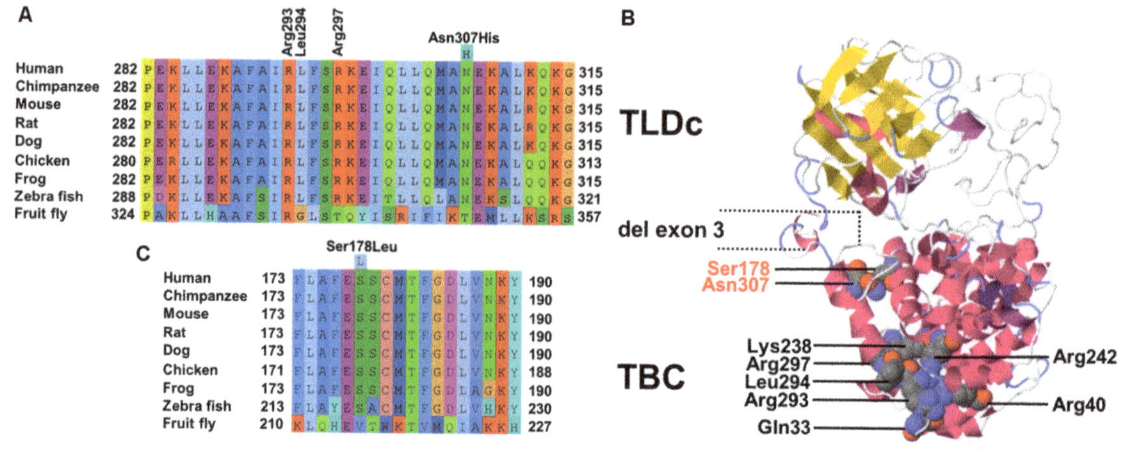

FIGURE 2 | (A) Cross-species multiple alignments of the α18 helix of TBC1D24 (p.282–315) reveal high conservation of a polar uncharged residue at p.Asn307. The positions of the coordinating residues (p.Arg293, p.Leu294, and p.Arg297) responsible for binding phosphoinositides phosphorylated at positions 4 and 5 derived from the crystal structure of *Drosophila Skywalker* are shown **(B)**. Phyre2 model of human TBC1D24 based on crystal structures of Skywalker (human TBC1D24 residues 21–310; PDB 5HJN) and the zebrafish TLDc domain-oxidation resistance protein 22 (residues 333–548; 4ACJ). Corey–Pauling–Koltun sphere representations of mutated p.Arg307 and p.Ser178 amino acid positions in ADHL and all residues that contribute to the binding pocket are shown. Coordinates of the in-frame deletion of exon 3 in the shorter isoform are indicated. **(C)** Cross-species multiple alignments of the α11 helix of TBC1D24 (p.173–190) containing p.Ser178.

(c.559C>T; p.Arg187Ter) and *CCNF* (c.109G>A; p.Glu37Lys) co-segregated with the disease in the Austrian family screened by WES and Sanger sequencing. Although *SYNE4* variations have to date only been associated with ARHL, heterozygous p.Arg187Ter has been previously identified in a sporadic case of HL (ClinVar RCV000213729) with a heterozygous pathogenic ADHL *COCH* variation (p.Cys542Tyr; Yuan et al., 2008). We, therefore, could not completely exclude p.Arg187Ter as a modifier or a secondary driver in the development of AD HL in a single family. Since one missense (p.Ser178Leu) variant in *TBC1D24* has previously been shown to cause ADHL with similar clinical characteristics seen in this study (Azaiez et al., 2014; Zhang et al., 2014), the p.Asn307His variation (ClinVar registration VCV000425556.1) shared by both families was considered the cause of disease.

TBC1D24 is a pleiotropic gene and variations cause both ARHL (DFNB86; MIM 614617), ADHL (DFNA65; MIM 616044), and several epilepsy syndromes such as AR DOORS (deafness, onychodystrophy, osteodystrophy, mental retardation, and seizures) syndrome (MIM 220500), AR early infantile epileptic encephalopathy-16 (MIM 615338) and AR familial infantile myoclonic epilepsy (MIM 605021; Mucha et al., 2017). To date, pathomechanistic investigations on TBC1D24 variations have been hampered by a lack of genotype-phenotype correlation when analyzing homozygous and compound heterozygous AR variants (Bakhchane et al., 2015; Aprile et al., 2019). Missense variations in the TBC domain and a truncating frameshift variation in the TLDc domain are known to cause prelingual-onset ARHL (Rehman et al., 2014; Bakhchane et al., 2015; Danial-Farran et al., 2018). Heterozygous carriers of the truncating variant are without symptoms (Azaiez et al., 2014; Rehman et al., 2017).

TBC1D24 is expressed in a broad range of tissues, and expression levels are highest in the brain (proteinatlas.org). In the auditory pathway, TBC1D24 is expressed in spiral ganglion cells, stereocilia and the cell bodies of IHC and OHC (Azaiez et al., 2014; Rehman et al., 2014; Zhang et al., 2014) although differences between murine and human expression patterns are still to be clarified. Tbc1d24 expression was reported in the SHIELD database in FACS-sorted supporting cells und HC from E16 to P7 and in spiral ganglion neurons from E12 to P15 but not in adult (P25-P30) IHC and OHC. In the Mouse Cochlea Gene Database, tbc1d24 expression was detected in whole cochleae of 9-week old mice. The 559-residue TBC1D24 protein contains an *N*-terminal Tre2-Bub2-Cdc16 (TBC) domain present in Rab GTPase-activating proteins (Rab GAPs), a domain linkage region, and a C-terminal TLDc domain with no known function but often found in TBC and lysine motif (LysM) domain-containing proteins (Corbett et al., 2010). A shorter 553-residue isoform (**Figure 2B**) generated by in-frame deletion of exon 3 (residues 322–327) is expressed in non-neural tissues (Guven and Tolun, 2013). Even though the presence of a TBC domain may indicate a role in vesicle trafficking, it is unknown whether TBC1D24 has Rab GAP activity as it lacks highly conserved residues pivotal for GTP hydrolysis (Pan et al., 2006; Hutagalung and Novick, 2011; Fischer et al., 2016). Recently, a lipid-binding pocket in TBC1D24 that binds phosphoinositides phosphorylated at positions 4 and 5 was identified from the crystal structure of the *Drosophila* ortholog Skywalker (human TBC1D24 equivalent residues 1–311) with the human TBC1D24 coordinates p.Gln33, p.Arg40, p.Lys238, p.Arg242, p.Arg293, p.Leu294 and p.Arg297 (Fischer et al., 2016). We, therefore, modeled human TBC1D24 on the Skywalker (residues 21–310; 5HJN) and the zebrafish TLDc domain-oxidation resistance protein 22 (residues 333–548; 4ACJ) crystal structures using Phyre[2] (Kelley et al., 2015). Three binding-pocket equivalent residues (p.Arg293, p.Leu294, and p.Arg297) are located with p.Asn307 in α18 (**Figure 2A**). It is therefore conceivable that the p.Asn307His variant disturbs the integrity of the binding pocket. Interestingly, the wildtype model predicts an interaction between p.Ser178 (α11) and p.Asn307 (α18), the sole residues associated with ADHL to date, at interhelix proximity of 6.8 Å (**Figure 2B**). This proximity and interaction may be indicative of a novel genotype-phenotype correlation in DFNA65. An adjacent glutamic acid residue to p.Ser178 in α11 (**Figure 2C**) could also potentially interact with p.307 positively charged residue variants in α18.

In summary, we identify a second variation (p. Asn307His) in *TBC1D24* that causes ADHL. By generating a TBC protein model on the crystal structure of *Drosophila* Skywalker, we show that p. Asn307 is within predicted α-helix 18 that contains three residues involved in forming a lipid-binding pocket in Skywalker. In this model, p. Asn307 is in close interhelix proximity to p.Ser178 in α11, the single position identified to date to cause ADHL. Therefore, this is the first report of a probable genotype-phenotype correlation for *TBC1D24*-caused disease. The identification of potential interactions may not only enable the development of novel personalized therapies for HL but also has implications for genetic counseling. This is further illustrated by a report of pathogenicity for a negatively charged variation at codon 307 (p.Asn307Asp) that, in conjunction with an α18 missense variant c.845C>G (p.Pro282Arg), causes AR focal seizures, developmental delays, malignant migrating partial seizures of infancy, and hippocampal atrophy (Appavu et al., 2016).

AUTHOR CONTRIBUTIONS

EA, KF, TL, WG, JE-D, and TP: conceptualization. MK, JW, MS, AF, FL, JN, CS, TL, KF, and TP: methodology. JE-D, SA, JW, EA, AF, FL, JN, TL, and TP: data analysis. MS, SA, EA, FL, TL, CS, and WG: resources. SA, AF, KF, TL, and TP: data curation. AF, FL, TL, EA, and TP: preparation of the manuscript. WG, TL, and TP: supervision. JE-D, AF, MK, KF, CS, TL, and TP: project administration. WG, KF, CS, TL, and TP: funding acquisition. All authors have critically read and agreed to the published version of the manuscript. All authors contributed to the article and approved the submitted version.

ACKNOWLEDGMENTS

We thank the families for their invaluable participation in this study. The data that support the findings of this study are available from the corresponding author upon reasonable request. This article is dedicated to the memory of Professor Maria Bitner-Glindzicz.

REFERENCES

Appavu, B., Guido-Estrada, N., Lindstrom, K., Grebe, T., Kerrigan, J. F., and Troester, M. (2016). Electroclinical phenotypes and outcomes in TBC1D24-related epilepsy. *Epileptic Disord.* 18, 324–328. doi: 10.1684/epd.2016.0849

Aprile, D., Fruscione, F., Baldassari, S., Fadda, M., Ferrante, D., Falace, A., et al. (2019). TBC1D24 regulates axonal outgrowth and membrane trafficking at the growth cone in rodent and human neurons. *Cell Death Differ.* 26, 2464–2478. doi: 10.1038/s41418-019-0313-x

Azaiez, H., Booth, K. T., Bu, F., Huygen, P., Shibata, S. B., Shearer, A. E., et al. (2014). TBC1D24 mutation causes autosomal-dominant nonsyndromic hearing loss. *Hum. Mutat.* 35, 819–823. doi: 10.1002/humu.22557

Bakhchane, A., Charif, M., Salime, S., Boulouiz, R., Nahili, H., Roky, R., et al. (2015). Recessive TBC1D24 mutations are frequent in moroccan non-syndromic hearing loss pedigrees. *PLoS One* 10:e0138072. doi: 10.1371/journal.pone.0138072

Corbett, M. A., Bahlo, M., Jolly, L., Afawi, Z., Gardner, A. E., Oliver, K. L., et al. (2010). A focal epilepsy and intellectual disability syndrome is due to a mutation in TBC1D24. *Am. J. Hum. Genet.* 87, 371–375. doi: 10.1016/j.ajhg.2010.08.001

Danial-Farran, N., Brownstein, Z., Gulsuner, S., Tammer, L., Khayat, M., Aleme, O., et al. (2018). Genetics of hearing loss in the arab population of northern israel. *Eur. J. Hum. Genet.* 26, 1840–1847. doi: 10.1038/s41431-018-0218-z

Fischer, B., Lüthy, K., Paesmans, J., De Koninck, C., Maes, I., Swerts, J., et al. (2016). Skywalker-TBC1D24 has a lipid-binding pocket mutated in epilepsy and required for synaptic function. *Nat. Struct. Mol. Biol.* 23, 965–973. doi: 10.1038/nsmb.3297

Guven, A., and Tolun, A. (2013). TBC1D24 truncating mutation resulting in severe neurodegeneration. *J. Med. Genet.* 50, 199–202. doi: 10.1136/jmedgenet-2012-101313

Hutagalung, A. H., and Novick, P. J. (2011). Role of Rab GTPases in membrane traffic and cell physiology. *Physiol. Rev.* 91, 119–149. doi: 10.1152/physrev.00059.2009

Kelley, L. A., Mezulis, S., Yates, C. M., Wass, M. N., and Sternberg, M. J. (2015). The phyre2 web portal for protein modeling, prediction and analysis. *Nature Protoc.* 10, 845–858. doi: 10.1038/nprot.2015.053

Lek, M., Karczewski, K. J., Minikel, E. V., Samocha, K. E., Banks, E., Fennell, T., et al. (2016). Analysis of protein-coding genetic variation in 60,706 humans. *Nature* 536, 285–291. doi: 10.1038/nature19057

Li, H., and Durbin, R. (2009). Fast and accurate short read alignment with burrows-wheeler transform. *Bioinformatics* 25, 1754–1760. doi: 10.1093/bioinformatics/btp324

Liu, H., Pecka, J. L., Zhang, Q., Soukup, G. A., Beisel, K. W., and He, D. Z. (2014). Characterization of transcriptomes of cochlear inner and outer hair cells. *J. Neurosci.* 34, 11085–11095. doi: 10.1523/JNEUROSCI.1690-14.2014

Lu, C. C., Appler, J. M., Houseman, E. A., and Goodrich, L. V. (2011). Developmental profiling of spiral ganglion neurons reveals insights into auditory circuit assembly. *J. Neurosci.* 31, 10903–10918. doi: 10.1523/JNEUROSCI.2358-11.2011

Mckenna, A., Hanna, M., Banks, E., Sivachenko, A., Cibulskis, K., Kernytsky, A., et al. (2010). The Genome Analysis Toolkit: a MapReduce framework for analyzing next-generation DNA sequencing data. *Genome Res.* 20, 1297–1303. doi: 10.1101/gr.107524.110

Mucha, B. E., Hennekam, R. C. M., Sisodiya, S., and Campeau, P. M. (2017). "TBC1D24-related disorders," in *GeneReviews[(R)]*, eds M. P. Adam, H. H. Ardinger, R. A. Pagon, S. E. Wallace, L. J. H. Bean, K. Stephens, et al. (Seattle, WA: University of Washington, Seattle), 1993–2020.

Oza, A. M., Distefano, M. T., Hemphill, S. E., Cushman, B. J., Grant, A. R., Siegert, R. K., et al. (2018). Expert specification of the ACMG/AMP variant interpretation guidelines for genetic hearing loss. *Hum. Mutat.* 39, 1593–1613. doi: 10.1002/humu.23630

Pan, X., Eathiraj, S., Munson, M., and Lambright, D. G. (2006). TBC-domain GAPs for Rab GTPases accelerate GTP hydrolysis by a dual-finger mechanism. *Nature* 442, 303–306. doi: 10.1038/nature04847

Rehman, A. U., Friedman, T. B., and Griffith, A. J. (2017). Unresolved questions regarding human hereditary deafness. *Oral Dis.* 23, 551–558. doi: 10.1111/odi.12516

Rehman, A. U., Santos-Cortez, R. L. P., Morell, R. J., Drummond, M. C., Ito, T., Lee, K., et al. (2014). Mutations in TBC1D24, a gene associated with epilepsy, also cause nonsyndromic deafness DFNB86. *Am. J. Hum. Genet.* 94, 144–152. doi: 10.1016/j.ajhg.2013.12.004

Scheffer, D. I., Shen, J., Corey, D. P., and Chen, Z. Y. (2015). Gene expression by mouse inner ear hair cells during development. *J. Neurosci.* 35, 6366–6380. doi: 10.1523/JNEUROSCI.5126-14.2015

Yuan, H. J., Han, D. Y., Sun, Q., Yan, D., Sun, H. J., Tao, R., et al. (2008). Novel mutations in the vWFA2 domain of COCH in two chinese DFNA9 families. *Clin. Genet.* 73, 391–394. doi: 10.1111/j.1399-0004.2008.00972.x

Zhang, L., Hu, L., Chai, Y., Pang, X., Yang, T., and Wu, H. (2014). A dominant mutation in the stereocilia-expressing gene TBC1D24 is a probable cause for nonsyndromic hearing impairment. *Hum. Mutat.* 35, 814–818. doi: 10.1002/humu.22558

12

Protective Effects of N[1]-Methylnicotinamide against High-Fat Diet- and Age-Induced Hearing Loss *via* Moderate Overexpression of Sirtuin 1 Protein

Toru Miwa [1,2]*

[1] *Department of Otolaryngology and Head and Neck Surgery, Kitano Hospital, Tazuke Kofukai Medical Research Institute, Osaka, Japan,* [2] *Department of Otolaryngology and Head and Neck Surgery, Graduate of School of Medicine, Kyoto University, Kyoto, Japan*

***Correspondence:**
Toru Miwa
t-miwa@kitano-hp.or.jp

Age-related hearing loss (ARHL) is the most common form of hearing loss and the predominant neurodegenerative disease associated with aging. *Sirtuin 1 (SIRT1)* is associated with the most complex physiological processes, including metabolism, cancer onset, and aging. SIRT1 protein levels are enhanced by the conversion of nicotinamide to N[1]-methylnicotinamide (MNAM), independent of its mRNA levels. Moreover, MNAM has implications in increased longevity achieved through its mitohormetic effects. Nicotinamide N-methyltransferase (Nnmt) is an enzyme involved in MNAM metabolism, and its level increases under caloric restriction (CR) conditions. The CR condition has implications in delaying ARHL onset. In this study, we aimed to determine the relationship between diet, hearing function, SIRT1 and SIRT3 expression levels in the inner ear, and cochlear morphology. Mice fed with a high-fat diet (HFD), HFD + 1% MNAM, and low-fat diet (LFD) were monitored for age-related auditory-evoked brainstem responses, and changes in cochlear histology, metabolism, and protein and mRNA expressions were analyzed. Our results revealed that the HFD- and aging-mediated downregulated expression of SIRT1 and SIRT3 promoted hearing loss that was obfuscated by MNAM supplementation-induced upregulated expression of cochlear SIRT1 and SIRT3. Thus, our results suggest that MNAM can be used as a therapeutic agent for preventing ARHL.

Keywords: hearing loss, sirtuin 1, N[1]-methylnicotinamide, high-fat diet, auditory brain stem responses

---

Abbreviations: ARHL, age-related hearing loss; NAD+, nicotinamide adenine dinucleotide; MNAM, N[1]-methylnicotinamide, HFD, high-fat diet; LFD, low-fat diet; SIRT, Sirtuins; Nnmt, nicotinamide N-methyltransferase; NaM, nicotinamide; CR, caloric restriction; PFA, paraformaldehyde; EDTA, ethylenediaminetetraacetic acid; PBS, phosphate-buffered saline; Tuj1, anti-beta III tubulin; SGCs, spiral ganglion cells; GAPDH, glyceraldehyde-3-phosphate dehydrogenase; cDNA, complementary DNA; ANOVA, analysis of variance; ABR, auditory brainstem responses; SLi, spiral ligament cells; OC, the organ of Corti; WB, western blotting; ELISA, enzyme-linked immunosorbent assay.

INTRODUCTION

Age-related hearing loss (ARHL) is a multifactorial disease that results from a combination of genetic predispositions and effects of the aging process, including a plethora of insults to the auditory organ throughout an individual's lifetime (Gates and Mills, 2005; Yamasoba et al., 2013). ARHL can be prevented by improving the health and quality of life in elderly individuals; however, thus far, no preventive measures have been outlined.

Sirtuins (Sirt) are a family of nicotinamide adenine dinucleotide (NAD^+)-dependent protein deacetylases that are known to extend the lifespan of lower organisms (Finkel et al., 2009). *Sirt1* expression plays critical roles in mammalian health and disease development and is often associated with the most complex physiological processes, including metabolism, the onset of cancer, and aging (Revollo and Li, 2013). At the cellular level, *Sirt1* controls deoxyribose nucleic acid (DNA) repair and apoptosis, circadian clocks, inflammatory pathways, insulin secretion, and mitochondrial biogenesis (Haigis and Sinclair, 2010; Chalkiadaki and Guarente, 2012). It also modulates apoptosis in response to oxidative and genotoxic stress in neurodegenerative diseases and ARHL (Someya et al., 2009; Donmez and Outeiro, 2013). Additionally, *Sirt1* may act as a sensor for metabolic adaptation to nutritional states since it is regulated by the availability of its substrate, NAD^+. Thus, the enzymes involved in the NAD^+ metabolic pathways may regulate metabolism through *Sirt1* (Chalkiadaki and Guarente, 2012). Nicotinamide N-methyltransferase (Nnmt) is an example of such an enzyme and regulates adipose tissue energy expenditure partly through induction of global changes in histone methylation and increased NAD^+ content (Kraus et al., 2014). Nnmt methylates nicotinamide (NAM), a form of vitamin B3, to produce N^1-methylnicotinamide (MNAM; schema, **Figure 1**). In humans, the expression of MNAM positively correlates with insulin resistance (Kannt et al., 2015). Additionally, MNAM possesses anti-inflammatory and antithrombotic properties and increases lifespan through the exertion of mitohormetic effects (Schmeisser et al., 2013). Both Nnmt and MNAM increase SIRT1 protein expression independently of its mRNA levels. SIRT1 is necessary for the exhibition of the metabolic effects of Nnmt and MNAM. Moreover, Nnmt and MNAM regulate the ubiquitin-proteasome degradation of SIRT1. Interestingly, expression of Nnmt is increased in B6 mice under the caloric restriction (CR) condition. This may promote SIRT3 expression, which is a mitochondrial Sirt that activates the glutathione-mediated mitochondrial antioxidant defense system. Thereby, several metabolic effects of CR may be mediated *via* Nnmt and SIRT3 expression enhancement (Someya et al., 2010). Thus, CR has implications in extending the lifespan and in the onset-delay of age-related diseases such as ARHL in mammals (Someya et al., 2010). Conversely, consumption of a high-fat diet (HFD) causes a decrease in SIRT1 expression (Wang et al., 2011; Chalkiadaki and Guarente, 2012) and damages metabolic changes such as glucose intolerance, insulin resistance, hepatic lipid accumulation and inflammation, and macrophage accumulation in the adipose tissue. This results in enhanced mitochondrial function, shortening of the lifespan (Chalkiadaki and Guarente, 2012), and early onset of ARHL in C57BL/6 (B6) and CBA/J mice (Le Prell et al., 2011; Du et al., 2012). Furthermore, elevated hearing thresholds during aging and a significant reduction in SIRT1 expression have been observed in the cochlea and auditory cortex of B6 mice (Keithley et al., 2004; Xiong et al., 2014). Hong et al. (2015) revealed the beneficial effects of dietary MNAM supplementation in B6 mice fed with an HFD as well as in humans. They reported that MNAM increased SIRT1 protein expression *in vivo* (Pfluger et al., 2008) and led to the exertion of systemic effects, such as significant lowering of serum cholesterol levels and changes in the lipoprotein profile (Hong et al., 2015). As it has been previously demonstrated that MNAM increases SIRT1 protein expression levels (Hong et al., 2015), these findings have led to the development of SIRT activators as a potential strategy to delay aging and age-related diseases in humans. However, use of a prevention therapy *via* MNAM supplementation for the delay of ARHL has not been reported. Therefore, we investigated its expression and roles in hearing function and the associated morphological changes in the cochlea using HFD, HFD + 1% MNAM (HFD-MNAM), and low-fat diet (LFD) aging B6 mice.

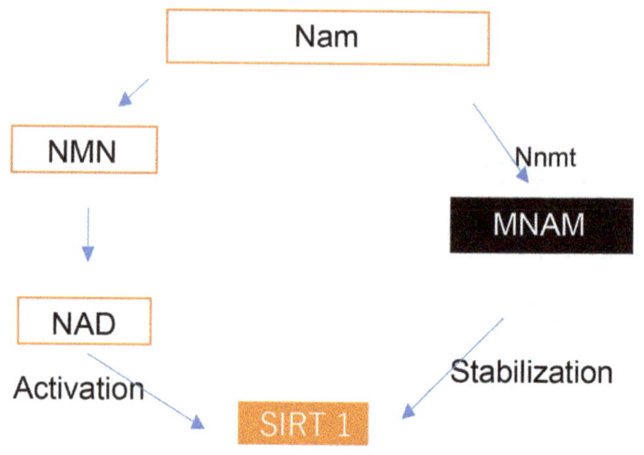

FIGURE 1 | Cascade of Sirt1 activation. SIRT 1, Sirtuin 1; Nam, nicotinamide; NMN, nicotinamide mononucleotide; NAD, nicotinamide adenine dinucleotide; Nnmt, nicotinamide N-methyltransferase; MNAM, N^1-methylnicotinamide.

MATERIALS AND METHODS

Animals

Thirty normal, 4-week-old, male B6 mice (*Mus musculus)* were purchased from Kyudo Company Limited (Kumamoto, Japan) and were randomly allocated into the following experimental groups: the HFD group, HFD-MNAM group, or LFD group (10 mice/group); subsequently, each group was further divided into the following subgroups (five mice/subgroup): 3-month-old and 6-month-old mice groups (**Figure 2**). Each subgroup was defined as YHFD, YHFD-MNAM, and YLFD for the 3-month-old mice groups and OHFD, OHFD-MNAM, and OLFD for the 6-month-old mice groups. The only criterion used was a matched group mean weight. The animals were housed

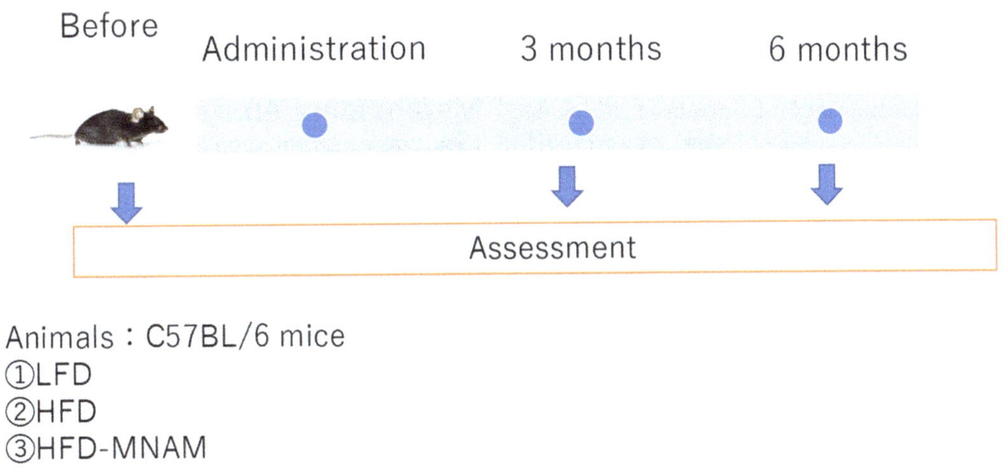

FIGURE 2 | Schedule of experiments. LFD, low-fat diet; HFD, high-fat diet; HFD-MNAM, high-fat diet plus 1% N^1-methylnicotinamide.

in an air-conditioned room maintained at a temperature of approximately 25°C with an approximate humidity of 50%. After 1 week of acclimatization, the mice were fed with an irradiated LFD (Low-Fat Diet 32, CLEA Japan Inc., Tokyo, Japan), HFD (High-Fat Diet 32, CLEA Japan Inc.), or HFD supplemented with 1% MNAM (TCI America, Portland, OR, USA). HFD + 1% MNAM was prepared by grinding the feed in a blender and by mixing powdered MNAM at 1% wt./wt. The concentration of MNAM was determined by the previous study (Hong et al., 2015) and our preliminary study (data not shown). The mice were housed group-wise with each type of food and water available *ad libitum*. A fresh diet was prepared weekly. The LFD, HFD, and HFD + 1% MNAM amounts were adjusted appropriately based on the weight of mice. All animal experiments were approved by the Committee on the Use and Care of Animals (Kumamoto University, Japan) and were performed according to accepted veterinary standards (Number: H30-079).

Body Weight and Blood Examination

Body weights were measured at baseline (pre-treatment) and 3 and 6 months after the commencement of the experiment. A venous blood sample was obtained from the tail and was measured using a complete clinical chemistry analyzer (BioMajesty™ JCA-BM6050, JEOL Limited, Tokyo, Japan) 6 months after experiment initiation.

The mice were euthanized by cervical dislocation and were fixed *via* cardiac perfusion using 4% paraformaldehyde (PFA) in phosphate-buffered saline (PBS), and the inner ears were dissected from the adult temporal bones and decalcified in 0.5 M ethylenediaminetetraacetic acid (EDTA)/PBS. The tissues were embedded in the optimal cutting temperature medium (Sakura Finetek Japan, Tokyo, Japan) and were serially cryosectioned at a thickness of 12 μm for further examination.

Immunohistochemistry

For the detection of antigens, the following primary antibodies and dilutions were used: anti-SIRT1 (1:100; cat. no. 13161-1-AP; Proteintech, Rosemont, IL, USA), anti-SIRT3 (1:200; cat. no. orb247889; Biorbyt, Cambridge, United Kingdom), anti-Na, K-ATPase 1 alpha1 (1:200; cat. no. NB300-146; Novus, Centennial, CO, USA), and anti-Connexin26 (1:200; cat. no. 710500; Life Technologies, Carlsbad, CA, USA). Fluorophore-conjugated secondary antibodies were used at a dilution of 1:500. Primary antibody labeling was performed at 4°C overnight after blocking in 10% goat or donkey serum for 10 min in PBS. Secondary antibody labeling was performed at 25°C for 1 h. Hoechst 33258 dye (Molecular Probes, Eugene, OR, USA) was used for 10 min to perform nuclear staining. The samples were examined under the BZ-9000 fluorescence microscope (Keyence, Osaka, Japan).

Hair Cell Count

To study the surface morphology of the cochleae, the mice were fixed *via* cardiac perfusion with PFA/PBS under anesthesia, and the bony capsule and lateral wall of the cochlea were removed. Texas Red-X phalloidin (1:100; Molecular Probes) was applied for 30 min, and the surface morphology of the cochleae was examined under the BZ-9000 fluorescence microscope (Keyence). Five randomly selected surface images of the organ of Corti (OCs) in every turn of the cochlea were acquired at a 40× magnification in each group. The numbers of outer hair cells (OHC) and inner hair cells (IHC) in a 140-μm basal segment of the basilar membrane were calculated in each group. Only the hair cells with an intact stereocilia bundle and a cuticular plate were counted in every turn of the cochlea as per previously described methods (Miwa et al., 2020). A second researcher confirmed the accuracy of the measurements.

Spiral Ganglion Cell Count

To assess the number of spiral ganglion cells (SGCs), the samples on the slides were labeled with the anti-beta III tubulin (Tuj1) antibody (1:200; MMS-435P, Covance, Princeton, NJ, USA), and the nuclei were counterstained using Hoechst 33258 dye (Molecular Probes). Three randomly selected images were acquired in every turn of the cochlea in each group. We classified the cells that were positive for both Tuj-1 and Hoechst staining in Rosenthal's canal as SGCs. We counted the SGCs at the basal, in the middle, and at the apical turns in three randomly selected sections per cochlea and marked the counted cells on the images to avoid double counting using the ImageJ software (NIH, Framingham, MA, USA) as per previously described protocols (Yamada et al., 2015). The accuracy of the analysis was confirmed by an independent second researcher.

Measurement of the Thickness of the Stria Vascularis

The average thickness of the stria vascularis was measured by analyzing the images of the sections containing the midmodiolar region using the ImageJ software (NIH) as per previously described methods (Miwa et al., 2019, 2020).

ELISA

Each cochlear sample was homogenized using the Sonifier S-250A analog ultrasonic processor (Branson, Danbury, CT, USA). Protein concentrations were measured using a bicinchoninic acid protein assay kit (Thermo Fisher Scientific, Rockford, IL, USA) and were adjusted at the same concentration. Tissue lysates were assayed by using a mouse enzyme-linked immunosorbent assay (ELISA) SIRT1 kit (ab206983; Abcam, Cambridge, United Kingdom) for single protein quantification by following the manufacturer's instructions. The plates were read on the Multiskan FC microplate reader (Thermo Fisher Scientific) at 450 nm.

Western Blotting (WB) Analysis

To confirm the results of the ELISA technique, the same lysates were separated by performing 12.5% sodium dodecyl sulfate-polyacrylamide gel electrophoresis and were detected using the following primary antibodies: anti-SIRT1 (1:1,000; Proteintech), horseradish peroxidase-conjugated secondary antibodies (Bio-Rad, Hercules, CA, USA) against primary antibodies, and horseradish peroxidase-conjugated anti-β-actin (PM053-7; MBL, Nagoya, Japan) at a dilution of 1:5,000. The signals were visualized using an electrochemiluminescence system (Bio-Rad). The detected bands were analyzed using the ImageJ software (NIH); β-actin was used as the internal loading control.

Real-Time Quantitative Reverse Transcription-Polymerase Chain Reaction (qRT-PCR)

Using a microRNA extraction kit (QIAGEN, Valencia, CA, USA), total RNA was extracted from each sample, quantified using the GeneQuant100 system (GE Healthcare, Amersham, UK), and diluted as required to achieve uniform concentrations. Complementary DNA (cDNA) was then synthesized using the One-Step PrimeScript RT-PCR Kit (Takara Bio, Otsu, Japan) according to the manufacturer's instructions using primers for *Sirt1* and glyceraldehyde-3-phosphate dehydrogenase (*GAPDH*) (Applied Bionics, Foster City, CA, USA). The targets were amplified using the Takara Dice TP960 system by subjecting the samples to over 40 cycles of denaturation at 95°C for 15 s and by annealing them at 60°C for 1 min. Relative gene expression was calculated by generating a standard curve and was normalized to the *GAPDH* expression signal.

Metabolome Analysis

Each mouse cochlear sample was dissected and washed using PBS and then preserved at −80°C until extraction. Metabolites were extracted using methanol containing hexamethylenetetramine internal standard solution 1 at 25°C. The metabolome was analyzed using gas chromatography coupled with mass spectrometry (Shimadzu Company, Tokyo, Japan). Peak detection was performed using the multivariate data analysis software (Travers MS, Reifycs Inc., Tokyo, Japan) in a three-step manner; first, mass values were detected within each spectrum. In the second step, a chromatogram was constructed for each of the mass values which spanned over a certain time range. Finally, deconvolution algorithms were applied to each chromatogram to recognize the actual chromatographic peaks. The average peak height for each metabolite was used for analysis, and the relative amounts of the metabolites were quantified. Heat map analysis, enrichment analysis, principal component analysis (PCA), and pathway analysis, including the TCA cycle, were performed using MetaboAnalyst[1] (Pang et al., 2020).

Auditory Thresholds

Before the commencement of the study, we examined the Preyer reflex and examined whether all mice possessed normal hearing abilities (Böhmer, 1988). We assessed the hearing thresholds in the 3-month-old and 6-month-old mice subgroups after the MNAM treatment by evaluating the auditory brainstem responses (ABR) (System 3; Tucker–Davis Technologies, Alachua, FL, USA) as per previously described protocols (Miwa et al., 2019). The animals were anesthetized as per the methods described above. Electrodes were placed beneath the pinna of the test ear and at the vertex below the surface of the skin. The ground electrode was placed under the contralateral ear. Auditory thresholds were measured at 4, 8, 12, 20, and 32 kHz by measuring the ABRs (15-ms duration, 1-ms rise/fall time, and tone burst). For each recording, an average of 512 sweeps was calculated. The stimulus levels near the threshold were varied in 10-dB steps, and the threshold was defined as the lowest level at which waves in the ABR could be clearly detected by visual inspection.

Statistical Analysis

The data are presented as mean ± standard deviation. A one-way analysis of variance (ANOVA) along with *ad hoc* Tukey–Kramer test (for all quantification experiments) was performed for the statistical analyses. $P \leq 0.05$ was considered significant. All statistical analyses were performed using EZR (Saitama Medical Center, Jichi Medical University, Saitama, Japan), which is a graphical user interface of R (The R Foundation for Statistical Computing, Vienna, Austria). Precisely, it is a modified version of the R commander that has been designed to include statistical functions that are frequently used in biostatistics.

[1] http://www.metaboanalyst.ca/

RESULTS

HFD-Fed Mice Exhibit Marked Increase in Body Weight, Serum Cholesterol, Triglyceride, and Blood Glucose Levels

There were no differences in water and food consumption among the three groups. The bodyweight of the LFD-fed mice steadily increased throughout the 6-month observation period. The HFD-fed mice exhibited considerable weight gain (**Supplementary Figures 1A,B**) as expected. Although considerable differences were not observed among the YHFD, YHFD-MNAM, and YLFD groups, the body weights of the OHFD mice markedly increased compared with both the OLFD mice and OHFD-MNAM mice groups (**Supplementary Figures 1A,B**).

Differences in the results of blood analysis across all groups during the study period are presented in **Supplementary Figure 1C**. The alanine aminotransferase levels in the OHFD mice were markedly higher than those in the other two groups (**Supplementary Figure 1C**). More sustained effects were observed on the lipid and cholesterol levels in this group. The OHFD mice presented with significantly higher serum cholesterol and triglyceride levels compared with the other groups, probably because the LFD and MNAM supplementation included with the HFD prevented such increases in these groups (**Supplementary Figure 1C**). Blood glucose levels in these mice were markedly higher than those in the other two groups (**Supplementary Figure 1C**).

HFD-Fed Mice Present With Severe Hearing Loss

ABR, an objective electrophysiological measure of hearing function, was used to monitor the progression of ARHL. The ABR recordings revealed that the YHFD and OHFD B6 mice developed severe hearing loss compared with the other two groups (**Figure 3A** and **Supplementary Figures 2A–C**). The average thresholds exhibited by the YHFD mice were markedly higher than those exhibited by the YLFD mice and the YHFD-MNAM mice at all examined frequencies (**Figure 3A** and **Supplementary Figures 2A–C**). The average thresholds exhibited by the OHFD mice were markedly higher than those exhibited by both the OLFD mice and OHFD-MNAM mice at all examined frequencies except for 32 kHz (**Figure 3A** and **Supplementary Figures 2A–C**).

The Cochlea of HFD-Fed Mice Exhibit Alterations Indicating Hearing Loss and These Cochlear Alterations Are Absent in Mice Supplemented With MNAM

To validate the ABR hearing test results, we performed histological analysis on cochlear tissue sections. There was no apparent OHC loss, IHC loss, or SGC loss in any of the turns in the YHFD, YHFD-MNAM, and YLFD mice (**Figures 3B–E**). However, the OHFD mice exhibited a remarkable loss of OHCs and IHCs in all cochlear turns compared to the OLFD mice (**Figures 3B,C**). Moreover, in the OHFD-MNAM mice, the prevention of OHC and IHC loss was observed in all turns except for the basal turn (**Figures 3B,C**). The OHFD mice showed remarkable loss of SGCs in all cochlear turns except for the basal turn compared with the OLFD mice (**Figures 3D,E**). In the OHFD-MNAM mice, the prevention of SGC loss was observed in all turns (**Figures 3D,E**).

The cochlea of YHFD mice showed slight degeneration of spiral ligament (SLi) cells (types II, IV, and V: Na, K-ATPase alpha 1 expression, type I: Cx26 expression) compared with the YLFD mice (**Figures 4A–C**). This degeneration of the SLi cells was not observed in the YHFD-MNAM mice (**Figures 3A–C**). Moreover, these SLi cells exhibited greater degeneration in the cochlea of OHFD mice compared with the OLFD mice (**Figures 4A–C**). Furthermore, this degeneration of the SLi cells was absent in the OHFD-MNAM mice (**Figures 4A–C**). The thickness of the stria vascularis was neither markedly different between YHFD, YLFD, and YHFD-MNAM mice nor was it different between OHFD, OHFD-MNAM, and OLFD mice (**Supplementary Figure 3**).

MNAM-Treated HFD-Fed Mice Exhibit Higher Cochlear SIRT1 Protein Expression Compared With HFD-Fed Mice

Using immunostaining assays, we determined whether cochlear SIRT1 levels increased with MNAM supplementation. Immunohistochemistry results revealed that the SIRT1 protein was present in the cochlea of YLFD mice, especially in types I, II, and V of SLi cells, OCs, including OHCs and IHCs, and SGCs (**Figures 5A,B**). In the OLFD mice, SIRT1 continued to be expressed and was well preserved in the OCs; however, it was decreased in the SLi cells and SGCs when compared with the YLFD mice (**Figure 5B**). The cochlea of the YHFD mice showed decreased SIRT1 expression in the OCs and SGCs **Figures 5A,B**), whereas, SIRT1 expression was not detected in the SLi cells, OCs, or SGC cochlea of the OHFD mice (**Figure 5B**), probably because the majority of the SLi cells, OHCs, IHCs, and SGCs was missing in these cochleae. Conversely, SIRT1 expression was preserved in the SLi cells, OCs, and SGCs of the YHFD-MNAM and OHFD-MNAM mice (**Figure 5B**). Moreover, immunostaining results revealed that SIRT3 expression followed the SIRT1 expression pattern in the inner ear (**Supplementary Figure 4**).

Further, to confirm these immunostaining results, we analyzed SIRT1 protein levels in inner ear tissues using WB analysis and ELISA. With aging, SIRT1 protein expression in the cochlea of OLFD mice was noticeably decreased (**Figures 5C,D**). SIRT1 protein expression in the OHFD mice was lower than that in the OLFD mice (**Figures 5C,D**). OHFD-MNAM mice demonstrated higher SIRT1 protein levels than the OHFD mice (**Figures 5C,D**), indicating that MNAM treatment prevented the decrease in SIRT1 protein levels in the cochlea of these mice. Although the mRNA expression of SIRT1 decreased with age in OHFD, OHFD-MNAM, and OLFD (**Figure 5E**), the decrease was not markedly different between the groups, even in OHFD, OHFD-MNAM, and OLFD mice (**Figure 5E**).

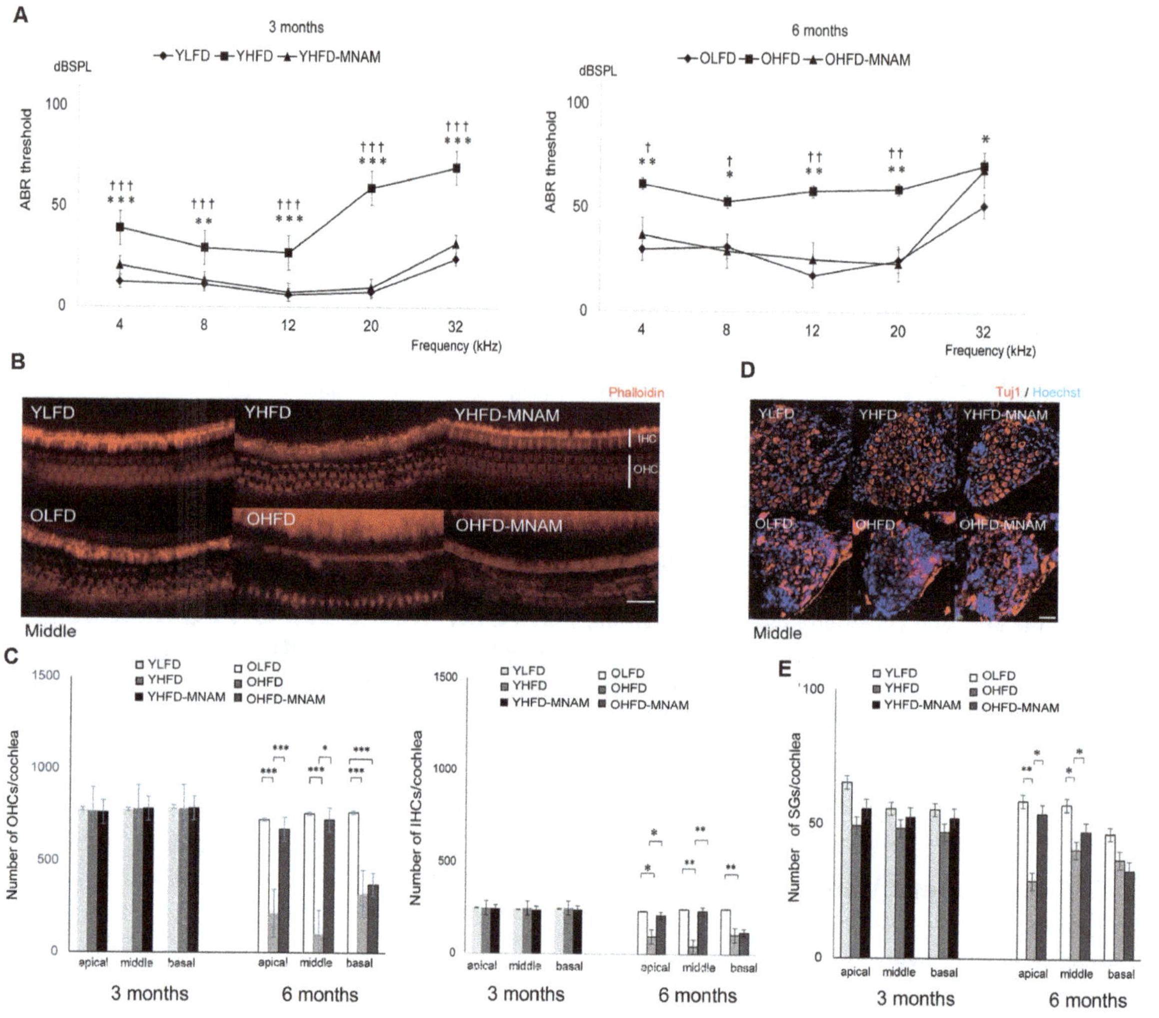

FIGURE 3 | The onset of age-related hearing loss (ARHL) and effect of MNAM supplementation on ARHL: developmental changes in auditory thresholds, hair cell counts, and spiral ganglion cell counts in the three tested mice groups. **(A)** The ABR recording results at 3 and 6 months after commencement of the experiment. All groups developed age-related hearing loss at 6 months, rather than at 3 months (YLFD: p = at 4 kHz, p = at 8 kHz, p = at 12 kHz, p = at 20 kHz, and p = at 32 kHz, YHFD: p = at 4 kHz, p = at 8 kHz, p = at 12 kHz, p = at 20 kHz, and p = at 32 kHz, YHFD-MNAM: p = at 4 kHz, p = at 8 kHz, p = at 12 kHz, p = at 20 kHz, and p = at 32 kHz). The YHFD and OHFD developed severe hearing loss compared with the YLFD and OLFD mice (YHFD vs. YLFD: $p < 0.001$ at 4 kHz, $p = 0.006$ at 8 kHz, $p < 0.001$ at 12 kHz, $p < 0.001$ at 20 kHz, and $p < 0.001$ at 32 kHz, OHFD vs. OLFD: $p = 0.003$ at 4 kHz, $p = 0.01$ at 8 kHz, $p = 0.003$ at 12 kHz, $p = 0.003$ at 20 kHz, and $p = 0.03$ at 32 kHz). All groups, $n = 5$, $^{*}p < 0.05$, $^{**}p < 0.01$, $^{***}p < 0.001$. In the YHFD-MNAM and OHFD-MNAM groups, hearing loss was prevented markedly compared with the YHFD and YLFD groups (YHFD-MNAM vs. YLFD-MNAM: $p < 0.001$ at 4 kHz, $p = 0.004$ at 8 kHz, $p < 0.001$ at 12 kHz, $p < 0.001$ at 20 kHz, and $p < 0.001$ at 32 kHz, OHFD-MNAM vs. OLFD: $p = 0.01$ at 4 kHz, $p = 0.04$ at 8 kHz, $p = 0.006$ at 12 kHz, $p = 0.005$ at 20 kHz, and $p = 0.40$ at 32 kHz). All groups, $n = 5$, $^{\dagger}p < 0.05$, $^{\dagger\dagger}p < 0.01$, $^{\dagger\dagger\dagger}p < 0.001$. **(B)** Phalloidin-staining of the HCs in a surface preparation in the middle turn at 3 and 6 months after experiment initiation. The OHFD mice developed greater OHC and IHC loss than the other two groups. The OHFD-MNAM mice exhibited lower OHC and IHC loss compared with the OHFD mice. **(C)** The OHC and IHC counts in all turns at 3 and 6 months after commencement of the experiment. The YHFD mice did not develop OHC and IHC loss, compared to the other two groups (YLFD; OHC: $p = 0.10$ at apical, $p = 0.09$ in the middle, $p = 0.13$ at basal, IHC: $p = 0.78$ at apical, $p = 0.61$ in the middle, $p = 0.43$ at basal, YHFD-MNAM; OHC: $p = 0.63$ at apical, $p = 0.10$ in the middle, $p = 0.62$ at basal, IHC: $p = 0.34$ at apical, $p = 0.23$ in the middle, $p = 0.41$ at basal). The OHFD mice developed greater OHC and IHC loss than the other two groups (OLFD; OHC: $p < 0.001$ in all turns, IHC: $p = 0.04$ at apical, $p = 0.008$ in the middle, $p = 0.002$ at basal, OHFD-MNAM mice; OHC: $p < 0.001$ at apical, $p = 0.01$ in the middle, $p = 0.67$ at basal, IHC: $p = 0.04$ at apical, $p = 0.009$ in the middle, $p = 0.29$ at basal). All groups, $n = 5$, $^{*}p < 0.05$, $^{**}p < 0.01$, $^{***}p < 0.001$. **(D)** The immunostaining of the SGCs using the anti-Tuj1 antibody in the middle turn at 3 and 6 months after commencement of the experiment. The OHFD mice developed greater SGC loss than the other two groups. The OHFD-MNAM mice exhibited lower SGC loss compared with the OHFD mice. **(E)** The SGC counts in all turns at 3 and 6 months after commencement of the experiment. There were no significant differences in SGC numbers between YLFD and YHFD ($p = 0.09$ at apical, $p = 0.28$ in the middle, $p = 0.10$ at basal), and between YHFD and YHFD-MNAM mice ($p = 0.31$ at apical, $p = 0.30$ in the middle, $p = 0.07$ at basal). The OHFD mice developed greater SGC loss than the OLFD mice, except for the basal turn ($p = 0.002$ at apical, $p = 0.03$ in the middle, $p = 0.07$ at basal). The OHFD-MNAM mice exhibited less SGC loss than the OHFD mice ($p = 0.01$ at apical, $p = 0.01$ in the middle, $p = 0.21$ at basal). All groups, $n = 5$, $^{*}p < 0.05$, $^{**}p < 0.01$, $^{***}p < 0.001$ (Bars: 100 μm; YLFD, low-fat diet-fed 3-month-old mice; OLFD, low-fat diet-fed 6-month-old mice; YHFD, high-fat diet-fed 3-month-old mice; OHFD, high-fat diet-fed 6-month-old mice; YHFD-MNAM, high-fat diet plus 1% N^1-methylnicotinamide-fed 3-month-old mice; OHFD-MNAM, high-fat diet plus 1% N^1-methylnicotinamide-fed 6-month-old mice; OHCs, outer hair cells; IHCs, inner hair cells; SGCs, spiral ganglion cells; anti-Tuj1, anti-beta III tubulin).

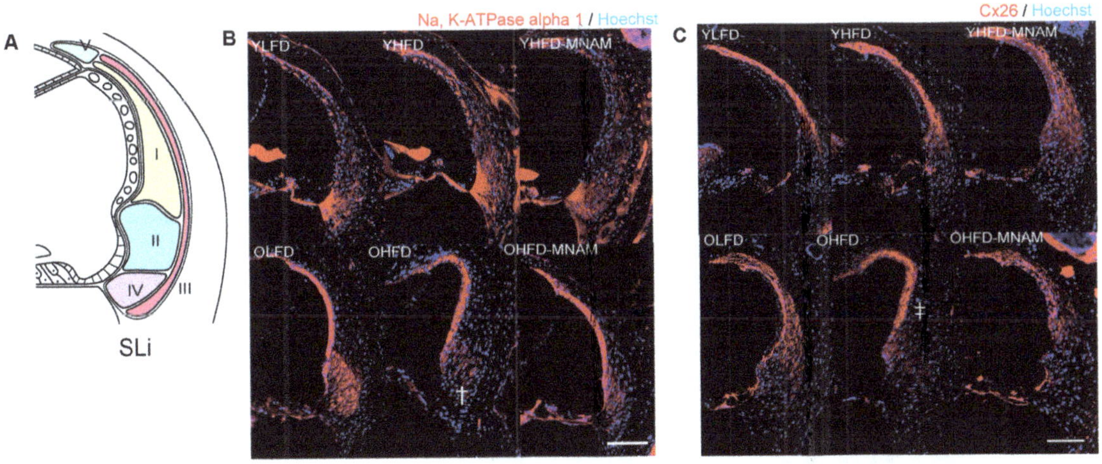

FIGURE 4 | Morphological analysis of the spiral ligament (SLi): age-related SLi alterations are observed in OHFD mice. **(A)** The schema of the SLi. The fibrocytes of SLi are divided into five types. **(B)** The immunostaining of types II and IV in the SLi using an anti-Na, K-ATPase alpha 1 antibody at 6 months after experiment initiation. The dagger symbol indicates a decrease in Na, K-ATPase alpha 1 expression in the cochlea of OHFD mice after the commencement of the experiment. **(C)** The immunostaining of type I and V cells in the SLi using the anti-Cx26 antibody at 3 and 6 months after experiment initiation. The double dagger symbol indicates a decrease in Cx26 expression in the cochlea of the OHFD mice after the commencement of the experiment (Bars: 100 μm, YLFD, low-fat diet-fed 3 month old mice; OLFD, low-fat diet-fed 6-month-old mice; YHFD, high-fat diet-fed 3-month-old mice; OHFD, high-fat diet-fed 6-month-old mice; YHFD-MNAM, high-fat diet plus 1% N[1]-methylnicotinamide-fed 3-month-old mice; OHFD-MNAM, high-fat diet plus 1% N[1]-methylnicotinamide-fed 6-month-old mice; OCs, the organ of Corti; SGC, spiral ganglion cells; SLi, spiral ligament; SV, stria vascularis).

Metabolome Analysis Reveals Differential Modulation of Various Metabolic Pathways in the Different Diet-Fed Mice Groups

A metabolome enrichment analysis revealed that the metabolic pathways related to methylhistidine metabolism, trehalose degradation, vitamin B6 metabolism, and the mitochondrial beta-oxidation of short-chain saturated fatty acids were remarkably activated in the cochlea of OLFD compared to YLFD mice (**Figure 6A**, **Supplementary Figure 5A**). Furthermore, the metabolic pathways related to glycolysis and aging were markedly activated in the cochlea of YHFD compared to YLFD mice (**Figure 6B**, **Supplementary Figure 5B**). Conversely, insulin resistance, obesity, non-alcoholic steatohepatitis, and aging pathways were remarkably activated in the cochlea of OHFD compared to OLFD mice (**Figure 6C**, **Supplementary Figure 5C**). Further, we analyzed the differences in the metabolic pathways activated in the cochlea of YHFD and YHFD-MNAM mice. We found that the metabolic pathways related to sphingolipid metabolism, fatty acid metabolism, thiamine metabolism, ethanol degradation, mitochondrial beta-oxidation of short-chain saturated fatty acids, and riboflavin metabolism were selectively activated in the cochlea of YHFD-MNAM compared to YHFD mice (**Figure 6D**, **Supplementary Figure 5D**). Moreover, pathways related to nicotine and nicotinamide metabolism, purine metabolism, fructose, and mannose degradation, and tryptophan metabolism showed increased activation in the cochlea of OHFD-MNAM compared to that of OHFD mice (**Figure 6E**, **Supplementary Figure 5E**). Pathway analysis revealed that the TCA cycle was activated with a high-fat diet and aging, however, there were slight differences between OHFD and OHFD-MNAM (**Supplementary Figures 5A–E**). Additionally, MNAM expression in OHFD mice decreased compared to that in YHFD mice. MNAM expression in YHFD-MNAM and OHFD-MNAM exhibited a marked increase compared to other groups (**Figure 6F**).

DISCUSSION

HFD-Fed Mice Exhibit ARHL and Decreased SIRT1 and SIRT3 Expression Levels

The increase in ABR thresholds associated with aging was markedly accelerated in the YHFD B6 mice compared with the YLFD mice. In OHFD B6 mice, there was a more remarkable loss of OHCs, IHCs, and SGCs in all cochlear turns as well as a loss of SLi cells (types I, II, V) as compared with the OLFD mice (**Figures 3, 4**). These results suggest that HFD accelerates ARHL progression in B6 mice. These observations are consistent with results of previous studies, conducted using CBA/CaJ (Vasilyeva et al., 2009) and CD/1 mice (Hwang et al., 2013), which have reported that HFD induces oxidative stress, mitochondrial damage, and cellular apoptosis in the inner ear (Hwang et al., 2013). Conversely, Fujita et al. (2015) stated that ARHL was suppressed in HFD B6 mice. They speculated that the nutrients in the HFD (HFD32) were different from those present in a normal diet (CE-2); particularly, the level of the antioxidant and anti-inflammatory vitamin E (Jiang, 2014) is three times higher in HFD compared with a normal diet. They suggested that a combination therapy including antioxidants and vitamin E could reduce a noise-induced hearing loss (Le Prell et al., 2011) and prevent ARHL in B6 mice (Heman-Ackah et al., 2010). Here, LFD rather than a CE-2

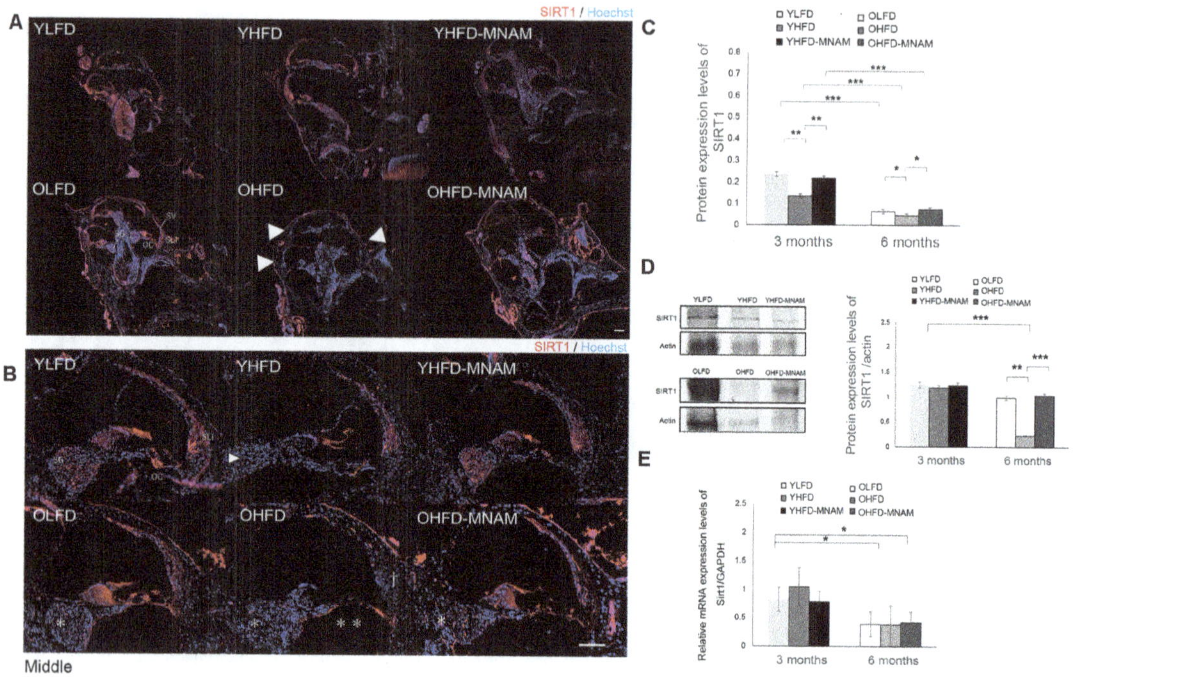

FIGURE 5 | SIRT1 expression in the cochlea: the age-related SIRT1 downregulation of expression observed in OHFD mice is absent in OHFD-MNAM mice. **(A)** SIRT1 staining (red) of the whole cochlea at 3 and 6 months after commencement of the experiment. SIRT1 is prominently localized in the OCs, SGCs, and type II and IV SLi cells in all turns within the cochlea. The arrowheads indicate a decrease in SIRT1 expression in the cochlea of the OHFD mice. **(B)** SIRT1 staining (red) of the middle turn of the cochlea at 3 and 6 months after commencement of the experiment. The arrowhead indicates a decrease in SIRT1 expression in the SGCs in the cochlea of the YHFD mice after experiment initiation. The asterisks indicate a decrease in SIRT1 expression in the SGCs in the cochlea of the OHFD mice after experiment initiation. The double asterisk indicates a decrease in SIRT1 expression in the OCs in the cochlea of the OHFD mice after experiment initiation. The dagger symbol indicates a decrease in SIRT1 expression in the SLi in the cochlea of the OHFD mice after experiment initiation. **(C)** The SIRT1 protein expression in the cochlea quantitatively analyzed using ELISA at 3 and 6 months after commencement of the experiment. The SIRT1 protein expression analyzed *via* ELISA decreased with aging ($p < 0.001$ in each group). The YHFD and OHFD groups exhibited a decrease in the SIRT1 protein expression compared with the YLFD and OLFD groups ($p = 0.002$ and $p = 0.04$). In the YHFD-MNAM and OHFD-MNAM, decrease in the SIRT1 protein expression was lower than that in the YHFD and OHFD groups ($p = 0.004$ and $p = 0.01$; All groups, $n = 5$; *$p < 0.05$, **$p < 0.01$, ***$p < 0.001$). **(D)** The SIRT1 protein expression in the cochlea quantitatively analyzed using WB analysis at 3 and 6 months after commencement of the experiment. β-actin expression was used as a reference. The OHFD mice exhibited a greater decrease in the SIRT1 protein expression compared to the OLFD mice ($p = 0.001$). In the OHFD-MNAM group, decrease in the SIRT1 protein expression was less than that in the OHFD group ($p < 0.001$; All groups, $n = 5$; **$p < 0.01$, ***$p < 0.001$). **(E)** *Sirt1* mRNA expression in the cochlea quantitatively analyzed using qRT-PCR at 3 and 6 months after commencement of the experiment. *GAPDH* expression was used as a reference. *Sirt1* mRNA expression analyzed *via* ELISA decreased with aging ($p = 0.03$ in the YLFD and OLFD, $p = 0.02$ in the YHFD and OHFD, $p = 0.04$ in the YHFD-MNAM and OHFD-MNAM). The YHFD and OHFD mice did not exhibit a decrease in *Sirt1* mRNA expression compared with the YLFD and OLFD groups ($p = 0.14$ and $p = 0.49$). In the YHFD-MNAM and OHFD-MNAM groups, there were no decreases in *Sirt1* mRNA expression compared with those in the YHFD and OHFD groups ($p = 0.11$ and $p = 0.45$; Bars: 100 µm; *Sirt1*, Sirtuin 1; YLFD, low-fat diet-fed 3-month-old mice; OLFD, low-fat diet-fed 6-month-old mice; YHFD, high-fat diet-fed 3-month-old mice; OHFD, high-fat diet-fed 6-month-old mice; YHFD-MNAM, high-fat diet plus 1% N^1-methylnicotinamide-fed 3-month-old mice; OHFD-MNAM, high-fat diet plus 1% N^1-methylnicotinamide-fed 6-month-old mice; OCs, the organ of Corti; SGCs, spiral ganglion cells; SLi, spiral ligament; SV, stria vascularis; ELISA, enzyme-linked immunosorbent assay; GAPDH, glyceraldehyde-3-phosphate dehydrogenase; WB, western blotting; mRNA, messenger ribose nucleic acid; qRT-PCR, quantitative reverse transcription-polymerase chain reaction).

was used as control. LFD and HFD are similar in the nutrient constitution, except for fat composition. Our results revealed that HFD induced a decrease in the expression of SIRT1 and SIRT3 proteins and mRNA levels in the cochlear samples. Results from immunohistology showed that their expression was decreased in the OHCs, IHCs, SGCs, and SLi cells in the cochlea of the OHFD mice (**Figure 5** and **Supplementary Figure 4**). However, the SIRT1 and SIRT3 expression remained unaltered in the cochlea of the YHFD mice (**Figure 5** and **Supplementary Figure 4**). These results were consistent with those of previous studies (Xiong et al., 2014), confirming that the inhibition of SIRT1 led to an increase in apoptosis in the mouse inner ear cell line (HEI-OC1) (Xiong et al., 2015). Furthermore, the metabolome enrichment analysis revealed that the cochlear metabolic pathways related to glycolysis and aging showed markedly higher activation in YHFD mice compared with YLFD mice (**Figure 6B**). However, insulin resistance, obesity, non-alcoholic steatohepatitis, and aging-related cochlear pathways showed increased activation in OHFD mice compared with those in OLFD mice (**Figure 6C**). SIRT1 regulates central metabolic functions, such as lipogenesis, protein synthesis, gluconeogenesis, and metabolic homeostasis, through deacetylation. Stress, particularly factors such as CR and HFD, alter Sirtuin activity that leads to significant alterations of certain intracellular processes; activation of reparation processes, increase in DNA stability, and elevation of metabolic rate and cell lifespan are observed. Our cochlear metabolome analysis results, including heatmap, enrichment analysis, PCA, pathway analysis (TCA cycle), were consistent with those reported in previous studies conducted on the investigation of liver metabolic profiles (Hong et al., 2015). Thus, our results suggested that during aging, HFD led to a SIRT decrease and caused metabolic changes in the inner ear, leading to early ARHL progression in B6 mice.

MNAM Supplementation Increases SIRT1 and SIRT3 Expression Levels in the Cochlea and Suppresses ARHL in C57BL/6 Mice

We found that dietary MNAM supplementation exerted beneficial effects associated with the prevention of ARHL progression. MNAM protected the sensory organs and the lateral wall in the cochlea from damage in OHFD B6 mice. In OHFD-MNAM mice, the loss of OHCs, IHC, SGCs, and SLi cells (types I, II, IV, and V) was prevented in all cochlear turns except at the basal turn (**Figures 3, 4**), indicating protection conferred against HFD-related stress. MNAM exerted this protective effect by increasing the SIRT1 and SIRT3 protein expression levels in the cochlea. Immunostaining results revealed that SIRT1 and SIRT3 protein expression levels were detected in the OHCs, IHCs, SGCs, and SLi cells in YHFD-MNAM and OHFD-MNAM mice (**Figure 5** and **Supplementary Figure 4**). However, this was not detected in the cochlea of OHFD mice. WB analysis and ELISA revealed significantly increased SIRT1 protein expression levels in the OHFD-MNAM mice compared with the levels in the OHFD mice (**Figures 5C,D**). Interestingly, no differences in the mRNA expression levels were observed among the three groups by qRT-PCR (**Figure 5E**). These results indicate that MNAM increases the SIRT1 protein expression levels independently of its mRNA levels. This observation is consistent with those reported in previous studies (Hong et al., 2015). Further, our findings suggest that dietary MNAM supplementation may activate SIRT3 expression in the cochlea. Previous studies have demonstrated that the activation of SIRT3 *via* the NAD^+ precursor, nicotinamide riboside, conferred protection against noise-induced hearing loss (Brown et al., 2014). However, further analysis will be necessary to confirm this result, as we have not extensively examined the SIRT3 protein and mRNA expression levels in the cochlea.

Additionally, metabolome enrichment analyses revealed that the cochlear metabolic pathways related to insulin resistance, aging, non-alcoholic steatohepatitis, oxidative damage, and mitochondrial beta-oxidation were activated to a greater extent in YHFD mice than those in YHFD-MNAM mice. However, the cochlear metabolic pathways related to nicotine, mitochondrial beta-oxidation, glycolysis, aging, and oxidative damage were activated to a greater extent in the cochlea of OHFD mice as compared with those in OHFD-MNAM mice. Previous studies have suggested that MNAM regulates glucose, lipid, and cholesterol metabolism by stabilizing SIRT1 expression in the liver (Hong et al., 2015). Thus, our results suggest that MNAM supplementation provides beneficial effects on metabolic pathways in cochlear aging related to hearing function. Interestingly, the TCA cycle did not activate in OHFD-MNAM. Further studies are necessary.

Adequate SIRT1 Expression May Play a Key Role in ARHL

In summary, our results revealed that HFD consumption-mediated downregulated expression of SIRT1 and SIRT3 and aging together lead to hearing loss. Additionally, MNAM-mediated cochlear upregulation of SIRT1 and SIRT3 protein expression levels exerted a preventive effect against the HFD- and aging-induced hearing loss. A similar result was obtained in a recent study conducted by the International Mouse Phenotyping Consortium. Their study demonstrated that young mice with homozygous *Sirt1* knockout mutation exhibited significantly increased ABR thresholds compared with B6 control mice[2]. However, conversely, Han et al. (2016) have reported that in hetero *Sirt1* transgenic B6 mice, the SIRT1 half deficiency reduces the age-related oxidative damage of the OHCs and SGCs while delaying the early onset of ARHL. This effect is caused by the enhancement of cochlear Foxo3a mediated oxidative stress resistance. They hypothesized that since homozygous *Sirt1* mutant mice infrequently survived postnatally and were small in size presenting with developmental defects, it might be possible that the MRC Harwell study reflected higher ABR thresholds due to developmental defects present in the inner ear and/or central nervous system (Cheng et al., 2003). However, Alcendor et al. (2007) reported that while *Sirt1* overexpression increased apoptotic cell death in the heart and decreased cardiac function in mice, *Sirt1* inhibition protected rat cortical neurons against oxidative stress (Li et al., 2008). The same study reported that the moderate heart-specific overexpression of *Sirt1* protected the heart from oxidative stress induced by paraquat and increased catalase expression in mice (Alcendor et al., 2007). Thus, current reports on the roles of Sirtuins in extending health-span and lifespan are controversial.

Therefore, we speculated that "minimum" expression levels of SIRT1 were crucial for the prevention of ARHL progression. In agreement with this hypothesis, our results revealed that the decrease in SIRT1 expression levels induced *via* HFD consumption and aging in B6 aged mice resulted in ARHL. Furthermore, moderate SIRT1 expression levels induced *via* MNAM supplementation in HFD-fed and aged B6 mice did not lead to ARHL. However, a previous report has suggested that the half expression of SIRT1 did not lead to ARHL (Xiong et al., 2014), whereas the lack of SIRT1 expression led to hearing loss. Considering these findings together, we suggest that SIRT1 may act as a pro-aging molecule in the cochlear cells of B6 mice. However, there are no reports on the mechanism by which a moderate inner-ear-specific overexpression of SIRT1 influences the progression of ARHL. Further research is warranted to

[2]http://www.mousephenotype.org/phenoview/?gid = 363&qeid = MP:0004738 &ctrl = 2357729&pt = 0.0001

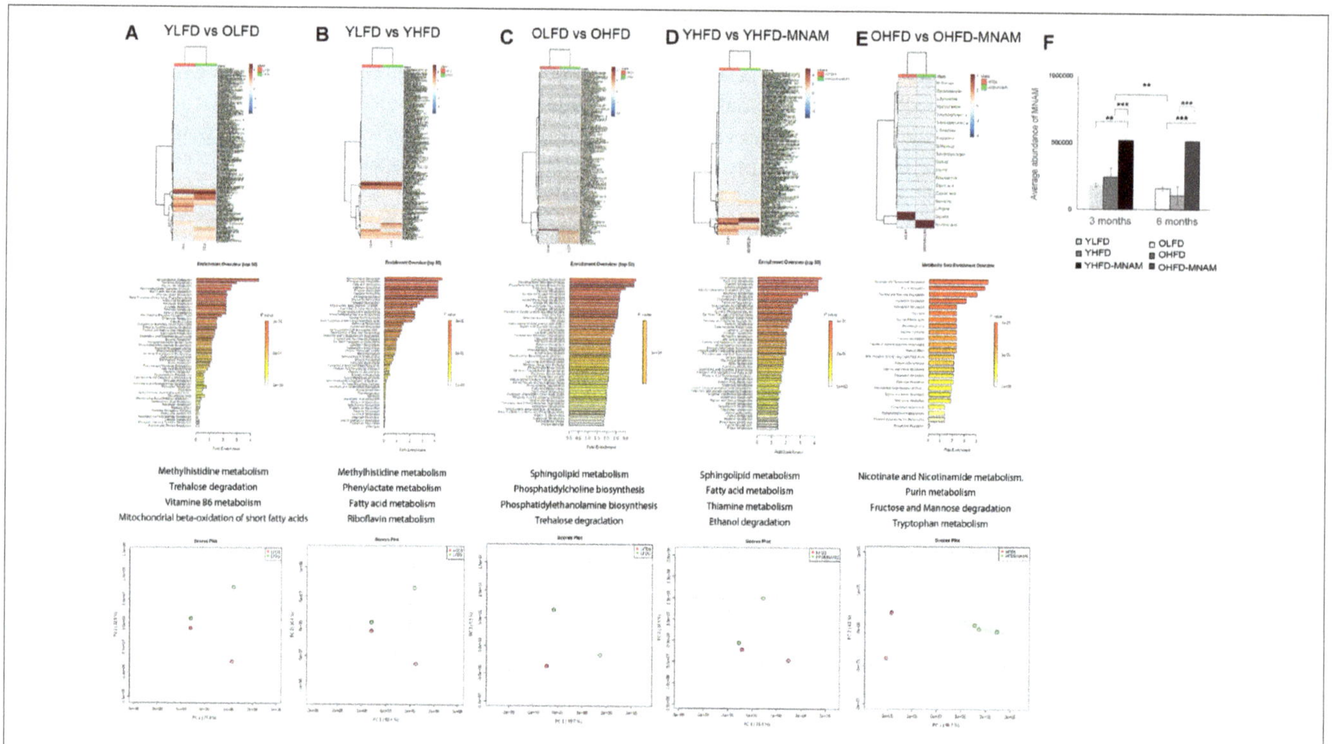

FIGURE 6 | Metabolome heatmap, enrichment analysis, and principal component analysis (PCA). **(A)** Comparison between the cochlea of the YLFD and OLFD mice. The metabolic pathways related to methylhistidine metabolism, trehalose degradation, vitamin B6 metabolism, and the mitochondrial beta-oxidation of short-chain saturated fatty acids were activated in the cochlea of the OLFD mice. **(B)** Comparison between the cochlea of the YLFD and YHFD mice. The metabolic pathways related to glycolysis and aging were activated in the cochlea of the YHFD mice. **(C)** Comparison between the cochlea of the OLFD and OHFD mice. The metabolic pathways related to insulin resistance, obesity, non-alcoholic steatohepatitis, and aging showed greater activation in the cochlea of the OHFD mice. **(D)** Comparison between the cochlea of the YHFD and YHFD-MNAM mice. The metabolic pathways related to sphingolipid metabolism, fatty acid metabolism, thiamine metabolism, ethanol degradation, the mitochondrial beta-oxidation of short-chain saturated fatty acids, and riboflavin metabolism showed greater activation in the cochlea of the YHFD-MNAM mice. **(E)** Comparison between the cochlea of the OHFD and OHFD-MNAM mice. The metabolic pathways related to nicotine and nicotinamide metabolism, purine metabolism, fructose, and mannose degradation and tryptophan metabolism showed greater activation in the cochlea of the OHFD-MNAM mice. **(F)** MNAM metabolomic analysis peaks in the cochlea at 3 and 6 months after the commencement of the experiment. MNAM expression in both YHFD and OHFD decreased with aging ($p = 0.002$). MNAM expression in YHFD-MNAM increased compared to the expression in YLFD and YHFD ($p = 0.001$ and $p < 0.001$, respectively). MNAM expression in OHFD-MNAM increased compared to the expression in OLFD and OHFD ($p < 0.001$ and $p < 0.001$, respectively). YLFD, low-fat diet-fed 3-month-old mice; OLFD, low-fat diet-fed 6-month-old mice; YHFD, high-fat diet-fed 3-month-old mice; OHFD, high-fat diet-fed 6-month-old mice; YHFD-MNAM, high-fat diet plus 1% N^1-methylnicotinamide-fed 3-month-old mice; OHFD-MNAM, a high-fat diet plus 1% N^1-methylnicotinamide-fed 6-month-old mice. $^{**}p < 0.01$, $^{***}p < 0.001$.

elucidate the relationship between the level of SIRT1 expression in the cochlea and the development of ARHL.

A limitation of our present study is that the progression of hearing loss was enhanced by HFD consumption. With an LFD consumption, there were no effects of MNAM on hearing loss detected in a preliminary study. Therefore, an HFD was selected for this study. HFD-fed mice might not be an appropriate model for studying ARHL. The overexpression of SIRT1 in the cochlea induced *via* MNAM supplementation or a genetic modification should be demonstrated in LFD-fed and aging B6 mice. Further research using an LFD ARHL mouse model is necessary. Additionally, our results may also be interpreted to suggest that MNAM solely acts as a preventive agent against ARHL. The etiologies of ARHL are due to multiple factors. Our study may have other signaling involved. Furthermore, our study showed that MNAM supplementation failed to prevent changes in the cochlear basal turn leading to ARHL. Differential MNAM concentration distribution in the cochlear turns may explain the lack of ARHL prevention in the basal turn. Studies measuring MNAM concentration in each cochlear turn may provide more evidence.

AUTHOR CONTRIBUTIONS

TM designed the research studies, conducted the experiments, acquired the data, analyzed the data, and wrote the manuscript.

ACKNOWLEDGMENTS

I thank Kyoko Tachii, Miho Kataoka, and Ryosei Minoda for their assistance with the technical experiments at various stages of this research project. Additionally, I thank Wiley's editing service for editing the manuscript for language and for formatting it.

REFERENCES

Alcendor, R. R., Gao, S., Zhai, P., Zablocki, D., Holle, E., Yu, X., et al. (2007). Sirt1 regulates aging and resistance to oxidative stress in the heart. *Circ. Res.* 100, 1512–1521. doi: 10.1161/01.RES.0000267723.65696.4a

Böhmer, A. (1988). The Preyer reflex--an easy estimate of hearing function in guinea pigs. *Acta Otolaryngol.* 106, 368–372. doi: 10.1515/cclm-2021-0170

Brown, K. D., Maqsood, S., Huang, J. Y., Pan, Y., Harkcom, W., Li, W., et al. (2014). Activation of Sirt3 by the NAD$^+$ precursor nicotinamide riboside protects from noise-induced hearing loss. *Cell Metab.* 20, 1059–1068. doi: 10.1016/j.cmet.2014.11.003

Chalkiadaki, A., and Guarente, L. (2012). High-fat diet triggers inflammation-induced cleavage of Sirt1 in adipose tissue to promote metabolic dysfunction. *Cell Metab.* 16, 180–188. doi: 10.1016/j.cmet.2012.07.003

Cheng, H.-L., Mostoslavsky, R., Saito, S., Manis, J. P., Gu, Y., Patel, P., et al. (2003). Developmental defects and p53 hyperacetylation in Sir2 homolog (Sirt1)-deficient mice. *Proc. Natl. Acad. Sci. U S A* 100, 10794–10799. doi: 10.1073/pnas.1934713100

Donmez, G., and Outeiro, T. F. (2013). Sirt1 and Sirt2: emerging targets in neurodegeneration. *EMBO Mol. Med.* 5, 344–352. doi: 10.1002/emmm.201302451

Du, Z., Yang, Y., Hu, Y., Sun, Y., Zhang, S., Peng, W., et al. (2012). A long-term high-fat diet increases oxidative stress, mitochondrial damage and apoptosis in the inner ear of D-galactose-induced aging rats. *Hear. Res.* 287, 15–24. doi: 10.1016/j.heares.2012.04.012

Finkel, T., Deng, C.-X., and Mostoslavsky, R. (2009). Recent progress in the biology and physiology of Sirtuins. *Nature* 460, 587–591. doi: 10.1038/nature08197

Fujita, T., Yamashita, D., Uehara, N., Inokuchi, G., Hasegawa, S., Otsuki, N., et al. (2015). A high-fat diet delays age-related hearing loss progression in C57BL/6J mice. *PLoS One* 10:e0117547. doi: 10.1371/journal.pone.0117547

Gates, G. A., and Mills, J. H. (2005). Presbycusis. *Lancet* 366, 1111–1120. doi: 10.1016/S0140-6736(05)67423-5

Haigis, M. C., and Sinclair, D. A. (2010). Mammalian sirtuins: biological insights and disease relevance. *Annu. Rev. Pathol.* 5, 253–295. doi: 10.1146/annurev.pathol.4.110807.092250

Han, C., Linser, P., Park, H. J., Kim, M. J., White, K., Vann, J. M., et al. (2016). Sirt1 deficiency protects cochlear cells and delays the early onset of age-related hearing loss in C57BL/6 mice. *Neurobiol. Aging* 43, 58–71. doi: 10.1016/j.neurobiolaging.2016.03.023

Heman-Ackah, S. E., Juhn, S. K., Huang, T. C., and Wiedmann, T. S. (2010). A combination antioxidant therapy prevents age-related hearing loss in C57BL/6 mice. *Otolaryngol. Head Neck Surg.* 143, 429–434. doi: 10.1016/j.otohns.2010.04.266

Hong, S., Moreno-Navarrete, J. M., Wei, X., Kikukawa, Y., Tzameli, I., Prasad, D., et al. (2015). Nicotinamide N-methyltransferase regulates hepatic nutrient metabolism through Sirt1 protein stabilization. *Nat. Med.* 21, 887–894. doi: 10.1038/nm.3882

Hwang, J.-H., Hsu, C.-J., Yu, W.-H., Liu, T.-C., and Yang, W.-S. (2013). Diet-induced obesity exacerbates auditory degeneration *via* hypoxia, inflammation, and apoptosis signaling pathways in CD/1 mice. *PLoS One* 8:e60730. doi: 10.1371/journal.pone.0060730

Jiang, Q. (2014). Natural forms of vitamin E: metabolism, antioxidant and anti-inflammatory activities and their role in disease prevention and therapy. *Free Radic. Biol. Med.* 72, 76–90. doi: 10.1016/j.freeradbiomed.2014.03.035

Kannt, A., Pfenninger, A., Teichert, L., Tönjes, A., Dietrich, A., Schön, M. R., et al. (2015). Association of nicotinamide-N-methyltransferase mRNA expression in human adipose tissue and the plasma concentration of its product, 1-methylnicotinamide, with insulin resistance. *Diabetologia* 58, 799–808. doi: 10.1007/s00125-014-3490-7

Keithley, E. M., Canto, C., Zheng, Q. Y., Fischel-Ghodsian, N., and Johnson, K. R. (2004). Age-related hearing loss and the ahl locus in mice. *Hear. Res.* 188, 21–28. doi: 10.1016/S0378-5955(03)00365-4

Kraus, D., Yang, Q., Kong, D., Banks, A. S., Zhang, L., Rodgers, J. T., et al. (2014). Nicotinamide N-methyltransferase knockdown protects against diet-induced obesity. *Nature* 508, 258–262. doi: 10.1038/nature13198

Le Prell, C. G., Gagnon, P. M., Bennett, D. C., and Ohlemiller, K. K. (2011). Nutrient-enhanced diet reduces noise-induced damage to the inner ear and hearing loss. *Transl. Res.* 158, 38–53. doi: 10.1016/j.trsl.2011.02.006

Li, Y., Xu, W., McBurney, M. W., and Longo, V. D. (2008). Sirt1 inhibition reduces IGF-I/IRS-2/Ras/ERK1/2 signaling and protects neurons. *Cell Metab.* 8, 38–48. doi: 10.1016/j.cmet.2008.05.004

Miwa, T., Minoda, R., Ishikawa, Y., Kajii, T., Orita, Y., and Ohyama, T. (2019). Role of Dach1 revealed using a novel inner ear-specific Dach1-knockdown mouse model. *Biol. Open* 8:bio043612. doi: 10.1242/bio.043612

Miwa, T., Ohta, K., Ito, N., Hattori, S., Miyakawa, T., Takeo, T., et al. (2020). Tsukushi is essential for the development of the inner ear. *Mol. Brain* 13:29. doi: 10.1186/s13041-020-00570-z

Pang, Z., Chong, J., Li, S., and Xia, J. (2020). MetaboAnalystR 3.0: toward an optimized workflow for global metabolomics. *Metabolites* 10:E186. doi: 10.3390/metabo10050186

Pfluger, P. T., Herranz, D., Velasco-Miguel, S., Serrano, M., and Tschöp, M. H. (2008). Sirt1 protects against high-fat diet induced metabolic damage. *Proc. Natl. Acad. Sci. U S A* 105, 9793–9798. doi: 10.1073/pnas.0802917105

Revollo, J. R., and Li, X. (2013). The ways and means that fine tune Sirt1 activity. *Trends Biochem. Sci.* 38, 160–167. doi: 10.1016/j.tibs.2012.12.004

Schmeisser, K., Mansfeld, J., Kuhlow, D., Weimer, S., Priebe, S., Heiland, I., et al. (2013). Role of Sirtuins in lifespan regulation is linked to methylation of nicotinamide. *Nat. Chem. Biol.* 9, 693–700. doi: 10.1038/nchembio.1352

Someya, S., Xu, J., Kondo, K., Ding, D., Salvi, R. J., Yamasoba, T., et al. (2009). Age-related hearing loss in C57BL/6J mice is mediated by Bak-dependent mitochondrial apoptosis. *Proc. Natl. Acad. Sci. U S A* 106, 19432–19437. doi: 10.1073/pnas.0908786106

Someya, S., Yu, W., Hallows, W. C., Xu, J., Vann, J. M., Leeuwenburgh, C., et al. (2010). Sirt3 mediates reduction of oxidative damage and prevention of age-related hearing loss under caloric restriction. *Cell* 143, 802–812. doi: 10.1016/j.cell.2010.10.002

Vasilyeva, O. N., Frisina, S. T., Zhu, X., Walton, J. P., and Frisina, R. D. (2009). Interactions of hearing loss and diabetes mellitus in the middle age CBA/CaJ mouse model of presbycusis. *Hear. Res.* 249, 44–53. doi: 10.1016/j.heares.2009.01.007

Wang, R.-H., Kim, H.-S., Xiao, C., Xu, X., Gavrilova, O., and Deng, C.-X. (2011). Hepatic Sirt1 deficiency in mice impairs mTorc2/Akt signaling and results in hyperglycemia, oxidative damage and insulin resistance. *J. Clin. Invest.* 121, 4477–4490. doi: 10.1172/JCI46243

Xiong, H., Dai, M., Ou, Y., Pang, J., Yang, H., Huang, Q., et al. (2014). Sirt1 expression in the cochlea and auditory cortex of a mouse model of age-related hearing loss. *Exp. Gerontol.* 51, 8–14. doi: 10.1016/j.exger.2013.12.006

Xiong, H., Pang, J., Yang, H., Dai, M., Liu, Y., Ou, Y., et al. (2015). Activation of miR-34a/Sirt1/p53 signaling contributes to cochlear hair cell apoptosis: implications for age-related hearing loss. *Neurobiol. Aging* 36, 1692–1701. doi: 10.1016/j.neurobiolaging.2014.12.034

Yamada, T., Minoda, R., Miwa, T., Ise, M., Takeda, H., and Yumoto, E. (2015). Neurogenesis of the spiral ganglion cells in the cochlea requires the transcriptional cofactor TIS21. *Neurosci. Lett.* 584, 265–269. doi: 10.1016/j.neulet.2014.10.001

Yamasoba, T., Lin, F. R., Someya, S., Kashio, A., Sakamoto, T., and Kondo, K. (2013). Current concepts in age-related hearing loss: epidemiology and mechanistic pathways. *Hear. Res.* 303, 30–38. doi: 10.1016/j.heares.2013.01.021

Xiong, H., Pang, J., Yang, H., Dai, M., Liu, Y., Ou, Y., et al. (2015). Activation of miR-34a/Sirt1/p53 signaling contributes to cochlear hair cell apoptosis: implications for age-related hearing loss. *Neurobiol. Aging* 36, 1692–1701. doi: 10.1016/j.neurobiolaging.2014.12.034

Yamada, T., Minoda, R., Miwa, T., Ise, M., Takeda, H., and Yumoto, E. (2015). Neurogenesis of the spiral ganglion cells in the cochlea requires the transcriptional cofactor TIS21. *Neurosci. Lett.* 584, 265–269. doi: 10.1016/j.neulet.2014.10.001

Yamasoba, T., Lin, F. R., Someya, S., Kashio, A., Sakamoto, T., and Kondo, K. (2013). Current concepts in age-related hearing loss: epidemiology and mechanistic pathways. *Hear. Res.* 303, 30–38. doi: 10.1016/j.heares.2013.01.021

13

Local Cisplatin Delivery in Mouse Reliably Models Sensorineural Ototoxicity without Systemic Adverse Effects

German Nacher-Soler[1], Sébastien Lenglet[2], Marta Coelho[1], Aurélien Thomas[2,3], François Voruz[1,4], Karl-Heinz Krause[5], Pascal Senn[1,4†] and Francis Rousset[1†]*

[1] *The Inner Ear and Olfaction Lab, Department of Pathology and Immunology, Faculty of Medicine, University of Geneva, Geneva, Switzerland,* [2] *Forensic Toxicology and Chemistry Unit, University Centre for Legal Medicine, Geneva University Hospital, Geneva, Switzerland,* [3] *Faculty Unit of Toxicology, University Centre of Legal Medicine, Lausanne University Hospital, Lausanne, Switzerland,* [4] *Department of Clinical Neurosciences, Service of ORL & Head and Neck Surgery, University Hospital of Geneva, Geneva, Switzerland,* [5] *Department of Pathology and Immunology, Faculty of Medicine, University of Geneva, Geneva, Switzerland*

***Correspondence:**
German Nacher-Soler
German.NacherSoler@unige.ch

† *These authors share last authorship*

Cisplatin is a lifesaving chemotherapeutic drug with marked ototoxic adverse effects. Cisplatin-induced hearing loss affects a significant part of cancer-surviving patients and is an unmet clinical need with important socioeconomic consequences. Unfortunately, in current preclinical animal models of cisplatin ototoxicity, which are mainly based on systemic delivery, important morbidity is observed, leading to premature death. This methodology not only raises obvious animal welfare concerns but also increases the number of animals used in ototoxicity studies to compensate for dropouts related to early death. To overcome these important limitations, we developed a local delivery model based on the application of a cisplatin solution directly into the otic bulla through a retroauricular approach. The local delivery model reliably induced significant hearing loss with a mean threshold shift ranging from 10 to 30 dB, strongly affecting the high frequencies (22 and 32 kHz). Importantly, mice did not show visible stress or distress indicators and no significant morbidity in comparison with a traditional systemic delivery control group of mice injected intraperitoneally with 10 mg/kg cisplatin, where significant weight loss >10% in all treated animals (without any recovery) led to premature abortion of experiments on day 3. Mass spectrometry confirmed the absence of relevant systemic uptake after local delivery, with platinum accumulation restricted to the cochlea, whereas important platinum concentrations were detected in the liver and kidney of the systemic cisplatin group. A clear correlation between the cochlear platinum concentration and the auditory threshold shift was observed. Immunohistochemistry revealed statistically significant loss of outer hair cells in the basal and apical turns of the cochlea and an important and statistically significant loss of auditory neurons and synapses in all cochlear regions. In conclusion, local cisplatin delivery induces robust hearing loss with minimal morbidity, thereby offering a reliable rodent model for human cisplatin ototoxicity, reducing the number of animals required and showing improved animal welfare compared with traditional systemic models.

Keywords: refinement, animal welfare, middle ear delivery, cisplatin ototoxicity, cochlea, mass spectrometry

INTRODUCTION

Hearing loss (HL) is the most common neurosensory deficit in humans, with over 5% of the worldwide population affected (WHO, March 2020 report), recognized as a major and growing socioeconomic burden leading to cognitive decline, depression, and social isolation (Panza et al., 2015; Rutherford et al., 2018).

Cisplatin (*cis*-diaminedichloroplatinum) is a widely used lifesaving chemotherapy used against different types of cancers, including carcinomas, germ cell tumors, lymphomas, and sarcomas (Dasari and Tchounwou, 2014). Cisplatin harbors antitumor effect through DNA alkylation, interfering with DNA replication and repair mechanisms, ultimately leading to apoptosis in proliferating cells (Basu and Krishnamurthy, 2010). Therefore, the antitumor effect of cisplatin is largely unspecific, leading to important systemic adverse effects including nephrotoxicity (Miller et al., 2010), neurotoxicity, myelosuppression, and ototoxicity (Dasari and Tchounwou, 2014). Cisplatin-related ototoxicity is characterized by irreversible damage to the cochlea leading to permanent sensorineural HL affecting primarily high frequencies, often in combination with tinnitus (Mujica-Mota et al., 2013). The incidence and severity of cisplatin-induced ototoxicity in humans vary widely in the literature, ranging from 12.5 to 100% in children and 26–100% in adults, depending on the HL criteria used for analysis (Landier, 2016). In a retrospective analysis of a large collection of 401 adults treated with cisplatin in Geneva's University Hospital, significant HL was found in 20% of cases, among whom 60% experienced tinnitus.

Nowadays, no preventive treatment is available to limit the adverse effects of cisplatin on hearing, and its related ototoxicity remains an unmet clinical need, although it is the only clinically relevant acute hearing insult that is foreseeable. Cisplatin ototoxicity conceptually offers a unique window for preventive HL treatment before or simultaneous to the administration of the chemotherapeutic. Addressing and potentially preventing cisplatin ototoxicity requires a deeper understanding of its molecular consequences on the cochlea. However, so far, the development of novel therapies is limited by the lack of a robust and 3R (replace, reduce, and refine principles) compatible preclinical model. The mouse is the most common mammalian model specie, combining short generation time, easy breeding, and relatively low housing costs. Furthermore, the mouse model allows in-depth characterization of putative target genes, as numerous knockout animals are available. Unfortunately, cisplatin HL is difficult to reproduce in a mouse model, as important systemic toxicity generally arises before the onset of mild to moderate ototoxicity. Current mouse models to study ototoxic adverse effects of cisplatin consist of intraperitoneal (IP) cisplatin injection of a single high dose (e.g., Parham, 2011; Naples et al., 2020) or lower doses in a repeated fashion (Breglio et al., 2017; Fernandez et al., 2019; DeBacker et al., 2020). However, in such models, strong toxicity and animal distress are observed, including important weight loss and ataxia, raising important and prohibitive ethical concerns. Because of systemic toxicity and morbidity, many animals are sacrificed before obtaining valid and reproducible results, also limiting the scientific value of the model. Recently, a more clinically relevant model was described consisting of several cycles of serial low doses of cisplatin injections with intercalated resting periods, for a total of 40 days (Breglio et al., 2017; Fernandez et al., 2019). In these studies, the cisplatin treatment was accompanied by a supplementary high-calorie diet and extensive care such as daily injection of saline to overcome the kidney toxicity. This model was reported to produce robust HL; however, it also led to important weight loss (20–30% compared with untreated controls of the same age), morbidity, and costs.

To address the limitations mentioned earlier, we set out to develop a robust and scientifically relevant HL model with minimal morbidity and mortality, in line with 3R principles based on local delivery of cisplatin into the middle ear *via* retroauricular access to the otic bulla. The surgical approach, inspired by previous studies (Stevens et al., 2015; Mulazimoglu et al., 2017), was atraumatic on mouse hearing and did not lead to any signs of morbidity or stress on operated animals. More importantly, this method led to a robust increase of hearing thresholds in cisplatin delivered ears. Mass spectrometry data showed important accumulation of platinum (Pt) in the operated ear but not in other organs such as the kidney, liver, or in the contralateral ear, which could be safely used as an internal control for hearing threshold comparison and histology. With this minimally invasive method, we also demonstrated a strong correlation between the Pt concentration in the cochlea and the extent of HL. This new preclinical model will not only improve animal welfare and experiment reproducibility but will also provide a model to study long-term consequences of cisplatin exposure on the hearing system, as mice will be able to survive longer and in better condition. We believe that the model is a timely and relevant development, as new and promising otoprotective compounds and preventive strategies are waiting to be tested in preclinical trials.

MATERIALS AND METHODS

The main aim of the study is to develop a robust and scientifically relevant HL model with minimal morbidity and mortality, in line with the 3R principles. To do so, a strict animal morbidity evaluation was conducted, comparing the new model with a currently used systemic approach. Secondly, we aim to describe the cisplatin correlation with HL using mass spectrometry analysis. The described protocols were executed in compliance with the Swiss regulations and the Animal Research: Reporting of *in vivo* Experiments guidelines.

Animal Experimentation

A total of $n = 52$ male and female C57BL/6 mice were used in this study. To avoid age-related HL interferences with the results, the experiments were carried out on young adult mice aged 6 to 8 weeks. The complete research protocol was approved by the local veterinary office and the Commission for Animal Experimentation of the Canton of Geneva ("Commission cantonale pour les expériences sur les animaux"), Switzerland, authorization number GE/149/18.

Animals were blindly assigned into saline 0.9% (control), local cisplatin delivery (5 mM), and IP systemic injection (10 mg/kg) groups, ensuring equal sex distribution. Cisplatin reagent was prepared after resuspension of *cis*-diamineplatinum (II) dichloride (Sigma-Aldrich, 479306) in saline 0.9%, for a final concentration of 5 mM. Animals assigned to the systemic delivery group received a single IP injection of cisplatin (10 mg/kg). As a comparison, systemically injected animals received approximately 0.210 mg of cisplatin (considering an average weight of 21 g), whereas the local delivery group (on average) received 0.012 mg of cisplatin locally.

Animals were anesthetized by an IP injection (dose of 10 µl/g) of ketamine (10%) and xylazine (5%) for the auditory testing and for the surgical procedure. If necessary, 10% ketamine solution was injected intramuscularly (dose 5 µl/g) to elongate the anesthesia and surgery time. During both procedures, the depth of anesthesia was checked every 30 min by testing the pedal withdrawal reflex. Additionally, analgesia was applied during and after the surgery by local injection (1.2 µl/g) of lidocaine and epinephrine (0.5%) to decrease post-surgery discomfort. The animal condition was monitored daily until day 7, recording an animal welfare score sheet.

At the day 7- or 14-time point after local delivery, animals were sacrificed by cervical dislocation under ketamine–xylazine anesthesia followed by decapitation to proceed with the histological and mass spectrometry protocols. Although similar time points were planned for animals receiving cisplatin systemically, the experiment was aborted at day 3, following humane endpoint (15% loss of weight).

Animal Care Score Sheet

Following the 3R principles, the discomfort and morbidity evaluation was assessed by the design and recording of a score sheet for each experimental subject. The score sheet includes the most relevant variables on rodent welfare, such as weight (general health indicator), piloerection, ataxia, wound condition (infection and sutures condition), and behavior (reaction to manipulation and social interaction). The scoring system was set from 0 (normal condition) to 3 (high severity). Level 1 animals were routinely evaluated, whereas level 2 subjects received analgesia and were closely monitored. Level 3 animals were sacrificed according to Swiss animal welfare legislation. Animal weight and behavior were monitored and evaluated every day, from treatment to death.

Retroauricular Surgical Approach

All surgeries were performed on the animal right ear with a Wild Heerbrug laparoscopy microscope (M655), maintaining the left ear (contralateral) as an internal control. Each animal underwent surgery and treatment only once. Animals were anesthetized, and the surgical procedure started once the proper anesthesia depth was achieved (after the stapedial reflex) and after local analgesia. The animal was placed upon a heating pad, covered with a sterilized cover, in a lateral position allowing access to the right ear. The surgical area was sterilized with 70% alcohol, and the fur was locally shaved with a scalpel. We proceeded with a retroauricular skin incision behind the ear canal (**Figure 1A**) to access the middle ear of the mice (**Figure 1B**). The overlying fascia was carefully dissected, allowing us to identify the great auricular nerve, which was used as a reference to identify and retract the cervical trapezius muscle. After the retraction, the bulla bone is identified as located under the facial nerve (**Figure 1C**). The remaining tissue in the bulla surface was set aside to localize the injection site within the bulla. The bulla was drilled in a posterior-dorsal position to avoid any potential damage during the procedure, using a 25G needle (**Figure 1D**). Our surgical design allowed the direct contact of the tested solutions with the cochlear round window, facilitating the diffusion into the cochlea. A 20-µl GELoader tip (Eppendorf) was used to deliver the experimental solution through the bulla opening. During 15 min, the bulla was refilled eight times with cisplatin 5 mM or saline 0.9%, maintaining a constant volume of solution into the middle ear, compensating the Eustachian tube drainage. After each 2-µl refill, the solution overflow was removed with a sterilized synthetic surgical sponge (FST, 18105-03).

At the end of the treatment protocol, the bulla space was rinsed three times with 3 µl of saline 0.9% and dried with a synthetic surgical sponge to remove the tested experimental solution from the middle ear. Then, a piece of tissue was disposed of in the bulla opening and sealed with cyanoacrylate glue. Finally, the retroauricular incision was closed by a skin suture. Analgesia was applied locally to reduce post-surgery discomfort. At the end of the surgery, the mice rested upon a heating pad until full recovery.

Auditory Testing

Animals were anesthetized and placed upon a heating pad to maintain body temperature. All subjects were auditory tested at two time points, the day before the surgery (D0) and 7 (D7) or 14 days (D14) after the local delivery procedure, to measure hearing thresholds. Animals receiving cisplatin systemically were tested at D0 and 3 days after the injection (D3). Auditory brainstem response (ABR) measurements were conducted in a soundproof chamber (IAC Acoustics, IL, United States). Pt electrodes were placed subcutaneously on the forehead of the mouse (+), on the mastoid of the recorded ear (−), and the reference electrode on the back of the mouse. ABRs were recorded after unilateral stimulation through a custom-made earplug adapter with 100-µs clicks or 3-ms tone pipes (2.0 to 32 kHz at a resolution of two steps per octave). The electrical wave outcome was averaged over 128 stimulus repetitions. For the stimulus generation and recording of responses, a multifunction IO-Card (National Instruments, Austin, TX, United States) was used. The sound pressure level (SPL) was controlled with an attenuator and amplifier (Otoconsult, Frankfurt, Germany). Furthermore, the sound pressure was calibrated online before each measurement with a microphone probe system (Bruel&Kjaer 4191) placed near the animals' ears. Recorded signals were amplified and bandpass filtered (80 dB; 0.2–3.0 kHz) using a filter/amplifier unit (Otoconsult, Frankfurt, Germany). For all frequencies, ABRs were analyzed from 0 to 80 dB SPL in 5 dB steps. The hearing threshold was visually

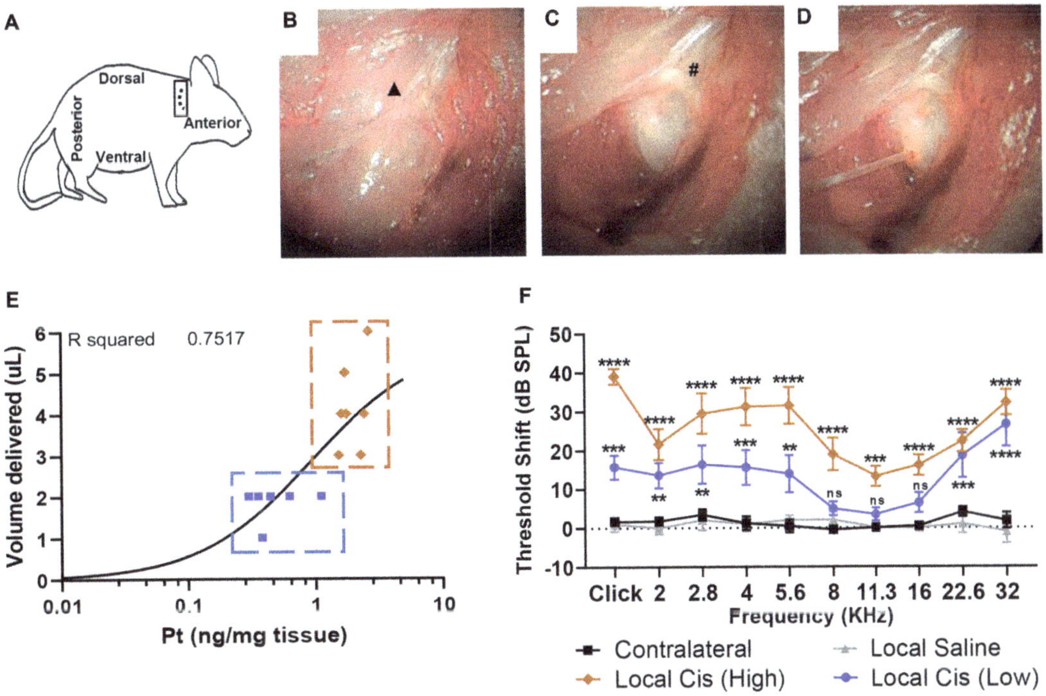

FIGURE 1 | Minimally invasive, retroauricular approach for local cisplatin delivery. To access retroauricular position of bulla, mouse is placed in lateral position, with right ear upward. An incision is made retroauricularly **(A)**. After skin retraction, cervical trapezius muscle and great auricular nerve (▲) are exposed **(B)**. After careful dissection of connective tissue, bulla bone and facial nerve (#) are identified **(C)**. Access hole is drilled in a posterior-dorsal position, minimizing risk for cochlear damage. A 0.3-mm diameter cannula is placed into bulla aperture **(D)** to deliver 2–5 μl of solution. Finally, a piece of tissue and cyanoacrylate glue are used to occlude the opening. **(E)** Correlation plot (n = 13) between cisplatin (5 mM) volume delivered (limited by bulla size) and Pt fixation. Animals with a volume of cisplatin <3 μl were classified in "low cisplatin" subgroup (blue), whereas animals with a volume of cisplatin ≥3 μl were classified in "high cisplatin" subgroup (orange). **(F)** Permanent threshold shift, measured by unilateral auditory brainstem response (ABR), in cisplatin-treated animals (5 mM, n = 13) was recorded 7 days after local delivery in comparison with delivery of saline solution (n = 5) and contralateral untreated ears. Cisplatin treated animal data were represented following "high" (orange) and "low" (blue) subclassification defined on **(E)**. The confidence interval for both statistics was set as 95% (a = 0.05); **p < 0.01; ***p < 0.005; ****p < 0.0005.

defined as the lowest SPL showing a conserved wave pattern. At the end of the ABR recording, mice were placed in a recovery cage upon a heating pad until consciousness recover.

Threshold shifts were determined as the difference between the post (D7) and presurgery (D0) ABR hearing threshold, providing paired values for all analyzed frequencies in each animal.

Cochlea Dissection and Histology

At the end of the experiment (D7 ABR), mice were sacrificed for cochlear histology. After the sagittal cut of the skull, the brain and brainstem were removed, and both temporal bones were immersed in 2.5 ml of ice-cold Hanks' balanced salt solution in a 35-mm Petri dish. The cochleas were extracted under a stereomicroscope (Nikkon, Japan). The dissection procedure allowed the evaluation of the inner ear and middle ear integrity, permitting the evaluation of any possible mechanical damages induced by the surgical approach.

For Pt titration by mass spectrometry, cochleas were weighed on a precision scale, frozen on liquid nitrogen, and conserved at −80°C until analysis. For histology (cytocochleograms and mid-modiolar cuts), cochleas were fixed in 4% formol overnight at room temperature and decalcified for 48 h under sonication (ultrasonic USE 33 decalcification machine, Medite, 03-3300-00) in USEDECALC solution (Medite commercial solution). Finally, decalcified cochleas were microdissected to perform cytocochleograms and immunostaining or embedded in paraffin for mid-modiolar cuts and hematoxylin–eosin staining.

Mass Spectrometry Analysis

Non-decalcified cochleas (conserved at −80°C) were used on the mass spectrometry analysis. Additionally, to evaluate the cisplatin systemic toxicity, kidney and liver samples were collected as representative tissues. The Pt concentration (LabKings, Hilversum, Netherlands) was measured in the collected mouse tissues (cochlea, liver, and kidney) by inductively coupled plasma mass spectrometry (ICP MS 7800 series; Agilent, Tokyo, Japan). As previously described (Vorobiev et al., 2019), before analysis, the mouse tissues were weighed and mineralized in Suprapur nitric acid (HNO_3) 65% (Merck, Darmstadt, Germany) at 80°C for 1 h. The samples, blanks, and calibration curves were diluted in a solution containing HNO_3 2%, butanol 1% (VWR, Fontenay-sous-Bois, France), and Triton 0.5% (Sigma, Buchs, Switzerland) in ultrapure water (resistivity greater than 18.2 MΩ cm) (Vorobiev et al., 2019). An external calibration curve in HNO_3 65% was prepared by monitoring the 195 Pt isotope with a dwell time of 300 ms in no-gas mode (without collision cell). Internal standards (rhodium and indium; Agilent, Basel, Switzerland) were added at 10 μg/L to the analytical calibration solutions, analytical blanks, and samples. The raw data were acquired using MassHunter software (Agilent, Tokyo, Japan).

Immunohistochemistry and Microscopy

Decalcified cochleas were microdissected under a binocular microscope (Nikkon, Japan). The bony cochlear wall was removed to uncover the auditory sensory epithelium (organ of Corti), which was separated from the stria vascularis and modiolus. The organ of Corti was divided then into three main sections, the basal, medial, and apical turns, and mounted as cytocochleograms.

The collected organs of Corti were permeabilized [3% Triton-X 100 in phosphate-buffered saline (PBS) 1×] for 30 min at room temperature. After three washing steps with PBS, the samples were placed in blocking solution (2% bovine serum albumin, 0.01% Triton-X 100, in PBS) for 30 min and posteriorly incubated with primary antibodies against Myosin 7a (polyclonal rabbit anti-Myosin 7a, Proteus) and CtBP2 (monoclonal mouse anti-CtBP2, BD Bioscience) (1:200 in blocking solution). Primary antibodies were incubated overnight at 4°C with a 10-rpm agitation on a gyratory rocker (Stuart SSM3). The following day, samples were rinsed three times with PBS and incubated with the secondary antibodies (goat anti-mouse Alexa 555, goat anti-rabbit 488, Life Technologies) (1:500 in blocking solution) for 2 h with a 10-rpm agitation at room temperature. Afterward, samples were washed three times with PBS, placed in glass slides, and mounted with Fluoroshield reagent containing 4′,6-diamidino-2-phenylindole (Sigma).

The image acquisition was performed with a confocal laser-scanning microscope (Zeiss LSM700), using a Plan-Neofluar 20X/0.50 and a Plan-Apochromat 63X/1.4 (Oil) objectives. Images were recorded with a CCD camera (Leica Microsystems) and analyzed with the open-source software FIJI (ImageJ).

Mid-Modiolar Cuts and Hematoxylin–Eosin Staining

Decalcified cochleas were dehydrated and embedded in paraffin as previously described (Rousset et al., 2020). Mid-modiolar cuts of 5 μm were processed and loaded onto gelatin-coated slides. The Harris' hematoxylin/eosin staining was performed on five non-consecutive mid-modiolar slides of each cochlea. A Zeiss Axioskop-2, equipped with an AxioCam HRc camera, was used to acquire images from the Rosenthal's canal corresponding to the basal, medial, and apical turns. Quantification of the spiral ganglion neurons was performed with the open-source software FIJI (ImageJ).

Image Processing and Analysis for Quantitative Cochlear Cytology

Pictures from cytocochleograms and mid-modiolar cuts were analyzed with the open-source software FIJI (ImageJ). Confocal 10–15-μm z-stack images (0.7 μm steps) were recorded with a 63X objective to quantify the synapses (Ctbp2) in each cochlear turn. The resulting files were reconstructed as two-dimensional images to allow accurate ribbon quantification from the whole sample depth. For each sample section (apical, medial, and basal turns), the number of ribbon synapses of two independent representative areas of 13–15 inner hair cells (IHCs) was analyzed and averaged. Artificial color images were assembled to facilitate analysis and visualization. Hair cell quantification was performed on 20X magnification pictures using the MyoVIIa and 4′,6-diamidino-2-phenylindole markers. IHC and outer hair cell (OHC) populations were counted in two representative areas of 100 μm for each cochlear turn, recording the HC survival average.

The spiral ganglion neuron density was determined by nuclear quantification of Rosenthal's canal population. Mid-modiolar single z-stack pictures (hematoxylin–eosin) were recorded from five non-consecutive 5-μm sections of each cochlear turn. The number of nuclei was determined manually and normalized to Rosenthal's canal total area (square millimeter). The measured densities were averaged for the basal, medial, and apical turns.

Statistics

All data were analyzed using the GraphPad Prism software (version 8.4.3). A two-way analysis of variance test (without repeated measures) followed by Bonferroni multiple comparison correction was used during ABR comparison and histological evaluation (cytocochleograms and synapses). For the comparison of Pt concentration in the liver, kidney, and cochlea by mass spectrometry, Brown–Forsythe and Welch analysis of variance tests with Dunnett's multiple comparison correction were used. *T*-test unpaired with Welch's correction was used on the spiral ganglion neuron population comparison. The confidence interval for both statistics was set as 95% ($\alpha = 0.05$); $^{*}p < 0.05$, $^{**}p < 0.01$, $^{***}p < 0.005$, $^{****}p < 0.0005$. The least-squares regression approach was used for the Pt/HL correlation and R squared measure.

RESULTS

Development of a Preclinical Model of Cisplatin Ototoxicity With Robust Hearing Loss

To develop a preclinical model of cisplatin ototoxicity compatible with the animal welfare legislation in Switzerland, we applied a cisplatin solution (5 mM) directly into the mouse otic bulla through a retroauricular approach (**Figure 1**). We performed a retroauricular skin incision behind the ear canal (**Figure 1A**) to access the mice's middle ear [**Figures 1B, C**; see also the *Materials and methods* section for a detailed description (*Retroauricular surgical approach*)]. A 25G opening was drilled on the bulla and repeatedly refilled to maintain a constant volume for 15 min (**Figure 1D**). During the surgery, we observed important variability of the bulla size across animals, and therefore, differences in the middle ear injected cisplatin volume, ranging from 1 to 6 μl (usually 2–4 μl) (**Figure 1E**). We also observed a correlation between the amount of Pt retained in the cochlea and the volume of cisplatin delivered in the tympanic bulla ($r^2 = 0.7517$). Based on the volume of cisplatin delivered, we defined two groups of cisplatin-treated animals. Animals receiving a volume of cisplatin <3 μl were classified in the "low cisplatin delivery" group (**Figure 1E**; blue), whereas animals injected with a volume of cisplatin ≥3 μl were defined as the "high cisplatin delivery" group (**Figure 1E**; orange). Seven days after the local delivery of cisplatin solution, we observed a significant elevation of click- and pure-tone-evoked hearing thresholds at all tested frequencies in the high cisplatin group (**Figure 1F**; orange). We also observed significant HL at most tested frequencies (**Figure 1**; blue) in the low cisplatin group, although the elevation of hearing threshold was overall milder. However, no HL was observed in sham-operated (saline) and non-operated, contralateral ears (**Figure 1F**; gray and black). Consistently, we observed a significant decrease of the click-evoked ABR wave 1 amplitude only after local delivery of cisplatin (averaging high and low cisplatin data) but not saline (**Supplementary Figure 1**). We reported comparable ABR threshold shifts 7 and 14 days after local cisplatin delivery, suggesting that the damage induced at D7 is already maximal (**Supplementary Figure 2A**). However, animals receiving repeated doses of cisplatin had, on average, higher hearing threshold shifts as compared with mice receiving a single local dose of cisplatin (without refilling) (**Supplementary Figure 2B**).

Local Delivery of Cisplatin Decreases Hair Cell Numbers in the Mouse Cochlea

Similar to what is observed in systemic models (Fernandez et al., 2019), local delivery of cisplatin primarily affected the OHC population (**Figures 2C, E**). However, no significant loss of IHC could be observed after local cisplatin treatment (**Figure 2D1**), compared with the non-operated contralateral (**Figure 2A**) or sham-operated (saline) (**Figure 2B**). The extent of sensory epithelium damages varied from only a few missing OHC on the low cisplatin group (**Supplementary Figure 3**) to almost complete HC disruption on the high cisplatin group (**Supplementary Figure 4**). On average, consistent with the ABR's hearing thresholds, hair cell apoptosis was more prominent in basal (**Figures 2C1, E1**) and apical turns (**Figures 2C3, E3**), whereas a milder effect was observed in the medial turn (**Figures 2C2, E2**). Importantly, no relevant hair cell loss was related to the surgical approach, as the saline group exhibited similar HC numbers comparable with the contralateral or untreated cochleas from the cisplatin group (**Figures 2B, D, E**).

Local Delivery of Cisplatin Leads to Auditory Neuropathy

Cisplatin is a potent neurotoxic drug, and loss of auditory neurons (auditory neuropathy) has been previously described in systemic cisplatin mice models (Liu et al., 2019). After local cisplatin delivery, we observed a significant decrease in the auditory neuron density compared with the contralateral cochleae (**Figure 3A**). Animal receiving "low volume" of cisplatin exhibited only minor loss of auditory neurons and minor morphological changes (**Supplementary Figure 3**), whereas more pronounced effects could be observed in "high volume" animals (**Supplementary Figure 4**). Overall, the decrease in the number of auditory neurons was statistically significant in all cochlear turns (**Figure 3C**), resulting in the presence of apoptotic bodies (**Figure 3B**, arrows). Therefore, the described local delivery model also recapitulates the cisplatin neurotoxicity observed in conventional systemic models.

Cisplatin Drastically Decreases the Number of Presynaptic Ribbons

The number of auditory neurons synapsing with a single IHC is critical for hearing perception in noisy environments (Kujawa and Liberman, 2015). The stronger effect of local cisplatin treatment was observed on the auditory synapse (**Figure 4**). Indeed, both animals receiving local low and high volumes of cisplatin exhibited a dramatic decrease in the CtBP2 positive signal for presynaptic vesicles (**Supplementary Figures 3, 4**). Remarkably, even animals receiving a low amount of cisplatin and where no sensory cell loss could be seen, exhibited a reduced number of auditory synapses, with a prominent effect on the basal and apical turns (**Supplementary Figure 3**). These data suggest that the auditory synapse is the most vulnerable part of the cochlea with respect to cisplatin ototoxicity and are consistent with the reported amplitude decrease of the ABR wave I (**Supplementary Figure 1**). Overall, cisplatin-treated cochleae showed a dramatic decrease in the number of synapses compared with the contralateral and saline conditions. This synaptic loss was significant in the basal, medial, and apical turns (**Figures 4C1–C3,D**) compared with the non-operated contralateral ear (**Figure 4A**) and with the sham-operated animals (**Figure 4B**).

Absence of Systemic Recirculation and Associated Morbidity After Cisplatin Local Delivery

Cisplatin accumulation in the liver and kidney is the main cause leading to the systemic toxicity observed in previously established models (Breglio et al., 2017). The cisplatin local delivery model was compared with the systemic model (IP, 10 mg/kg) with respect to general welfare (as assessed by weight measurement and score sheet) and in respect to the Pt retention in the cochlea, kidney, and liver (**Figure 5**). Animals injected IP with 10 mg/kg of cisplatin exhibited important accumulation of Pt in the kidney, liver, and cochlea (**Figure 5A**). Seven days after local delivery of cisplatin, we reported a strong Pt accumulation in cochleae of the high cisplatin group, above the levels observed on the systemic delivery, and a significant accumulation on the low cisplatin group (below the systemic levels); however, no significant Pt amount was detected in liver and kidney. Importantly, we did not observe any signs of systemic toxicity such as piloerection, ataxia, or any distress behavior in operated animals (not shown). Consistently, no weight differences were observed between the saline and cisplatin groups, and all the animals significantly overcame the presurgery weight by day 7, without any supplementary diet (**Figure 5B**). In contrast,

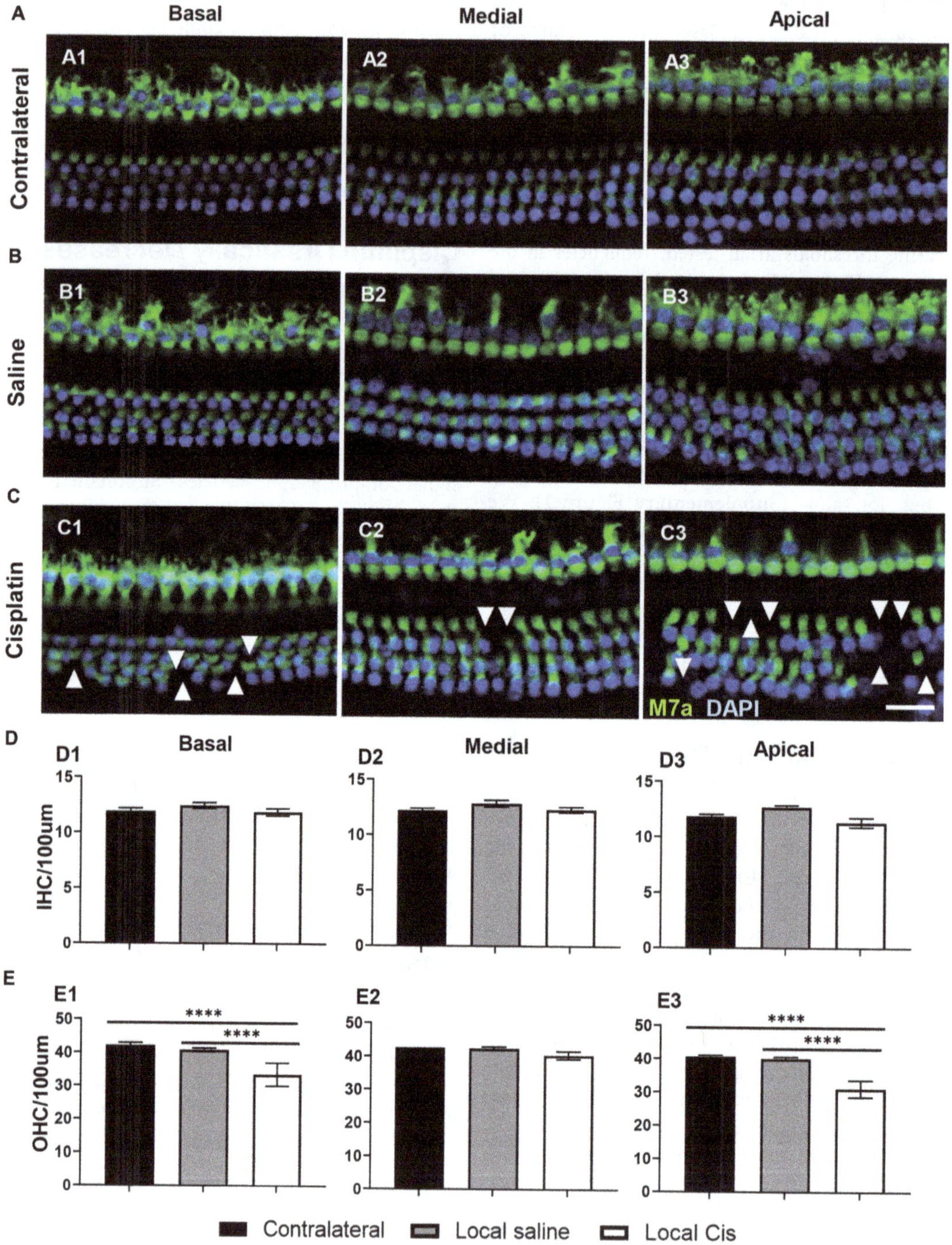

FIGURE 2 | Effects of cisplatin local delivery on IHC and OHC viability. Cytocochleogram showing both IHC and OHC, quantified in a representative area of 100-μm length from basal, medial, and apical cochlear turns, in **(A)** contralateral, **(B)** saline, and **(C)** local-cisplatin (5 mM) cochleae. Samples were stained for 4′,6-diamidino-2-phenylindole (blue) and myosin VIIa (green). **(D)** Bar graphs show number of IHC/100 μm area in **(D1)** basal, **(D2)** medial, and **(D3)** apical turns of cochlea (without subgroup distinction). **(E)** Bar graphs show number of OHC/100 μm area in **(E1)** basal, **(E2)** medial, and **(E3)** apical turns of cochlea (without subgroup distinction). White arrows indicate missing hair cells. Scale bar: 20 μm. *n* = 15. The confidence interval for both statistics was set as 95% (*a* = 0.05); ****$p < 0.0005$.

mice receiving 10 mg/kg of cisplatin IP (which is usually lower than most of the systemic protocols) lost approximately 15% of weight after only 3 days, leading to premature sacrifice. Unfortunately, in the systemic model, no significant effect of cisplatin on hearing could be observed 3 days after the cisplatin injection (**Figure 5C**), demonstrating that the cisplatin systemic adverse effects occur before the onset of HL. ABR threshold shifts of local cisplatin delivery, already shown in **Figure 1**, are

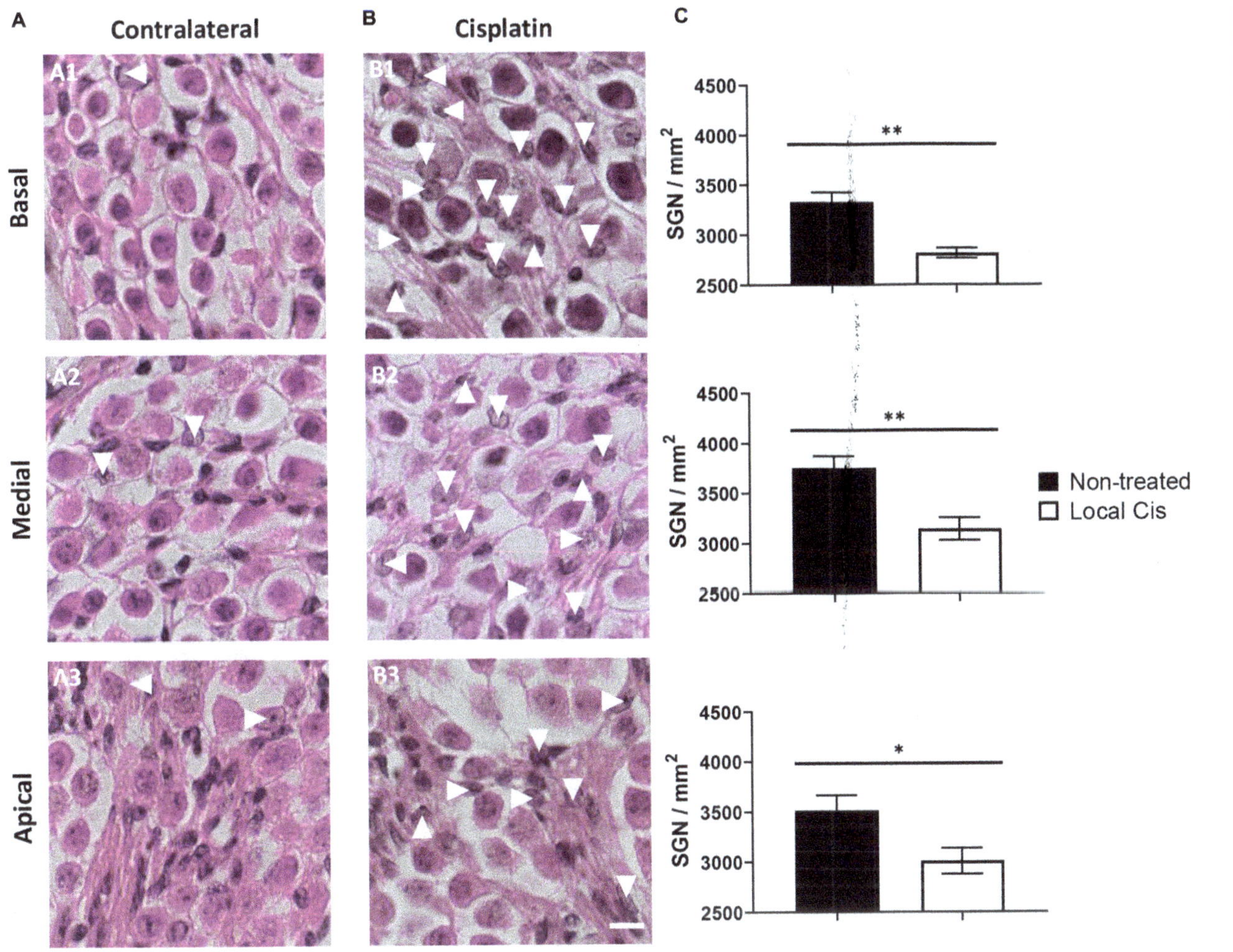

FIGURE 3 | Local delivery of cisplatin effect on auditory neuron viability. **(A,B)** Mid-modiolar histology of mouse cochlea treated with local-cisplatin (5 mM) **(B)** or contralateral cochlea **(A)** showing spiral ganglion. Spiral ganglion neurons in basal **(A1,B1)**, medial **(A2,B2)**, and apical **(A3,B3)** turns were quantified and normalized with size of counting area (in square millimeter). **(C)** Bar graph showing density of auditory neurons. Arrows indicate apoptotic or missing auditory neurons (without subgroup distinction). Scale bar: 10 μm. *n* = 15. The confidence interval for both statistics was set as 95% (a = 0.05); $^*p < 0.05$; $^{**}p < 0.01$.

also displayed in **Figure 5C** for the purpose of comparison. In the local cisplatin model, a dose–response curve could be obtained between the amount of Pt retained in the cochlea and the extent of HL, resulting in a robust correlation (R^2 = 0.8848) (**Figure 5D**). In the systemic model, although a significant amount of Pt was found in the cochlea, no significant HL could be observed, rendering impossible a dose–response comparison. The comparison with the local model is, however, difficult given the premature termination of the experiment at day 3.

DISCUSSION

A preclinical mouse model of local cisplatin delivery into the otic bulla *via* retroauricular approach has been introduced to study ototoxic HL without relevant systemic adverse effects. The model is relevant, as the main functional and morphological consequences of cisplatin treatment in the cochlea can be robustly induced through local delivery, in line with the ototoxic effects reported after systemic delivery (Sheth et al., 2017). The local delivery model has the main advantage of greatly reducing mortality and morbidity of experimental animals compared with similar studies based on systemic cisplatin delivery, in line with the 3R principles (Parham, 2011; Fernandez et al., 2019). This is not only of relevance for the well-being of the animals, but because more animals survive and are able to live longer, long-term effects of cisplatin on the cochlea can be studied, which has not been possible to this extent in systemic models. In addition, depending on the volume of cisplatin delivered, groups with different severity of HL can be defined and studied, ranging from auditory synaptopathy to sensorineural affection.

In this study, the retroauricular route was chosen in front of the intratympanic delivery procedure, as this approach allows repeated delivery during the same surgical procedure, without increasing the risk of middle ear overpressure and without perforation of the tympanic membrane. Indeed, the

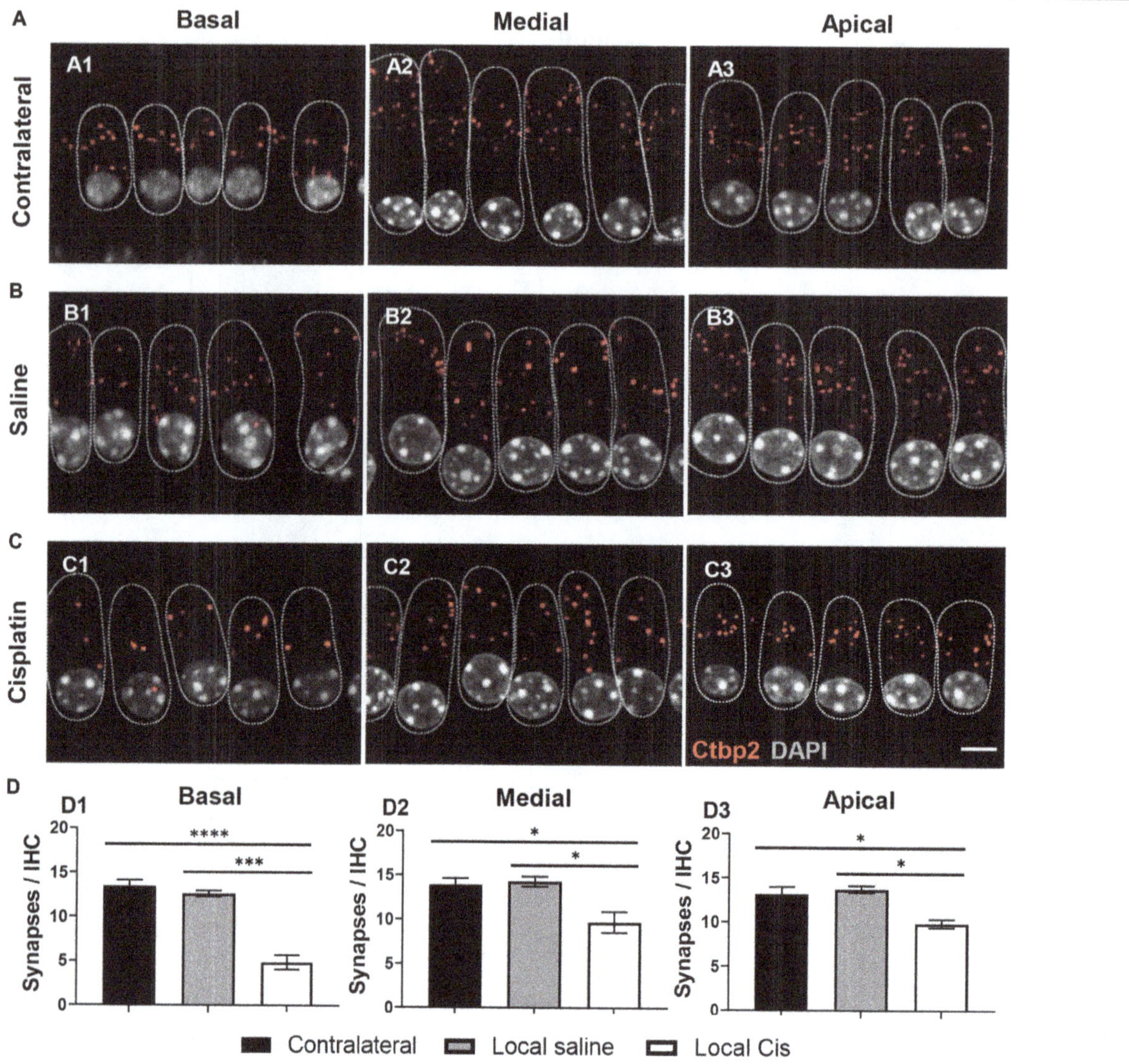

FIGURE 4 | Effect of cisplatin local delivery on number of synapses/IHC. IHC from **(A)** contralateral, **(B)** saline, and **(C)** local-cisplatin (5 mM) cochleas were stained with DAPI (nucleus, white), Ctbp2 (ribbon synapsis, red dots), and myosin VIIa (HCs, substituted by dotted lines to facilitate visualization). **(A1–C1)** Basal, **(A2–C2)** medial, and **(A3–C3)** apical cochlear turns. **(D)** Bar graphs show number of presynaptic ribbons/IHC in apical **(D1)**, medial **(D2)**, and basal **(D3)** turns of cochlea (without subgroup distinction). MyoVIIa staining was replaced with a dotted line, highlighting IHC area, to facilitate Ctbp2 visualization. Scale bar: 5 μm. $n = 11$. The confidence interval for both statistics was set as 95% ($a = 0.05$); $^{*}p < 0.05$; $^{***}p < 0.005$; $^{****}p < 0.0005$.

retroauricular approach was completely atraumatic on the mice's hearing. The possibility of conductive HL induced by the surgery was excluded as the sham-operated animal had completely normal hearing (**Figure 1F**), as was also demonstrated in previous studies with similar approaches (Stevens et al., 2015; Murillo-Cuesta et al., 2017; Rousset et al., 2019).

In the cochlea, the hallmarks of cisplatin ototoxicity can be evoked after local cisplatin treatment, namely predominant outer hair cell loss, loss of auditory neurons, and robust HL. In addition, the more recently discovered loss of synaptic connections between inner hair cells and auditory neurons can be reliably induced. This is of relevance for modeling another typical outcome in cisplatin-treated patients, the hidden HL phenomenon, cursing with tinnitus, and decreased speech perception in the presence of only mild, or absent, measurable HL (El Charif et al., 2019). By reducing the dose of local cisplatin delivered, a hidden HL situation can be adequately modeled through local delivery (**Supplementary Figure 3**).

Cisplatin has a predominant effect on the patient's high frequencies (Liberman et al., 2013). This pattern of HL is generally well reproduced on current systemic injected animal models (Fernandez et al., 2019). In the local delivery model, the hearing threshold elevation, as well as the histological features, was also markedly enhanced in the basal cochlear turn in both local cisplatin subgroups, showing similar threshold shifts between low and high volume delivered. These results reinforce the current hypothesis, suggesting this cochlear area is more susceptible to damages even with low doses of cisplatin

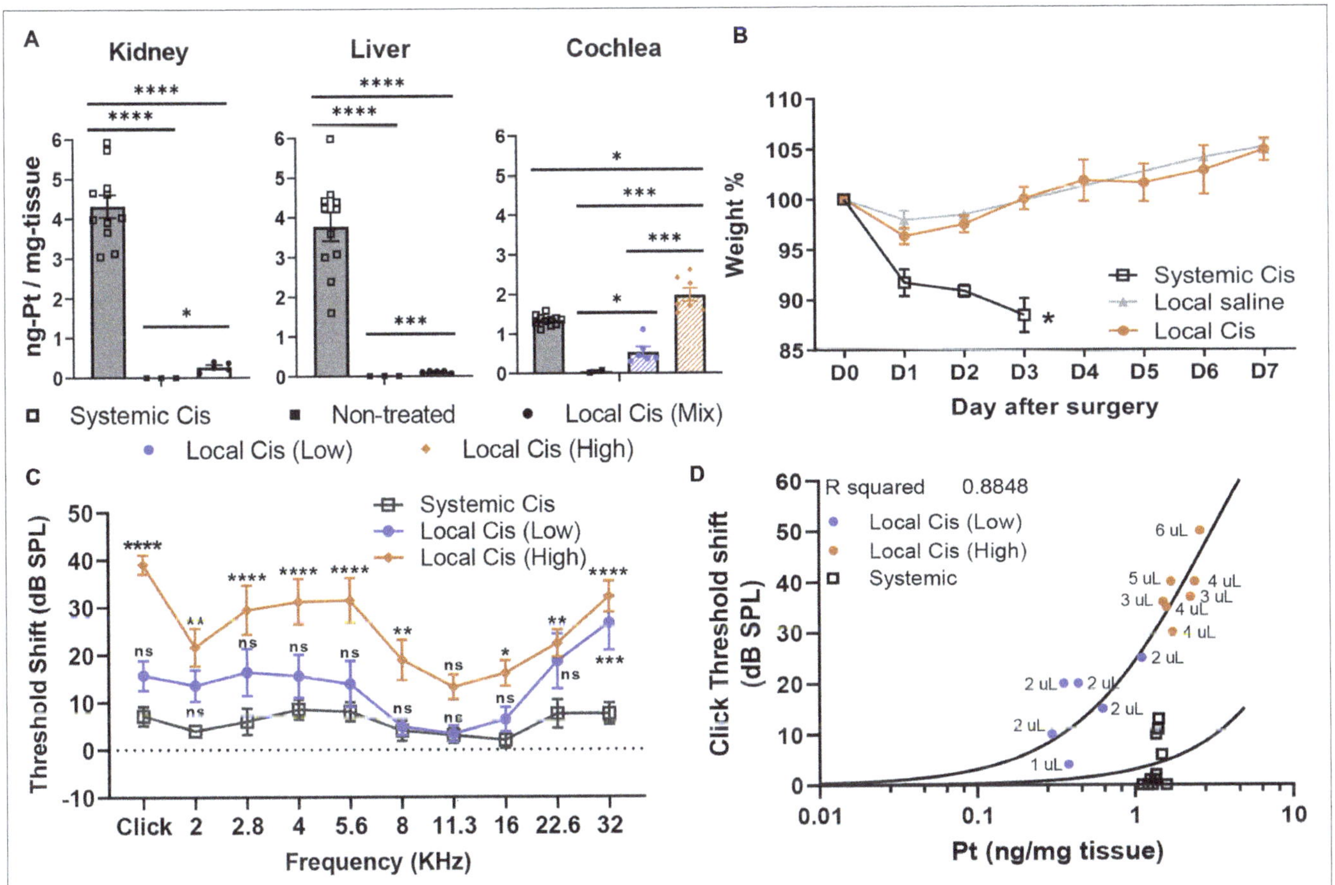

FIGURE 5 | Comparison of systemic *vs.* local cisplatin delivery. **(A)** Comparison of platinum concentration (ng-Pt/mg-tissue) (n = 26) in kidney, liver, and cochlea of control (non-injected), IP (10 mg/kg) cisplatin-injected, and cisplatin (5 mM) trans bulla-delivered mice. Mice delivered with cisplatin retroauricularly were divided into two groups according to volume delivered. Group receiving ≥3 µl of cisplatin solution is denominated as "high" cisplatin (orange), and group receiving <3 µl is "low" cisplatin (blue). **(B)** Posttreatment weight evolution. Systemic delivery of 10 mg/kg cisplatin led to weight loss > 10% and early sacrifice at D3, whereas local delivery only mildly affected weight (<5%) in first 2 days post-intervention. Presurgery weight (D0) was set as 100%. **(C)** Local delivery permanent threshold shift dataset (from **Figure 1**), as calculated from unilateral auditory brainstem response (ABR), in "high" (orange) and "low" (blue) volume cisplatin-treated animals (n = 13), is reused for comparison with hearing threshold shifts of animals receiving systemic cisplatin delivery (10 mg/kg). **(D)** Correlation plot between click-evoked hearing threshold shifts and Pt titer 7 days after local cisplatin delivery [5-mM cisplatin (n = 13)] and 3 days after systemic delivery (IP 10 mg/kg). Associated to each dot, bulla volume value is displayed (microliters). The confidence interval for both statistics was set as 95% (a = 0.05); *p < 0.05; **p < 0.01; ***p < 0.005; ****p < 0.0005.

(Arora et al., 2009). However, the cisplatin local delivery effects were not only limited to high frequencies. Indeed, in the high cisplatin group, significant elevation of the hearing thresholds was observed all along the tonotopic axis (**Figures 1F, 5C**). By comparison, the systemic cisplatin group exhibited evident signs of morbidity without significant effect on hearing and resulted in the premature sacrifice of the animals on day 3 (**Figure 5C**).

Differences in the pattern of HL observed between systemic and local delivery models (**Figure 5C**) could be explained by the cisplatin entry route. The stria vascularis could be the main entry point for systemic cisplatin delivery (through the vasculature) (Karasawa and Steyger, 2015). However, in the local delivery model, the mass spectrometry data showed only residual amounts of Pt in the analyzed organs compared with the systemic approach, including the liver, kidney, or even in the contralateral ear (**Figure 5A**), excluding important cisplatin diffusion through the vasculature. Most likely, cisplatin delivered locally predominantly diffuses from the otic bulla directly into the cochlea through the round window membrane or directly reaching the modiolus through the cochlear bone (Mikulec et al., 2009). Direct diffusion of cisplatin to the modiolus is indeed an interesting hypothesis that could explain the predominant effect on auditory neurons and the relatively milder effect on the sensory epithelium but requires further validation. Nevertheless, the pattern of HL observed on the systemic group (**Figure 5C**), although significantly lower, showed similarities with the local model, with stronger effects on the 22.6–32 kHz frequencies, but also on the tested frequencies between 2.8 and 5.6 kHz.

Although all animals in the 5-mM cisplatin local delivery group were injected following the same exact protocol (see *Materials and methods*), we observed differences in the Pt (cisplatin) retention in the cochlea between animals. Initially, we correlated this apparent high variability with the animal sex. However, we did not observe such sex difference in the Pt cochlear concentration at D3 after the systemic injection (data not shown), excluding a sex-related protection mechanism hypothesis, previously suggested (Park et al., 2019). Nevertheless, we believed that anatomical variations, as previously reported for the human cochlea (Braga et al., 2019), could explain the different cisplatin concentrations observed between animals. Accordingly, we observed a correlation between the tympanic bulla volume capacity (size) and the cochlear Pt concentration (R^2 = 0.7517) (**Figure 1E**) and thus the extent of HL (R^2 = 0.8848) (**Figure 5D**), explaining the observed variability. This intrinsic variability allowed us to recapitulate the effect of low and high cisplatin doses on the hearing system.

Cisplatin concentrations in the cochlea were slightly superior when delivered through the local delivery approach, on the high local group, compared with the systemic route (**Figure 5A**). However, the difference in the HL incidence between groups was rather considerable (**Figure 5C**). However, we must be cautious with the interpretations of these results, as IP injected animals already lost 15% of their weight 72 h after the injection and were immediately sacrificed. The animals in the local delivery groups (low and high volume delivered) were sacrificed 1 week after the injection, at the end of the experimental design. In the systemic group, the observed effect on the hearing thresholds was probably still incomplete due to the early sacrifice time (D3), rendering a direct comparison between both models difficult. Alternatively, these differences could be explained following a different penetration profile of cisplatin in the inner ear when delivered locally or systemically (see above).

Interestingly, following the different cisplatin (Pt) fixation rates depending on the bulla size, we observed a strong correlation (R^2 = 0.8848) between the Pt concentration retained in the cochlea and the hearing threshold shift (click threshold, **Figure 5D**). Hence, from the extent of HL observed, our model allows accurate prediction of the Pt concentration retained in the cochlea. Such a correlation is important and demonstrated that even when low doses of cisplatin are retained in the cochlea, a significant effect on the animal hearing is observed. Similarly, a correlation plot comparison representing HL and Pt could be used to identify new therapeutical targets following local delivery on knockout models. This approach can be implemented to preliminarily evaluate candidate targets, reducing the number of animals deployed for systemic evaluation and therefore reducing the associated morbidity of these studies, in line with the 3R principles.

CONCLUSION

The presented preclinical model of local delivery of cisplatin to the cochlea adequately models the known changes in inner ear morphology and function after the ototoxic insult without inducing relevant morbidity, in line with 3R principles. In numerous countries, animal welfare regulation is not compatible with current systemic cisplatin preclinical models, which generally lead to important loss of weight, morbidity, and mortality before reaching significant ototoxic effects. Due to the unchanged life expectancy of locally treated animals, the long-term effects of cisplatin ototoxicity can now be adequately addressed. Furthermore, local delivery HL–Pt correlation comparison can be used to preliminary evaluate new therapeutic targets, significantly reducing the animals intended for systemic cisplatin evaluation. Taken together, the local delivery model offers many advantages and will, at least in our laboratory, be used to identify genetic targets for drug-based otoprotection and to further evaluate the possibility of gene therapy-based prevention of cisplatin-induced HL in preclinical studies (Waissbluth et al., 2012).

AUTHOR CONTRIBUTIONS

FR, PS, and K-HK conceived the project. GN-S, PS, and FR conceived and planned the experiments. GN-S carried out the experiments and surgeries. GN-S analyzed the data. FR supervised the data curation. GN-S and FR drafted the manuscript and designed the figures. PS finalized the manuscript writing. SL carried out the mass spectrometry analysis. MC worked out the technical details and sample preparation. AT supervised the mass spectrometry analysis. FV contributed to the project design. All authors discussed the results and contributed to the final manuscript.

ACKNOWLEDGMENTS

We would like to thank the Clinical Pathology Service of the University of Geneva for the reagents and materials provided during cochlear decalcification.

REFERENCES

Arora, R., Thakur, J. S., Azad, R. K., Mohindroo, N. K., Sharma, D. R., and Seam, R. K. (2009). Cisplatin-based chemotherapy: add high-frequency audiometry in the regimen. *Indian J. Cancer* 46, 311–317. doi: 10.4103/0019-509x.55551

Basu, A., and Krishnamurthy, S. (2010). Cellular responses to cisplatin-induced DNA damage. *J. Nucleic Acids* 2010:201367.

Braga, J., Samir, C., Risser, L., Dumoncel, J., Descouens, D., Thackeray, J. F., et al. (2019). Cochlear shape reveals that the human organ of hearing is sex-typed from birth. *Sci. Rep.* 9:10889.

Breglio, A. M., Rusheen, A. E., Shide, E. D., Fernandez, K. A., Spielbauer, K. K., McLachlin, K. M., et al. (2017). Cisplatin is retained in the cochlea indefinitely following chemotherapy. *Nat. Commun.* 8:1654.

Dasari, S., and Tchounwou, P. B. (2014). Cisplatin in cancer therapy: molecular mechanisms of action. *Eur. J. Pharmacol.* 740, 364–378. doi: 10.1016/j.ejphar.2014.07.025

DeBacker, J. R., Harrison, R. T., and Bielefeld, E. C. (2020). Cisplatin-induced threshold shift in the CBA/CaJ, C57BL/6J, BALB/cJ mouse models of hearing loss. *Hear. Res.* 387, 107878. doi: 10.1016/j.heares.2019.107878

El Charif, O., Mapes, B., Trendowski, M. R., Wheeler, H. E., Wing, C., Dinh, P. C. Jr., et al. (2019). Clinical and genome-wide analysis of cisplatin-induced tinnitus implicates novel ototoxic mechanisms. *Clin. Cancer Res.* 25, 4104–4116. doi: 10.1158/1078-0432.ccr-18-3179

Fernandez, K., Wafa, T., Fitzgerald, T. S., and Cunningham, L. L. (2019). An optimized, clinically relevant mouse model of cisplatin-induced ototoxicity. *Hear. Res.* 375, 66–74. doi: 10.1016/j.heares.2019.02.006

Karasawa, T., and Steyger, P. S. (2015). An integrated view of cisplatin-induced nephrotoxicity and ototoxicity. *Toxicol. Lett.* 237, 219–227. doi: 10.1016/j.toxlet.2015.06.012

Kujawa, S. G., and Liberman, M. C. (2015). Synaptopathy in the noise-exposed and aging cochlea: primary neural degeneration in acquired sensorineural hearing loss. *Hear. Res.* 330(Pt B), 191–199. doi: 10.1016/j.heares.2015.02.009

Landier, W. (2016). Ototoxicity and cancer therapy. *Cancer* 122, 1647–1658. doi: 10.1002/cncr.29779

Liberman, P. H., Schultz, C., Goffi-Gomez, M. V., and Lopes, L. F. (2013). Speech recognition and frequency of hearing loss in patients treated for cancer in childhood. *Pediatr. Blood Cancer* 60, 1709–1713. doi: 10.1002/pbc.24560

Liu, W., Xu, X., Fan, Z., Sun, G., Han, Y., Zhang, D., et al. (2019). Wnt signaling activates TP53 induced glycolysis and apoptosis regulator and protects against cisplatin-induced spiral ganglion neuron damage in the mouse cochlea. *Antioxid. Redox Signal.* 30, 1389–1410. doi: 10.1089/ars.2017.7288

Mikulec, A. A., Plontke, S. K., Hartsock, J. J., and Salt, A. N. (2009). Entry of substances into perilymph through the bone of the otic capsule after intratympanic applications in guinea pigs: implications for local drug delivery in humans. *Otol. Neurotol.* 30, 131–138. doi: 10.1097/mao.0b013e318191bff8

Miller, R. P., Tadagavadi, R. K., Ramesh, G., and Reeves, W. B. (2010). Mechanisms of cisplatin nephrotoxicity. *Toxins (Basel)* 2, 2490–2518. doi: 10.3390/toxins2112490

Mujica-Mota, M., Waissbluth, S., and Daniel, S. J. (2013). Characteristics of radiation-induced sensorineural hearing loss in head and neck cancer: a systematic review. *Head Neck* 35, 1662–1668. doi: 10.1002/hed.23201

Mulazimoglu, S., Ocak, E., Kaygusuz, G., and Gokcan, M. K. (2017). Retroauricular approach for targeted cochlear therapy experiments in wistar albino rats. *Balkan Med. J.* 34, 200–205. doi: 10.4274/balkanmedj.2016.0226

Murillo-Cuesta, S., Vallecillo, N., Cediel, R., Celaya, A. M., Lassaletta, L., Varela-Nieto, I., et al. (2017). A comparative study of drug delivery methods targeted to the mouse inner ear: bullostomy versus transtympanic injection. *J. Vis. Exp.* 121:54951.

Naples, J. G., Ruckenstein, M. J., Singh, J., Cox, B. C., and Li, D. (2020). Intratympanic diltiazem-chitosan hydrogel as an otoprotectant against cisplatin-induced ototoxicity in a mouse model. *Otol. Neurotol.* 41, 115–122. doi: 10.1097/mao.0000000000002417

Panza, F., Solfrizzi, V., and Logroscino, G. (2015). Age-related hearing impairment-a risk factor and frailty marker for dementia and AD. *Nat. Rev. Neurol.* 11, 166–175. doi: 10.1038/nrneurol.2015.12

Parham, K. (2011). Can intratympanic dexamethasone protect against cisplatin ototoxicity in mice with age-related hearing loss? *Otolaryngol. Head Neck Surg.* 145, 635–640. doi: 10.1177/0194599811409304

Park, H. J., Kim, M. J., Rothenberger, C., Kumar, A., Sampson, E. M., Ding, D., et al. (2019). GSTA4 mediates reduction of cisplatin ototoxicity in female mice. *Nat. Commun.* 10:4150.

Rousset, F., Kokje, V. B. C., Coelho, M. D. C., Mugnier, T., Belissa, E., Gabriel, D., et al. (2019). Poly-lactic acid-based biopolymer formulations are safe for sustained intratympanic dexamethasone delivery. *Otol. Neurotol.* 40, e739–e746.

Rousset, F., Nacher-Soler, G., Coelho, M., Ilmjarv, S., Kokje, V. B. C., Marteyn, A., et al. (2020). Redox activation of excitatory pathways in auditory neurons as mechanism of age-related hearing loss. *Redox Biol.* 30:101434. doi: 10.1016/j.redox.2020.101434

Rutherford, B. R., Brewster, K., Golub, J. S., Kim, A. H., and Roose, S. P. (2018). Sensation and psychiatry: linking age-related hearing loss to late-life depression and cognitive decline. *Am. J. Psychiatry* 175, 215–224. doi: 10.1176/appi.ajp.2017.17040423

Sheth, S., Mukherjea, D., Rybak, L. P., and Ramkumar, V. (2017). Mechanisms of cisplatin-induced ototoxicity and otoprotection. *Front. Cell. Neurosci.* 11:338. doi: 10.3389/fncel.2017.00338

Stevens, S. M., Brown, L. N., Ezell, P. C., and Lang, H. (2015). The mouse round-window approach for ototoxic agent delivery: a rapid and reliable technique for inducing cochlear cell degeneration. *J. Vis. Exp.* 105:53131.

Vorobiev, V., Babic, A., Crowe, L. A., Van De Looij, Y., Lenglet, S., Thomas, A., et al. (2019). Pharmacokinetics and biodistribution study of self-assembled Gd-micelles demonstrating blood-pool contrast enhancement for MRI. *Int. J. Pharm.* 568:118496. doi: 10.1016/j.ijpharm.2019.118496

Waissbluth, S., Pitaro, J., and Daniel, S. J. (2012). Gene therapy for cisplatin-induced ototoxicity: a systematic review of in vitro and experimental animal studies. *Otol. Neurotol.* 33, 302–310. doi: 10.1097/mao.0b013e318248ee66

14

Initiation of Supporting Cell Activation for Hair Cell Regeneration in the Avian Auditory Epithelium: An Explant Culture Model

Mami Matsunaga[1], *Tomoko Kita*[1], *Ryosuke Yamamoto*[1], *Norio Yamamoto*[1], *Takayuki Okano*[1], *Koichi Omori*[1], *Satoko Sakamoto*[2] *and Takayuki Nakagawa*[1]*

[1]*Department of Otolaryngology, Head and Neck Surgery, Graduate School of Medicine, Kyoto University, Kyoto, Japan,*
[2]*Medical Innovation Center, Kyoto University, Kyoto, Japan*

***Correspondence:**
Takayuki Nakagawa
tnakagawa@ent.kuhp.kyoto-u.ac.jp

Sensorineural hearing loss is a common disability often caused by the loss of sensory hair cells in the cochlea. Hair cell (HCs) regeneration has long been the main target for the development of novel therapeutics for sensorineural hearing loss. In the mammalian cochlea, hair cell regeneration is limited, but the auditory epithelia of non-mammalian organisms retain the capacity for hair cell regeneration. In the avian basilar papilla (BP), supporting cells (SCs), which give rise to regenerated hair cells, are usually quiescent. Hair cell loss induces both direct transdifferentiation and mitotic division of supporting cells. Here, we established an explant culture model for hair cell regeneration in chick basilar papillae and validated it for investigating the initial phase of hair cell regeneration. The histological assessment demonstrated hair cell regeneration *via* direct transdifferentiation of supporting cells. Labeling with 5-ethynyl-2′-deoxyuridine (EdU) revealed the occurrence of mitotic division in the supporting cells at specific locations in the basilar papillae, while no EdU labeling was observed in newly generated hair cells. RNA sequencing indicated alterations in known signaling pathways associated with hair cell regeneration, consistent with previous findings. Also, unbiased analyses of RNA sequencing data revealed novel genes and signaling pathways that may be related to the induction of supporting cell activation in the chick basilar papillae. These results indicate the advantages of our explant culture model of the chick basilar papillae for exploring the molecular mechanisms of hair cell regeneration.

Keywords: atoh1, basilar papilla, regeneration, hair cell, supporting cell, transdifferentiation, type 1 interferon

---

Abbreviations: ANOVA, analysis of variance; BMP, bone morphogenetic protein; BP, basilar papilla; CCN, cellular communication network factor; DAMP, damage-associated molecular pattern; DAPI, 4′,6-diamidino-2-phenylindole; DEG, differentially expressed gene; EdU, 5-ethynyl-2′-deoxyuridine; FGF, fibroblast growth factor; GO, gene ontology; HC, hair cell; IFN, interferon; ISH, *in situ* hybridization; JAK, Janus kinase; PBS, phosphate-buffered saline; PRR, pattern recognition receptor; qPCR, quantitative real-time polymerase chain reaction; RNA-seq, RNA sequencing; SC, supporting cell; SFP, superior fibrocartilaginous plate; SM, streptomycin; STAT, signal transducer and activator of transduction; TF, transcriptional factor.

INTRODUCTION

The mammalian cochlea cannot regenerate hair cells (HCs) after birth (Bohne et al., 1976; Hawkins et al., 1976; Oesterle et al., 2008). Recent studies have revealed that supporting cells (SCs) are capable of generating new HCs *in vitro* (White et al., 2006; Oshima et al., 2007; Sinkkonen et al., 2011). Furthermore, neonatal mammalian cochlear SCs were found to be capable of HC regeneration through direct transdifferentiation and mitotic division under certain conditions (Cox et al., 2014), similar to the avian basilar papilla (BP) SCs. Direct transdifferentiation of SCs can be induced by genetic or pharmacological inhibition of Notch signaling (Yamamoto et al., 2006; Doetzlhofer et al., 2009) or by ectopic expression of Atoh1 (Zheng and Gao, 2003; Kelly et al., 2012; Liu et al., 2012). However, studies on adult animals have shown only limited recovery of hearing ability (Mizutari et al., 2013; Tona et al., 2014). More recently, manipulation of MYC and NOTCH induced HC regeneration *via* SC proliferation in the adult mice (Shu et al., 2019), and *Hes1* modulation in adult guinea pigs resulted in HC restoration (Du et al., 2018). In contrast to mammals, the regenerative capacity of avian BPs is robust and capable of restoring cellular patterning and function (Saunders and Salvi, 2008; Saunders, 2010). Moreover, the potential for HC regeneration is present in the BP throughout the life of the animal, but in an undamaged animal, no spontaneous replacement of HCs occurs in the BP. Previously, analyses of transcriptomic profiles during BP development focused on major signaling pathways, including Notch (Daudet and Lewis, 2005; Daudet et al., 2007; Thiede et al., 2014; Petrovic et al., 2014), fibroblast growth factor (FGF; Bermingham-McDonogh et al., 2001; Jacques et al., 2012a), and Wnt signaling (Sienknecht and Fekete, 2008; Munnamalai et al., 2017). However, there is limited information regarding the molecular pathways and their interactions during HC regeneration in chick BPs compared to that in the zebrafish (Kniss et al., 2016; Denans et al., 2019). More recently, a road map of molecular events during the development of mouse cochlear sensory epithelia has been reported using single-cell ribonucleic acid (RNA) sequencing (RNA-seq; Kolla et al., 2020). These findings provide valuable information for the development of novel strategies for the promotion of HC regeneration in adult mammalian cochleae.

In the avian BP, no HC replacement by SCs has been observed under homeostatic conditions. Once HC loss is induced, the regenerative process is initiated immediately. There are two modes for HC regeneration in the avian BP: direct transdifferentiation of SCs and division of SCs, followed by differentiation into HCs. The former is the predominant process for HC regeneration (Stone and Cotanche, 2007) and can also be induced in adult mammalian cochleae, although with limited capacity (Hori et al., 2007; Mizutari et al., 2013; Tona et al., 2014). On the other hand, in the lateral line of the zebrafish, the primary route for HC regeneration is the mitotic regeneration of SCs (Kniss et al., 2016; Denans et al., 2019). Hence, understanding the precise mechanisms for HC regeneration in chick BPs, especially direct transdifferentiation of SCs, may contribute to a better understanding of the molecular and cellular pathways involved in the regenerative potential of mammalian HCs.

Our ultimate goal is to explore novel strategies for inducing SC activation for HC regeneration in mammalian cochleae. Therefore, we focused on the signals that trigger SC activation in the initial phase of HC regeneration in chick BPs by using an explant culture model for HC regeneration after ototoxic insult. Explant culture systems of chick BPs have been employed for decades to figure out mechanisms for HC regeneration (Oesterle et al., 1993; Stone et al., 1996; Warchol and Corwin, 1996). We examined the temporal and spatial characteristics of the cellular events using our explant culture model. Based on the time course of cellular events in cultured BPs, we defined specific time points for sampling and performed bulk RNA-seq to characterize the initial phase of HC regeneration.

MATERIALS AND METHODS

Animals

Post-hatched 1-day-old male Momiji (*Gallus domesticus*) chicks were purchased from Goto Furan-Jo (Gifu, Japan) and placed in the experimental room, which was maintained at a temperature of approximately 23°C, in the box in which they were transported, less than 3 h after delivery. All animal procedures were performed following the National Institutes of Health (NIH; Bethesda, MD, USA) Guide for the Care and Use of Laboratory Animals (NIH Publications No. 8023, revised 1978) and were approved by the Animal Research Committee of Kyoto University Graduate School of Medicine (Med Kyo 20133).

BP Explant Culture

The BP explant culture was performed based on previous studies (Stone et al., 1996; Shang et al., 2010; Wan et al., 2020). The middle ear cavity was opened, followed by the extirpation of the cochlear duct. Cochlear ducts were placed in ice-cold sterile medium 199 (catalog #11150059, Thermo Fisher Scientific, Waltham, MA, USA). The tegmentum vasculosum was carefully removed from the cochlear duct. The remaining tissue containing the BP was cultured in a free-floating manner (submerged in the medium) in 500 μl Dulbecco's modified Eagle's medium with 4.5 g/l glucose (catalog #08459-35, Nacalai Tesque, Kyoto, Japan) supplemented with 1% fetal bovine serum (catalog #12389802, Thermo Fisher Scientific, Waltham, MA, USA) in 48-well plates (Iwaki Co. Limited, Tokyo, Japan). Culture media were changed every other day. The following antibiotics (Sigma–Aldrich, St. Louis, MO, USA) were also added to culture media: penicillin only, or penicillin/streptomycin (SM; 200 penicillin units per ml and 78 μM streptomycin, catalog #P4333). At the end of SM exposure, SM was washed out by changing the medium twice. For cell proliferation assay, BP explants were treated with 10 μM EdU during the whole culture duration (catalog #C10340, Thermo Fisher Scientific, Waltham, MA, USA). For pharmacological inhibition of the Janus kinase (JAK)/signal transducer and activator of transduction (STAT) signaling pathway, 10 μM ruxolitinib phosphate (catalog #CS-0326, Chem Scene LLC, Monmouth Junction, NJ, USA) was added to the media. The concentration of ruxolitinib phosphate was determined according to a previous publication (Febvre-James et al., 2018).

Immunohistochemistry

Immunofluorescence analyses were performed on whole-mount preparations or frozen sections of the chick cochlea duct. After fixation with 4% paraformaldehyde in phosphate-buffered saline (PBS) for 15 min at room temperature, dehydration was performed using 15% sucrose with 0.2 mM ethylenediaminetetraacetic acid in PBS overnight followed by 30% sucrose with 0.2 mM ethylenediaminetetraacetic acid at 4°C for the frozen section, as previously described (Bermingham-McDonogh et al., 2001). Cryostat-cut sections (10 μm in thickness) of Optimal Cutting Temperature (catalog #4583, OCT, Sakura Finetek Japan, Co., Ltd., Tokyo, Japan)-embedded frozen samples were mounted directly onto MAS-coated slides (catalog #SMAS-01, Matsunami Glass Inc., Osaka, Japan). The ensemble of sections collected from three to four BPs was distributed to almost 20 slides (7–9 sections per slide) for each experiment. Each slide contained a reliable representation of the entire length of the BP in a serial manner, which provided uniformity of treatment for cross-sections throughout the cochlear length.

Both the whole mount and section samples were incubated in blocking solution (1% bovine serum albumin and 5% normal goat serum in PBS) for 30 min at room temperature. Samples were incubated with primary antibodies in a blocking solution containing 0.2% Triton X-100 (Nacalai Tesque) overnight at 4°C, followed by incubation with the corresponding secondary antibodies for 1 h at room temperature. Mouse anti-myosin VIIa (2 μg/ml; catalog #138-1, Developmental Studies Hybridoma Bank, IA, USA) and rabbit anti-Sox2 (1:500; catalog #AB5603, Sigma–Aldrich, St. Louis, MO, USA) were the primary antibodies used, and Alexa Fluor 488-, 546-, or 647-conjugated anti-mouse or anti-rabbit IgG antibodies (Thermo Fisher Scientific, Waltham, MA, USA) were the secondary antibodies used. 4′,6-diamidino-2-phenylindole (DAPI, catalog #D1306, Thermo Fisher Scientific, Waltham, MA, USA) was used for nuclear counterstaining. After several washes with PBS, samples were mounted using Fluoromount-G (catalog #00-4958-02, Southern Biotech, Birmingham, AL, USA).

EdU staining was performed according to the Click-iT imaging kit instructions (catalog #C10340, Thermo Fisher Scientific, Waltham, MA, USA) after staining for myosin VIIa and Sox2. As regards the whole-mount preparation for EdU staining, the tectorial membrane was removed by treatment with 100 μg/ml subtilisin (catalog #P8038, Sigma–Aldrich, St. Louis, MO, USA) for 10 min at room temperature to expose the sensory epithelia before fixation. Counterstaining with DAPI was performed as the last step of EdU staining.

All fluorescence images were obtained using a TCS-SPE confocal microscope (equipped with 40×/1.15 objective, Leica Microsystems, Wetzlar, Germany). For the whole mount samples, the area around 40% of the distal end of each of the BP samples was used for quantitative analyses. Optical sections in the *xy*-field ("*z*-sections") were imaged and recorded at 4-μm intervals, with the span adjusted to include the HC and SC layers in the *xy*-field of view. The total BP length between the proximal portion and the distal portion was calculated using ImageJ software (NIH)[1].

In situ Hybridization

Frozen section samples for *in situ* hybridization (ISH) were prepared similarly to those for immunohistochemistry, with the following amendments: duration of fixation (4°C for 3–4 h), higher ethylenediaminetetraacetic acid concentration (333 mM) in 30% sucrose, and thicker sections (14 μm in thickness). All ISH experiments were performed using the RNAscope 2.5 HD Duplex Detection Kit (catalog #322430, Advanced Cell Diagnostics Inc., Hayward, CA, USA) on frozen section samples according to the manufacturer's instructions. On each individual section, five target mRNAs were examined: atonal homologl (*Atoh1*; #574081-C2 for ggATOH1, ACD), secreted frizzled-related protein 2 (*Sfrp2*; #837131-C2 for ggSFRP2), cysteine-rich angiogenic inducer 61 (*Cyr61*; #837121-C2 for ggCYR61), ribonucleotide reductase regulatory subunit M2 (*Rrm2*; #838951-C2 for ggRRM2), and interferon-alpha inducible protein 6 (*Ifi6*; #847081-C2 for ggIFI6). Both positive and negative control probes [#453961-C2 for ggUBC (ubiquitin C) or No.320751, ACD] were also labeled with alkaline phosphatase and red substrates for control purposes. The GenBank accession numbers and probe regions for each target probe are as follows: ggATOH1 (GenBank, XM_004941130.3; probe region, 107–1545), ggSFRP2 (GenBank NM_204773.1; probe region, 64–1019), ggCYR61 (GenBank NM_001031563.1; probe region, 498–1666), ggRRM2 (GenBank XM_001231544.5; probe region, 393–1843), and ggIFI6 (GenBank NM_001001296.5; probe region, 2–476). DAPI was used to stain the cell nuclei, and the slides were imaged using a BX50 microscope (Olympus, Tokyo, Japan) to acquire 20× and 40× bright-field and fluorescence images with DAPI filter from more than three BP samples for each time point.

Quantitative Real-Time Polymerase Chain Reaction

Total RNA for each sample was extracted pooled 10 BPs using the RNeasy Plus Micro kit (catalog # 74004, QIAGEN, Venlo, Netherlands) according to the manufacturer's protocol. DNase I treatment was performed using spin columns. RNA was reverse-transcribed using the SuperScript III First-Strand Synthesis System (catalog #N8080234, Thermo Fisher Scientific, Waltham, MA, USA). Quantitative real-time polymerase chain reaction (qPCR) was performed using a StepOnePlus Real-Time PCR system (Thermo Fisher Scientific, Waltham, MA, USA). cDNA was amplified using the Power SYBR Green PCR Master Mix (catalog #4367659, Thermo Fisher Scientific, Waltham, MA, USA). Target gene expression was normalized to hypoxanthine

[1]https://imagej.nih.gov/ij/

phosphoribosyltransferase 1 (*Hprt1*, Hassanpour et al., 2019). cDNA from the brain tissue of post-hatched 1-day-old chickens was used to generate standard curves for each gene. Relative quantification was performed using Real-Time PCR System Software v2.0, with the $2^{-\Delta\Delta CT}$ method (Thermo Fisher Scientific, Waltham, MA, USA). The following primers were used:

Hprt1 forward, 5′-GCACTATGACTCTACCGACTATTGC-3′
Hprt1 reverse, 5′-CAGTTCTGGGTTGATGAGGTT-3′
Atoh1 forward, 5′-AACAACGACAAGAAGCTCTCCAA-3′
Atoh1 reverse, 5′-GCGAGGGCGCTGATGTAG-3′
Ifi6 forward, 5′-GCGCGATGTTTCTATGGCTT-3′
Ifi6 reverse, 5′-TTGTCCCCAATCCAGCGTAT-3′

RNA Sequencing

At the end of the culture period, the surrounding tissues, such as the tectorial membrane, were removed from the sensory epithelium with thermolysin treatment (500 μg/ml in medium 199, catalog #T7902, Sigma–Aldrich, St. Louis, MO, USA) at 37°C for 30 min, followed by transfer of BPs to media supplemented with 5% fetal bovine serum. Over 1.72 μg (OD260/280, 0.82–1.70 in OD230/280) of total RNA was collected from 50 cultured BPs for each experimental group.

RNA-seq analysis was performed using the Illumina NovaSeq6000, PE150 by Novogene (Tianjin, China). Approximately 6 Gb of row read sequence data were obtained for each sample, and FASTQ files were analyzed using the following procedure: After exclusion of rRNA sequences using Bowtie2 (ver. 2.1.0; Langmead and Salzberg, 2012), data were mapped to the reference genome (GRCg6a/galgal6) using the STAR program with ENCODE options (ver. 2.7.1a; Dobin et al., 2013). Gene expression values [in transcripts per million (TPM)] were then calculated using RSEM (ver. 1.3.0; Li and Dewey, 2011). Differentially expressed genes (DEGs) were determined with DEseq2 (ver. 1.8.2; Love et al., 2014) and the weighted average difference (WAD) method (Kadota et al., 2008). We employed DEseq2 for normalization for raw read counts and determination threshold for WAD analyses. Initially, we listed genes that fulfilled the following characteristics: $p < 0.05$, fold change for normalized read counts >1.3 or <1/1.3, raw read counts ≥7, and TPM ≥1 in either of the compared conditions with DEseq2. Then we set thresholds for WAD analyses to cover the listed genes (**Supplementary Table 1**). Obtained DEG were clustered with k-means clustering ($k = 11$), followed by translation to human homologous genes (NCBI homoloGene database) and gene ontology (GO)/pathway analysis with Metascape[2] (date of analysis: 2020/8/27; Tripathi et al., 2015). For k-means clustering, we used z-score translated raw-read counts, and the parameter k was determined to reduce clusters with redundant expression profiles, starting from $k = 12$. Transcription factors (TFs) or co-factors were determined by the following GO terms: GO: 0005634 nucleus; GO: 0045892 negative regulation of transcription, DNA-templated; GO: 0045944 positive regulation of transcription from RNA polymerase II promoter' GO: 0044212 transcription regulatory region DNA binding; and GO: 0006351 transcriptions, DNA-templated.

Statistical Analysis

One-way analysis of variance (ANOVA) with a Tukey's *post hoc* test or Student's t-test was used to compare the counts and qPCR data between experimental groups with XLSTAT Basic (version; 2020.2.2.65342, Addinsoft Inc., New York, NY, USA). Data are expressed as mean ± standard deviation. Differences with $p < 0.05$ were considered statistically significant.

RESULTS

Time Course of HC Regeneration in the BP Explants

First, we examined the time course of HC regeneration in explant cultures of the post-hatched 1-day-old chick BP after ototoxic insult with SM. BP explants were exposed to SM for 48 h to induce HC damage, according to previous reports (Shang et al., 2010; Lewis et al., 2012, 2018). BP explants were then maintained in culture media without SM for a maximum of 144 h (**Figure 1A**). Samples were collected every 48 h [SM0 (before SM exposure), SM48, post-SM48, post-SM96, and post-SM144; $n = 3–5$] for histological analyses in the surface preparation (**Figure 1A**). HCs were identified by immunostaining for myosin VIIa and nuclear staining with DAPI. The number of HCs was manually counted in the two layers in the area 40% from the distal end of the BPs (**Figures 1B–G′**). Virtually no myosin VIIa-positive cells were observed in SM48 samples (**Figures 1D,D′**), indicating that 48 h exposure to SM caused a total loss of HCs in this region. Newly generated HCs were observed in post-SM48 samples that were incubated for an additional 48 h after SM treatment (**Figures 1E,E′**). Robust HCs were found in post-SM144 samples (**Figures 1G,G′**). Quantitative assessments revealed a significant loss of HCs in SM48 samples ($p < 0.0001$, one-way ANOVA with a Tukey's *post hoc* test) compared with that in SM0 samples as well as a significant increase in HC numbers in post-SM96 ($p = 0.035$, one-way ANOVA with a Tukey's *post hoc* test) and post-SM144 samples ($p = 0.004$, one-way ANOVA with a Tukey's *post hoc* test) compared to that in SM48 samples (**Figure 1H**). These findings demonstrate that HC regeneration occurred in explant cultures of post-hatched 1-day old chick BPs and that newly generated HCs already appeared 48 h after SM exposure (post SM48).

Time Points for Total HC Loss and the Emergence of Converting HCs

Next, we aimed to clarify the exact time points at which total HC loss occurred and at which newly generated HCs appeared in chick BP explant cultures. We prepared consecutive frozen sections of BP cultures that were collected at nine time-points ($n = 3$ for each) from SM0 to post-SM48 (**Figure 1I**), in which newly generated HCs were identified in whole mounts

[2]https://metascape.org/

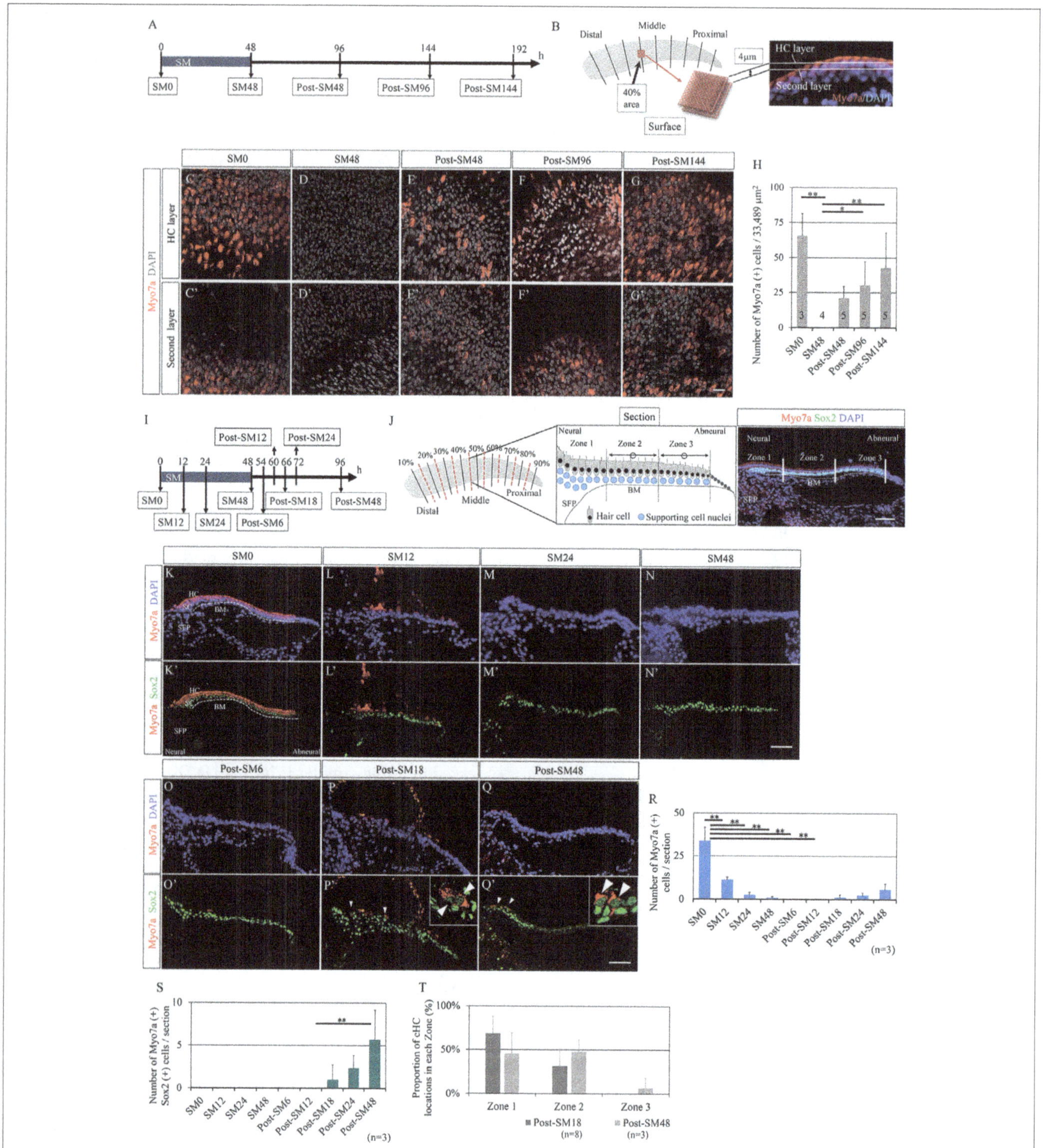

FIGURE 1 | Time course of hair cell regeneration in the basilar papilla explants. **(A)** Diagram of exposure to streptomycin (SM) and sampling time points. **(B)** Schematic drawing showing the observation area and two layers for counting hair cells (HCs) that are labeled with myosin VIIa (Myo7a) and nuclear staining with 4′,6-diamidino-2-phenylindole (DAPI). **(C–G′)** Representative images of immunostaining for Myo7a (red) and nuclear staining with DAPI (gray) in two layers at each sampling time point. In SM48 samples **(D,D′)**, virtually no HCs were observed, and newly generated HCs appeared from post-SM48 **(E,E′)**. Scale bar represents 20 μm. **(H)** Myo7a-positive cells as sums of two layers in the 40% area (33,489 μm²). Differences in the numbers of Myo7a-positive cells between SM0 and SM48, and between SM48 and post-SM96 or post-SM144 were statistically significant [*$p < 0.05$, **$p < 0.01$, analysis of variance (ANOVA) with a Tukey's *post hoc* test]. Bars represent standard deviations. **(I)** Diagram for sampling for the detailed analysis of HC loss and emerging new HCs. **(J)** Schematic drawing showing the preparation of serial frozen sections (red dotted lines). Three zones in a cross-section are shown in a schematic drawing as is a cross-sectional image stained for

(*Continued*)

FIGURE 1 | Continued
Myo7a, Sox2, and DAPI. From each sample, seven to eight sections were used for staining and quantification. The most neural zone adjacent to the superior fibrocartilaginous plate (SFP) is named Zone 1. The remaining sensory epithelia on the basilar membrane (BM) are divided equally into Zone 2 (neural side) and Zone 3 (abneural side). **(K′–Q′)** Representative images of immunostaining for Myo7a (red) and Sox2 (green) or nuclear staining with DAPI (blue). Arrowheads indicate converting HCs that are co-stained with Myo7a and Sox2. Dotted lines indicate the location of the basilar membrane (BM). The scale bar represents 50 μm. **(R)** Numbers of Myo7a-positive cells per section at each time point (**$p < 0.01$, ANOVA with a Tukey's *post hoc* test). **(S)** Numbers of Myo7a and Sox2 co-stained cells per section at each time point (**$p < 0.01$, ANOVA with a Tukey's *post hoc* test). **(T)** Proportions of converting hair cell locations in post-SM18 and post-SM48 samples. Bars in **(R–T)** represent standard deviations.

(**Figures 1E,E′**). From each BP culture, eight sections (0–20% from the distal end, 20–30%, 30–40%, 40–50%, 50–60%, 60–70%, 70–80%, 80%-the proximal end) were generated for histological analyses (**Figure 1J**). In a cross-section of BPs, we divided the sensory epithelium into three regions to validate the location of regenerated HCs (**Figure 1J**). In the current study, we defined myosin VIIa$^+$ and Sox2$^+$ double-positive cells as converting HCs. Immunostaining for myosin VIIa and Sox2 demonstrated dynamic changes in cell populations of BP explants (**Figures 1K–Q′**). Initially, myosin VIIa$^+$ cells disappeared at SM24 (**Figures 1M,M′**) myosin VIIa$^+$ cells, co-expressing Sox2 in their nuclei, reappeared from post-SM18 (**Figures 1P,P′**). Cells co-expressing myosin VIIa and Sox2 had a long and narrow shape (**Figures 1P′,Q′**), consistent with the morphological characteristics of converting HCs (Stone and Cotanche, 2007; Daudet et al., 2009). A quantitative assessment of myosin VIIa$^+$ cells demonstrated a precise time course of HC loss and regeneration (**Figure 1R**). A significant loss of HCs was observed at SM12 ($p < 0.0001$, one-way ANOVA with a Tukey's *post hoc* test) compared to that at SM0. Virtually no HCs existed in BPs from SM24 to post-SM12 (**Figure 1R**). The number of converting HCs that expressed both myosin VIIa and Sox2 increased over time (**Figure 1S**).

We also examined the location of the converting HCs in BPs. Zone 1 is the most neural-sided portion of BPs, namely the neural edge, which is adjacent to the superior fibrocartilaginous plate (SFP; **Figure 1J**). SFP is a cartilaginous tissue that is located over the cochlear ganglion and connects with the basilar membrane. The nerve fibers between the cochlear ganglion neurons and HCs run through the SFP. The sensory epithelium on the basilar membrane was divided into two equal parts: Zone 2 (neural side) and Zone 3 (abneural side; **Figure 1J**). In post-SM18 samples, converting HCs were observed only in Zones 1 and 2 (**Figure 1T**). In post-SM48, converting HCs were also found in Zone 3, but they were predominantly located in Zone 1 or 2 (**Figure 1T**). Nearly total HC loss was observed at SM24, and converting HCs first appeared in the neural half of BPs in post-SM18 samples.

Cell Division of SCs in BP Explants After HC Loss

Mitotic division of SCs could also be involved in the restoration of BPs, although the predominant mode of HC regeneration in chick BPs is reported to be direct transdifferentiation of SCs (Stone and Cotanche, 2007; Shang et al., 2010). Scheibinger et al. (2018) proposed three different behaviors of SCs during the process of HC regeneration in chick utricles: asymmetric division, direct transdifferentiation, and symmetric division for the replenishment of SCs. To evaluate the SC division and its contribution to HC regeneration in our culture model, we performed EdU labeling. EdU was added to the culture media throughout the culture period and sample collection was performed at SM24, SM48, and post-SM144 ($n = 3–7$; **Figure 2A**). In SM24 samples, EdU-positive cells were found in the neural edges of BPs (**Figures 2B,B′**). The distribution of EdU-positive cells in SM24 samples was sporadic. In SM48 samples, EdU-positive cells were distributed in the neural edges of BPs (**Figures 2C,C′**). Besides, EdU-labeled cells were also found in the SFP (**Figures 2C,C′**). The distribution of EdU-positive cells was not sporadic at SM48. Some EdU-positive cells were adjacent to other EdU-positive cells (**Figures 2C,C′**). In post-SM144 samples also, EdU labeling was found in the neural edges of BPs (**Figures 2D,D′**). Myosin VIIa-positive cells were observed in the neural edge of BPs of post-SM144 samples, but these cells did not exhibit EdU labeling (**Figures 2D,D′**). In both Zones 2 and 3, several myosin VIIa-positive cells were also identified, while no EdU labeling was found in myosin VIIa-positive cells (**Figures 2E,F**). Quantitative assessments of EdU-positive cells in BP cross-sections were performed according to the three separate zones of BPs (**Figure 1J**). All EdU-positive cells were located in Zone 1, the neural edge of BPs, in SM24, SM48, and post-SM144 samples (**Figure 2G**). Time-dependent increases in the number of EdU-positive cells were found ($p = 0.001$ by one-way ANOVA). Differences in the number of EdU-positive cells were statistically significant between SM24 and post-SM144 ($p = 0.001$ by Tukey's *post hoc* test) and between SM48 and post-SM144 ($p = 0.028$ by Tukey's *post hoc* test).

To confirm the absence of myosin VIIa-positive cells labeled with EdU, we also assessed for EdU-positive cells in the surface preparation of post-SM144 samples (**Figures 2H–I″**). In the area, 40% from the distal end of the BPs of post-SM144 samples, 26.5 ± 17.8 myosin VIIa-expressing cells, and 17.25 ± 6.2 EdU-positive cells were observed, while EdU incorporation was not observed in any myosin VIIa-expressing cells in the surface preparation (**Figure 2J**). These findings strongly suggest that myosin VIIa-positive cells in post-SM144 samples were generated through direct transdifferentiation of SCs. Altogether, SC division in the neural edge of BPs was initiated immediately after total HC loss, which may contribute to the replenishment of SCs, not the increase in myosin VIIa-positive cells.

Clustering DEGs in BPs in the Early Phase of HC Regeneration

To examine possible alterations in the expression levels of genes, we performed bulk RNA-seq of BP explants. Based on the time course of HC loss and the emergence of converting HCs in histological assessments, we set four time-points for sampling: SM0 (before SM exposure), SM24 (24-h exposure to SM, the time point for total HC loss), SM48 (48-h exposure to

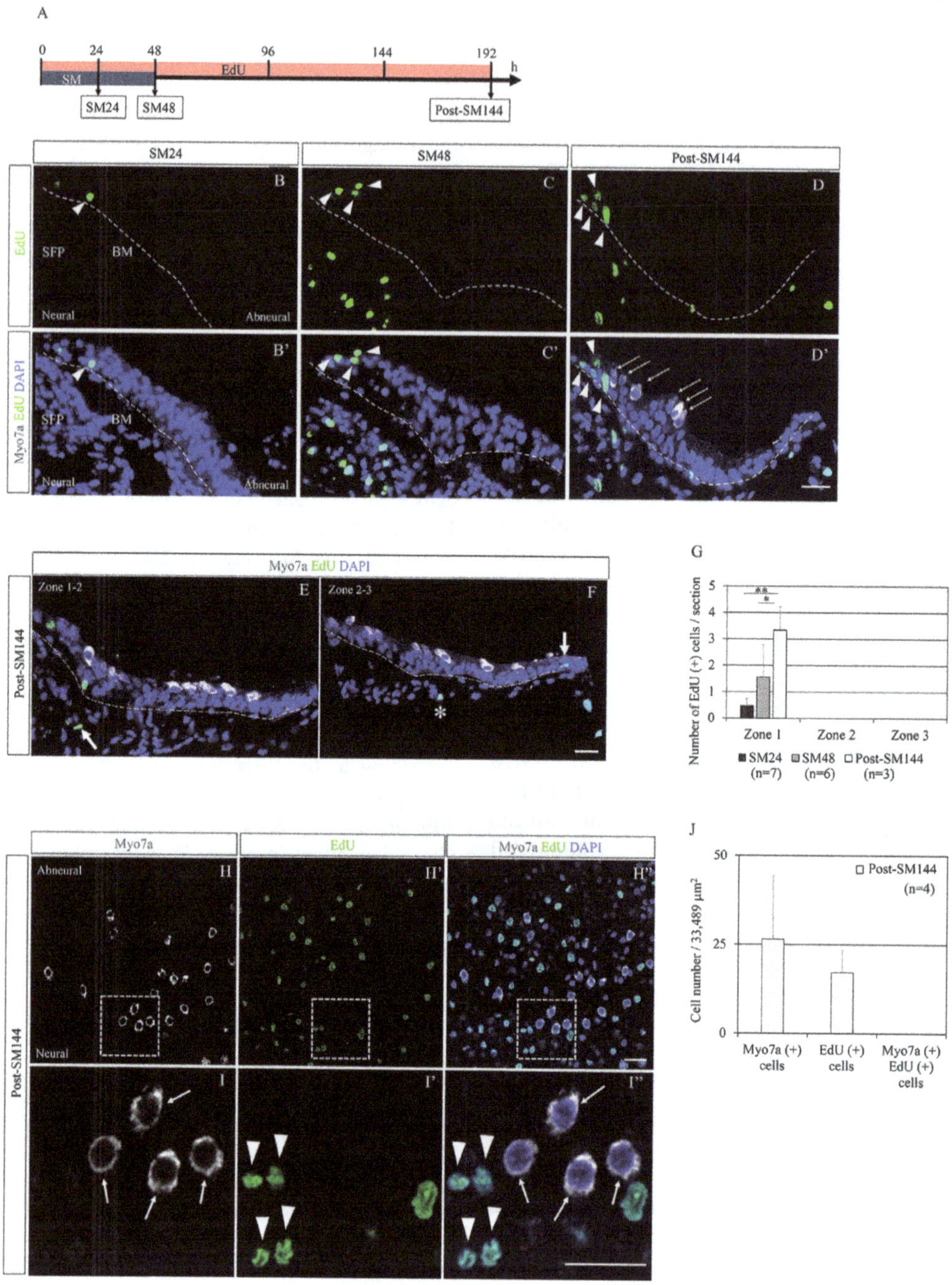

FIGURE 2 | Cell division of supporting cells in basilar papilla (BP) explants after hair cell (HC) loss and its contribution to HC regeneration. **(A)** Diagram of EdU labeling assay. **(B–D′)** Representative images of EdU labeling (green; arrowheads) in cross-sections of SM24, SM48, and post-SM144 samples. Nuclear staining with 4′,6-diamidino-2-phenylindole (DAPI) is shown as blue staining, and immunostaining for myosin VIIa (Myo7a; arrows) is shown as gray. Dotted lines indicate the location of the basilar membrane. Scale bar represents 20 μm. **(E,F)** Representative images of Myo7a-positive cells in Zones 2 and 3 in cross-sections of post-SM144 samples. Nuclear staining with DAPI is shown as blue staining, and immunostaining for Myo7a is shown as gray. Dotted lines indicate the location of the basilar membrane (BM). Scale bar represents 20 μm. An arrow in **(E)** indicates EdU labeling in the superior fibrocartilaginous plate (SFP). An arrow in **(F)** indicates EdU labeling in a hyaline cell, and an asterisk indicates EdU labeling a mesenchymal cell underneath the BM. Scale bar represents 20 μm. **(G)** The number of EdU-positive cells per section in Zones 1–3 in SM24, SM48, and post-SM144 samples. All EdU-labeled cells were found in Zone 1. Differences in the number of EdU-positive cells were statistically significant between SM24 and post-SM144 (**$p = 0.001$ by Tukey's *post hoc* test) and between SM48 and post-SM144 (*$p = 0.028$ by Tukey's *post hoc* test). Bars represent standard deviations. **(H–I″)** Representative images of EdU labeling in post-SM144 samples in surface preparation. Upper panels **(H–H″)** are low-magnification views, and lower panels **(I–I″)** show high-magnification views of the area within the dotted squares in the upper panels. Arrowheads indicate EdU labeling, and arrows indicate Myo7a-expressing cells. Scale bars represent 20 μm. **(J)** The number of Myo7a-positive cells, EdU-positive cells, or Myo7a and EdU double-positive cells in the area 40% from the distal end of the BPs of post-SM144 samples. Bars represent standard deviations.

SM, the endpoint of SM exposure), and post-SM6 (6 h after SM treatment, 12 h before the emergence of converting HCs; $n = 50$ for each time point; **Figure 3A**). We found a total of 19, 238 expressed genes in these four groups.

Among the 19,238 genes expressed in BPs, 1,219 genes were identified as DEGs ($p < 0.05$, fold change ≥ 1.3 or $\leq 1/1.3$, raw read counts ≥ 7, and TPM ≥ 1 in either of the compared conditions for DEseq2 followed by WAD). A remarkable number of DEGs were found between SM0 and SM24 (227 downregulated and 208 upregulated). Further changes were observed between SM24 and SM48 (83 downregulated and 397 upregulated), and between SM48 and post-SM6 (136 downregulated and 24 upregulated; **Figure 3B**). These findings indicate that dynamic changes occurred during and immediately after HC loss.

These 1,219 DEGs were divided into 11 clusters with K-means clustering (**Figure 3C**, **Supplementary Table 2**). Clusters 4, 6, and 9 included DEGs that were downregulated during the experimental time course (**Figure 3C**). Clusters 3 and 7 included upregulated DEGs from SM24, and Clusters 8, 10, and 11 included upregulated genes from SM48 (**Figure 3C**). Cluster 1 included DEGs showing temporal downregulation at SM48, Cluster 2 included DEGs showing temporal downregulation at SM24, and Cluster 5 included DEGs showing temporal upregulation at SM48 (**Figure 3C**). The human homologs of our DEGs (**Figure 3D**) were used to perform GO enrichment analysis using Metascape (**Figure 3E**). In Cluster 4, the following categories were enriched: "sensory perception of sound," "sensory organ development," and "chemical synaptic transmission." Cluster 7 was characterized by "NABA_CORE_MATRISOME," "extracellular structure organization," "response to growth factor," and "regulation of cell adhesion." Clusters 2, 8, and 11 exhibited a similar trend to Cluster 7. Cluster 3 was characterized by "cell division," "Aurora B pathway," and "positive regulation of cell cycle." These findings indicate that DEGs associated with the structure and function of the inner ear, especially those associated with HCs, were downregulated after SM treatment, indicating that such changes may reflect the degeneration of HCs. However, DEGs associated with tissue reorganization and cell proliferation were upregulated immediately after HC loss.

Among the 1, 219 DEGs, we identified 55 TFs and 34 TF co-factors according to GO terms (**Figure 3C**). TFs associated with HC differentiation was found in Cluster 9 (BARHL1), Cluster 4 (POU4F3, LHX3, GFI1), and Cluster 7 (ATOH1). Except for ATOH1, TFs associated with HC differentiation were downregulated, which may be related to the absence of HCs in SM24, SM48, and post-SM6 samples. Also, RNA-seq sampling was performed during the early phase of HC regeneration, during which converting HCs in BPs are still in the initial stage of differentiation. Therefore, HC differentiation genes may not have been upregulated during our observation period.

Alterations in Known Signaling Pathways in the Initial Phase of HC Regeneration

We attempted to illustrate trends of alterations in transcripts of known signaling pathways—Notch, FGF, Wnt, bone morphogenetic protein (BMP)/transforming growth factor-beta (TGFb), vascular endothelial growth factor (VEGF), and Yap—among the 1, 219 DEGs identified ($p < 0.05$, fold change ≥ 1.3 or $\leq 1/1.3$, raw read counts ≥ 7, and TPM ≥ 1 in either of the compared conditions for DEseq2 followed by WAD). The differentially expressed levels, compared to SM0 samples, are shown in **Figures 4A,L–P**. Among Notch signaling-associated genes, *Jag1, Dll1, Dll4, Atoh1, Hes6, Hes5, Heyl,* and *Lfng* tended to be upregulated (**Figure 4A**), consistent with previous observations of HC formation in developing chick BPs (Petrovic et al., 2014) and HC regeneration in mature chick BPs (Daudet et al., 2009). Among these genes, *Atoh1* is a fundamental component for the induction of HC formation or regeneration (Lewis et al., 2012; Petrovic et al., 2014). To determine the timing and levels of *Atoh1* upregulation, we examined alterations in *Atoh1* mRNA expression by qPCR (**Figure 4B**). For this purpose, BP samples that were exposed to SM for 12 h were prepared, in addition to the SM0, SM24, and SM48 samples ($n = 6$ for each). In SM12 samples, no significant elevation of *Atoh1* mRNA levels was found compared to SM0 samples ($p = 0.9999$, one-way ANOVA with a Tukey's *post hoc* test). SM24 and SM48 samples exhibited significant elevation compared to the SM0 or SM12 samples (fold change: 13.79 ± 4.24, $p = 0.0005$ for SM0 vs. SM24, fold change: 7.00 ± 2.15, $p = 0.002$ for SM12 vs. SM24, fold change: 18.30 ± 8.52, $p < 0$, 0001 for SM0 vs. SM48, fold change: 9.29 ± 4.32, $p < 0.0001$ for SM12 vs. SM48, one-way ANOVA with a Tukey's *post hoc* test; **Figure 4B**). ISH for *Atoh1* demonstrated a spatial pattern of SCs showing *Atoh1* upregulation (**Figures 4C–K′**). In SM0 samples, *Atoh1* expression was observed in a small number of SCs on the neural edge of the distal and middle portions of the BPs (**Figures 4C,D′**). In SM24 and SM48 samples, intense expression of *Atoh1* mRNA was observed on both the neural and abneural sides of BPs (**Figures 4F–K′**), which is similar to the pattern observed in the acute phase of damaged BPs *in vivo* (Cafaro et al., 2007; Lewis et al., 2018). These findings confirmed that *Atoh1* is upregulated in SCs immediately after total HC loss.

Besides the Notch signaling pathway, we monitored alterations in genes associated with the Wnt, FGF, BMP/TGFb, VEGF, and Yap signaling pathways (**Figures 4L–P**). Among Wnt signaling-associated genes, expression of two Wnt ligands, *Wnt4* and *Wnt11*, one frizzled receptor, *Fzd9*, and four secreted frizzled-related Wnt inhibitors, *Sfrp1, Sfrp2, Sfrp4,* and *Frzb*, exhibited a trend of upregulation (**Figure 4L**). Of these seven genes, *Sfrp2, Frzb*, and *Fzd9* have also been found to be upregulated from the early development stage of chick BPs and contribute to the specification of BPs (Sienknecht and Fekete, 2008). Among FGF signaling-related genes, *Fgfr2* was upregulated, while *Fgf3* and *Fgfbp1* were downregulated (**Figure 4M**). The expression of *Fgfr1* and *Fgfr3*, which are known to be expressed in the chick BP (Bermingham-McDonogh et al., 2001; Jacques et al., 2012a; Honda et al., 2018), exhibited no alteration (**Figure 4M**). Among BMP/TGFb signaling-associated genes, downregulation of *Bmp4* was observed (**Figure 4N**), which may be a consequence of HC loss as described previously (Lewis et al., 2018). Upregulation of *Tgfbi*, TGFb signaling

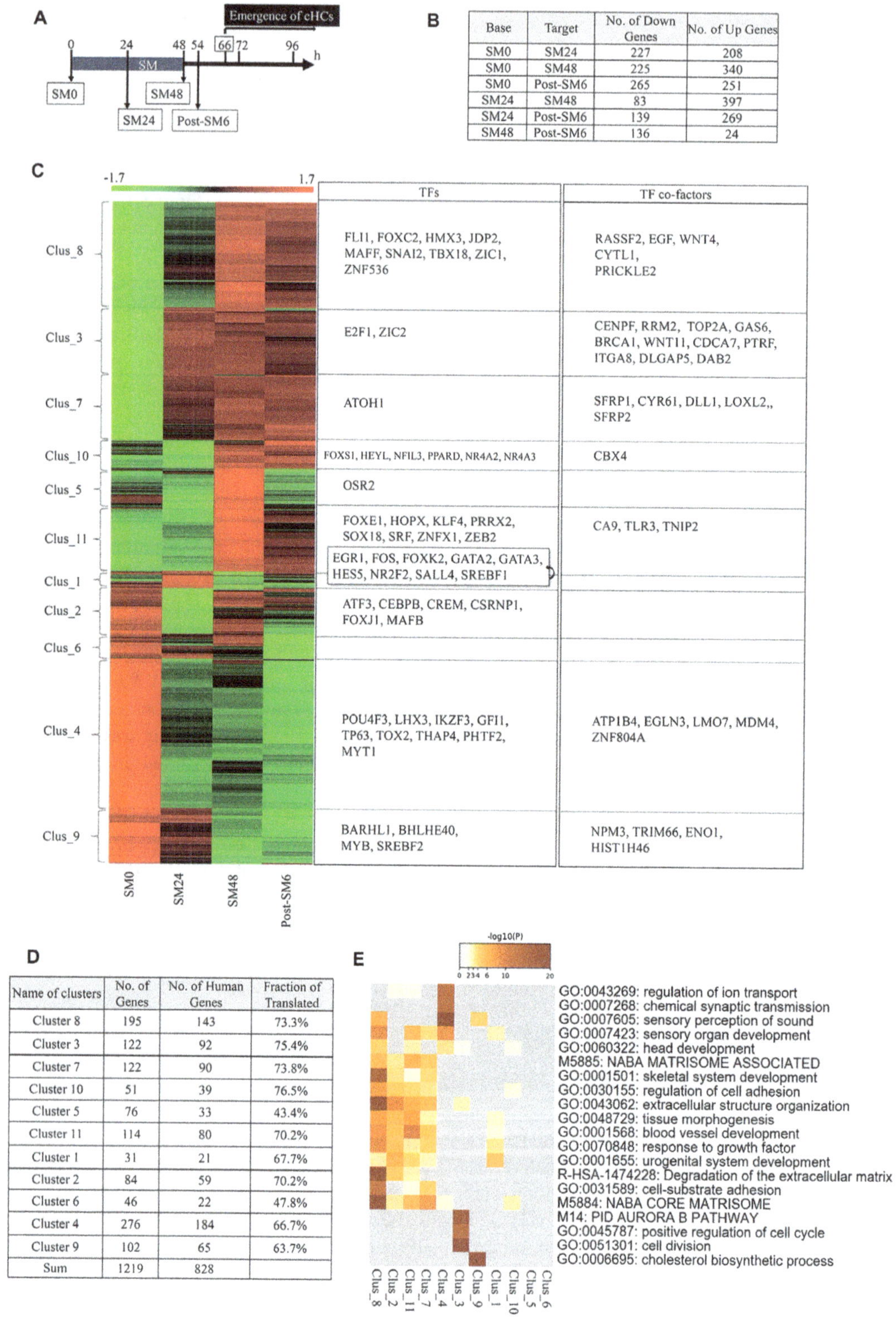

Base	Target	No. of Down Genes	No. of Up Genes
SM0	SM24	227	208
SM0	SM48	225	340
SM0	Post-SM6	265	251
SM24	SM48	83	397
SM24	Post-SM6	139	269
SM48	Post-SM6	136	24

Name of clusters	No. of Genes	No. of Human Genes	Fraction of Translated
Cluster 8	195	143	73.3%
Cluster 3	122	92	75.4%
Cluster 7	122	90	73.8%
Cluster 10	51	39	76.5%
Cluster 5	76	33	43.4%
Cluster 11	114	80	70.2%
Cluster 1	31	21	67.7%
Cluster 2	84	59	70.2%
Cluster 6	46	22	47.8%
Cluster 4	276	184	66.7%
Cluster 9	102	65	63.7%
Sum	1219	828	

FIGURE 3 | Differentially expressed genes (DEGs) in the basilar papilla (BP) explants during the initial phase of hair cell (HC) regeneration. **(A)** Diagram of sampling time points for RNA sequencing. Converting hair cells (cHCs) were observed at 66 h. **(B)** The number of differentially expressed genes (DEGs; $p < 0.05$, fold change for normalized read counts ≥ 1.3 or $\leq 1/1.3$, raw read counts ≥ 7, and TPM ≥ 1 in either of the compared conditions for DEseq2 followed by the weighted average difference (WAD) method) at each time point. **(C)** Heat map showing 11 clusters determined with K-means clustering and transcription factors (TFs) or TF co-factors in each cluster. **(D)** Numbers and ratios for the human homologs of DEGs in each cluster. **(E)** Metascape GO enrichment analysis of human homologs of DEGs for each cluster.

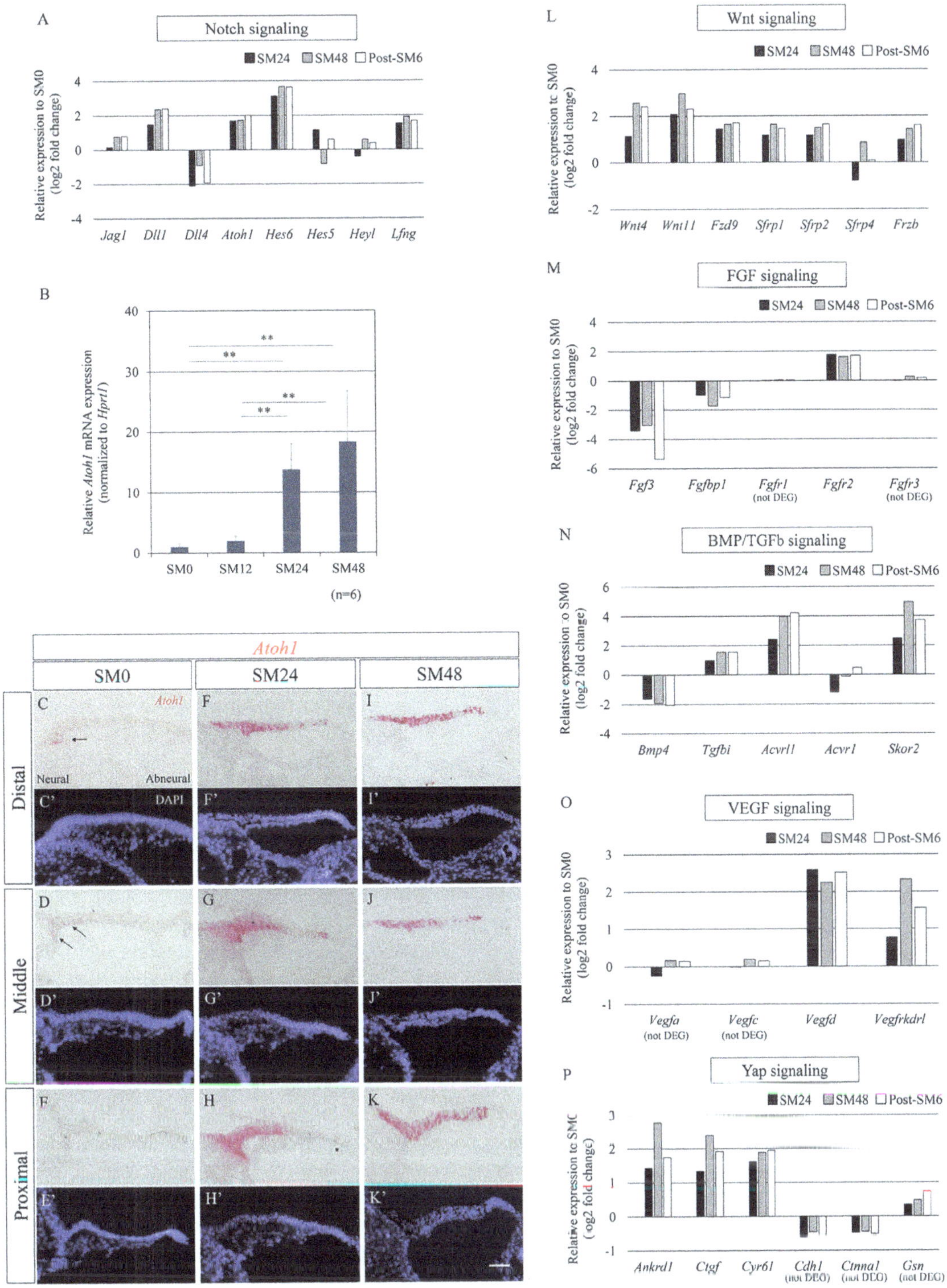

FIGURE 4 | Alterations in genes associated with known signaling pathways during the initial phase of hair cell (HC) regeneration. **(A)** Relative expression levels of differentially expressed genes (DEGs; $p < 0.05$, fold change for normalized read counts ≥ 1.3 or $\leq 1/1.3$, raw read counts ≥ 7, and TPM ≥ 1 in either of the compared conditions for DEseq2 followed by the WAD method) associated with Notch signaling compared to SM0 samples. **(B)** Relative mRNA expression levels of *Atoh1* by quantitative RT-PCR. *Atoh1* mRNA levels are expressed relative to *Hprt1*. $^{**}p < 0.01$, ANOVA with a Tukey's *post hoc* test. Bars represent standard deviations. **(C–K′)** *In situ* hybridization for *Atoh1* mRNA and nuclear staining with 4′,6-diamidino-2-phenylindole (DAPI) in the distal, middle, and proximal portions of the basilar papillae (BP). The intense expression of *Atoh1* was observed in SM24 and SM48 samples **(F–K′)**. Arrows indicate *Atoh1* expression in SM0 samples **(C,D)**. Scale bar represents 40 μm. **(L–P)** Relative expression levels of genes associated with Wnt **(L)**, fibroblast growth factor (FGF; **M**), bone morphogenetic protein (BMP)/Transforming growth factor-beta (TGFb; **N**), vascular endothelial growth factor (VEGF; **O**), and Yap signaling **(P)** compared to SM0 samples. Genes that did not pass our filter for differentially expressed genes are stated as (not DEG).

downstream, and *Acvrl1* and *Acvr1*, type 1 receptors of TGFb family ligands were observed, while *Skor2*, a TGFb antagonist was also upregulated (**Figure 4N**). In VEGF signaling, *Vegfd* and *Vegfrkdrl*, a VEGF signaling ligand and its receptor, were upregulated (**Figure 4O**), suggesting the activation of VEGF signaling in BPs. Three major YAP signaling downstream genes, *Ankrd1*, *Ctgf*, and *Cyr61*, were upregulated, while genes encoding inhibitors of Yap translocation to the nucleus, *Cdh1*, *Ctnna1*, and *Gsn*, were detectable, but not passed our filter for DEGs (**Figure 4P**), indicating the involvement of Yap signaling in the initial phase of HC regeneration in chick BPs.

Taken together, *Atoh1* upregulation immediately after total HC loss was observed in our explant culture model, similar to previous observations in chick BPs (Cafaro et al., 2007; Lewis et al., 2018). A trend showing upregulation of *Dll1* and *Hes6*, which are thought to be downstream of Atoh1 (Mulvaney and Dabdoub, 2012), suggested that the differentiation process to HCs had already been initiated in *Atoh1*-expressing SCs at SM24. Alterations in major signaling pathways associated with HC formation or regeneration suggested involvements of these signaling pathways in the early phase of HC regeneration in our culture model consistent with previous observations.

Expression Patterns of Upregulated Genes in the Early Phase of HC Regeneration

To explore the molecular events associated with the responses in SCs during initiation of HC regeneration, we focused on Clusters 3 and 7 that included DEGs upregulated from SM24. We chose two TF co-factors, *Sfrp2* (secreted frizzled-related protein 2) and *Cyr61* (cysteine-rich angiogenic inducer 61) from Cluster 7 and one TF co-factor, *Rrm2* (ribonucleotide reductase regulatory subunit M2) from Cluster 3 as the DEGs of interest (**Figure 3C**). SFRP2 is a soluble Wnt inhibitor that is expressed in developing BPs (Sienknecht and Fekete, 2008). CYR61 or cellular communication network factor (CCN) 1 is a member of the CCN family of matricellular proteins, and one of the Yap targets (Gnedeva et al., 2017). RRM2 is expressed during the late G1/early S phase when DNA replication occurs (Chabes et al., 2003, 2004).

Expression of *Sfrp2* in SM0 samples was observed in SCs, with broad distribution (**Figures 5A–A″**). The expression pattern of *Sfrp2* in SM0 samples was identical to that in the late embryonic stage of chick BPs (Sienknecht and Fekete, 2008). In SM24 and SM48 samples, *Sfrp2* expression was intense in SCs, especially in the neural half of BPs (**Figures 5B–C″**). No alteration in the distribution of *Sfrp2* was observed.

In SM0 samples, virtually no expression of *Cyr61* was observed in SCs in the distal or middle portion of BPs (**Figures 5D,D′**). *CYR 61* expression was found around the neural edge of BPs in the proximal portion (**Figure 5D″**). In SM24 and SM48 samples, intense expression was observed in and/or outside of the neural edges of BPs (**Figures 5E–F″**). Some SCs in the abneural portion of BPs showed *Cyr61* expression (**Figures 5E″,F′,F″**).

In SM0 samples, weak expression of *Rrm2* was observed in the neural edge of the middle and proximal portions (**Figures 5G′,G″**). In SM24 and SM48 samples, strong expression of *Rrm2* was found in and/or outside of the neural edge of BPs (**Figures 5H–I″**). Also, *Rrm2* expression was observed in the cells that were present in SFP (**Figures 5H,I″**). The distribution of *Rrm2* expression in SM24 and SM48 samples was identical to that of EdU-positive cells in SM48 samples (**Figures 2C,C′**).

Alterations in Type I Interferon Signaling-Associated Genes

To explore candidate signals for initiating activation of SCs after HC loss, we sought DEGs that were upregulated at SM24 compared to SM0 and downregulated at SM48 or post-SM6 compared to SM24. Consequently, only one DEG, IFI6, was identified in Cluster 3. *IFI6* is a type I interferon (IFN)-stimulated gene that is regulated by the JAK/ STAT signaling pathway (Friedman et al., 1984; Porter et al., 1988). The JAK/STAT signaling pathway is a key regulator of HC regeneration in zebrafish lateral lines (Liang et al., 2012). Bulk RNA-seq analysis of HC regeneration in chick BPs *in vivo* also demonstrated the involvement of JAK/STAT signaling (Jiang et al., 2018). Hence, we focused on type I IFN/JAK/STAT signaling.

Type I IFN/JAK/STAT signaling-associated genes are divided into three groups: type I IFN production, type I IFN receptors, and JAK/STAT signaling mediators of type I IFN/JAK/STAT signaling. Type I IFNs are secreted after recognition of damage-associated molecular patterns (DAMPs) and pathogen-associated molecular patterns by pattern recognition receptors (PRRs). We found 13 DEGs encoded molecules associated with the type I IFN/JAK/STAT signaling pathway (**Figure 6A**). As candidates of DAMPs, heat shock protein A family genes, *Hspa2* and *Hspa8* were identified. As *Hspa8* showed a trend of downregulation, *Hspa2* can be a candidate of DAMPs in our culture model. Among genes encoded PRRs, a trend for upregulation was observed in *Tlr2a* and *Tlr3* (**Figure 6A**). In downstream of type I IFN/JAK/STAT signaling, six IFN-stimulated genes (ISGs), and *Usp18*, which are included products of non-canonical JAK/STAT pathway, and three genes that are products of canonical JAK/STAT pathway were found in DEGs (**Figure 6A**). Two canonical JAK/STAT pathway-associated genes, *Socs1* and *Socs3* showed a trend of downregulation. As for type I IFNs and their receptors, *Ifnal2, Ifnal6, Ifnar1, and Ifnar2* were detectable in each time point, but did not pass our filter for DEGs. To confirm the alteration in *Ifi6* expression in BPs, we performed ISH (**Figures 6B–J′**). Virtually no expression was found in SM0 samples (**Figures 6B–D′**), while both the SM24 and SM48 samples exhibited intense expression in some SCs (**Figures 6E–J′**). SCs expressing *Ifi6* exhibited a scattered distribution in BPs and were frequently found in the neural half of BPs (**Figures 6E–J′**). These findings indicate the activation of non-canonical type I IFN/JAK/STAT signaling in SCs of damaged BPs.

To examine an effect of JAK/STAT signaling on *Atoh1* activation in SCs, we performed an experiment using pharmacological inhibition of JAK/STAT signaling (**Figure 6K**). Chick BP explants were cultured with SM and a JAK

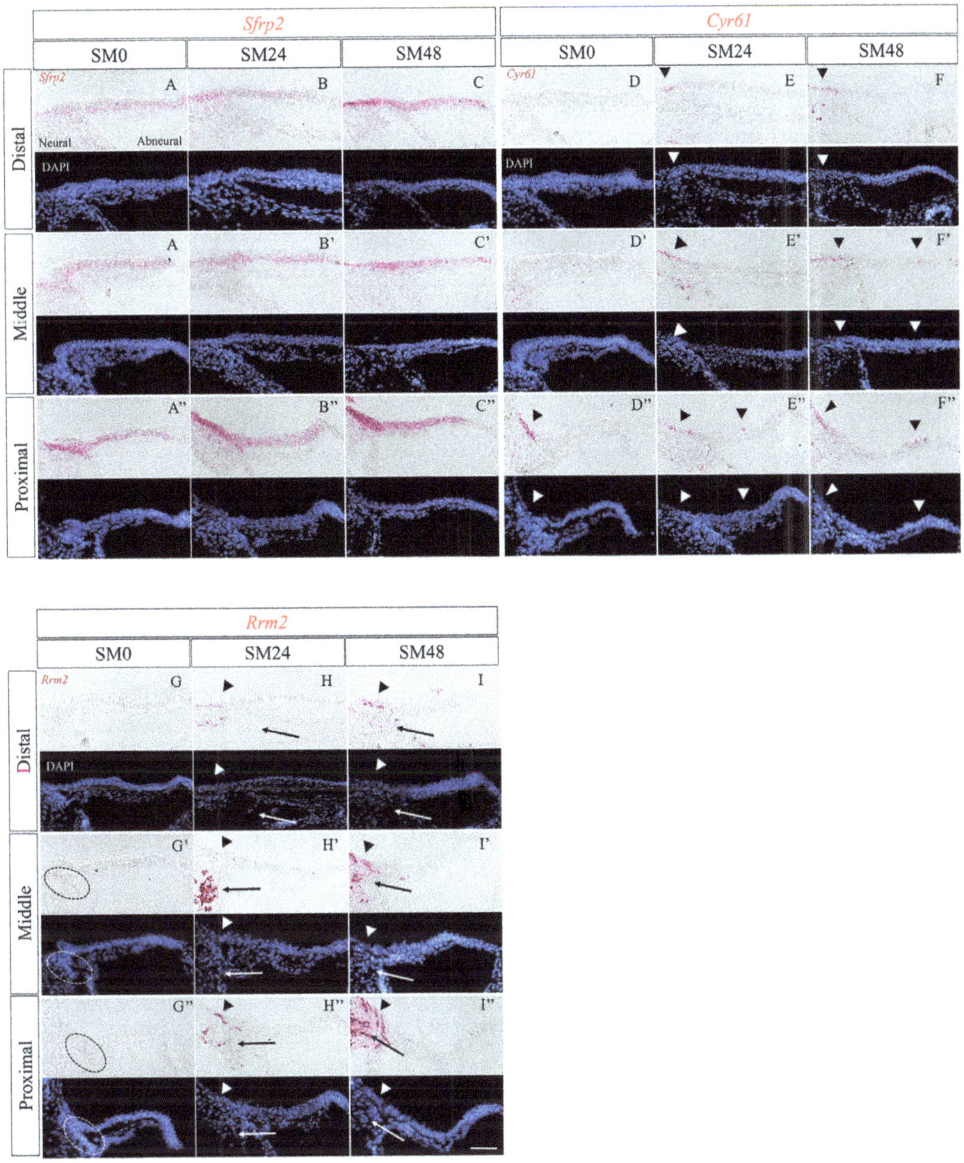

FIGURE 5 | The expression patterns of the newly identified genes in the basilar papilla (BP) in the early phase of hair cell (HC) regeneration. **(A–I″)** Representative images of *in situ* hybridization for *Sfrp2* **(A–C″)**, *Cyr61* **(D–F″)**, and *Rrm2* **(G–I″)** in BPs of SM0, SM24, and SM48 samples. Cells were counterstained with 4′,6-diamidino-2-phenylindole (DAPI). Arrowheads indicate the location of expressed cells in the BP (red). Dotted lines in **(G′,G″)** indicate *Rrm2* expression in SCs in the neural edge of SM0 samples. Arrows in **(H–I″)** indicate *Rrm2* expression in cells in the superior fibrocartilaginous plate (SFP). Scale bars represent 40 μm.

inhibitor, ruxolitinib phosphate for 24 h. Assessments by qPCR demonstrated a significant increase of *Ifi6* expression in SM24 samples that were incubated with SM alone compared with SM0 samples ($p = 0.002$ by Student's *t*-test; **Figure 6L**). Supplementation of ruxolitinib phosphate significantly attenuated *Ifi6* upregulation at 24 h after SM exposure ($p = 0.0459$ by Student's *t*-test; **Figure 6L**), indicating that a JAK inhibitor, ruxolitinib phosphate efficiently blocked JAK-STAT signaling in our explant cultures. The expression level of *Atoh1* was also increased in SM24 samples in comparison with SM0 samples ($p < 0.0001$ by Student's *t*-test; **Figure 6M**). Ruxolitinib phosphate treatment showed a trend to decrease *Atoh1* expression levels in comparison with SM24 samples, although the difference was not statistically significant ($p = 0.150$ by Student's *t* test; **Figure 6M**). These findings suggested that IFN/JAK/STAT signaling could be associated with *Atoh1* activation in SCs of chick BPs in response to SM-induced damage.

DISCUSSION

In the current study, we established a new chick BP model for HC regeneration using explant cultures. In our model, the generation of new HCs mainly occurred through direct transdifferentiation

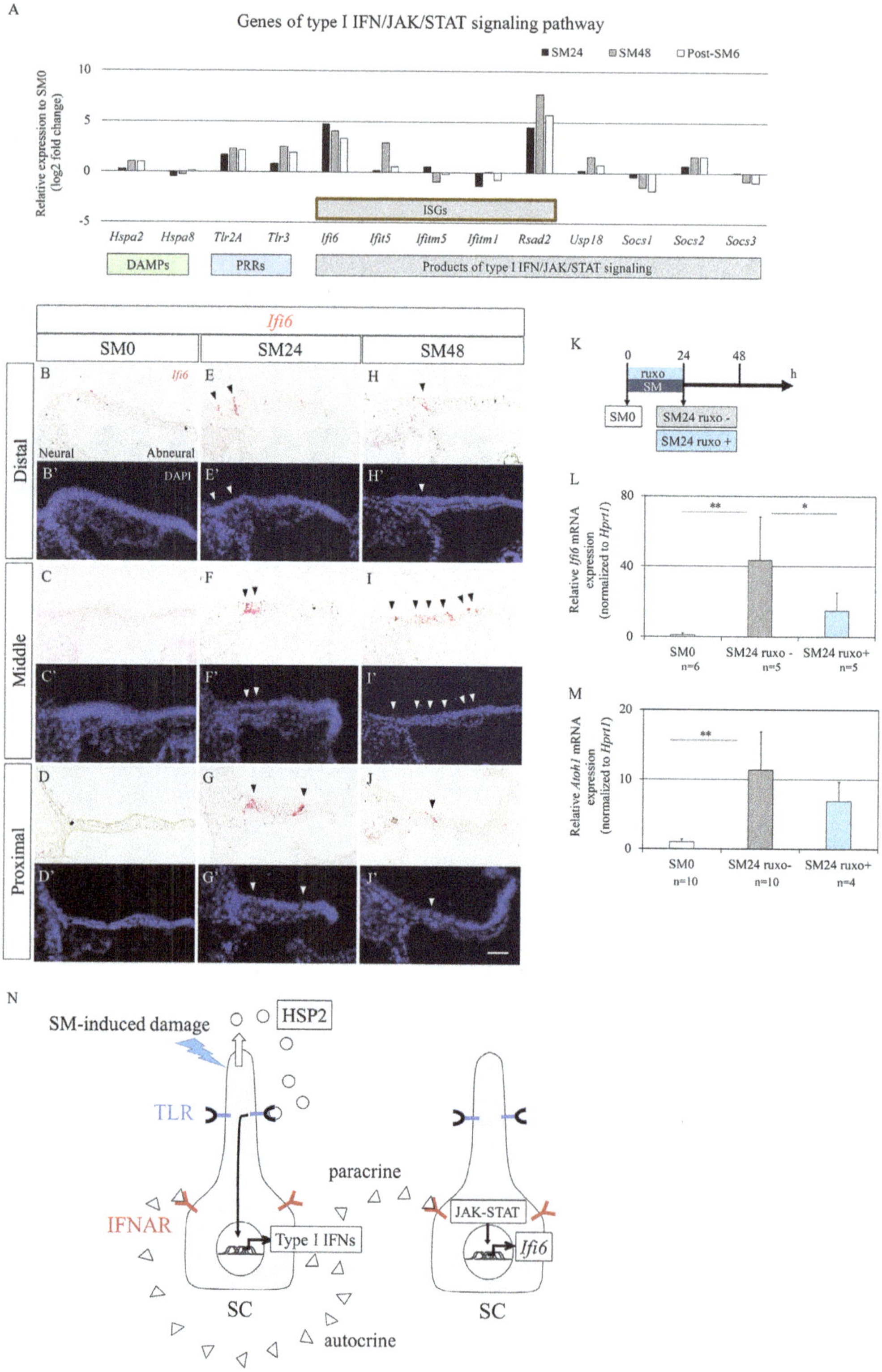

FIGURE 6 | Alterations in genes associated with type I interferon (IFN) signaling in basilar papilla (BP) explants. **(A)** mRNA expression levels ($\log_2$ fold changes) of differentially expressed genes ($p < 0.05$, fold change for normalized read counts ≥ 1.3 or $\leq 1/1.3$, raw read counts ≥ 7, and TPM ≥ 1 in either of the compared conditions for DEseq2 followed by the WAD method) associated with type I IFN/JAK/signal transducer and activator of transduction (STAT) signaling pathway relative to their expression levels at SM0. **(B–J')** Representative images of *in situ* hybridization for *Ifi6* mRNA expression and nuclear staining with 4',6-diamidino-2-phenylindole (DAPI) in the BP. Arrowheads indicate *Ifi6* mRNA expression. Scale bar represents 40 µm. **(K)** Diagram of exposure to streptomycin (SM) and ruxolitinib

(Continued)

FIGURE 6 | Continued
phosphate (ruxo) and sampling time points. **(L,M)** Relative mRNA expression levels of *Ifi6* **(L)** and *Atoh1* **(M)** by quantitative RT-PCR. *Ifi6* mRNA levels are expressed relative to *Hprt1* (**$p < 0.01$, *$p < 0.05$ by Student's *t*-test). Bars represent standard deviations. **(N)** Hypothetical model of type I IFN/JAK/STAT signaling regulation in chick BPs. Streptomycin (SM)-induced damages induce the secretion of heat shock protein 2 (HSP2) family from supporting cells (SCs), which activates Toll-like receptors (TLR) on SCs resulting in the production of type I IFNs. Type I IFNs activate interferon alpha and beta receptor subunits (IFNAR) on SCs in a paracrine or autocrine fashion leading to upregulation of IFN-stimulated genes including *Ifi6* through JAK/STAT signaling.

of SCs. Known molecular events in the initial phase of HC regeneration were also observed in our model. In particular, alterations in *Atoh1* expression observed in the present study are consistent with other similar observations in the early phase of HC regeneration in chick BPs (Cafaro et al., 2007; Lewis et al., 2012). Bulk RNA-seq during the initial phase of HC regeneration indicated several unique transcriptional responses associated with SC activation. Taken together, our BP explant culture model can be utilized to explore the mechanisms of SC activation in the initial phase of HC regeneration.

Two Different Responses of SCs During HC Loss

In addition to direct transdifferentiation of SCs, the mitotic division of SCs, another response of SCs after induction of HC loss, was also observed during the initial phase of HC regeneration in our model. However, myosin VIIa-positive cells did not show EdU incorporation during the culture period. These results strongly suggest that the mitotic division of SCs contributes to the replenishment of SCs in our model. However, it is also possible that SCs after mitotic division disappeared due to cell death during differentiation into HCs, or that several SC divisions resulted in EdU dilution to undetectable levels in newly generated HCs. Shang et al. (2010) demonstrated that a high concentration of bromodeoxyuridine, a traditional thymidine analog, affected HC differentiation of SCs incorporated bromodeoxyuridine, although it increased the labeling ratio of proliferating SCs, suggesting that EdU incorporation could prevent HC differentiation of SCs. Hence, EdU labeling used in the present study can affect SC differentiation into HCs. In present results, EdU labeling was limitedly observed in the neural edge of BPs, even in post-SM144 samples (**Figures 2D–G**), suggesting that SC division occurred only in the neural edge of BPs in our explant culture model. We assessed the expression of *Rrm2*, which is one of the DEGs identified by RNA-seq in the present study and is a marker for the late G1/early S phase of the cell cycle (Chabes et al., 2003, 2004). The results showed a similar distribution of *Rrm2* expression and EdU labeling (**Figures 5G–I″**), which supports our hypothesis that SC division occurred only in the neural edge of BPs. On the other hand, expression of *Atoh1* after HC loss was mainly observed in the neural half of BPs (**Figures 4C–K′**), indicating that SC activation in response to HC loss occurred in broader areas than did SC division. Also, converting HCs initially appeared in the neural half of BPs (**Figures 1P′,Q′,T**). These results indicate that two different responses of SCs, direct transdifferentiation to HCs and mitotic division, were induced simultaneously in the initial phase of HC regeneration. In the neural edge of BPs, two different types of SCs may be present based on their proliferative ability and cell fate.

Alterations in Known Signaling Pathways in the Early Phase of HC Regeneration

In the current study, we examined changes in the expression patterns of genes associated with the Notch, Wnt, FGF, BMP/TGFb, VEGF, and Yap signaling pathways in the initial phase of HC regeneration in our explant culture model. Previous studies have revealed the critical roles of these signaling pathways in the development and regeneration of auditory sensory epithelia (Schimmang, 2007; Atkinson et al., 2015; Ebeid and Huh, 2017; Gnedeva et al., 2017, 2020; Denans et al., 2019; Samarajeewa et al., 2019; Rudolf et al., 2020; Wan et al., 2020). Also, cross-talk between these signaling pathways has been reported (Millimaki et al., 2007; Sweet et al., 2011; Jacques et al., 2012b; Munnamalai and Fekete, 2016; Lewis et al., 2018).

Previous studies demonstrated that *Atoh1* was upregulated in SCs in two different phases of HC regeneration in chick BPs (Cafaro et al., 2007; Lewis et al., 2012). In the acute phase of damage, activated SC progenitors expressed *Atoh1*, which showed a broad distribution in BPs, in contrast with the restricted *Atoh1* expression in the later phase of SC differentiation into HCs (Cafaro et al., 2007). The upregulation of *Atoh1* observed in the present study is likely associated with the activation of SCs in response to HC loss, not with lateral inhibition associated with HC differentiation, because of other HC differentiation genes (*Pou4f3, Lhx3, Gfi1*, and *Barhl1*) were downregulated. On the other hand, a trend for the upregulation of *Dll1, Hes6*, and *Lfng* was observed in the present study, which is also consistent with previous findings in the acute phase of HC regeneration in chick BPs (Daudet et al., 2009). These results indicate that the process of SC differentiation into HCs has already been initiated. Taken together, the fate of some activated SCs was already determined as direct transdifferentiation to HCs, but the process of differentiation into HCs was still in the early phase during our observation period. A recent study demonstrates that transient activation of Notch signaling induces reprogramming of adult cochlear SCs in mice, leading to the enhancement of SC potential for transdifferentiation into HCs (Shu et al., 2019). As shown in the present and previous studies (Daudet et al., 2009), Notch signaling is upregulated in chick BP SCs before direct conversion to HCs. This indicates that manipulation of the pathways identified in the present study could affect the potential of mature mammalian SCs for transdifferentiation into HCs.

During the development of the inner ear in chicks, Wnt ligands mostly originate from non-sensory tissue domains, whereas the sensory primordia preferentially express frizzled receptors and/or secreted frizzled-related Wnt inhibitors (Sienknecht and Fekete, 2008). In the present study, a trend for the upregulation of secreted frizzled-related Wnt inhibitors, *Sfrp2* and *Frzb*, and a Frizzled receptor, *Fzd9*, was observed. These three genes are associated with the specification of BP during the early phase of development (Sienknecht and Fekete, 2008). In the late stage of development, *Sfrp2* is expressed in SCs in BPs (Sienknecht and Fekete, 2008). In the present study, ISH demonstrated that *Sfrp2* is expressed in SCs of BPs before SM exposure, consistent with a previous observation (Sienknecht and Fekete, 2008). After induction of total HC loss, *Sfrp2* expression increased, while no change in its distribution was observed. These results suggest the involvement of Wnt signaling in SC activation in the initial process of HC regeneration, similar to the development of chick BP HCs. However, further studies are required to reveal the distinct roles of these Wnt-associated genes in HC regeneration in BPs.

Among genes associated with FGF signaling, *Fgf3* downregulation was observed in the present study, which is reported in the process of HC regeneration in the lateral line neuromast in the zebrafish (Lush et al., 2019). In developing chick BP explants, pharmacological inhibition of FGF signaling results in the induction of direct SC transdifferentiation into HCs (Jacques et al., 2012a). Therefore, the *Fgf3* downregulation observed in the present study may explain the promotion of direct transdifferentiation of SCs. On the other hand, in the zebrafish lateral line, *Fgfr2* is also downregulated after HC loss (Lush et al., 2019), while in the present study, it was upregulated after HC loss. There are several differences in the roles of FGF signaling in HC formation and regeneration between species (Atkinson et al., 2015). The distinct roles of FGF signaling in the initiation of HC regeneration in chick BPs remain unclear, and further investigations are required.

A recent publication using a similar BP explant culture model to the present study demonstrated the involvement of VEGF signaling in the induction of SC proliferation in chick BPs (Wan et al., 2020). In the present study, the upregulation of VEGF signaling ligand and receptor was also found, suggesting that VEGF signaling is also related to SC proliferation observed in the present study. As upstream of VEGF signaling, a previous study (Hori et al., 2010) indicated possible roles of prostaglandin E signaling, which demonstrated that prostaglandin E induced VEGF secretion from mouse cochlear explants. Some genes encoded prostaglandin E synthase was detectable, but not passed our filter for DEGs, in the present data set of RNA-seq (**Supplementary Table 2**).

Recently, a couple of publications showed significant roles of Yap signaling in HC regeneration in the mouse utricle (Gnedeva et al., 2017; Rudolf et al., 2020) and the cochlea (Gnedeva et al., 2020). We identified the upregulation of Yap targets in our data set. Also, no upregulation in genes encoded inhibitors for Yap translocation into the nucleus was observed in the present study, suggesting that Yap signaling may also work in HC regeneration in chick BPs.

Newly Identified Genes Involved in the Early Phase of HC Regeneration

In the current study, we attempted to explore novel molecules involved in the initial process of HC regeneration using our explant culture model. Bulk RNA-seq of BP explant cultures during the initial phase of HC regeneration indicated the involvement of *Cyr61* and *Rrm2*, in the initiation of SC activation. Expressions of both *Cyr61* and *Rrm2* were upregulated in BPs after total HC loss in a specific region, the neural edge of BPs (**Figures 5D–I″**), where EdU labeling was specifically observed (**Figures 2C–D″**). CYR 61 is a CCN matricellular protein that regulates diverse cellular functions, including cell adhesion, migration, proliferation, differentiation, and survival in a cell-type- and context-dependent manner (Chen and Lau, 2009). Therefore, CYR61 may affect the induction of cell proliferation, particularly on SCs in the neural edge of BPs. Also, *Cyr61* expression around the neural edge of BPs suggests a possible involvement of Yap signaling in cell proliferation in this region. RRM2 is also expressed in retinal progenitor (Trimarchi et al., 2008) and neural progenitor cells (Habib et al., 2016). CCN proteins are reported to shape the microenvironment associated with fate determination of stem or progenitor cells (Chen and Lau, 2009; Zuo et al., 2010; Lukjanenko et al., 2019). Therefore, *Cyr61* and *Rrm2* expression in the neural edge of BPs in SM0 samples (**Figures 5D″,G′,G″**) may indicate the presence of progenitor-like cells in this specific location. Taken together, SCs in the neural edge of BPs may have different cell characteristics from SCs in other locations.

Samarajeewa et al. (2018) demonstrated that SC proliferation by Wnt activation in the early neonatal mouse cochlea is correlated with unique transcriptional responses that diminish with age. The upregulation of *Cyr61* and *Rrm2* occurs with such transcriptional changes, suggesting the involvement of these genes in the induction of SC proliferation in the neonatal mouse cochlea (Samarajeewa et al., 2018). Therefore, SC proliferation in the neonatal mouse cochlea and chick BP after damage may share the same signaling pathways. On the other hand, *Sfrp2* was downregulated in neonatal mouse cochleae after Wnt activation (Samarajeewa et al., 2018), in contrast to the present findings. Based on the spatial and temporal expression of *Sfrp2* in damaged chick BPs, *Sfrp2* may be associated with the differentiation of activated SCs rather than induction of SC division.

Possible Role of Type I IFN/JAK/STAT Signaling in the Initial Phase of HC Regeneration

In the current study, we focused on *IFI6*, one of the Cluster 3 genes, because it was the only gene upregulated at SM24 compared to SM0 and downregulated at post-SM6 compared to SM24. IFI6 is a type I IFN-stimulated gene that is regulated by the JAK/STAT signaling pathway (Friedman et al., 1984; Porter et al., 1988). Hence, we examined alterations in genes associated with the type I IFN/JAK/STAT signaling pathway and identified the upregulation of several genes associated with this signaling pathway. In present results, several targets of the non-canonical type I IFN/JAK/STAT signaling pathway showed a trend for upregulation, while those of the canonical signaling pathways exhibited a trend of downregulation. ISH demonstrated the expression of *Ifi6* in SCs in damaged BPs. These findings strongly suggested the involvement of non-canonical type I IFN/JAK/STAT signaling in the initial step for HC regeneration. Pharmacological inhibition of JAK-STAT signaling exhibited significant attenuation of *Ifi6* expression and a trend for attenuation of *Atoh1* activation. Altogether, non-canonical type I IFN/JAK/STAT signaling could be associated with the activation of some populations of SCs immediately after HC loss. In neural stem cells, IFN signaling induces dormant neural stem cell subpopulations to enter the primed state in response to ischemic injury (Llorens-Bobadilla et al., 2015). Therefore, the non-canonical type I IFN/JAK/STAT signaling could initiate alterations of SC states from dormant or quiescent to primed or activated.

The primary step of type I IFN/JAK/STAT signaling is the recognition of DAMPs by PRRs. There are two candidates for DAMPs in the initiation of this signaling in chick BP explant cultures, HC debris and heat shock protein A family proteins. SCs in vestibular epithelia have phagocytic activity in response to HC death (Bird et al., 2010; Monzack et al., 2015; Hirose et al., 2017). However, published studies suggest that nearly all HC debris is extruded from the luminal surface of BPs (Hirose et al., 2004; Warchol et al., 2012) and that little or no HC debris is detected in SCs in BPs (Warchol et al., 2012), indicating that phagocytosis of SCs may not be a mechanism for the initiation of type I IFN/JAK/STAT signaling in chick BPs. Rather than phagocytosis, the recognition of heat shock protein A family proteins as DAMPs through toll-like receptors (TLR) can be a mechanism for IFN production in chick BPs (**Figure 6N**). Upregulation of genes encoded heat shock protein A family proteins and TLR including *Tlr2a* was found in our data set. Also, the upregulation of HSP70 was found in mouse cochlear SCs after noise exposure (Gratton et al., 2011), and expression of adaptor proteins of type I IFN/JAK/STAT signaling in the mouse cochlea has been reported (Hayashi et al., 2013). HSP70 secreted from SCs contributes to the protection of HCs against aminoglycoside toxicity in mouse utricles (May et al., 2013).

Resident macrophages in the inner ear could be associated with type I IFN/JAK/STAT signaling in chick BPs. Migration of macrophages was observed in chick BP explants after HC injury (Warchol et al., 2012), suggesting a certain role of macrophages in processing dying HCs and/or in consecutive repair processes. However, migrated macrophages are located underneath the basilar membrane of chick BPs, and elimination of macrophages does not affect the capacity for HC regeneration in chick BP explants (Warchol et al., 2012). We, therefore, presume that SCs may play a central role in IFN production in response to SM injury in chick BPs. It may be worthy to investigate the roles of TLR in responses to SM-induced damage in chick BPs.

Comparisons of Changes in Gene Expressions Between Chick BP and Utricle Explant Cultures

To illustrate the differences and similarities in the early phase of HC regeneration between the chick BP and utricle, we referred to the data set GSE57134_CU_REGEN.txt.gz (Ku et al., 2014), in which bulk RNA-seq was performed to investigate HC regeneration processes in chick utricle explant cultures. For comparison between BP and utricle explants, we extracted the data of the early time-points from GSE57134_CU_REGEN.txt.gz, and compared changes of gene expression patterns between two time-points corresponding to SM24 and SM48 in the present study. Gene expression patterns in Notch and FGF signaling in the utricle showed similar trends to those of BPs observed in the present study. In other signaling pathways, we found two differences between BPs and utricles. One is changes in the expression levels of cell-cycle associated genes (*Cyr61* and *Rrm2*). They were saturated at SM24 in BPs in present results, while in the utricle, further remarkable increases were observed at SM48. This may be reflected the difference in the capacity for cell proliferation between two organs. Another is downstream of IFN/JAK/STAT signaling. In the BP, target genes of the non-canonical pathway were upregulated, while canonical pathway-downstream genes, *Socs1* and *Socs3*, showed a trend to increase in the utricle. Further studies are required to conclude this issue.

CONCLUSIONS

We established a chick BP explant culture model for HC regeneration. In our model, SC behaviors were divided into direct transdifferentiation to HCs and mitosis, indicating the heterogeneity of SCs in chick BPs. Transcriptomics at the single-cell level and/or Spatio-temporal transcriptomic analysis is required to clarify how SCs are activated after HC loss. Further, the present results indicate the involvement of type I IFN/JAK/STAT signaling in the initial step of HC regeneration in chick BPs. We believe that our explant culture model will contribute to exploring the molecular mechanisms of SC activation towards HC regeneration in chick BPs and the development of therapeutics for HC regeneration in the mammalian cochlea.

AUTHOR CONTRIBUTIONS

TN, TK, MM, and NY designed the study. MM and TK performed the laboratory experiments. RY, TO, KO, SS, and NY contributed to data analysis and critical discussion. MM, TK, and TN wrote the manuscript. All authors contributed to the article and approved the submitted version.

FUNDING

The study was partly supported by KAKENHI (Grants-in-Aid for Scientific Research (20K09708) to TN from the Japan

Society for the Promotion of Science, by AMED (Japan Agency for Medical Research and Development) under Grant (20lm0203013j0002) to TO, and by Boehringer Ingelheim Pharma GmbH. The funders had no role in study design, data collection, and analysis, decision to publish, or preparation of the manuscript.

ACKNOWLEDGMENTS

We thank J. S. Stone and her lab members (University of Washington, Seattle, WA, USA) for valuable advises regarding explant cultures of chick basilar papillae, K. Iida (Medical Research Support Center, Graduate School of Medicine Kyoto University, Kyoto, Japan) for bioinformatics analyses, A. Watanabe (Center for iPS Cell Research and Application, Kyoto University, Kyoto, Japan) for valuable discussion on experimental design, and Editage (https://www.editage.com) for English language editing.

SUPPLEMENTARY MATERIAL

SUPPLEMENTARY TABLE 1 | Thresholds for the weighted average difference (WAD) method.

SUPPLEMENTARY TABLE 2 | Transcripts per million (TPM) and row counts of expressed genes in chick basilar papilla explants at each time point.

REFERENCES

Atkinson, P. J., Huarcaya-Najarro, E., Sayyid, Z. N., and Cheng, A. G. (2015). Sensory hair cell development and regeneration: similarities and differences. *Development* 142, 1561–1571. doi: 10.1242/dev.114926

Bermingham-McDonogh, O., Stone, J. S., Reh, T. A., and Rubel, E. W. (2001). FGFR3 expression during development and regeneration of the chick inner ear sensory epithelia. *Dev. Biol.* 238, 247–259. doi: 10.1006/dbio.2001.0412

Bird, J. E., Daudet, N., Warchol, M. E., and Gale, J. E. (2010). Supporting cells eliminate dying sensory hair cells to maintain epithelial integrity in the avian inner ear. *J Neurosci.* 30, 12545–12556. doi: 10.1523/JNEUROSCI.3042-10.2010

Bohne, B. A., Ward, P. H., and Fernández, C. (1976). Irreversible inner ear damage from rock music. *Trans. Sect. Otolaryngol. Am. Acad. Ophthalmol. Otolaryngol.* 82, ORL50–ORL59.

Cafaro, J., Lee, G. S., and Stone, J. S. (2007). Atoh1 expression defines activated progenitors and differentiating hair cells during avian hair cell regeneration. *Dev. Dyn.* 236, 156–170. doi: 10.1002/dvdy.21023

Chabes, A. L., Björklund, S., and Thelander, L. (2004). S Phase-specific transcription of the mouse ribonucleotide reductase R2 gene requires both a proximal repressive E2F-binding site and an upstream promoter activating region. *J. Biol. Chem.* 279, 10796–10807. doi: 10.1074/jbc.M312482200

Chabes, A. L., Pfleger, C. M., Kirschner, M. W., and Thelander, L. (2003). Mouse ribonucleotide reductase R2 protein: a new target for anaphase-promoting complex-Cdh1-mediated proteolysis. *Proc. Natl. Acad. Sci. U S A* 100, 3925–3929. doi: 10.1073/pnas.0330774100

Chen, C. C., and Lau, L. F. (2009). Functions and mechanisms of action of CCN matricellular proteins. *Int. J. Biochem. Cell Biol.* 41, 771–783. doi: 10.1016/j.biocel.2008.07.025

Cox, B. C., Chai, R., Lenoir, A., Liu, Z., Zhang, L., Nguyen, D. H., et al. (2014). Spontaneous hair cell regeneration in the neonatal mouse cochlea *in vivo*. *Development* 141, 816–829. doi: 10.1242/dev.103036

Daudet, N., Ariza-McNaughton, L., and Lewis, J. (2007). Notch signalling is needed to maintain, but not to initiate, the formation of prosensory patches in the chick inner ear. *Development* 134, 2369–2378. doi: 10.1242/dev.001842

Daudet, N., Gibson, R., Shang, J., Bernard, A., Lewis, J., and Stone, J. (2009). Notch regulation of progenitor cell behavior in quiescent and regenerating auditory epithelium of mature birds. *Dev. Biol.* 326, 86–100. doi: 10.1016/j.ydbio.2008.10.033

Daudet, N., and Lewis, J. (2005). Two contrasting roles for notch activity in chick inner ear development: specification of prosensory patches and lateral inhibition of hair-cell differentiation. *Development* 132, 541–551. doi: 10.1242/dev.01589

Denans, N., Baek, S., and Piotrowski, T. (2019). Comparing sensory organs to define the path for hair cell regeneration. *Annu. Rev. Cell Dev. Biol.* 35, 567–589. doi: 10.1146/annurev-cellbio-100818-125503

Dobin, A., Davis, C. A., Schlesinger, F., Drenkow, J., Zaleski, C., Jha, S., et al. (2013). STAR: ultrafast universal RNA-seq aligner. *Bioinformatics* 29, 15–21. doi: 10.1093/bioinformatics/bts635

Doetzlhofer, A., Basch, M. L., Ohyama, T., Gessler, M., Groves, A. K., and Segil, N. (2009). Hey2 regulation by FGF provides a Notch-independent mechanism for maintaining pillar cell fate in the organ of Corti. *Dev. Cell* 16, 58–69. doi: 10.1016/j.devcel.2008.11.008

Du, X., Cai, Q., West, M. B., Youm, I., Huang, X., Li, W., et al. (2018). Regeneration of cochlear hair cells and hearing recovery through Hes1 modulation with siRNA nanoparticles in adult guinea pigs. *Mol. Ther.* 2, 1313–1326. doi: 10.1016/j.ymthe.2018.03.004

Ebeid, M., and Huh, S. H. (2017). FGF signaling: diverse roles during cochlear development. *BMB Rep.* 50, 487–495. doi: 10.5483/bmbrep.2017.50.10.164

Febvre-James, M., Lecureur, V., Augagneur, Y., Mayati, A., and Fardel, O. (2018). Repression of interferon β-regulated cytokines by the JAK1/2 inhibitor ruxolitinib in inflammatory human macrophages. *Int. Immunopharmacol.* 54, 354–365. doi: 10.1016/j.intimp.2017.11.032

Friedman, R. L., Manly, S. P., McMahon, M., Kerr, I. M., and Stark, G. R. (1984). Transcriptional and posttranscriptional regulation of interferon-induced gene expression in human cells. *Cell* 38, 745–755. doi: 10.1016/0092-8674(84)90270-8

Gnedeva, K., Jacobo, A., Salvi, J. D., Petelski, A. A., and Hudspeth, A. J. (2017). Elastic force restricts growth of the murine utricle. *eLife* 25:e25681. doi: 10.7554/eLife.25681

Gnedeva, K., Wang, X., McGovern, M. M., Barton, M., Tao, L., Trecek, T., et al. (2020). Organ of corti size is governed by Yap/Tead-mediated progenitor self-renewal. *Proc. Natl. Acad. Sci. U S A* 16, 13552–13561. doi: 10.1073/pnas.2000175117

Gratton, M. A., Eleftheriadou, A., Gracia, J., Verduzco, E., Martin, G. K., Lonsbury-Martin, B. L., et al. (2011). Noise-induced changes in gene expression in the cochleae of mice differing in their susceptibility to noise damage. *Hear. Res.* 277, 211–226. doi: 10.1016/j.heares.2010.12.014

Habib, N., Li, Y., Heidenreich, M., Swiech, L., Avraham-Davidi, I., Trombetta, J. J., et al. (2016). Div-Seq: single-nucleus RNA-Seq reveals dynamics of rare adult newborn neurons. *Science* 353, 925–928. doi: 10.1126/science.aad7038

Hassanpour, H., Aghajani, Z., Bahadoran, S., Farhadi, N., Nazari, H., and Kaewduangta, W. (2019). Identification of reliable reference genes for quantitative real-time PCR in ovary and uterus of laying hens under heat stress. *Stress* 22, 387–394. doi: 10.1080/10253890.2019.1574294

Hawkins, J. E., Johnsson, L. G., Stebbins, W. C., Moody, D. B., and Coombs, S. L. (1976). Hearing loss and cochlear pathology in monkeys after noise exposure. *Acta Otolaryngol.* 81, 337–343. doi: 10.3109/00016487609119971

Hayashi, Y., Onomoto, K., Narita, R., Yoneyama, M., Kato, H., Nakagawa, T., et al. (2013). Virus-induced expression of retinoic acid inducible gene-I and melanoma differentiation-associated gene 5 in the cochlear sensory epithelium. *Microbes Infect.* 15, 592–598. doi: 10.1016/j.micinf.2013.04.008

Hirose, K., Rutherford, M. A., and Warchol, M. E. (2017). Two cell populations participate in clearance of damaged hair cells from the sensory epithelia of the inner ear. *Hear. Res.* 352, 70–81. doi: 10.1016/j.heares.2017.04.006

Hirose, K., Westrum, L. E., Cunningham, D. E., and Rubel, E. W. (2004). Electron microscopy of degenerative changes in the chick basilar papilla after gentamicin exposure. *J. Comp. Neurol.* 470, 164–180. doi: 10.1002/cne.11046

Honda, A., Kita, T., Seshadri, S. V., Misaki, K., Ahmed, Z., Ladbury, J. E., et al. (2018). FGFR1-mediated protocadherin 15 loading mediates cargo specificity during intraflagellar transport in inner ear hair-cell kinocilia. *Proc. Natl. Acad. Sci. U S A* 14, 8388–8393. doi: 10.1073/pnas.1719861115

Hori, R., Nakagawa, T., Sakamoto, T., Matsuoka, Y., Takebayashi, S., and Ito, J. (2007). Pharmacological inhibition of Notch signaling in the mature guinea pig cochlea. *Neuroreport* 18, 1911–1914. doi: 10.1097/WNR.0b013e3282f213e0

Hori, R., Nakagawa, T., Yamamoto, N., Hamaguchi, K., and Ito, J. (2010). Role of prostaglandin E receptor subtypes EP2 and EP4 in autocrine and paracrine functions of vascular endothelial growth factor in the inner ear. *BMC Neurosci.* 11:35. doi: 10.1186/1471-2202-11-35

Jacques, B. E., Dabdoub, A., and Kelley, M. W. (2012a). Fgf signaling regulates development and transdifferentiation of hair cells and supporting cells in the basilar papilla. *Hear. Res.* 289, 27–39. doi: 10.1016/j.heares.2012.04.018

Jacques, B. E., Puligilla, C., Weichert, R. M., Ferrer-Vaquer, A., Hadjantonakis, A. K., Kelley, M. W., et al. (2012b). A dual function for canonical Wnt/β-catenin signaling in the developing mammalian cochlea. *Development* 139, 4395–4404. doi: 10.1242/dev.080358

Jiang, L., Xu, J., Jin, R., Bai, R., Zhang, M., Yang, S., et al. (2018). Transcriptomic analysis of chicken cochleae after gentamicin damage and the involvement of four signaling pathways (Notch, FGF, Wnt and BMP) in hair cell regeneration. *Hear. Res.* 361, 66–79. doi: 10.1016/j.heares.2018.01.004

Kadota, K., Nakai, Y., and Shimizu, K. (2008). A weighted average difference method for detecting differentially expressed genes from microarray data. *Algorithms Mol. Biol.* 3:8. doi: 10.1186/1748-7188-3-8

Kelly, M. C., Chang, Q., Pan, A., Lin, X., and Chen, P. (2012). Atoh1 directs the formation of sensory mosaics and induces cell proliferation in the postnatal mammalian cochlea *in vivo*. *J. Neurosci.* 32, 6699–6710. doi: 10.1523/JNEUROSCI.5420-11.2012

Kniss, J. S., Jiang, L., and Piotrowski, T. (2016). Insights into sensory hair cell regeneration from the zebrafish lateral line. *Curr. Opin. Genet. Dev.* 40, 32–40. doi: 10.1016/j.gde.2016.05.012

Kolla, L., Kelly, M. C., Mann, Z. F., Anaya-Rocha, A., Ellis, K., Lemons, A., et al. (2020). Characterization of the development of the mouse cochlear epithelium at the single cell level. *Nat. Commun.* 11:2389. doi: 10.1038/s41467-020-16113-y

Ku, Y. C., Renaud, N. A., Veile, R. A., Helms, C., Voelker, C. C. J., Warchol, M. E., et al. (2014). The Transcriptome of utricle hair cell regeneration in the avian inner ear. *J. Neurosci.* 34, 3523–3535. doi: 10.1523/JNEUROSCI.2606-13.2014

Langmead, B., and Salzberg, S. L. (2012). Fast gapped-read alignment with Bowtie 2. *Nat. Methods* 9, 357–359. doi: 10.1038/nmeth.1923

Lewis, R. M., Hume, C. R., and Stone, J. S. (2012). Atoh1 expression and function during auditory hair cell regeneration in post-hatch chickens. *Hear. Res.* 289, 74–85. doi: 10.1016/j.heares.2012.04.008

Lewis, R. M., Keller, J. J., Wan, L., and Stone, J. S. (2018). Bone morphogenetic protein 4 antagonizes hair cell regeneration in the avian auditory epithelium. *Hear. Res.* 364, 1–11. doi: 10.1016/j.heares.2018.04.008

Li, B., and Dewey, C. N. (2011). RSEM: accurate transcript quantification from RNA-Seq data with or without a reference genome. *BMC Bioinformatics* 12:323. doi: 10.1186/1471-2105-12-323

Liang, J., Wang, D., Renaud, G., Wolfsberg, T. G., Wilson, A. F., and Burgess, S. M. (2012). The stat3/socs3a pathway is a key regulator of hair cell regeneration in zebrafish. [corrected]. *J. Neurosci.* 32, 10662–10673. doi: 10.1523/JNEUROSCI.5785-10.2012

Liu, Z., Dearman, J. A., Cox, B. C., Walters, B. J., Zhang, L., Ayrault, O., et al. (2012). Age-dependent *in vivo* conversion of mouse cochlear pillar and Deiters' cells to immature hair cells by Atoh1 ectopic expression. *J. Neurosci.* 32, 6600–6610. doi: 10.1523/JNEUROSCI.0818-12.2012

Llorens-Bobadilla, E., Zhao, S., Baser, A., Saiz-Castro, G., Zwadlo, K., and Martin-Villalba, A. (2015). Single-cell transcriptomics reveals a population of dormant neural stem cells that become activated upon brain injury. *Cell Stem Cell* 17, 329–340. doi: 10.1016/j.stem.2015.07.002

Love, M. I., Huber, W., and Anders, S. (2014). Moderated estimation of fold change and dispersion for RNA-seq data with DESeq2. *Genome Biol.* 15:550. doi: 10.1186/s13059-014-0550-8

Lukjanenko, L., Karaz, S., Stuelsatz, P., Gurriaran-Rodriguez, U., Michaud, J., Dammone, G., et al. (2019). Aging disrupts muscle stem cell function by impairing matricellular WISP1 secretion from fibro-adipogenic progenitors. *Cell Stem Cell* 24, 433.e7–446.e7. doi: 10.1016/j.stem.2018.12.014

Lush, M. E., Diaz, D. C., Koenecke, N., Baek, S., Boldt, H., St Peter, M.K., et al. (2019). scRNA-Seq reveals distinct stem cell populations that drive hair cell regeneration after loss of Fgf and Notch signaling. *eLife* 8:e44431. doi: 10.7554/eLife.44431

May, L. A., Kramarenko, I. I., Brandon, C. S., Voekel-Johnson, C., Roy, S., Truong, K., et al. (2013). Inner ear supporting cells protect hair cells by secreting HSP70. *J. Clin. Invest.* 123, 3577–3587. doi: 10.1172/JCI68480

Millimaki, B. B., Sweet, E. M., Dhason, M. S., and Riley, B. B. (2007). Zebrafish atoh1 genes: classic proneural activity in the inner ear and regulation by Fgf and Notch. *Development* 134, 295–305. doi: 10.1242/dev.02734

Mizutari, K., Michikawa, T., Saito, H., Okamoto, Y., Enomoto, C., Takebayashi, T., et al. (2013). Age-related hearing loss and the factors determining continued usage of hearing aids among elderly community-dwelling residents. *PLoS One* 8:e73622. doi: 10.1371/journal.pone.0073622

Monzack, E. L., May, L. A., Roy, S., Gale, J. E., and Cunningham, L. L. (2015). Live imaging the phagocytic activity of inner ear supporting cells in response to hair cell death. *Cell Death Differ.* 22, 1995–2005. doi: 10.1038/cdd.2015.48

Mulvaney, J., and Dabdoub, A. (2012). Atoh1, an essential transcription factor in neurogenesis and intestinal and inner ear development: function, regulation and context dependency. *J. Assoc. Res. Otolaryngol.* 13, 281–293. doi: 10.1007/s10162-012-0317-4

Munnamalai, V., and Fekete, D. M. (2016). Notch-Wnt-Bmp crosstalk regulates radial patterning in the mouse cochlea in a spatiotemporal manner. *Development* 143, 4003–4015. doi: 10.1242/dev.139469

Munnamalai, V., Sienknecht, U. J., Duncan, R. K., Scott, M. K., Thawani, A., Fantetti, K. N., et al. (2017). Wnt9a can influence cell fates and neural connectivity across the radial axis of the developing cochlea. *J. Neurosci.* 37, 8975–8988. doi: 10.1523/JNEUROSCI.1554-17.2017

Oesterle, E. C., Campbell, S., Taylor, R. R., Forge, A., and Hume, C. R. (2008). Sox2 and JAGGED1 expression in normal and drug-damaged adult mouse inner ear. *J. Assoc. Res. Otolaryngol.* 9, 65–89. doi: 10.1007/s10162-007-0106-7

Oesterle, E. C., Tuse, T. T., Reh, T. A., and Rubel, E. W. (1993). Hair cell regeneration in organ cultures of the postnatal chicken inner ear. *Hear Res.* 70, 85–108. doi: 10.1016/0378-5955(93)90054-5

Oshima, K., Grimm, C. M., Corrales, C. E., Senn, P., Martinez-Monedero, R., Géléoc, G. S., et al. (2007). Differential distribution of stem cells in the auditory and vestibular organs of the inner ear. *J. Assoc. Res. Otolaryngol.* 8, 18–31. doi: 10.1007/s10162-006-0058-3

Petrovic, J., Formosa-Jordan, P., Luna-Escalante, J. C., Abelló, G., Ibañes, M., Neves, J., et al. (2014). Ligand-dependent Notch signaling strength orchestrates lateral induction and lateral inhibition in the developing inner ear. *Development* 141, 2313–2324. doi: 10.1242/dev.108100

Porter, A. C., Chernajovsky, Y., Dale, T. C., Gilbert, C. S., Stark, G. R., and Kerr, I. M. (1988). Interferon response element of the human gene 6-16. *EMBO J.* 7, 85–92.

Rudolf, M. A., Andreeva, A., Kozlowski, M. M., Kim, C. E., Moskowitz, B. A., Anaya-Rocha, A., et al. (2020). YAP mediates hair cell regeneration in balance organs of chickens, but LATS kinases suppress its activity in mice. *J. Neurosci.* 13, 3915–3932. doi: 10.1523/JNEUROSCI.0306-20.2020

Samarajeewa, A., Jacques, B. E., and Dabdoub, A. (2019). Therapeutic potential of wnt and notch signaling and epigenetic regulation in mammalian sensory hair cell regeneration. *Mol. Ther.* 27, 904–911. doi: 10.1016/j.ymthe.2019.03.017

Samarajeewa, A., Lenz, D. R., Xie, L., Chiang, H., Kirchner, R., Mulvaney, J. F., et al. (2018). Transcriptional response to Wnt activation regulates the regenerative capacity of the mammalian cochlea. *Development* 145:dev166579. doi: 10.1242/dev.166579

Saunders, J. C. (2010). The role of hair cell regeneration in an avian model of inner ear injury and repair from acoustic trauma. *ILAR J.* 51, 326–337. doi: 10.1093/ilar.51.4.326

Saunders, J. C., and Salvi, R. J. (2008). "Recovery of function in the avian auditory system after ototrauma," in *Hair Cell Regeneration, Repair and Protection*, eds R. J. Salvi, A. N. Popper, and R. R. Fay (New York, NY: Springer), 77–116.

Scheibinger, M., Ellwanger, D. C., Corrales, C. E., Stone, J. S., and Heller, S. (2018). Aminoglycoside damage and hair cell regeneration in the chicken utricle. *J. Assoc. Res. Otolaryngol.* 19, 17–29. doi: 10.1007/s10162-017-0646-4

Schimmang, T. (2007). Expression and functions of FGF ligands during early otic development. *Int. J. Dev. Biol.* 51, 473–481. doi: 10.1387/ijdb.072334ts

Shang, J., Cafaro, J., Nehmer, R., and Stone, J. (2010). Supporting cell division is not required for regeneration of auditory hair cells after ototoxic injury *in vitro*. *J. Assoc. Res. Otolaryngol.* 11, 203–222. doi: 10.1007/s10162-009-0206-7

Shu, Y., Li, W., Huang, M., Quan, Y. Z., Scheffer, D., Tian, C., et al. (2019). Renewed proliferation in adult mouse cochlea and regeneration of hair cells. *Nat. Commun.* 10:5530. doi: 10.1038/s41467-019-13157-7

Sienknecht, U. J., and Fekete, D. M. (2008). Comprehensive Wnt-related gene expression during cochlear duct development in chicken. *J. Comp. Neurol.* 510, 378–395. doi: 10.1002/cne.21791

Sinkkonen, S. T., Chai, R., Jan, T. A., Hartman, B. H., Laske, R. D., Gahlen, F., et al. (2011). Intrinsic regenerative potential of murine cochlear supporting cells. *Sci. Rep.* 1:26. doi: 10.1038/srep00026

Stone, J. S., and Cotanche, D. A. (2007). Hair cell regeneration in the avian auditory epithelium. *Int. J. Dev. Biol.* 51, 633–647. doi: 10.1387/ijdb.072408js

Stone, J. S., Leano, S. G., Baker, L. P., and Rubel, E. W. (1996). Hair cell differentiation in chick cochlear epithelium after aminoglycoside toxicity: *in vivo* and *in vitro* observations. *J. Neurosci.* 16, 6157–6174. doi: 10.1523/JNEUROSCI.16-19-06157.1996

Sweet, E. M., Vemaraju, S., and Riley, B. B. (2011). Sox2 and Fgf interact with Atoh1 to promote sensory competence throughout the zebrafish inner ear. *Dev. Biol.* 358, 113–121. doi: 10.1016/j.ydbio.2011.07.019

Thiede, B. R., Mann, Z. F., Chang, W., Ku, Y. C., Son, Y. K., Lovett, M., et al. (2014). Retinoic acid signalling regulates the development of tonotopically patterned hair cells in the chicken cochlea. *Nat. Commun.* 20:3840. doi: 10.1038/ncomms4840

Tona, Y., Hamaguchi, K., Ishikawa, M., Miyoshi, T., Yamamoto, N., Yamahara, K., et al. (2014). Therapeutic potential of a γ-secretase inhibitor for hearing restoration in a guinea pig model with noise-induced hearing loss. *BMC Neurosci.* 15:66. doi: 10.1186/1471-2202-15-66

Trimarchi, J. M., Stadler, M. B., and Cepko, C. L. (2008). Individual retinal progenitor cells display extensive heterogeneity of gene expression. *PLoS One* 3:e1588. doi: 10.1371/journal.pone.0001588

Tripathi, S., Pohl, M. O., Zhou, Y., Rodriguez-Frandsen, A., Wang, G., Stein, D. A., et al. (2015). Meta- and orthogonal integration of influenza "omics" data defines a role for ubr4 in virus budding. *Cell Host Microbe* 18, 723–735. doi: 10.1016/j.chom.2015.11.002

Wan, L., Lovett, M., Warchol, M. E., and Stone, J. S. (2020). Vascular endothelial growth factor is required for regeneration of auditory hair cells in the avian inner ear. *Hear. Res.* 385:107839. doi: 10.1016/j.heares.2019.107839

Warchol, M. E., and Corwin, J. T. (1996). Regenerative proliferation in organ cultures of the avian cochlea: identification of the initial progenitors and determination of the latency of the proliferative response. *J. Neurosci.* 16, 5466–5477. doi: 10.1523/JNEUROSCI.16-17-05466.1996

Warchol, M. E., Schwendener, R. A., and Hirose, K. (2012). Depletion of resident macrophages does not alter sensory regeneration in the avian cochlea. *PLoS One* 7:e51574. doi: 10.1371/journal.pone.0051574

White, P. M., Doetzlhofer, A., Lee, Y. S., Groves, A. K., and Segil, N. (2006). Mammalian cochlear supporting cells can divide and trans-differentiate into hair cells. *Nature* 441, 984–987. doi: 10.1038/nature04849

Yamamoto, N., Tanigaki, K., Tsuji, M., Yabe, D., Ito, J., and Honjo, T. (2006). Inhibition of Notch/RBP-J signaling induces hair cell formation in neonate mouse cochleas. *J. Mol. Med.* 84, 37–45. doi: 10.1007/s00109-005-0706-9

Zheng, J. L., and Gao, W. Q. (2003). Overexpression of Math1 induces robust production of extra hair cells in postnatal rat inner ears. *Nat. Neurosci.* 3, 580–586. doi: 10.1038/75753

Zuo, G. W., Kohls, C. D., He, B. C., Chen, L., Zhang, W., Shi, Q., et al. (2010). The CCN proteins: important signaling mediators in stem cell differentiation and tumorigenesis. *Histol. Histopathol.* 25, 795–806. doi: 10.14670/HH-25.795

15

Transcription Factor Reprogramming in the Inner Ear: Turning on Cell Fate Switches to Regenerate Sensory Hair Cells

*Amrita A. Iyer[1,2] and Andrew K. Groves[1,2,3]**

[1]*Department of Molecular and Human Genetics, Baylor College of Medicine, Houston, TX, United States,* [2]*Program in Genetics & Genomics, Houston, TX, United States,* [3]*Department of Neuroscience, Baylor College of Medicine, Houston, TX, United States*

Correspondence:
Andrew K. Groves
akgroves@bcm.edu

Non-mammalian vertebrates can restore their auditory and vestibular hair cells naturally by triggering the regeneration of adjacent supporting cells. The transcription factor ATOH1 is a key regulator of hair cell development and regeneration in the inner ear. Following the death of hair cells, supporting cells upregulate ATOH1 and give rise to new hair cells. However, in the mature mammalian cochlea, such natural regeneration of hair cells is largely absent. Transcription factor reprogramming has been used in many tissues to convert one cell type into another, with the long-term hope of achieving tissue regeneration. Reprogramming transcription factors work by altering the transcriptomic and epigenetic landscapes in a target cell, resulting in a fate change to the desired cell type. Several studies have shown that ATOH1 is capable of reprogramming cochlear non-sensory tissue into cells resembling hair cells in young animals. However, the reprogramming ability of ATOH1 is lost with age, implying that the potency of individual hair cell-specific transcription factors may be reduced or lost over time by mechanisms that are still not clear. To circumvent this, combinations of key hair cell transcription factors have been used to promote hair cell regeneration in older animals. In this review, we summarize recent findings that have identified and studied these reprogramming factor combinations for hair cell regeneration. Finally, we discuss the important questions that emerge from these findings, particularly the feasibility of therapeutic strategies using reprogramming factors to restore human hearing in the future.

Keywords: transcription factors, reprogramming, pioneer factor, inner ear, hair cell, regeneration

INTRODUCTION

Hearing loss is a globally prevalent disorder characterized by one or a combination of loss of inner ear hair cells, malfunction, or degeneration of components critical to hearing such as the stria vascularis, or loss of spiral ganglion neurons or their synaptic connections with hair cells. In practice, assistive devices such as hearing aids, cochlear implants, and auditory brainstem implants are the only current options available to help manage hearing loss, but these cannot fully restore hearing. Regeneration of inner ear hair cells by supporting cells or other non-sensory cells has been an attractive possibility for hearing restoration since its discovery as a naturally occurring phenomenon in non-mammalian vertebrates (Corwin and Cotanche, 1988; Ryals and Rubel, 1988; Cotanche, 1999). Supporting cells can either directly transdifferentiate or re-enter the cell cycle and divide to yield new hair cells. Since then, efforts to translate this phenomenon to mammals have gained traction, intending to treat human hearing loss.

One of several interventions explored is the ectopic expression of hair cell-specific transcription factors such as ATOH1 to reprogram non-sensory inner ear cells into hair cells. Studies over the past 20 years have shown that ATOH1 successfully reprograms non-sensory cells adjacent to the organ of Corti to form hair cells in the neonatal mouse cochlea, and a small number of studies have reported a similar result in older animals, although at far lower efficiency (Kelly et al., 2012; Lee S. et al., 2020). This age-dependent decline in the reprogramming ability of ATOH1 led to a search for additional transcription factors to reprogram older cochlear cells into hair cells. In this review, we focus on the potential for transcription factor reprogramming in the adult inner ear. We also discuss the potential of different cochlear cell types to serve as reprogramming reservoirs within the mammalian inner ear.

CELLULAR REPROGRAMMING: TOWARDS A PLURIPOTENT CELL FATE

What we now refer to as cellular reprogramming was first demonstrated by John Gurdon through the process of somatic cell nuclear transfer in frogs in the 1950s. His experiments showed that nuclei from tadpole intestinal epithelial cells led to the development of a normal tadpole when transferred to an enucleated egg (Gurdon, 1962). Following this, virus-mediated cell fusion experiments coupled with microsurgical removal of zygotic pronuclei were carried out in mice. When donor nuclei were introduced into enucleated mouse zygotes, the resulting embryos developed comparably normally to those derived from unmanipulated zygotes (McGrath and Solter, 1983). Cloning experiments in sheep demonstrated that donor nuclei from fetal and adult mammary gland cells could produce healthy embryos when transferred into unfertilized eggs (Willadsen, 1986; Wilmut et al., 1997). Though the field lacked a detailed molecular and genetic understanding of reprogramming at that point, these experiments provided definitive evidence for the presence of factors in the egg cytoplasm that were capable of restoring the chromatin of a differentiated cell to something resembling its original pluripotent state (DiBerardino et al., 1984).

Although the experiments described above relied on cytoplasmic factors to elicit reprogramming, the known ability of transcription factors to drive cell fate conversion led to the search for transcription factors that could reprogram differentiated cells back to a pluripotent state. A unique cocktail of transcription factors in pluripotent embryonic stem cells—OCT4, SOX2, KLF4, and C-MYC (designated the OSKM/Yamanaka factors after the laboratory that first identified them)—was demonstrated to reprogram mouse embryonic and adult fibroblasts into a "pre-differentiated" or pluripotent stem cell state (Takahashi and Yamanaka, 2006). The cells that were induced to become pluripotent after reprogramming became known as induced pluripotent stem cells (iPSCs). Cultured iPSCs expressed specific pluripotency markers and possessed embryonic stem cell-like morphology and growth characteristics. When transplanted into immunocompromised nude mice these cells gave rise to cell types from all three germ layers, confirming their pluripotent properties (Takahashi and Yamanaka, 2006). Human iPSCs were generated using the same four OSKM factors by Yamanaka's group the following year (Takahashi et al., 2007).

Another transcription factor combination comprising SOX2, OCT4, NANOG, and LIN28 was discovered to yield "fate irreversible" pluripotent stem cells (in previous cases, most of the iPSCs reverted to their original fate after 2–3 generations) from human dermal fibroblast cells (Yu et al., 2007; Tanabe et al., 2013). Furthermore, it was shown that NKX-3, a transiently expressed homeobox transcription factor endogenously activated OCT4 and was essential for iPSC reprogramming of mouse and human cells (Mai et al., 2018). The addition of small molecules like Valproic acid (VPA), a histone deacetylase (HDAC) inhibitor, together with OSKM factors improved reprogramming efficiency in mouse fibroblasts by 100-fold (Huangfu et al., 2008). The same study showed that VPA was also successful as a replacement for *c-Myc*, an oncogene whose overexpression in iPSCs was a cause of concern due to its potential tumorigenicity. It was then established that a set of seven small-molecule compounds, namely Valproic acid (VPA, an HDAC inhibitor), FSK (Forskolin, an adenylyl cyclase activator), CHIR (Aminopyramidine derivative, a GSK-3 beta inhibitor), 616452 (a TGF-beta receptor inhibitor), Tranyl (a histone demethylation inhibitor), DZNep (adenosine analog, an EZH2 inhibitor) and TTNPB (Retinoic acid analog, a retinoic acid pathway activator) could replace all four transcription factors to successfully reprogram mouse somatic cells into pluripotent stem cells (Hou et al., 2013).

Mechanistic studies in mouse fibroblasts showed that the induction of pluripotency begins with the repression of fibroblast-specific marker genes, followed by the endogenous expression of the transcription factor genes, *Oct4*, *Sox2*, and *Klf4* (OKS) that are sufficient for a self-sustaining pluripotency state, along with the upregulation of telomerase. Exogenous expression of the OKS factors alone was found to enable multiple somatic cell types to reprogram to an iPSC fate (Maherali et al., 2007; Brambrink et al., 2008; Stadtfeld et al., 2008). OCT4 and SOX2 are known to interact with each other cooperatively to activate OCT/SOX-specific enhancers in genes like *Fbx15* and *Nanog* to maintain pluripotency in mouse embryonic stem cells (Tokuzawa et al., 2003; Masui et al., 2007). Further, it was shown experimentally that NANOG recruits RNA polymerase II and promotes the expression of *Esrrb* that is critical for pluripotency fate in multiple cell phases (pre iPSC, partially/incompletely reprogrammed iPSCs, and developing embryonic stem cells) (Festuccia et al., 2012). Interactome studies showed that almost all pluripotency genes lie within the gene regulatory networks of OCT4, SOX2, and NANOG (Wang et al., 2006). The reprogramming mechanisms of C-MYC include the recruitment of several chromatin remodelers (p400, Ini1, Tip48/49), ubiquitin ligases (Fbw7, Skp2), and histone acetyltransferases (Tip60, p300,

GCN5; Adhikary and Eilers, 2005). Within iPSCs, C-MYC predominantly maintains lineage-specific transcription factor genes in a bivalent state (in conjunction with H3K27 methylation marks and the SUZ12 subunit of the PcG repressor complex), altering H3K27 and H3K4 methylation status of target gene promoters for their repression or expression, respectively (Mikkelsen et al., 2007).

iPSC reprogramming is known to suffer from unpredictable and low efficiencies, resulting in heterogeneous populations of iPSCs (Stadtfeld and Hochedlinger, 2010). In human somatic cells, combined single-cell analysis of transcription and chromatin accessibility during reprogramming showed that a switch from gene regulatory networks controlled by FOSL1 to networks regulated by TEAD4 can drive cells towards a pluripotent cell state (Xing et al., 2020). The application of single-cell RNA sequencing and ATAC sequencing to study these reprogrammed heterogenous populations continues to advance our understanding of reprogramming efficiency-associated roadblocks.

The *in vivo* introduction of pluripotency genes adds challenges associated with the negative effects of their genomic integration and continued overexpression. Several pluripotency genes especially *Oct-4*, *Nanog*, *Gdf3*, and *Stella* are known to be expressed in germline tumors (Clark et al., 2004). OCT4 inhibits cellular differentiation resulting in dysplasia of epithelial tissue which supports the notion that a progenitor phase precedes tumorigenesis in adult tissue (Hochedlinger et al., 2005). When applying combinations of reprogramming factors in any tissue, the reprogrammed cell transitions through multiple potential progenitor phases which could lead to malignancy. Recent studies have employed a more transient overexpression model to address tumorigenicity issues. For example, mouse skeletal muscle was regenerated after injury with no tumorigenicity when OSKM factors were transiently overexpressed using plasmids (De Lázaro et al., 2019). Another study showed that transient overexpression of the OSKMLN reprogramming factors through mRNA cocktails improved the progression of aging in progeroid mice (Sarkar et al., 2020). Chromatin remodeling-based modifications for tissue reprogramming through CRISPR/Cas9 targeting have been reviewed recently (Martinez-Redondo and Izpisua Belmonte, 2020). In particular, CRISPR-based strategies devised to have no detectable off-target effects have been proposed for long-term applications (Akcakaya et al., 2018). Incorporating techniques that enhance safety and retain the efficacy of reprogramming is an important consideration when aiming to ultimately treat human disease.

DNA methylation is a heritable epigenetic modifier that controls cell fates. It is promoted by DNA methyltransferases (DNMT1, DNMT3a, DNMT3b) which catalyze the addition of a methyl group to the cytosine residue at specific DNA loci (Hon et al., 2009). DNA methylation at the promoter and enhancer regions of genes prevents the binding of transcription factors, resulting in gene repression (Xie et al., 2013). During the process of differentiation, promoter and enhancer regions of pluripotency genes are hypermethylated as they are down-regulated, allowing for the expression of differentiation genes and the adoption of unique cell fates. Additionally, differential methylation of lineage-specifying gene enhancers results in the production of functionally diverse cell types within the same tissue. For example, a study of adult skin and hematopoietic stem cell differentiation revealed locus-specific methylation changes in different cell types, often associated with the repression in a particular cell type of transcription factors specific for other cell types in that lineage (Bock et al., 2012). Analysis of DNA methylation during reprogramming can be used to identify the fidelity of the reprogramming mechanism—for example, a genome-wide DNA methylation analysis showed that the promoters of *Oct4*, *Nanog*, and *Dnmt3b* were unmethylated in ES cells but partially methylated in iPS cells, providing markers to differentiate between them (Deng et al., 2009). Another study compared the regions of DNA hypo- and hypermethylation between iPSCs and parental fibroblasts to find that complete reprogramming requires extensive DNA methylation alterations (Doi et al., 2009). iPSCs were also found to possess residual DNA methylation marks from the parental cell type with a tendency to re-differentiate (Kim et al., 2010; Polo et al., 2010). Incompletely reprogrammed iPSCs were unable to reactivate pluripotency genes due to persistent hypermethylation of pluripotency gene promoters and incomplete repression of cell type-specific transcription factors (Mikkelsen et al., 2008). Studies of methylation during reprogramming have also been helped by recent advances in sequencing platforms that have enabled the study of cell methylomes at single-nucleotide resolution employing MethylCseq (Lister and Ecker, 2009).

DIRECT CELLULAR REPROGRAMMING: TOWARDS A SPECIFIC CELL FATE

Transcription factors are capable of reprogramming one differentiated cell type into another directly without the need to actively induce an intermediate pluripotent stem cell fate. This process is termed direct cellular reprogramming or direct transdifferentiation. Initial cell fusion experiments between human amniocytes and mouse muscle cells showed activation of a muscle cell-specific genetic program in the resultant heterokaryons (Blau et al., 1983). In mice, ectopic expression of *MyoD* in fibroblasts successfully transdifferentiated them into myoblasts (Davis et al., 1987). Its identification came about through a subtraction-hybridization method for cDNAs of genes differentially expressed in myoblasts and not in the mesodermal stem cell line C3H10T1/2. When *MyoD* cDNA was ectopically expressed in 10T1/2 cells, it resulted in stable clones of myogenic cells that were competent enough to undergo further myogenesis. These early results showed the feasibility of direct reprogramming, and we describe recent examples of this strategy in the following sections.

Recent Attempts at Direct Cellular Reprogramming in the Nervous System, Pancreas, and Heart

Initial attempts to promote direct transdifferentiation of one cell type to another through transcription factor reprogramming used a strategy similar to that used for identifying the OSKM factors—the screening of an initial pool of transcription factors to identify combinations that could promote conversion. In these direct reprogramming efforts, the starting pool of transcription factors was selected based on their known roles in the differentiation of the desired cell type. For example, a transcription factor cocktail comprising ASCL1, BRN2, and MYT1L was identified to be the most efficient for transdifferentiating mouse embryonic and postnatal fibroblasts into induced neurons (Vierbuchen et al., 2010). This combination was identified from a pool of 19 transcription factors implicated in neuronal development. ASCL1, BRN2, and MYT1L in conjunction with NEUROD1 were also able to transdifferentiate human fetal and adult fibroblasts into induced neurons (Pang et al., 2011). Further efforts with different transcription factor combinations were able to generate specific types of neurons. For example, a combination of FOXG1, SOX2, ASCL1, DLX5, and LHX6 transdifferentiated mouse fibroblasts into specific GABAergic neurons (Colasante et al., 2015). ASCL1, BRN3B, ISL1, and SOX4 converted human and mouse embryonic fibroblasts into retinal ganglion cell-like neurons (Wang et al., 2020). Additionally, small molecules and microRNAs have been used to improve the transdifferentiation efficiency of fibroblasts to neurons. For example, porcine fibroblasts were efficiently converted into induced neurons with a combination of transcription factor ASCL1 and microRNAs miR9/9* and miR124 (Habekost et al., 2020). These microRNAs repress the SWI/SNF-like BAF chromatin remodeling complex and enable induced neurons to exit the progenitor state to continue differentiating (Yoo et al., 2011).

Outside the nervous system, directed transdifferentiation has been attempted to produce cell types as part of future regenerative therapies. For example, the generation of insulin-producing pancreatic beta cells has been considered as a treatment option for patients with Type1 diabetes. The transcription factors PDX1, NEUROG3, and MAFA (PNM factors) were identified to be essential during embryonic beta-cell development (reviewed by Zhu et al., 2017). Overexpression of this cocktail through adenoviral gene delivery methods in adult somatic cells of exocrine origin, liver duct, intestine (duodenum, jejunum) and gall bladder epithelium transdifferentiated them into insulin-producing beta cell-like cells (Zhou et al., 2008; Banga et al., 2012, 2014; Hickey et al., 2013; Chen et al., 2014). Moreover, the addition of PAX4 to the PNM factor cocktail transdifferentiated human pancreatic exocrine cells into beta cell-like cells that showed potent glucose-regulating effects when transplanted into diabetic mice (Lima et al., 2016).

In the heart, cardiomyocyte regeneration is a therapeutic option to treat coronary artery disease. A screening approach using cardiomyocyte-specific promoter-driven reporter expression, FACS, and gene expression analysis showed that three transcription factors, GATA4, MEF2C, and TBX5 (GMT factors) transdifferentiated cardiac and dermal fibroblasts into induced cardiomyocytes (Ieda et al., 2010). In human fibroblasts derived from neonatal skin, fetal heart, or embryonic stem cells, the GMT factors plus ESSRG, MESP1, Myocardin, and ZFPM2 enhanced the global expression of cardiac genes and overall transdifferentiation efficiency (Fu et al., 2013).

Mechanisms of Direct Cellular Reprogramming

Transcription factors play a multitude of genetic and epigenetic roles within cells to bring about transdifferentiation. For example, ASCL1, a proneural bHLH transcription factor is known to play the role of an "on target" pioneer factor, meaning it binds directly to all its targets and initiates gene expression by altering chromatin conformation. Alternatively, BRN2 is recruited genome-wide by ASCL1 for binding and expressing proneural genes. MYT1L on the other hand activates gene expression in open chromatin regions by enhancing the H3K27ac and H3K4me status through KMT2B, a methyltransferase (Wapinski et al., 2013; Barbagiovanni et al., 2018). In the case of pancreatic beta-cell regeneration, it was found that PDX1 initiated the pancreatic gene expression program, specification of endocrine lineage, and maturation of beta cells (Holland et al., 2002). NEUROG3 enabled cells to take up an endocrine fate by suppressing exocrine specific genes and MAFA activates insulin expression by binding to a conserved insulin enhancer element RIPE3b/C1-A2 (Matsuoka et al., 2004; Wang et al., 2010). *Mef2c* overexpression in fibroblasts initiates the switching on of genes necessary for the formation of cardiac structures, and synthesis of contractile proteins (Dodou et al., 2004). GATA4 binds to and promotes the acetylation of H3K27 loci of cardiac genes that further results in active chromatin regions especially at the enhancers for transcription (He et al., 2014). TBX5 binds to both GATA4 and MEF2C to form unique pairs that repress non-cardiac genes in both developing and induced cardiomyocytes (Steimle and Moskowitz, 2016).

DNA methylation also plays a role in silencing non-specific gene memory signatures during direct reprogramming. During fibroblast reprogramming into induced neurons, accumulation of mCH and mCG hypermethylation marks serves a repressive function to silence fibroblast and myogenic fates (Luo et al., 2019). In sensory organs such as the retina, DNA methyltransferases (*Dnmt1, Dnmt3a, Dnmt3b*) are expressed in abundance during embryonic ages and co-operate during the formation of photoreceptors and retinal neurons in the mammalian eye (Singh et al., 2017). The expression pattern of DNMTs at postnatal ages reveals their role in the differential remodeling of cell types such as cones and rods (Nasonkin et al., 2011). Conditional knockdown of *Dnmt1* led to the aberrant apicobasal polarity of retinal pigment epithelium and neural retina differentiation (Nasonkin et al., 2013). The DNA methylation status of developing embryonic and post-natal cochlear sensory epithelia of mice has been established through whole-genome bisulfite sequencing (Yizhar-Barnea et al., 2018). In a rat aging model, hypermethylation of Connexin 26 promoter regions resulted in low expression levels and concomitant age-related hearing loss (Wu et al., 2014). Currently, there is no data on DNA methylation studies concerning hair cell reprogramming in the inner ear.

Mechanisms of Direct Cellular Reprogramming by Pioneer Factors

A comparison of individual transcription factors highlight the fact that a select group, namely pioneer factors, has a significantly higher reprogramming ability. Pioneer factors are unique in their interactions with unmarked (no histone modifications), silent chromatin to induce transcription of genes (Zaret and Carroll, 2011; Iwafuchi-Doi and Zaret, 2014, 2016). They do this by recruiting other cofactors (activators or repressors) that by themselves are unable to interact with the silent chromatin (Gualdi et al., 1996; Carroll et al., 2005; Sekiya and Zaret, 2007). The transcription factors OCT4, SOX2, KLF-4, three of the four Yamanaka factors for pluripotency are known pioneer factors (Soufi et al., 2012, 2015). Similarly, ASCL1 in neuronal reprogramming, FOXA2 resulting from Neurogenin-3 regulation during pancreatic beta-cell reprogramming, and GATA4 in cardiac reprogramming are all pioneer factors (Bossard and Zaret, 1998; Ejarque et al., 2013; Wapinski et al., 2013). This suggests that many successful reprogramming factor combinations require pioneer factor activity for efficiently driving and establishing cell fate changes in a target cell type (Morris, 2016). Fine-tuning overexpression strategies while introducing these factors into target cells need to be explored thoroughly for obtaining completely reprogrammed cells.

Selection and Optimization of Transcription Factors for Direct Cellular Reprogramming

A complete understanding of the reprogramming potential of the ~2,000 currently identified transcription factors by testing them individually and in combinations on approximately 250 different cell types would be an arduous trial and error-based experimental ordeal. The development of meticulous computational approaches involving several algorithms, databases, experimental results, and prediction programs (summarized in **Table 1**) have helped identify many "reprogramming factor/s—cell type" pairs for subsequent *in vitro* and *in vivo* testing. Transdifferentiation of multiple cell types like neurons, immune cells, pancreatic beta cells, cardiac muscle cells, and fibroblasts have been promoted for addressing cardiac and neurodegenerative diseases (Graf and Enver, 2009; Vierbuchen et al., 2010; Ladewig et al., 2013; Morris and Daley, 2013; Morris, 2016).

The above examples shed light on the therapeutic applications of reprogramming factor overexpression. Despite all the promising data on reprogramming, there are certain recurrent themes on its limitations that need to be addressed. First, in almost all cases of reprogramming the resultant cells are found to be immature at several levels (all studies summarized above mention this aspect as a caveat). A specific example is that in macrophages obtained from reprogrammed fibroblasts, there is residual fibroblast gene expression, instability, and de-differentiation once the reprogramming factor expression ceases (Feng et al., 2008). Thorough reasoning and analysis into why this may be the case has shed some light on the fact that target cells may pass through a series of intermediate phases during reprogramming (pluripotent, multipotent, and precursor; Bar-Nur et al., 2015; Maza et al., 2015; Morris, 2016). These observations suggest the fidelity of reprogramming factors in truly "direct" cell fate conversions may be improbable, inefficient, and may require the transient acquisition of progenitor or stem cell states for efficient conversion.

Considerations of Direct Cellular Reprogramming in the Inner Ear

In addition to the above considerations that have been discovered during reprogramming studies, the inner ear poses several challenges concerning reprogramming outcomes and their success rates. Employing reprogramming factors to convert iPSCs or fibroblasts *in vitro* into hair cells that may be eventually transplanted, is possible in many tissues where the cellular organization is not paramount, but unlikely to succeed in the inner ear where the precise number and location of sensory cells is crucial to their function, and the mechanical properties of the cochlea. Alternatively, the reprogramming of abundantly available cells that serve as a reservoir within the inner ear tissue, such as supporting cells of the organ of Corti or the adjacent non-sensory cells of the inner and outer sulci may also be attempted. Many non-sensory cell reservoirs exist within the mammalian inner ear and show evidence for their responsiveness to transcription factor-mediated reprogramming into induced hair cells. We discuss these transcription factors and the cell types capable of being reprogrammed in further sections.

TRANSCRIPTIONAL CONTROL OF HAIR CELL REGENERATION IN NON-MAMMALIAN VERTEBRATES

Non-mammalian vertebrates such as fish, birds, and amphibians are known to regenerate hair cells in response to noise or chemical damage, as well as replacing hair cells through physiological turnover under normal, undamaged conditions (Cotanche, 1987; Cruz et al., 1987; Corwin and Cotanche, 1988; Ryals and Rubel, 1988; Lippe et al., 1991; Lombarte et al., 1993; Taylor and Forge, 2005; Smith et al., 2006). This regeneration process can occur by asymmetric division of supporting cells to give rise to hair cells, as well as direct transdifferentiation of supporting cells into hair cells in the absence of cell division (Adler and Raphael, 1996; Roberson et al., 1996; Baird et al., 2000). Zebrafish and chicken are useful non-mammalian vertebrate models to study the inner ear, owing to the conservation of inner ear development genes between these species and mammals (Gates et al., 1999; Barbazuk et al., 2000; Chan et al., 2009). Additionally, delineating the molecular and genetic differences between a regenerating and non-regenerating system may shed light on potential strategies to regenerate hair cells in mammals.

The proneural family of transcription factor genes was found to be important for the generation of neurons, and also cells that differentiated into sensory organs (Ghysen and Dambly-Chaudiere, 1989; Bertrand et al., 2002). bHLH transcription factors include the proneural genes *atoh1*, *neurog1-3*, and *neurod1* (Murre et al., 1989). In zebrafish, the *atoh1* homologs *atoh1a* and *atoh1b* are required for hair cell development

TABLE 1 | Computational approaches developed to predict transcription factor/s (TF) suitable for reprogramming one somatic cell type to another.

No.	Model type	Approach incorporated	Validation status	Reference
1.	Expression reversal based	Data-driven approach. Representation and analysis of gene expression data as gene pairs. Identification of each gene's strength in cell type reversal based on calculated normalizations.	No new experimental validation available	Heinäniemi et al. (2013)
2.	Polycomb repression TF model	A data-driven approach using ChIP seq and RNA seq data. The model predicts that all those TFs strongly polycomb repressed in the source cell and highly expressed in target cells are reprogramming factors for that cell pair.	No new experimental validation available	Davis and Eddy (2013)
3.	TF Cross repression model	The model predicts the reprogramming effect of unique gene set perturbations based on their influence on the stability of cell fate-specific gene networks. No prior knowledge of candidate genes/pathways was considered.	No new experimental validation available	Crespo and del Sol (2013)
4.	Epigenetic landscape mathematical model	Employing 63 cell fates and 1337 TFs from mouse microarray gene expression data, a predictive epigenetic model was built to identify hybrid cell fates, known reprogramming factors, new factors that could reprogram specific cell types.	No new experimental validation available.	Lang et al. (2014)
5.	CellNet	Gene regulatory network-based approach to compare engineered cells to target cells. New reprogramming factors were identified to uncover transitionary cellular programs and enhance the quality of engineered cells to mimic target cells.	CellNet results were tested on the conversion of B cells into macrophages. A new intestinal program was identified and fine-tuned in mouse fibroblasts reprogrammed to hepatic cells.	Morris et al. (2014)
6.	Candidate core TF atlas	An entropy-based method used to identify and build an atlas of candidate core TFs across a range of human cell types.	Results obtained from this model were tested on the conversion of human fibroblasts into induced retinal pigment epithelial-like cells.	D'Alessio et al. (2015)
7.	Mogrify	Integration of gene expression data and regulatory network information to predict reprogramming factors. A method applicable to diverse sets of TFs and cell types.	Results tested on the induction of keratinocytes from dermal fibroblasts, induction of microvascular endothelial cells from keratinocytes.	Rackham et al. (2016) and Ouyang et al. (2019)
8.	Stem cell differentiation model	Exclusive stem cell differentiation factor prediction model based on gene regulatory networks.	Results tested on neural stem cells. Overexpression of RUNX2 and ESR1 reprogrammed neural stem cells to neuronal and astrocyte cell fate, respectively.	Okawa et al. (2016)

(Millimaki et al., 2007). Expression of *atoh1a* in support cells along with disruption of Notch signaling gave rise to supernumerary hair cells that eventually did not survive (Itoh and Chitnis, 2001; Itoh et al., 2003). In addition to *atoh1a*, another proneural factor, *neurod*, was found to be expressed in the zebrafish lateral line. Loss of function of either *atoh1a* or *neurod* resulted in the loss of hair cells (Sarrazin et al., 2006). In the chicken inner ear, ATOH1 is involved in hair cell development and regeneration, just as in zebrafish. Hair cells require sensory lineage specification by SOX2 and subsequent differentiation driven by ATOH1 (Neves et al., 2012). Regeneration of hair cells in the basilar papilla of birds occurs only in the event of hair cell death or damage and occurs by supporting cells transdifferentiating into hair cells, either directly or after re-entering the cell cycle (Tsue et al., 1994). This process is mediated by upregulation of ATOH1 in supporting cells (Cafaro et al., 2007)—for example, 15% of supporting cells labeled by a BrdU pulse given 4 days after deafening expressed ATOH1 within 2 h of the pulse. These early studies confirmed the conservation and importance of ATOH1 homologs in the development and regeneration of vertebrate auditory hair cells.

Independent studies in zebrafish and chicken identified additional factors important for hair cell regeneration. For example, *sox2*, a known pluripotency transcription factor, was shown to be involved in the regulation of hair cell regeneration in zebrafish (Millimaki et al., 2010). Overexpression of a combination of *sox2* and *atoh1a* resulted in an enhanced number of ectopic hair cells in the zebrafish lateral line compared to either one alone (Sweet et al., 2011). A bulk RNA-seq analysis performed on support cells and mantle cells (a stem cell population in the zebrafish lateral line) showed that the Notch and Fgf signaling pathways were significantly downregulated in early hair cell regeneration (Jiang et al., 2014). In chicken, a large-scale gene expression analysis study focusing on identifying differentially expressed genes in regenerating utricles identified 15 transcription factors whose expression correlated with regeneration (Ku et al., 2014). These included functionally unique genes like BTG1 that appear to promote hair cell differentiation but negatively regulate proliferation (Rouault et al., 1992; Rodier et al., 1999), and factors that had not previously been associated with regeneration such as IRF-1 and CITED4. Among highly expressed transcription factors were targets of the Notch signaling pathway, including MAMLD1, RBPJ, the ID family genes (ID1, ID4, ID2), ATOH1, and HEYL (Ku et al., 2014).

HAIR CELL REGENERATION IN MAMMALS

The cochlea of neonatal mammals possesses a limited capacity for spontaneous hair cell regeneration in response to hair cell death. Newborn mouse supporting cells respond to signals from dying hair cells and regenerate new hair cells through mitotic division or direct transdifferentiation (Cox et al., 2014). Mechanistic studies have shown Wnt, Notch, and ERBB2 signaling pathways to be essential for spontaneous hair cell regeneration in neonatal mice (Hu et al., 2016; Ni et al., 2016; Zhang et al., 2018). Specific manipulations involving these signaling pathways have been explored for mammalian hair cell regeneration. For example, Wnt pathway activation or Beta-catenin overexpression led to the proliferation of hair cell progenitors that differentiated eventually into hair cells (Chai et al., 2012; Shi et al., 2014). Inhibition of the Notch pathway is known to upregulate ATOH1 in neonatal supporting cells, enabling their transdifferentiation into hair cells (Korrapati et al., 2013; Mizutari et al., 2013). Although such attempts were successful in regenerating hair cells in young, pre-hearing animals, their ability to achieve similar results in older animals failed. To regenerate hair cells in older animals, the overexpression of transcription factors to reprogram nonsensory inner ear cells into hair cells is a promising approach. We discuss a variety of non-sensory cell types that are potential targets for reprogramming in the mammalian cochlea.

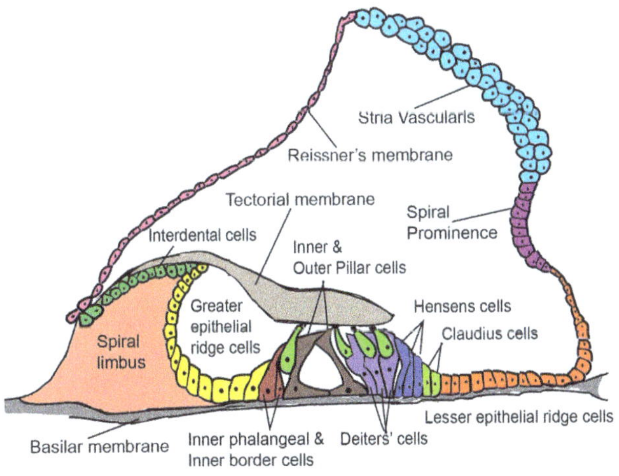

FIGURE 1 | Schematic cross-sectional view of the postnatal mammalian organ of Corti, denoting some structural features and a variety of cell types of interest for *in vivo* hair cell reprogramming.

Inner Ear Non-sensory Cells: Potential Targets for Transcription Factor Reprogramming

The various non-sensory cell types of the mammalian cochlea are indicated in **Figure 1**. Supporting cells lie adjacent to hair cells in the organ of Corti and are the most suitable for hair cell regeneration through transcription factor reprogramming. Developmentally, supporting cells and hair cells arise from common progenitors in the sensory patch of the cochlea. The differentiation and patterning of the two cell types are influenced by the expression of several genes and signaling pathway members, such as Notch signaling (reviewed by Basch et al., 2016). Supporting cells are broadly classified into inner border cells, inner phalangeal cells, pillar cells (inner and outer), Hensen cells, Deiters' cells, and Claudius cells (Raphael and Altschuler, 2003). Previous studies have shown that supporting cell-specific damage results in the regeneration of inner border and phalangeal cells but not pillar or Deiters' cells in neonatal mice (Mellado Lagarde et al., 2013, 2014).

Greater epithelial ridge (GER) cells are columnar cells lying adjacent to the inner hair cell layer of the organ of Corti. They are a transient population of cells occurring in neonatal animals and undergo thyroid hormone-dependent remodeling between 1 and 2 weeks of age (Sharlin et al., 2011; Peeters et al., 2015). This remodeling involving programmed cell death and cell shape changes, creates the inner sulcus, a cavity filled with short cuboidal epithelial cells that promote free movement of hair cell stereocilia against the tectorial membrane during sound transduction (Hinojosa, 1977; Kamiya et al., 2001). The physiological plasticity of GER cells that enable their remodeling into the inner sulcus has also been exploited to regenerate hair cells through the ectopic expression of *Atoh1* in the neonatal mouse cochlea (Kelly et al., 2012), which we discuss further below.

Interdental cells are present medial to the GER region and are the point of attachment for the tectorial membrane. The interdental cells secrete components of the tectorial membrane matrix and are involved in K^+ recycling for hair cell function (Lim, 1972; Spicer et al., 1999). Lesser epithelial ridge (LER) cells lie adjacent to the outer hair cells, comprise the Hensen's and Claudius supporting cell types, are lateral to the organ of Corti, and eventually form the outer sulcus region. When *Atoh1* is induced in cochlear LER cells *in vitro*, they differentiate into hair cell-like cells (Zhai et al., 2005). Interestingly, the GER, LER, and interdental cells arise from the same pool of *Eya1*$^+$ multipotent progenitors that give rise to hair cells and supporting cells during inner ear development (Xu et al., 2017). Currently, there are no *in vivo* reprogramming attempts targeting the LER and interdental cells for hair cell regeneration.

ATOH1–Inner Ear Development, Context-Dependence, and Reprogramming

The mammalian inner ear is derived from an ectodermal thickening named the otic placode, developing on either side of the embryonic hindbrain. The transient expression of the *Sox2* transcription factor in a specific population of cells in the cochlear duct marks the prosensory domain followed by the expression of *p27kip1* that drives sensory cells to become post-mitotic (Lee, 2006). The ATOH1 transcription factor is then expressed in a cluster of prosensory cells and a hair cell differentiation program is initiated (Bermingham et al., 1999; Woods et al., 2004; Driver et al., 2013). Simultaneously, the expression of Notch ligands is induced in these nascent hair cells, thereby inhibiting a hair cell fate in adjacent cells through lateral inhibition (Lanford et al., 1999; Kiernan et al., 2005). The *Atoh1* promoter regions in these adjacent cells undergo rapid repression through induction of Hes/Hey genes, causing them to adopt a supporting cell fate (Abdolazimi et al., 2016). Three-dimensional live imaging of ATOH1 activity in cochlear explants showed that hair cell induction occurs with the formation of inner hair cells (medial) followed by that of outer hair cells (lateral) (Tateya et al., 2019). In mammals, hair cell differentiation starts near the base and ends at the apex of the cochlea. After this initial developmental phase, ATOH1 is also necessary for the survival and proper function of hair cells (Pan et al., 2012; Cai et al., 2013; Chonko et al., 2013).

ATOH1 plays the most important role in hair cell fate specification, implicating it as a master regulator (a single factor determining a unique cell fate). ATOH1 independently recognizes and binds to specific E-box motifs in the promoter and enhancer regions of its targets (Powell et al., 2008). However, the set of targets it regulates is variable between ATOH1-expressing cell types, implying that ATOH1 acts in a context-dependent fashion to promote cellular differentiation. Transcriptomic characterization of neonatal hair cells has identified hair cell-specific ATOH1 target genes of which a small number overlap with those found in ChIP-seq data from the cerebellum and intestine (Cai et al., 2015). Several mechanisms may promote the specificity of ATOH1's targets in hair cells. First, the transient expression of *Sox2*, a pioneer factor ahead of *Atoh1* which is unique to hair cell differentiation, results in a changing chromatin landscape enhancing chromatin accessibility for ATOH1 to bind to its targets in hair cell progenitors (Kempfle et al., 2016). Second, differential control of ATOH1 activity through the phosphorylation of a serine moiety in its bHLH domain which acts as a switch to control ATOH1's DNA binding ability in a variable manner across tissues (Quan et al., 2016; Xie et al., 2017). Third, within the inner ear hair cells, ATOH1's expression is tightly temporally regulated by a series of histone modifications of its promoter and enhancer regions H3K4me3/H3K27me3, H3K9ac and H3K9me3. These marks enable ATOH1 to rapidly and dynamically transition from a poised to an active state during hair cell specification, and to render the ATOH1 locus in a repressive state postnatally in supporting cells (Stojanova et al., 2015).

The importance of *Atoh1*'s expression in hair cell development made it an excellent candidate for reprogramming to promote hair cell regeneration. *Atoh1* overexpression in postnatal cochlear and utricle explants from rat inner ears transdifferentiated nonsensory cells into ectopic hair cells (Zheng and Gao, 2000; Shou et al., 2003). Mouse embryonic stem cells transdifferentiated *in vitro* into hair cell-like cells (expressing cochlear hair cell markers) in response to ectopic expression of *Atoh1* (Ouji et al., 2013). A transcriptomic study showed that induced multipotent otic progenitors showed a profound "pro hair cell" effect compared to mouse embryonic stem cells in response to *Atoh1* overexpression (Ebeid et al., 2017). Early *in vivo* ATOH1 gene therapy studies employing adenoviral gene delivery methods in normal and deafened adult guinea pig cochleae showed regeneration of hair cells and improvement of hearing thresholds (Kawamoto et al., 2003; Izumikawa et al., 2005). However, these studies also highlight several confounding aspects, such as tissue damage in response to viral inoculation into the endolymph. Initial *in vivo* studies in the neonatal mouse cochlea, which investigated the effect of ATOH1 on reprogramming non-sensory cells into hair cells, employed transgenic mice harboring an inducible *Atoh1* transgene. Histological analysis post-overexpression showed that the greater epithelial ridge cells, as well as a small percentage of pillar and Deiters' cells, could be reprogrammed to hair cells (Kelly et al., 2012; Liu et al., 2012). Among supporting cells, the efficiency of ATOH1 reprogramming was much better when targeted to the inner phalangeal and border cells in the neonatal mouse cochlea, but virtually non-existent in Deiters' or pillar cells. The ectopic hair cells expressed several hair cell-specific markers and showed minimal synaptic density (Liu et al., 2014). However, the competence of these cells to become hair cells in response to ATOH1 alone declined rapidly with age, challenging the feasibility of employing this strategy for hair cell regeneration in older animals (Kelly et al., 2012; Liu et al., 2012). This prompted the search for other transcription factors in addition to ATOH1 that could enhance reprogramming efficiency for auditory hair cell regeneration, by analogy to the direct reprogramming studies in other tissues that we described earlier in the review.

Hair Cell Reprogramming Strategies Employing ATOH1 in Combination With Other Reprogramming Partners

ATOH1 and POU4F3

The POU-IV domain transcription factor, POU4F3 (also BRN-3C) is a downstream target of ATOH1 and is induced after the onset of *Atoh1* expression in inner ear hair cells [validated computationally and through ChIP experiments by Masuda et al. (2011, 2012)]. ATOH1 regulates *Pou4f3* expression synergistically with GATA3, MYC, and TFE2 (Ikeda et al., 2015). POU4F3 plays a major role in the maturation and survival of hair cells (Xiang et al., 1998). Deletion of *Pou4f3* in the mouse inner ear leads to severe morphological deficits and apoptosis of hair cells (Xiang et al., 1997, 1998). A combination of ATOH1, POU4F3, and GATA3 was able to reprogram mature supporting cells into hair cell-like cells in the adult cochlea. This study also provided evidence for the *p27kip1* gene playing a critical role in preventing ATOH1 mediated transdifferentiation of supporting cells by down-regulating GATA3 in mature cochlear supporting cells (Walters et al., 2017), although whether the P27 protein is functioning in this context as a cyclin-dependent kinase inhibitor or mediating an additional function is not clear.

ATOH1 and GFI1

GFI1 (Growth factor independent 1) is a zinc-finger transcription factor expressed in hair cells and cochlear neurons during development (Wallis et al., 2003). Loss of function studies in mice has shown that GFI1 does not disrupt hair cell specification but affects later-stage morphology and survival of hair cells. In *Gfi1* null mice, outer hair cells followed by inner hair cells undergo apoptosis that is complete by 2 weeks of age, although vestibular hair cells survive, albeit in an abnormal condition (Wallis et al., 2003; Hertzano et al., 2004). An *in vivo* translatome analysis performed using *Gfi1Cre;RiboTag* mice showed that in the absence of GFI1, neuronal fate genes such as *Pou4f1* were upregulated in hair cells (Matern et al., 2020). Hence, GFI1 may play a dual role in fine-tuning hair cell differentiation by repressing non-hair cell genes (particularly neuronal genes), in addition to enabling the expression of hair cell-specific genes. *In vivo* studies employing a hair cell damage model (*Pou4f3DTR*) in adult mice showed that adenoviral delivery of ATOH1 and GFI1 together post hair cell ablation in the organ of Corti led to the transdifferentiation of supporting cells to give rise to hair cells at a significantly higher efficiency than ATOH1 alone (Lee S. et al., 2020).

ATOH1 and ISL1

Islet-1 (ISL1) is a LIM domain transcription factor and like ATOH1, ISL1 behaves in a context-dependent manner in neuronal and non-neuronal tissue types (Hobert and Westphal, 2000). It is an early marker of both the prosensory domain and spiral ganglion neuron in the developing otic placode (Radde-Gallwitz et al., 2004; Huang et al., 2013), but is also expressed transiently in hair cells (Cai et al., 2015). Early overexpression of *Isl1* in the inner ear results in an age-related hearing loss phenotype in mice (Chumak et al., 2016). However, overexpression of *Isl1* in postnatal mouse cochlear hair cells specifically protects them from damage due to age or noise with no functional anomaly (Huang et al., 2013). Ectopic co-expression of both *Atoh1* and *Isl1* in neonatal cochlear explants *in vitro* and neonatal mice *in vivo* resulted in a significantly higher number of reprogrammed hair cells as compared to overexpression of *Atoh1* alone (Yamashita et al., 2018).

ATOH1, GFI1, and POU4F3

In vitro studies in mouse embryonic stem cells and chick otic epithelial cells showed that overexpressing *Atoh1* alone drove them to adopt a neuronal fate (Costa et al., 2015). In contrast, a combination of ATOH1, POU4F3, and GFI1 induced many hair cell genes when misexpressed in mouse embryonic stem cells. These induced hair cells expressed characteristic markers, possessed hair bundle-like projections and their transcriptome indicated elements of a hair cell signature (Costa et al., 2015). The GAP factors together with another transcription factor, SIX1, reprogrammed mouse embryonic fibroblasts and adult tail-tip fibroblasts *in vitro* into induced hair cells. In addition to what was seen in the previous study, these induced hair cells possessed a hair cell-like epigenetic profile, electrophysiological properties, expression of transduction channel proteins, and sensitivity to ototoxins (Menendez et al., 2020).

Thoughts on Additional Reprogramming Factors—SOX2, GATA3, EYA1, and SIX1

In addition to the above reprogramming factor combinations, SOX2, GATA3, EYA1, and SIX1 are additional reprogramming factor candidates whose combinatorial overexpression shows promise to induce hair cells, based on their expression pattern and co-operativity. For example, analysis of open chromatin regions of prosensory cells indicated that binding sites for SOX2, GATA3, and SIX1 were highly enriched, implying these genes play a critical downstream role for hair cell differentiation (Wilkerson et al., 2019). The transient expression of SOX2 preceding ATOH1's hair cell specification role is governed by the activity of SIX1 that in turn downregulates SOX2 (Zhang et al., 2017). SIX1 was found to be a hair cell selector gene that governs the sequence of events for hair cell differentiation. It does so by occupying enhancer regions of its target genes which are transcribed, and physically interacting and synergizing with the GFI1, ATOH1, and POU4F3 factors and GATA3 (Li et al., 2020). The interaction of EYA1 and SIX1 is necessary in addition to SOX2 expression for the induction of ATOH1 in the developing mouse cochlea (Ahmed et al., 2012). *In vivo* analysis of GATA3's role in the prosensory domain indicate its involvement in *Atoh1* upregulation and spiral ganglion neuron development (Duncan and Fritzsch, 2013). These factors have the potential to supplement the GFI1/ATOH1/POU4F3 factors and thereby enable fine-tuning of hair cell reprogramming efficiency.

CONCLUSION AND FUTURE PERSPECTIVES

Successful reprogramming of non-sensory cells into hair cells (summarized in **Figure 2**) in the mammalian inner ear is a promising approach to restore auditory function. Reprogramming factors that have been shown to drive cells towards a hair cell fate when overexpressed together include ATOH1, GFI1, POU4F3, and SIX1. Selective inclusion of other factors and perturbations of critical pathways like Notch, Wnt, and Fgf signaling may be necessary, in addition to epigenetic remodeling of the target cell population to make their chromatin more accessible to reprogramming factors. There is a good chance that an optimal reprogramming factor code may differ slightly between different "starter" cell types that have to be reprogrammed into hair cells. Supporting cells remain the target cells of choice for reprogramming based on their proximity to hair cells. However, just as in non-mammalian vertebrates, replacement of the reprogrammed supporting cells will be necessary to preserve normal cochlear mechanics. We discuss these, some additional questions, and the challenges of hair cell reprogramming below.

To What Extent Are Reprogrammed Hair Cells Functional, and Can They Restore Function in the Damaged Auditory or Vestibular System?

Most reprogramming studies to date have evaluated the reprogramming outcome primarily from a genetic and protein expression perspective with less focus on hair cells, and overall auditory or vestibular function. Testing the mechanotransduction ability of reprogrammed hair cells through electrophysiological studies is an important assay for individual reprogrammed hair cell function. Moreover, it is also essential to evaluate the higher-order functional consequences of reprogramming through audiological and/or vestibular testing. In this regard, it is notable that regenerative reprogramming of vestibular hair cells in the mouse utricle has recently been shown to restore aspects of vestibular function over several months (Sayyid et al., 2019).

For How Long Do Reprogrammed Cells Survive, and Are They a Long-Term Solution to Hearing or Balance Defects?

The survival and maturation of reprogrammed hair cells are necessary for long-term auditory function. From prior studies and our unpublished data, we know that reprogrammed hair cells derived from supporting cells and GER cells do not survive for more than a few weeks *in vivo* in the mammalian cochlea. Even within this time frame, reprogrammed hair cells lack certain intricate developmental features like planar cell polarity and frequency tuning properties, as seen by the haphazard, non-directional stereocilia arrangement, which could be due to defects in individual cells, or disorganization caused by excess hair cell production (Kelly et al., 2012). Future reprogramming studies need to focus on maximizing the extent of hair cell maturation and survival to aim for long-term function. A striking example of the consequences of suboptimal hair cell differentiation on survival was recently observed in mice carrying a single point mutation of *Atoh1*. The Atoh1S193A variant in the bHLH domain does not appear to affect transcription in reporter assays, yet this mutation causes progressive cochlear hair cell degeneration (Xie et al., 2017).

Can Reprogramming Generate Hair Cell Subtypes?

Hair cells can be divided broadly into inner and outer hair cells of the auditory system, and type I and II hair cells in the vestibular system. Moreover, regional differences are known to exist in a given inner ear sensory organ, such as the significant differences in cell and hair bundle size along the tonotopic axis of the cochlea. At present, it is not clear when each type of hair cell is specified, what signals are responsible for subtype specification, and whether current reprogramming cocktails favor one hair cell subtype over another, as has been seen with current protocols that generate largely vestibular hair cells in embryonic stem cell- or iPS cell-derived organoids (Longworth-Mills et al., 2016; Koehler et al., 2017). There may be a need for other reprogramming factors that will play a "subtype specification" role. For example, INSM1 is a zinc finger transcription factor family member unique in expression to outer hair cells of the mammalian cochlea (Lorenzen et al., 2015). *Insm1* deletion in the neonatal cochlea leads to the expression of inner hair cell-specific genes in outer hair cells (Wiwatpanit et al., 2018). Similarly, IKZF2/Helios is another outer hair cell transcription factor whose overexpression upregulates outer hair cell-specific genes and confers electromotility characteristics to target cells (Chessum et al., 2018). In the vestibular system, EMX2 is a transcription factor known for its role in controlling hair bundle orientation across the line of polarity reversal in the mouse utricle (Jiang et al., 2017).

Will Prolonged Overexpression of Reprogramming Factors Pose Long-Term Challenges Post Hair Cell Reprogramming?

During the development of the mouse organ of Corti, the expression of some hair cell transcription factors such as ATOH1 are transient, and some are present in progenitor cells before restricting to hair cells. Current *in vivo* hair cell reprogramming strategies generally drive constant expression of reprogramming factors, and so it is possible that the persistence of factors whose expression is normally downregulated in hair cells may compromise their mature function or may hold the reprogrammed hair cells in a permanently immature state. More studies are required to determine whether this will impede regeneration driven by reprogramming. Recent advances in the delivery of encapsulated RNA or DNA editing molecules or fusion of proteins to cell-penetrating peptides may offer a way to transiently deliver reprogramming factors to the ear (Takeda et al., 2016; Gao et al., 2018).

What Are the Consequences of Losing Reprogrammed Cells as They Convert Into Hair Cells?

Inner border and inner phalangeal cells lie adjacent to inner hair cells and exhibit higher plasticity towards reprogramming

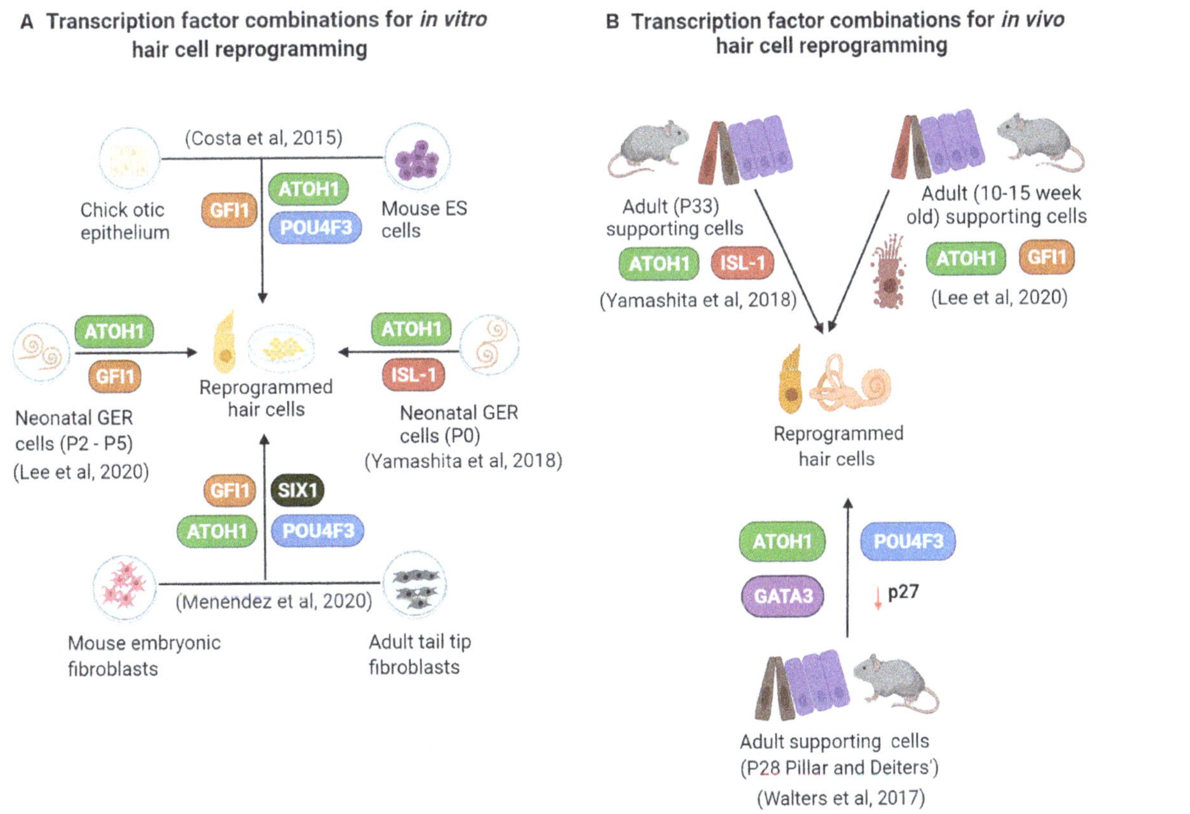

FIGURE 2 | A summary of some current *in vitro* **(A)** and *in vivo* **(B)** reprogramming studies employing overexpression of different transcription factor combinations.

as opposed to Hensen cells, Deiters' cells, and Claudius cells that lie adjacent to outer hair cells (Liu et al., 2014; **Figure 1**). The question of why some supporting cells are harder to reprogram as compared to others, even in early postnatal ages remains unanswered. Nevertheless, supporting cell reprogramming is the most optimal regeneration strategy given their physical proximity to hair cells. However, the loss of supporting cells by transdifferentiation without supporting cell division will pose a challenge for the hearing function, as studies have shown that supporting cell loss disrupts auditory function (reviewed by Wan et al., 2013). Similarly, the timely remodeling of GER cells into the inner sulcus is another critical event that ensures correct auditory function, and any change in GER remodeling may affect hearing directly (Peeters et al., 2015). So, evaluating the long-term loss of these cell types and/or considerations to regenerate these cells is essential.

How Efficient Is the Reprogramming Process From the Perspective of Upregulated Hair Cell Gene Regulatory Networks and Silenced Target Cell Gene Networks?

Detailed gene expression and gene regulatory network analyses are necessary to fully understand the reprogramming efficiency of a transcription factor cocktail as a target cell transitions from its original fate to a specific final fate. For example, single-cell mapping studies for delineating cell reprogramming identity and lineage (Biddy et al., 2018). However, the complexity of the reprogramming process and the fact that it is influenced by variables such as age and epigenetic state make this testing more challenging in comparison to the functional studies required above. Epigenetic landscapes of both the target cell and the reprogrammed cell are controlled by specific transcription factor combinations used in reprogramming. As mentioned earlier, cell types respond more completely to reprogramming when a pioneer factor is overexpressed along with other transcription factors (Morris, 2016). A detailed understanding of how pioneer factors like POU4F3 and SOX2 alter the epigenetic landscapes of the target cell towards that of hair cells can be determined through ATAC sequencing experiments. With the advent of newer high-throughput technologies and bioinformatics pipelines, addressing reprogramming efficiency will become more tractable in the future, leading to better strategies to drive reprogramming and regeneration in the inner ear.

What is the Best *In vivo* Gene Delivery Strategy for Hair Cell Reprogramming Employing Transcription Factors?

The application of reprogramming factors as a therapeutic strategy for hair cell regeneration requires optimal gene delivery *in vivo*. Like the retina, the inner ear is an attractive tissue for targeted therapies as it is relatively well-enclosed and isolated from the central nervous system and circulatory system. For inner ear-specific therapies, various anatomical routes have been tested, including approaches through the posterior semicircular canal, round window, and cochleostomy (reviewed by Ahmed et al., 2017). Non-viral methods of gene delivery through cationic lipid nanoparticles (to deliver Cas9 guide RNA lipid complexes specific for *Tmc1* allele) have been successful in reducing hearing loss in mice (Gao et al., 2018). Other modes of delivering genes, proteins, drugs, and siRNAs molecules include hydrogel encapsulation, exosomes, PLGA nanoparticles, and supra-particles (reviewed in Ma et al., 2019). The limitation of these unique delivery systems is that not all regions of the inner ear can be accessed and that restricts the scope of its application for treatment. However, the transient nature of these treatments may reduce the potential negative consequences of over-expressing transcription factors for extended periods.

Gene delivery through viral methods includes the use of adenovirus, adeno-associated-virus, lentivirus, and exosome-associated adenoviruses. Studies in animal models have shown that adeno-associated viruses are effective in targeting hair cells for hearing loss gene therapy (Landegger et al., 2017; Akil et al., 2019; Isgrig et al., 2019; Nist-Lund et al., 2019). AAVs were found to have low overall toxicity due to minimal immune response to it by the host and low rate of host genome integration (Nakai et al., 2001). Genetically engineered and improvised AAV9-PHP.B was found to be efficient for targeting hair cells in the organ of Corti in mice and primates (György et al., 2019; Lee J. et al., 2020). Though not tested directly, similar technologies will likely be effective in targeting non-sensory and supporting cells for hair cell reprogramming.

AUTHOR CONTRIBUTIONS

Both authors wrote and edited the manuscript. AI prepared the figures. All authors contributed to the article and approved the submitted version.

ACKNOWLEDGMENTS

We thank Ms. Abhinaya Anand and BioRender.com for helping create the illustrations for this review.

REFERENCES

Abdolazimi, Y., Stojanova, Z., and Segil, N. (2016). Selection of cell fate in the organ of Corti involves the integration of Hes/Hey signaling at the Atoh1 promoter. *Development* 143, 841–850. doi: 10.1242/dev.129320

Adhikary, S., and Eilers, M. (2005). Transcriptional regulation and transformation by Myc proteins. *Nat. Rev. Mol. Cell Biol.* 6, 635–645. doi: 10.1038/nrm1703

Adler, H. J., and Raphael, Y. (1996). New hair cells arise from supporting cell conversion in the acoustically damaged chick inner ear. *Neurosci. Lett.* 205, 17–20. doi: 10.1016/0304-3940(96)12367-3

Ahmed, H., Shubina-Oleinik, O., and Holt, J. R. (2017). Emerging gene therapies for genetic hearing loss. *J. Assoc. Res. Otolaryngol.* 18, 649–670. doi: 10.1007/s10162-017-0634-8

Ahmed, M., Wong, E. Y. M., Sun, J., Xu, J., Wang, F., and Xu, P.-X. (2012). Eya1-Six1 interaction is sufficient to induce hair cell fate in the cochlea by activating Atoh1 expression in cooperation with Sox2. *Dev. Cell* 22, 377–390. doi: 10.1016/j.devcel.2011.12.006

Akcakaya, P., Bobbin, M. L., Guo, J. A., Malagon-Lopez, J., Clement, K., Garcia, S. P., et al. (2018). *in vivo* CRISPR editing with no detectable genome-wide off-target mutations. *Nature* 561, 416–419. doi: 10.1038/s41586-018-0500-9

Akil, O., Dyka, F., Calvet, C., Emptoz, A., Lahlou, G., Nouaille, S., et al. (2019). Dual AAV-mediated gene therapy restores hearing in a DFNB9 mouse model. *Proc. Natl. Acad. Sci. U S A* 116, 4496–4501. doi: 10.1073/pnas.1817537116

Baird, R. A., Burton, M. D., Fashena, D. S., and Naeger, R. A. (2000). Hair cell recovery in mitotically blocked cultures of the bullfrog saccule. *Proc. Natl. Acad. Sci. U S A* 97, 11722–11729. doi: 10.1073/pnas.97.22.11722

Banga, A., Akinci, E., Greder, L. V., Dutton, J. R., and Slack, J. M. W. (2012). *in vivo* reprogramming of Sox9+ cells in the liver to insulin-secreting ducts. *Proc. Natl. Acad. Sci. U S A* 109, 15336–15341. doi: 10.1073/pnas.1201701109

Banga, A., Greder, L. V., Dutton, J. R., and Slack, J. M. W. (2014). Stable insulin-secreting ducts formed by reprogramming of cells in the liver using a three-gene cocktail and a PPAR agonist. *Gene Ther.* 21, 19–27. doi: 10.1038/gt.2013.50

Barbagiovanni, G., Germain, P.-L., Zech, M., Atashpaz, S., Lo Riso, P., D'Antonio-Chronowska, A., et al. (2018). KMT2B is selectively required for neuronal transdifferentiation and its loss exposes dystonia candidate genes. *Cell Rep.* 25, 988–1001. doi: 10.1016/j.celrep.2018.09.067

Barbazuk, W. B., Korf, I., Kadavi, C., Heyen, J., Tate, S., Wun, E., et al. (2000). The syntenic relationship of the zebrafish and human genomes. *Genome Res.* 10, 1351–1358. doi: 10.1101/gr.144700

Bar-Nur, O., Verheul, C., Sommer, A. G., Brumbaugh, J., Schwarz, B. A., Lipchina, I., et al. (2015). Lineage conversion induced by pluripotency factors involves transient passage through an iPSC stage. *Nat. Biotechnol.* 33, 761–768. doi: 10.1038/nbt.3247

Basch, M. L., Brown, R. M. II., Jen, H.-I., and Groves, A. K. (2016). Where hearing starts: the development of the mammalian cochlea. *J. Anat.* 228, 233–254. doi: 10.1111/joa.12314

Bermingham, N. A., Hassan, B. A., Price, S. D., Vollrath, M. A., Ben-Arie, N., Eatock, R. A., et al. (1999). Math1: an essential gene for the generation of inner ear hair cells. *Science* 284, 1837–1841. doi: 10.1126/science.284.5421.1837

Bertrand, N., Castro, D. S., and Guillemot, F. (2002). Proneural genes and the specification of neural cell types. *Nat. Rev. Neurosci.* 3, 517–530. doi: 10.1038/nrn874

Biddy, B. A., Kong, W., Kamimoto, K., Guo, C., Waye, S. E., Sun, T., et al. (2018). Single-cell mapping of lineage and identity in direct reprogramming. *Nature* 564, 219–224. doi: 10.1038/s41586-018-0744-4

Blau, H. M., Chiu, C.-P., and Webster, C. (1983). Cytoplasmic activation of human nuclear genes in stable heterocaryons. *Cell* 32, 1171–1180. doi: 10.1016/0092-8674(83)90300-8

Bock, C., Beerman, I., Lien, W.-H., Smith, Z. D., Gu, H., Boyle, P., et al. (2012). DNA methylation dynamics during *in vivo* differentiation of blood and skin stem cells. *Mol. Cell* 47, 633–647. doi: 10.1016/j.molcel.2012.06.019

Bossard, P., and Zaret, K. S. (1998). GATA transcription factors as potentiators of gut endoderm differentiation. *Development* 125, 4909–4917.

Brambrink, T., Foreman, R., Welstead, G. G., Lengner, C. J., Wernig, M., Suh, H., et al. (2008). Sequential expression of pluripotency markers during direct reprogramming of mouse somatic cells. *Cell Stem Cell* 2, 151–159. doi: 10.1016/j.stem.2008.01.004

Cafaro, J., Lee, G. S., and Stone, J. S. (2007). Atoh1 expression defines activated progenitors and differentiating hair cells during avian hair cell regeneration. *Dev. Dyn.* 236, 156–170. doi: 10.1002/dvdy.21023

Cai, T., Jen, H.-I., Kang, H., Klisch, T. J., Zoghbi, H. Y., and Groves, A. K. (2015). Characterization of the transcriptome of nascent hair cells and identification of direct targets of the atoh1 transcription factor. *J. Neurosci.* 35, 5870–5883. doi: 10.1523/JNEUROSCI.5083-14.2015

Cai, T., Seymour, M. L., Zhang, H., Pereira, F. A., and Groves, A. K. (2013). Conditional deletion of Atoh1 reveals distinct critical periods for survival and function of hair cells in the organ of Corti. *J. Neurosci.* 33, 10110–10122. doi: 10.1523/JNEUROSCI.5606-12.2013

Carroll, J. S., Liu, X. S., Brodsky, A. S., Li, W., Meyer, C. A., Szary, A. J., et al. (2005). Chromosome-wide mapping of estrogen receptor binding reveals long-range regulation requiring the forkhead protein FoxA1. *Cell* 122, 33–43. doi: 10.1016/j.cell.2005.05.008

Chai, R., Kuo, B., Wang, T., Liaw, E. J., Xia, A., Jan, T. A., et al. (2012). Wnt signaling induces proliferation of sensory precursors in the postnatal mouse cochlea. *Proc. Natl. Acad. Sci. U S A* 109, 8167–8172. doi: 10.1073/pnas.1202774109

Chan, E. T., Quon, G. T., Chua, G., Babak, T., Trochesset, M., Zirngibl, R. A., et al. (2009). Conservation of core gene expression in vertebrate tissues. *J. Biol.* 8:33. doi: 10.1186/jbiol130

Chen, Y.-J., Finkbeiner, S. R., Weinblatt, D., Emmett, M. J., Tameire, F., Yousefi, M., et al. (2014). De novo formation of insulin-producing "neo-β cell islets" from intestinal crypts. *Cell Rep.* 6, 1046–1058. doi: 10.1016/j.celrep.2014.02.013

Chessum, L., Matern, M. S., Kelly, M. C., Johnson, S. L., Ogawa, Y., Milon, B., et al. (2018). Helios is a key transcriptional regulator of outer hair cell maturation. *Nature* 563, 696–700. doi: 10.1038/s41586-018-0728-4

Chonko, K. T., Jahan, I., Stone, J., Wright, M. C., Fujiyama, T., Hoshino, M., et al. (2013). Atoh1 directs hair cell differentiation and survival in the late embryonic mouse inner ear. *Dev. Biol.* 381, 401–410. doi: 10.1016/j.ydbio.2013.06.022

Chumak, T., Bohuslavova, R., Macova, I., Dodd, N., Buckiova, D., Fritzsch, B., et al. (2016). Deterioration of the medial olivocochlear efferent system accelerates age-related hearing loss in Pax2-Isl1 transgenic mice. *Mol. Neurobiol.* 53, 2368–2383. doi: 10.1007/s12035-015-9215-1

Clark, A. T., Rodriguez, R. T., Bodnar, M. S., Abeyta, M. J., Cedars, M. I., Turek, P. J., et al. (2004). Human STELLAR, NANOG, and GDF3 genes are expressed in pluripotent cells and map to chromosome 12p13, a hotspot for teratocarcinoma. *Stem Cells* 22, 169–179. doi: 10.1634/stemcells.22-2-169

Colasante, G., Lignani, G., Rubio, A., Medrihan, L., Yekhlef, L., Sessa, A., et al. (2015). Rapid conversion of fibroblasts into functional forebrain GABAergic interneurons by direct genetic reprogramming. *Cell Stem Cell* 17, 719–734. doi: 10.1016/j.stem.2015.09.002

Corwin, J., and Cotanche, D. (1988). Regeneration of sensory hair cells after acoustic trauma. *Science* 240, 1772–1774. doi: 10.1126/science.3381100

Costa, A., Sanchez-Guardado, L., Juniat, S., Gale, J. E., Daudet, N., and Henrique, D. (2015). Generation of sensory hair cells by genetic programming with a combination of transcription factors. *Development* 142, 1948–1959. doi: 10.1242/dev.119149

Cotanche, D. A. (1987). Regeneration of hair cell stereociliary bundles in the chick cochlea following severe acoustic trauma. *Hear. Res.* 30, 181–195. doi: 10.1016/0378-5955(87)90135-3

Cotanche, D. A. (1999). Structural recovery from sound and aminoglycoside damage in the avian cochlea. *Audiol. Neurotol.* 4, 271–285. doi: 10.1159/000013852

Cox, B. C., Chai, R., Lenoir, A., Liu, Z., Zhang, L., Nguyen, D.-H., et al. (2014). Spontaneous hair cell regeneration in the neonatal mouse cochlea *in vivo*. *Development* 141, 816–829. doi: 10.1242/dev.103036

Crespo, I., and del Sol, A. (2013). A general strategy for cellular reprogramming: the importance of transcription factor cross-repression. *Stem Cells* 31, 2127–2135. doi: 10.1002/stem.1473

Cruz, R. M., Lambert, P. R., and Rubel, E. W. (1987). Light microscopic evidence of hair cell regeneration after gentamicin toxicity in chick cochlea. *Arch. Otolaryngol. Head Neck Surg.* 113, 1058–1062. doi: 10.1001/archotol.1987.01860100036017

D'Alessio, A. C., Fan, Z. P., Wert, K. J., Baranov, P., Cohen, M. A., Saini, J. S., et al. (2015). A systematic approach to identify candidate transcription factors that control cell identity. *Stem Cell Rep.* 5, 763–775. doi: 10.1016/j.stemcr.2015.09.016

Davis, F. P., and Eddy, S. R. (2013). Transcription factors that convert adult cell identity are differentially polycomb repressed. *PLoS One* 8:e63407. doi: 10.1371/journal.pone.0063407

Davis, R. L., Weintraub, H., and Lassar, A. B. (1987). Expression of a single transfected cDNA converts fibroblasts to myoblasts. *Cell* 51, 987–1000. doi: 10.1016/0092-8674(87)90585-x

De Lázaro, I., Yilmazer, A., Nam, Y., Qubisi, S., Razak, F. M. A., Degens, H., et al. (2019). Non-viral, tumor-free induction of transient cell reprogramming in mouse skeletal muscle to enhance tissue regeneration. *Mol. Ther.* 27, 59–75. doi: 10.1016/j.ymthe.2018.10.014

Deng, J., Shoemaker, R., Xie, B., Gore, A., LeProust, E. M., Antosiewicz-Bourget, J., et al. (2009). Targeted bisulfite sequencing reveals changes in DNA methylation associated with nuclear reprogramming. *Nat. Biotechnol.* 27, 353–360. doi: 10.1038/nbt.1530

DiBerardino, M., Hoffner, N., and Etkin, L. (1984). Activation of dormant genes in specialized cells. *Science* 224, 946–952. doi: 10.1126/science.6719127

Dodou, E., Verzi, M. P., Anderson, J. P., Xu, S.-M., and Black, B. L. (2004). Mef2c is a direct transcriptional target of ISL1 and GATA factors in the anterior heart field during mouse embryonic development. *Development* 131, 3931–3942. doi: 10.1242/dev.01256

Doi, A., Park, I.-H., Wen, B., Murakami, P., Aryee, M. J., Irizarry, R., et al. (2009). Differential methylation of tissue- and cancer-specific CpG island shores distinguishes human induced pluripotent stem cells, embryonic stem cells and fibroblasts. *Nat. Genet.* 41, 1350–1353. doi: 10.1038/ng.471

Driver, E. C., Sillers, L., Coate, T. M., Rose, M. F., and Kelley, M. W. (2013). The Atoh1-lineage gives rise to hair cells and supporting cells within the mammalian cochlea. *Dev. Biol.* 376, 86–98. doi: 10.1016/j.ydbio.2013.01.005

Duncan, J. S., and Fritzsch, B. (2013). Continued expression of GATA3 is necessary for cochlear neurosensory development. *PLoS One* 8:e62046. doi: 10.1371/journal.pone.0062046

Ebeid, M., Sripal, P., Pecka, J., Beisel, K. W., Kwan, K., and Soukup, G. A. (2017). Transcriptome-wide comparison of the impact of Atoh1 and miR-183 family on pluripotent stem cells and multipotent otic progenitor cells. *PLoS One* 12:e0180855. doi: 10.1371/journal.pone.0180855

Ejarque, M., Cervantes, S., Pujadas, G., Tutusaus, A., Sanchez, L., and Gasa, R. (2013). Neurogenin3 cooperates with Foxa2 to autoactivate its own expression. *J. Biol. Chem.* 288, 11705–11717. doi: 10.1074/jbc.M112.388173

Feng, R., Desbordes, S. C., Xie, H., Tillo, E. S., Pixley, F., Stanley, E. R., et al. (2008). PU.1 and C/EBP convert fibroblasts into macrophage-like cells. *Proc. Natl. Acad. Sci. U S A* 105, 6057–6062. doi: 10.1073/pnas.0711961105

Festuccia, N., Osorno, R., Halbritter, F., Karwacki-Neisius, V., Navarro, P., Colby, D., et al. (2012). Esrrb is a direct nanog target gene that can substitute for nanog function in pluripotent cells. *Cell Stem Cell* 11, 477–490. doi: 10.1016/j.stem.2012.08.002

Fu, J.-D., Stone, N. R., Liu, L., Spencer, C. I., Qian, L., Hayashi, Y., et al. (2013). Direct reprogramming of human fibroblasts toward a cardiomyocyte-like state. *Stem Cell Rep.* 1, 235–247. doi: 10.1016/j.stemcr.2013.07.005

Gao, X., Tao, Y., Lamas, V., Huang, M., Yeh, W.-H., Pan, B., et al. (2018). Treatment of autosomal dominant hearing loss by *in vivo* delivery of genome editing agents. *Nature* 553, 217–221. doi: 10.1038/nature25164

Gates, M. A., Kim, L., Egan, E. S., Cardozo, T., Sirotkin, H. I., Dougan, S. T., et al. (1999). A genetic linkage map for zebrafish: comparative analysis and localization of genes and expressed sequences. *Genome Res.* 9, 334–347.

Ghysen, A., and Dambly-Chaudiere, C. (1989). Genesis of the *Drosophila* peripheral nervous system. *Trends Genet.* 5, 251–255. doi: 10.1016/0168-9525(89)90097-8

Graf, T., and Enver, T. (2009). Forcing cells to change lineages. *Nature* 462, 587–594. doi: 10.1038/nature08533

Gualdi, R., Bossard, P., Zheng, M., Hamada, Y., Coleman, J. R., and Zaret, K. S. (1996). Hepatic specification of the gut endoderm *in vitro*: cell signaling and transcriptional control. *Genes Dev.* 10, 1670–1682. doi: 10.1101/gad.10.13.1670

Gurdon, J. B. (1962). The developmental capacity of nuclei taken from intestinal epithelium cells of feeding tadpoles. *J. Embryol. Exp. Morphol.* 10, 622–640.

György, B., Meijer, E. J., Ivanchenko, M. V., Tenneson, K., Emond, F., Hanlon, K. S., et al. (2019). Gene transfer with AAV9-PHP.B rescues hearing in a mouse model of usher syndrome 3A and transduces hair cells in a non-human primate. *Mol. Ther. Methods Clin. Dev.* 13, 1–13. doi: 10.1016/j.omtm.2018.11.003

Habekost, M., Jørgensen, A. L., Qvist, P., and Denham, M. (2020). MicroRNAs and Ascl1 facilitate direct conversion of porcine fibroblasts into induced neurons. *Stem Cell Res.* 48:101984. doi: 10.1016/j.scr.2020.101984

He, A., Gu, F., Hu, Y., Ma, Q., Yi Ye, L., Akiyama, J. A., et al. (2014). Dynamic GATA4 enhancers shape the chromatin landscape central to heart development and disease. *Nat. Commun.* 5:4907. doi: 10.1038/ncomms5907

Heinäniemi, M., Nykter, M., Kramer, R., Wienecke-Baldacchino, A., Sinkkonen, L., Zhou, J. X., et al. (2013). Gene-pair expression signatures reveal lineage control. *Nat. Methods* 10, 577–583. doi: 10.1038/nmeth.2445

Hertzano, R., Montcouquiol, M., Rashi-Elkeles, S., Elkon, R., Yücel, R., Frankel, W. N., et al. (2004). Transcription profiling of inner ears from Pou4f3ddl/ddl identifies Gfi1 as a target of the Pou4f3 deafness gene. *Hum. Mol. Genet.* 13, 2143–2153. doi: 10.1093/hmg/ddh218

Hickey, R. D., Galivo, F., Schug, J., Brehm, M. A., Haft, A., Wang, Y., et al. (2013). Generation of islet-like cells from mouse gall bladder by direct *ex vivo* reprogramming. *Stem Cell Res.* 11, 503–515. doi: 10.1016/j.scr.2013.02.005

Hinojosa, R. (1977). A note on development of corti's organ. *Acta Otolaryngol.* 84, 238–251. doi: 10.3109/00016487709123963

Hobert, O., and Westphal, H. (2000). Functions of LIM-homeobox genes. *Trends Genet.* 16, 75–83. doi: 10.1016/s0168-9525(99)01883-1

Hochedlinger, K., Yamada, Y., Beard, C., and Jaenisch, R. (2005). Ectopic expression of Oct-4 blocks progenitor-cell differentiation and causes dysplasia in epithelial tissues. *Cell* 121, 465–477. doi: 10.1016/j.cell.2005.02.018

Holland, A. M., Hale, M. A., Kagami, H., Hammer, R. E., and MacDonald, R. J. (2002). Experimental control of pancreatic development and maintenance. *Proc. Natl. Acad. Sci. U S A* 99, 12236–12241. doi: 10.1073/pnas.192255099

Hon, G., Wang, W., and Ren, B. (2009). Discovery and annotation of functional chromatin signatures in the human genome. *PLoS Comput. Biol.* 5:e1000566. doi: 10.1371/journal.pcbi.1000566

Hou, P., Li, Y., Zhang, X., Liu, C., Guan, J., Li, H., et al. (2013). Pluripotent stem cells induced from mouse somatic cells by small-molecule compounds. *Science* 341, 651–654. doi: 10.1126/science.1239278

Hu, L., Lu, J., Chiang, H., Wu, H., Edge, A. S. B., and Shi, F. (2016). Diphtheria toxin-induced cell death triggers Wnt-dependent hair cell regeneration in neonatal mice. *J. Neurosci.* 36, 9479–9489. doi: 10.1523/JNEUROSCI.2447-15.2016

Huang, M., Kantardzhieva, A., Scheffer, D., Liberman, M. C., and Chen, Z.-Y. (2013). Hair cell overexpression of Islet1 reduces age-related and noise-induced hearing loss. *J. Neurosci.* 33, 15086–15094. doi: 10.1523/JNEUROSCI.1489-13.2013

Huangfu, D., Maehr, R., Guo, W., Eijkelenboom, A., Snitow, M., Chen, A. E., et al. (2008). Induction of pluripotent stem cells by defined factors is greatly improved by small-molecule compounds. *Nat. Biotechnol.* 26, 795–797. doi: 10.1038/nbt1418

Ieda, M., Fu, J.-D., Delgado-Olguin, P., Vedantham, V., Hayashi, Y., Bruneau, B. G., et al. (2010). Direct reprogramming of fibroblasts into functional cardiomyocytes by defined factors. *Cell* 142, 375–386. doi: 10.1016/j.cell.2010.07.002

Ikeda, R., Pak, K., Chavez, E., and Ryan, A. F. (2015). Transcription factors with conserved binding sites near ATOH1 on the POU4F3 gene enhance the induction of cochlear hair cells. *Mol. Neurobiol.* 51, 672–684. doi: 10.1007/s12035-014-8801-y

Isgrig, K., McDougald, D. S., Zhu, J., Wang, H. J., Bennett, J., and Chien, W. W. (2019). AAV2.7m8 is a powerful viral vector for inner ear gene therapy. *Nat. Commun.* 10:427. doi: 10.1038/s41467-018-08243-1

Itoh, M., and Chitnis, A. B. (2001). Expression of proneural and neurogenic genes in the zebrafish lateral line primordium correlates with selection of hair cell fate in neuromasts. *Mech. Dev.* 102, 263–266. doi: 10.1016/s0925-4773(01)00308-2

Itoh, M., Kim, C.-H., Palardy, G., Oda, T., Jiang, Y.-J., Maust, D., et al. (2003). Mind bomb is a ubiquitin ligase that is essential for efficient activation of notch signaling by delta. *Dev. Cell* 4, 67–82. doi: 10.1016/s1534-5807(02)00409-4

Iwafuchi-Doi, M., and Zaret, K. S. (2014). Pioneer transcription factors in cell reprogramming. *Genes Dev.* 28, 2679–2692. doi: 10.1101/gad.253443.114

Iwafuchi-Doi, M., and Zaret, K. S. (2016). Cell fate control by pioneer transcription factors. *Development* 143, 1833–1837. doi: 10.1242/dev.133900

Izumikawa, M., Minoda, R., Kawamoto, K., Abrashkin, K. A., Swiderski, D. L., Dolan, D. F., et al. (2005). Auditory hair cell replacement and hearing improvement by Atoh1 gene therapy in deaf mammals. *Nat. Med.* 11, 271–276. doi: 10.1038/nm1193

Jiang, L., Romero-Carvajal, A., Haug, J. S., Seidel, C. W., and Piotrowski, T. (2014). Gene-expression analysis of hair cell regeneration in the zebrafish lateral line. *Proc. Natl. Acad. Sci. U S A* 111, E1383–E1392. doi: 10.1073/pnas.1402898111

Jiang, T., Kindt, K., and Wu, D. K. (2017). Transcription factor Emx2 controls stereociliary bundle orientation of sensory hair cells. *Elife* 6:e23661. doi: 10.7554/eLife.23661

Kamiya, K., Takahashi, K., Kitamura, K., Momoi, T., and Yoshikawa, Y. (2001). Mitosis and apoptosis in postnatal auditory system of the C3H/He strain. *Brain Res.* 901, 296–302. doi: 10.1016/s0006-8993(01)02300-9

Kawamoto, K., Ishimoto, S.-I., Minoda, R., Brough, D. E., and Raphael, Y. (2003). Math1 gene transfer generates new cochlear hair cells in mature guinea pigs *in vivo*. *J. Neurosci.* 23, 4395–4400. doi: 10.1523/JNEUROSCI.23-11-04395.2003

Kelly, M. C., Chang, Q., Pan, A., Lin, X., and Chen, P. (2012). Atoh1 directs the formation of sensory mosaics and induces cell proliferation in the postnatal mammalian cochlea *in vivo*. *J. Neurosci.* 32, 6699–6710. doi: 10.1523/JNEUROSCI.5420-11.2012

Kempfle, J. S., Turban, J. L., and Edge, A. S. B. (2016). Sox2 in the differentiation of cochlear progenitor cells. *Sci. Rep.* 6:23293. doi: 10.1038/srep23293

Kiernan, A. E., Cordes, R., Kopan, R., Gossler, A., and Gridley, T. (2005). The Notch ligands DLL1 and JAG2 act synergistically to regulate hair cell development in the mammalian inner ear. *Development* 132, 4353–4362. doi: 10.1242/dev.02002

Kim, K., Doi, A., Wen, B., Ng, K., Zhao, R., Cahan, P., et al. (2010). Epigenetic memory in induced pluripotent stem cells. *Nature* 467, 285–290. doi: 10.1038/nature09342

Koehler, K. R., Nie, J., Longworth-Mills, E., Liu, X.-P., Lee, J., Holt, J. R., et al. (2017). Generation of inner ear organoids containing functional hair cells from human pluripotent stem cells. *Nat. Biotechnol.* 35, 583–589. doi: 10.1038/nbt.3840

Korrapati, S., Roux, I., Glowatzki, E., and Doetzlhofer, A. (2013). Notch signaling limits supporting cell plasticity in the hair cell-damaged early postnatal murine cochlea. *PLoS One* 8:e73276. doi: 10.1371/journal.pone.0073276

Ku, Y.-C., Renaud, N. A., Veile, R. A., Helms, C., Voelker, C. C. J., Warchol, M. E., et al. (2014). The transcriptome of utricle hair cell regeneration in the avian inner ear. *J. Neurosci.* 34, 3523–3535. doi: 10.1523/JNEUROSCI.2606-13.2014

Ladewig, J., Koch, P., and Brüstle, O. (2013). Leveling Waddington: the emergence of direct programming and the loss of cell fate hierarchies. *Nat. Rev. Mol. Cell Biol.* 14, 225–236. doi: 10.1038/nrm3543

Landegger, L. D., Pan, B., Askew, C., Wassmer, S. J., Gluck, S. D., Galvin, A., et al. (2017). A synthetic AAV vector enables safe and efficient gene transfer to the mammalian inner ear. *Nat. Biotechnol.* 35, 280–284. doi: 10.1038/nbt.3781

Lanford, P. J., Lan, Y., Jiang, R., Lindsell, C., Weinmaster, G., Gridley, T., et al. (1999). Notch signaling pathway mediates hair cell development in mammalian cochlea. *Nat. Genet.* 21, 289–292. doi: 10.1038/6804

Lang, A. H., Li, H., Collins, J. J., and Mehta, P. (2014). Epigenetic landscapes explain partially reprogrammed cells and identify key reprogramming genes. *PLoS Comput. Biol.* 10:e1003734. doi: 10.1371/journal.pcbi.1003734

Lee, Y.-S. (2006). A morphogenetic wave of p27Kip1 transcription directs cell cycle exit during organ of Corti development. *Development* 133, 2817–2826. doi: 10.1242/dev.02453

Lee, J., Nist-Lund, C., Solanes, P., Goldberg, H., Wu, J., Pan, B., et al. (2020). Efficient viral transduction in mouse inner ear hair cells with utricle injection and AAV9-PHP.B. *Hear. Res.* 394:107882. doi: 10.1016/j.heares.2020.107882

Lee, S., Song, J.-J., Beyer, L. A., Swiderski, D. L., Prieskorn, D. M., Acar, M., et al. (2020). Combinatorial Atoh1 and Gfi1 induction enhances hair cell regeneration in the adult cochlea. *Sci. Rep.* 10:21397. doi: 10.1038/s41598-020-78167-8

Li, J., Zhang, T., Ramakrishnan, A., Fritzsch, B., Xu, J., Wong, E. Y. M., et al. (2020). Dynamic changes in cis-regulatory occupancy by Six1 and its cooperative interactions with distinct cofactors drive lineage-specific gene expression programs during progressive differentiation of the auditory sensory epithelium. *Nucleic Acids Res.* 48, 2880–2896. doi: 10.1093/nar/gkaa012

Lim, D. J. (1972). Fine morphology of the tectorial membrane: its relationship to the organ of corti. *Arch. Otolaryngol.* 96, 199–215. doi: 10.1001/archotol.1972.00770090321001

Lima, M. J., Muir, K. R., Docherty, H. M., McGowan, N. W. A., Forbes, S., Heremans, Y., et al. (2016). Generation of functional β-like cells from human exocrine pancreas. *PLoS One* 11:e0156204. doi: 10.1371/journal.pone.0156204

Lippe, W. R., Westbrook, E. W., and Ryals, B. M. (1991). Hair cell regeneration in the chicken cochlea following aminoglycoside toxicity. *Hear. Res.* 56, 203–210. doi: 10.1016/0378-5955(91)90171-5

Lister, R., and Ecker, J. R. (2009). Finding the fifth base: genome-wide sequencing of cytosine methylation. *Genome Res.* 19, 959–966. doi: 10.1101/gr.083451.108

Liu, Z., Dearman, J. A., Cox, B. C., Walters, B. J., Zhang, L., Ayrault, O., et al. (2012). Age-dependent *in vivo* conversion of mouse cochlear pillar and deiters' cells to immature hair cells by atoh1 ectopic expression. *J. Neurosci.* 32, 6600–6610. doi: 10.1523/JNEUROSCI.0818-12.2012

Liu, Z., Fang, J., Dearman, J., Zhang, L., and Zuo, J. (2014). *in vivo* generation of immature inner hair cells in neonatal mouse cochleae by ectopic atoh1 expression. *PLoS One* 9:e89377. doi: 10.1371/journal.pone.0089377

Lombarte, A., Yan, H. Y., Popper, A. N., Chang, J. S., and Platt, C. (1993). Damage and regeneration of hair cell ciliary bundles in a fish ear following treatment with gentamicin. *Hear. Res.* 64, 166–174. doi: 10.1016/0378-5955(93)90002-i

Longworth-Mills, E., Koehler, K. R., and Hashino, E. (2016). Generating inner ear organoids from mouse embryonic stem cells. *Methods Mol. Biol.* 1341, 391–406. doi: 10.1007/7651_2015_215

Lorenzen, S. M., Duggan, A., Osipovich, A. B., Magnuson, M. A., and Garcia-Añoveros, J. (2015). Insm1 promotes neurogenic proliferation in delaminated otic progenitors. *Mech. Dev.* 138, 233–245. doi: 10.1016/j.mod.2015.11.001

Luo, C., Lee, Q. Y., Wapinski, O., Castanon, R., Nery, J. R., Mall, M., et al. (2019). Global DNA methylation remodeling during direct reprogramming of fibroblasts to neurons. *Elife* 8:e40197. doi: 10.7554/eLife.40197

Ma, Y., Wise, A. K., Shepherd, R. K., and Richardson, R. T. (2019). New molecular therapies for the treatment of hearing loss. *Pharmacol. Ther.* 200, 190–209. doi: 10.1016/j.pharmthera.2019.05.003

Maherali, N., Sridharan, R., Xie, W., Utikal, J., Eminli, S., Arnold, K., et al. (2007). Directly reprogrammed fibroblasts show global epigenetic remodeling and widespread tissue contribution. *Cell Stem Cell* 1, 55–70. doi: 10.1016/j.stem.2007.05.014

Mai, T., Markov, G. J., Brady, J. J., Palla, A., Zeng, H., Sebastiano, V., et al. (2018). NKX3-1 is required for induced pluripotent stem cell reprogramming and can replace OCT4 in mouse and human iPSC induction. *Nat. Cell Biol.* 20, 900–908. doi: 10.1038/s41556-018-0136-x

Martinez-Redondo, P., and Izpisua Belmonte, J. C. (2020). Tailored chromatin modulation to promote tissue regeneration. *Semin. Cell Dev. Biol.* 97, 3–15. doi: 10.1016/j.semcdb.2019.04.015

Masuda, M., Dulon, D., Pak, K., Mullen, L. M., Li, Y., Erkman, L., et al. (2011). Regulation of POU4F3 gene expression in hair cells by 5′ DNA in mice. *Neuroscience* 197, 48–64. doi: 10.1016/j.neuroscience.2011.09.033

Masuda, M., Pak, K., Chavez, E., and Ryan, A. F. (2012). TFE2 and GATA3 enhance induction of POU4F3 and myosin VIIa positive cells in nonsensory cochlear epithelium by ATOH1. *Dev. Biol.* 372, 68–80. doi: 10.1016/j.ydbio.2012.09.002

Masui, S., Nakatake, Y., Toyooka, Y., Shimosato, D., Yagi, R., Takahashi, K., et al. (2007). Pluripotency governed by Sox2 *via* regulation of Oct3/4 expression in mouse embryonic stem cells. *Nat. Cell Biol.* 9, 625–635. doi: 10.1038/ncb1589

Matern, M. S., Milon, B., Lipford, E. L., McMurray, M., Ogawa, Y., Tkaczuk, A., et al. (2020). GFI1 functions to repress neuronal gene expression in the developing inner ear hair cells. *Development* 147:dev186015. doi: 10.1242/dev.186015

Matsuoka, T.-A., Artner, I., Henderson, E., Means, A., Sander, M., and Stein, R. (2004). The MafA transcription factor appears to be responsible for tissue-specific expression of insulin. *Proc. Natl. Acad. Sci. U S A* 101, 2930–2933. doi: 10.1073/pnas.0306233101

Maza, I., Caspi, I., Zviran, A., Chomsky, E., Rais, Y., Viukov, S., et al. (2015). Transient acquisition of pluripotency during somatic cell transdifferentiation with iPSC reprogramming factors. *Nat. Biotechnol.* 33, 769–774. doi: 10.1038/nbt.3270

McGrath, J., and Solter, D. (1983). Nuclear transplantation in the mouse embryo by microsurgery and cell fusion. *Science* 220, 1300–1302. doi: 10.1126/science.6857250

Mellado Lagarde, M. M., Cox, B. C., Fang, J., Taylor, R., Forge, A., and Zuo, J. (2013). Selective ablation of pillar and deiters' cells severely affects cochlear postnatal development and hearing in mice. *J. Neurosci.* 33, 1564–1576. doi: 10.1523/JNEUROSCI.3088-12.2013

Mellado Lagarde, M. M., Wan, G., Zhang, L., Gigliello, A. R., McInnis, J. J., Zhang, Y., et al. (2014). Spontaneous regeneration of cochlear supporting cells after neonatal ablation ensures hearing in the adult mouse. *Proc. Natl. Acad. Sci. U S A* 111, 16919–16924. doi: 10.1073/pnas.1408064111

Menendez, L., Trecek, T., Gopalakrishnan, S., Tao, L., Markowitz, A. L., Yu, H. V., et al. (2020). Generation of inner ear hair cells by direct lineage conversion of primary somatic cells. *Elife* 9:e55249. doi: 10.7554/eLife.55249

Mikkelsen, T. S., Hanna, J., Zhang, X., Ku, M., Wernig, M., Schorderet, P., et al. (2008). Dissecting direct reprogramming through integrative genomic analysis. *Nature* 454, 49–55. doi: 10.1038/nature07056

Mikkelsen, T. S., Ku, M., Jaffe, D. B., Issac, B., Lieberman, E., Giannoukos, G., et al. (2007). Genome-wide maps of chromatin state in pluripotent and lineage-committed cells. *Nature* 448, 553–560. doi: 10.1038/nature06008

Millimaki, B. B., Sweet, E. M., Dhason, M. S., and Riley, B. B. (2007). Zebrafish atoh1 genes: classic proneural activity in the inner ear and regulation by Fgf and Notch. *Development* 134, 295–305. doi: 10.1242/dev.02734

Millimaki, B. B., Sweet, E. M., and Riley, B. B. (2010). Sox2 is required for maintenance and regeneration, but not initial development, of hair cells in the zebrafish inner ear. *Dev. Biol.* 338, 262–269. doi: 10.1016/j.ydbio.2009.12.011

Mizutari, K., Fujioka, M., Hosoya, M., Bramhall, N., Okano, H. J., Okano, H., et al. (2013). Notch inhibition induces cochlear hair cell regeneration and recovery of hearing after acoustic trauma. *Neuron* 77, 58–69. doi: 10.1016/j.neuron.2012.10.032

Morris, S. A. (2016). Direct lineage reprogramming *via* pioneer factors; a detour through developmental gene regulatory networks. *Development* 143, 2696–2705. doi: 10.1242/dev.138263

Morris, S. A., Cahan, P., Li, H., Zhao, A. M., San Roman, A. K., Shivdasani, R. A., et al. (2014). Dissecting engineered cell types and enhancing cell fate conversion *via* CellNet. *Cell* 158, 889–902. doi: 10.1016/j.cell.2014.07.021

Morris, S. A., and Daley, G. Q. (2013). A blueprint for engineering cell fate: current technologies to reprogram cell identity. *Cell Res.* 23, 33–48. doi: 10.1038/cr.2013.1

Murre, C., McCaw, P. S., and Baltimore, D. (1989). A new DNA binding and dimerization motif in immunoglobulin enhancer binding, daughterless, MyoD, and myc proteins. *Cell* 56, 777–783. doi: 10.1016/0092-8674(89)90682-x

Nakai, H., Yant, S. R., Storm, T. A., Fuess, S., Meuse, L., and Kay, M. A. (2001). Extrachromosomal recombinant adeno-associated virus vector genomes are primarily responsible for stable liver transduction *in vivo*. *J. Virol.* 75, 6969–6976. doi: 10.1128/JVI.75.15.6969-6976.2001

Nasonkin, I. O., Lazo, K., Hambright, D., Brooks, M., Fariss, R., and Swaroop, A. (2011). Distinct nuclear localization patterns of DNA methyltransferases in developing and mature mammalian retina. *J. Comp. Neurol.* 519, 1914–1930. doi: 10.1002/cne.22613

Nasonkin, I. O., Merbs, S. L., Lazo, K., Oliver, V. F., Brooks, M., Patel, K., et al. (2013). Conditional knockdown of DNA methyltransferase 1 reveals a key role of retinal pigment epithelium integrity in photoreceptor outer segment morphogenesis. *Development* 140, 1330–1341. doi: 10.1242/dev.086603

Neves, J., Uchikawa, M., Bigas, A., and Giraldez, F. (2012). The prosensory function of Sox2 in the chicken inner ear relies on the direct regulation of Atoh1. *PLoS One* 7:e30871. doi: 10.1371/journal.pone.0030871

Ni, W., Zeng, S., Li, W., Chen, Y., Zhang, S., Tang, M., et al. (2016). Wnt activation followed by Notch inhibition promotes mitotic hair cell regeneration in the postnatal mouse cochlea. *Oncotarget* 7, 66754–66768. doi: 10.18632/oncotarget.11479

Nist-Lund, C. A., Pan, B., Patterson, A., Asai, Y., Chen, T., Zhou, W., et al. (2019). Improved TMC1 gene therapy restores hearing and balance in mice with genetic inner ear disorders. *Nat. Commun.* 10:236. doi: 10.1038/s41467-018-08264-w

Okawa, S., Nicklas, S., Zickenrott, S., Schwamborn, J. C., and del Sol, A. (2016). A generalized gene-regulatory network model of stem cell differentiation for predicting lineage specifiers. *Stem Cell Rep.* 7, 307–315. doi: 10.1016/j.stemcr.2016.07.014

Ouji, Y., Ishizaka, S., Nakamura-Uchiyama, F., Wanaka, A., and Yoshikawa, M. (2013). Induction of inner ear hair cell-like cells from Math1-transfected mouse ES cells. *Cell Death Dis.* 4:e700. doi: 10.1038/cddis.2013.230

Ouyang, J. F., Kamaraj, U. S., Polo, J. M., Gough, J., and Rackham, O. J. L. (2019). Molecular interaction networks to select factors for cell conversion. *Methods Mol. Biol.* 1975, 333–361. doi: 10.1007/978-1-4939-9224-9_16

Pan, N., Jahan, I., Kersigo, J., Duncan, J. S., Kopecky, B., and Fritzsch, B. (2012). A novel atoh1 "self-terminating" mouse model reveals the necessity of proper Atoh1 level and duration for hair cell differentiation and viability. *PLoS One* 7:e30358. doi: 10.1371/journal.pone.0030358

Pang, Z. P., Yang, N., Vierbuchen, T., Ostermeier, A., Fuentes, D. R., Yang, T. Q., et al. (2011). Induction of human neuronal cells by defined transcription factors. *Nature* 476, 220–223. doi: 10.1038/nature10202

Peeters, R. P., Ng, L., Ma, M., and Forrest, D. (2015). The timecourse of apoptotic cell death during postnatal remodeling of the mouse cochlea and its premature onset by triiodothyronine (T3). *Mol. Cell. Endocrinol.* 407, 1–8. doi: 10.1016/j.mce.2015.02.025

Polo, J. M., Liu, S., Figueroa, M. E., Kulalert, W., Eminli, S., Tan, K. Y., et al. (2010). Cell type of origin influences the molecular and functional properties of mouse induced pluripotent stem cells. *Nat. Biotechnol.* 28, 848–855. doi: 10.1038/nbt.1667

Powell, L. M., Deaton, A. M., Wear, M. A., and Jarman, A. P. (2008). Specificity of Atonal and Scute bHLH factors: analysis of cognate E box binding sites and the influence of Senseless. *Genes Cells* 13, 915–929. doi: 10.1111/j.1365-2443.2008.01217.x

Quan, X.-J., Yuan, L., Tiberi, L., Claeys, A., De Geest, N., Yan, J., et al. (2016). Post-translational control of the temporal dynamics of transcription factor activity regulates neurogenesis. *Cell* 164, 460–475. doi: 10.1016/j.cell.2015.12.048

Rackham, O. J. L., Firas, J., Fang, H., Oates, M. E., Holmes, M. L., Knaupp, A. S., et al. (2016). A predictive computational framework for direct reprogramming between human cell types. *Nat. Genet.* 48, 331–335. doi: 10.1038/ng.3487

Radde-Gallwitz, K., Pan, L., Gan, L., Lin, X., Segil, N., and Chen, P. (2004). Expression of Islet1 marks the sensory and neuronal lineages in the mammalian inner ear. *J. Comp. Neurol.* 477, 412–421. doi: 10.1002/cne.20257

Raphael, Y., and Altschuler, R. A. (2003). Structure and innervation of the cochlea. *Brain Res. Bull.* 60, 397–422. doi: 10.1016/s0361-9230(03)00047-9

Roberson, D. W., Kreig, C. S., and Rubel, E. W. (1996). Light microscopic evidence that direct transdifferentiation gives rise to new hair cells in regenerating avian auditory epithelium. *Audit. Neurosci.* 2, 195–205.

Rodier, A., Marchal-Victorion, S., Rochard, P., Casas, F., Cassar-Malek, I., Rouault, J.-P., et al. (1999). BTG1: a triiodothyronine target involved in the myogenic influence of the hormone. *Exp. Cell Res.* 249, 337–348. doi: 10.1006/excr.1999.4486

Rouault, J. P., Rimokh, R., Tessa, C., Paranhos, G., Ffrench, M., Duret, L., et al. (1992). BTG1, a member of a new family of antiproliferative genes. *EMBO J.* 11, 1663–1670. doi: 10.1002/j.1460-2075.1992.tb05213.x

Ryals, B., and Rubel, E. (1988). Hair cell regeneration after acoustic trauma in adult Coturnix quail. *Science* 240, 1774–1776. doi: 10.1126/science.3381101

Sarkar, T. J., Quarta, M., Mukherjee, S., Colville, A., Paine, P., Doan, L., et al. (2020). Transient non-integrative expression of nuclear reprogramming factors promotes multifaceted amelioration of aging in human cells. *Nat. Commun.* 11:1545. doi: 10.1038/s41467-020-15174-3

Sarrazin, A. F., Villablanca, E. J., Nuñez, V. A., Sandoval, P. C., Ghysen, A., and Allende, M. L. (2006). Proneural gene requirement for hair cell differentiation in the zebrafish lateral line. *Dev. Biol.* 295, 534–545. doi: 10.1016/j.ydbio.2006.03.037

Sayyid, Z. N., Wang, T., Chen, L., Jones, S. M., and Cheng, A. G. (2019). Atoh1 directs regeneration and functional recovery of the mature mouse vestibular system. *Cell Rep.* 28, 312.e4–324.e4. doi: 10.1016/j.celrep.2019.06.028

Sekiya, T., and Zaret, K. S. (2007). Repression by Groucho/TLE/Grg proteins: genomic site recruitment generates compacted chromatin *in vitro* and impairs activator binding *in vivo*. *Mol. Cell* 28, 291–303. doi: 10.1016/j.molcel.2007.10.002

Sharlin, D. S., Visser, T. J., and Forrest, D. (2011). Developmental and cell-specific expression of thyroid hormone transporters in the mouse cochlea. *Endocrinology* 152, 5053–5064. doi: 10.1210/en.2011-1372

Shi, F., Hu, L., Jacques, B. E., Mulvaney, J. F., Dabdoub, A., and Edge, A. S. B. (2014). β-catenin is required for hair-cell differentiation in the cochlea. *J. Neurosci.* 34, 6470–6479. doi: 10.1523/JNEUROSCI.4305-13.2014

Shou, J., Zheng, J. L., and Gao, W.-Q. (2003). Robust generation of new hair cells in the mature mammalian inner ear by adenoviral expression of Hath1. *Mol. Cell. Neurosci.* 23, 169–179. doi: 10.1016/s1044-7431(03)00066-6

Singh, R. K., Mallela, R. K., Hayes, A., Dunham, N. R., Hedden, M. E., Enke, R. A., et al. (2017). Dnmt1, Dnmt3a and Dnmt3b cooperate in photoreceptor and outer plexiform layer development in the mammalian retina. *Exp. Eye Res.* 159, 132–146. doi: 10.1016/j.exer.2016.11.014

Smith, M. E., Coffin, A. B., Miller, D. L., and Popper, A. N. (2006). Anatomical and functional recovery of the goldfish (Carassius auratus) ear following noise exposure. *J. Exp. Biol.* 209, 4193–4202. doi: 10.1242/jeb.02490

Soufi, A., Donahue, G., and Zaret, K. S. (2012). Facilitators and impediments of the pluripotency reprogramming factors' initial engagement with the genome. *Cell* 151, 994–1004. doi: 10.1016/j.cell.2012.09.045

Soufi, A., Garcia, M. F., Jaroszewicz, A., Osman, N., Pellegrini, M., and Zaret, K. S. (2015). Pioneer transcription factors target partial DNA motifs on nucleosomes to initiate reprogramming. *Cell* 161, 555–568. doi: 10.1016/j.cell.2015.03.017

Spicer, S. S., Salvi, R. J., and Schulte, B. A. (1999). Ablation of inner hair cells by carboplatin alters cells in the medial K+ flow route and disrupts tectorial membrane. *Hear. Res.* 136, 139–150. doi: 10.1016/s0378-5955(99)00118-5

Stadtfeld, M., and Hochedlinger, K. (2010). Induced pluripotency: history, mechanisms, and applications. *Genes Dev.* 24, 2239–2263. doi: 10.1101/gad.1963910

Stadtfeld, M., Maherali, N., Breault, D. T., and Hochedlinger, K. (2008). Defining molecular cornerstones during fibroblast to iPS cell reprogramming in mouse. *Cell Stem Cell* 2, 230–240. doi: 10.1016/j.stem.2008.02.001

Steimle, J. D., and Moskowitz, I. P. (2016). TBX5: a key regulator of heart development. *Curr. Top. Dev. Biol.* 122, 195–221. doi: 10.1016/bs.ctdb.2016.08.008

Stojanova, Z. P., Kwan, T., and Segil, N. (2015). Epigenetic regulation of Atoh1 guides hair cell development in the mammalian cochlea. *Development* 142, 3529–3536. doi: 10.1242/dev.126763

Sweet, E. M., Vemaraju, S., and Riley, B. B. (2011). Sox2 and Fgf interact with Atoh1 to promote sensory competence throughout the zebrafish inner ear. *Dev. Biol.* 358, 113–121. doi: 10.1016/j.ydbio.2011.07.019

Takahashi, K., Tanabe, K., Ohnuki, M., Narita, M., Ichisaka, T., Tomoda, K., et al. (2007). Induction of pluripotent stem cells from adult human fibroblasts by defined factors. *Cell* 131, 861–872. doi: 10.1016/j.cell.2007.11.019

Takahashi, K., and Yamanaka, S. (2006). Induction of pluripotent stem cells from mouse embryonic and adult fibroblast cultures by defined factors. *Cell* 126, 663–676. doi: 10.1016/j.cell.2006.07.024

Takeda, H., Kurioka, T., Kaitsuka, T., Tomizawa, K., Matsunobu, T., Hakim, F., et al. (2016). Protein transduction therapy into cochleae *via* the round window niche in guinea pigs. *Mol. Ther. Methods Clin. Dev.* 3:16055. doi: 10.1038/mtm.2016.55

Tanabe, K., Nakamura, M., Narita, M., Takahashi, K., and Yamanaka, S. (2013). Maturation, not initiation, is the major roadblock during reprogramming toward pluripotency from human fibroblasts. *Proc. Natl. Acad. Sci. U S A* 110, 12172–12179. doi: 10.1073/pnas.1310291110

Tateya, T., Sakamoto, S., Ishidate, F., Hirashima, T., Imayoshi, I., and Kageyama, R. (2019). Three-dimensional live imaging of Atoh1 reveals the dynamics of hair cell induction and organization in the developing cochlea. *Development* 146:dev177881. doi: 10.1242/dev.177881

Taylor, R. R., and Forge, A. (2005). Hair cell regeneration in sensory epithelia from the inner ear of a urodele amphibian. *J. Comp. Neurol.* 484, 105–120. doi: 10.1002/cne.20450

Tokuzawa, Y., Kaiho, E., Maruyama, M., Takahashi, K., Mitsui, K., Maeda, M., et al. (2003). Fbx15 is a novel target of Oct3/4 but is dispensable for embryonic stem cell self-renewal and mouse development. *Mol. Cell. Biol.* 23, 2699–2708. doi: 10.1128/mcb.23.8.2699-2708.2003

Tsue, T. T., Oesterle, E. C., and Rubel, E. W. (1994). Diffusible factors regulate hair cell regeneration in the avian inner ear. *Proc. Natl. Acad. Sci. U S A* 91, 1584–1588. doi: 10.1073/pnas.91.4.1584

Vierbuchen, T., Ostermeier, A., Pang, Z. P., Kokubu, Y., Südhof, T. C., and Wernig, M. (2010). Direct conversion of fibroblasts to functional neurons by defined factors. *Nature* 463, 1035–1041. doi: 10.1038/nature08797

Wallis, D., Hamblen, M., Zhou, Y., Venken, K. J. T., Schumacher, A., Leighton Grimes, H., et al. (2003). The zinc finger transcription factor Gfi1, implicated in lymphomagenesis, is required for inner ear hair cell differentiation and survival. *Development* 130, 221–232. doi: 10.1242/dev.00190

Walters, B. J., Coak, E., Dearman, J., Bailey, G., Yamashita, T., Kuo, B., et al. (2017). *in vivo* interplay between $p27^{Kip1}$, GATA3, ATOH1, and POU4F3 converts non-sensory cells to hair cells in adult mice. *Cell Rep.* 19, 307–320. doi: 10.1016/j.celrep.2017.03.044

Wan, G., Corfas, G., and Stone, J. S. (2013). Inner ear supporting cells: rethinking the silent majority. *Semin. Cell Dev. Biol.* 24, 448–459. doi: 10.1016/j.semcdb.2013.03.009

Wang, J., He, Q., Zhang, K., Sun, H., Zhang, G., Liang, H., et al. (2020). Quick commitment and efficient reprogramming route of direct induction of retinal ganglion cell-like neurons. *Stem Cell Rep.* 15, 1095–1110. doi: 10.1016/j.stemcr.2020.09.008

Wang, J., Rao, S., Chu, J., Shen, X., Levasseur, D. N., Theunissen, T. W., et al. (2006). A protein interaction network for pluripotency of embryonic stem cells. *Nature* 444, 364–368. doi: 10.1038/nature05284

Wang, S., Yan, J., Anderson, D. A., Xu, Y., Kanal, M. C., Cao, Z., et al. (2010). Neurog3 gene dosage regulates allocation of endocrine and exocrine cell fates in the developing mouse pancreas. *Dev. Biol.* 339, 26–37. doi: 10.1016/j.ydbio.2009.12.009

Wapinski, O. L., Vierbuchen, T., Qu, K., Lee, Q. Y., Chanda, S., Fuentes, D. R., et al. (2013). Hierarchical mechanisms for direct reprogramming of fibroblasts to neurons. *Cell* 155, 621–635. doi: 10.1016/j.cell.2013.09.028

Wilkerson, B. A., Chitsazan, A. D., VandenBosch, L. S., Wilken, M. S., Reh, T. A., and Bermingham-McDonogh, O. (2019). Open chromatin dynamics in prosensory cells of the embryonic mouse cochlea. *Sci. Rep.* 9:9060. doi: 10.1038/s41598-019-45515-2

Willadsen, S. M. (1986). Nuclear transplantation in sheep embryos. *Nature* 320, 63–65. doi: 10.1038/320063a0

Wilmut, I., Schnieke, A. E., McWhir, J., Kind, A. J., and Campbell, K. H. S. (1997). Viable offspring derived from fetal and adult mammalian cells. *Nature* 385, 810–813. doi: 10.1038/385810a0

Wiwatpanit, T., Lorenzen, S. M., Cantú, J. A., Foo, C. Z., Hogan, A. K., Márquez, F., et al. (2018). Trans-differentiation of outer hair cells into inner hair cells in the absence of INSM1. *Nature* 563, 691–695. doi: 10.1038/s41586-018-0570-8

Woods, C., Montcouquiol, M., and Kelley, M. W. (2004). Math1 regulates development of the sensory epithelium in the mammalian cochlea. *Nat. Neurosci.* 7, 1310–1318. doi: 10.1038/nn1349

Wu, X., Wang, Y., Sun, Y., Chen, S., Zhang, S., Shen, L., et al. (2014). Reduced expression of Connexin26 and its DNA promoter hypermethylation in the inner ear of mimetic aging rats induced by d-galactose. *Biochem. Biophys. Res. Commun.* 452, 340–346. doi: 10.1016/j.bbrc.2014.08.063

Xiang, M., Gao, W. Q., Hasson, T., and Shin, J. J. (1998). Requirement for Brn-3c in maturation and survival, but not in fate determination of inner ear hair cells. *Development* 125, 3935–3946.

Xiang, M., Gan, L., Li, D., Chen, Z.-Y., Zhou, L., O'Malley, B. W., et al. (1997). Essential role of POU-domain factor Brn-3c in auditory and vestibular hair cell development. *Proc. Natl. Acad. Sci. U S A* 94, 9445–9450. doi: 10.1073/pnas.94.17.9445

Xie, W. R., Jen, H.-I., Seymour, M. L., Yeh, S.-Y., Pereira, F. A., Groves, A. K., et al. (2017). An Atoh1-S193A phospho-mutant allele causes hearing deficits and motor impairment. *J. Neurosci.* 37, 8583–8594. doi: 10.1523/JNEUROSCI.0295-17.2017

Xie, W., Schultz, M. D., Lister, R., Hou, Z., Rajagopal, N., Ray, P., et al. (2013). Epigenomic analysis of multilineage differentiation of human embryonic stem cells. *Cell* 153, 1134–1148. doi: 10.1016/j.cell.2013.04.022

Xing, Q. R., El Farran, C. A., Gautam, P., Chuah, Y. S., Warrier, T., Toh, C. X. D., et al. (2020). Diversification of reprogramming trajectories revealed by parallel single-cell transcriptome and chromatin accessibility sequencing. *Sci. Adv.* 6:eaba1190. doi: 10.1126/sciadv.aba1190

Xu, J., Ueno, H., Xu, C. Y., Chen, B., Weissman, I. L., and Xu, P.-X. (2017). Identification of mouse cochlear progenitors that develop hair and supporting cells in the organ of Corti. *Nat. Commun.* 8:15046. doi: 10.1038/ncomms15046

Yamashita, T., Zheng, F., Finkelstein, D., Kellard, Z., Carter, R., Rosencrance, C. D., et al. (2018). High-resolution transcriptional dissection of *in vivo* Atoh1-mediated hair cell conversion in mature cochleae identifies Isl1 as a co-reprogramming factor. *PLoS Genet.* 14:e1007552. doi: 10.1371/journal.pgen.1007552

Yizhar-Barnea, O., Valensisi, C., Jayavelu, N. D., Kishore, K., Andrus, C., Koffler-Brill, T., et al. (2018). DNA methylation dynamics during embryonic development and postnatal maturation of the mouse auditory sensory epithelium. *Sci. Rep.* 8:17348. doi: 10.1038/s41598-018-35587-x

Yoo, A. S., Sun, A. X., Li, L., Shcheglovitov, A., Portmann, T., Li, Y., et al. (2011). MicroRNA-mediated conversion of human fibroblasts to neurons. *Nature* 476, 228–231. doi: 10.1038/nature10323

Yu, J., Vodyanik, M. A., Smuga-Otto, K., Antosiewicz-Bourget, J., Frane, J. L., Tian, S., et al. (2007). Induced pluripotent stem cell lines derived from human somatic cells. *Science* 318, 1917–1920. doi: 10.1126/science.1151526

Zaret, K. S., and Carroll, J. S. (2011). Pioneer transcription factors: establishing competence for gene expression. *Genes Dev.* 25, 2227–2241. doi: 10.1101/gad.176826.111

Zhai, S., Shi, L., Wang, B., Zheng, G., Song, W., Hu, Y., et al. (2005). Isolation and culture of hair cell progenitors from postnatal rat cochleae. *J. Neurobiol.* 65, 282–293. doi: 10.1002/neu.20190

Zhang, J., Wang, Q., Abdul-Aziz, D., Mattiacio, J., Edge, A. S. B., and White, P. M. (2018). ERBB2 signaling drives supporting cell proliferation *in vitro* and apparent supernumerary hair cell formation *in vivo* in the neonatal mouse cochlea. *Eur. J. Neurosci.* 48, 3299–3316. doi: 10.1111/ejn.14183

Zhang, T., Xu, J., Maire, P., and Xu, P.-X. (2017). Six1 is essential for differentiation and patterning of the mammalian auditory sensory epithelium. *PLoS Genet.* 13:e1006967. doi: 10.1371/journal.pgen.1006967

Zheng, J. L., and Gao, W.-Q. (2000). Overexpression of Math1 induces robust production of extra hair cells in postnatal rat inner ears. *Nat. Neurosci.* 3, 580–586. doi: 10.1038/75753

Zhou, Q., Brown, J., Kanarek, A., Rajagopal, J., and Melton, D. A. (2008). *in vivo* reprogramming of adult pancreatic exocrine cells to β-cells. *Nature* 455, 627–632. doi: 10.1038/nature07314

Zhu, Y., Liu, Q., Zhou, Z., and Ikeda, Y. (2017). PDX1, Neurogenin-3, and MAFA: critical transcription regulators for β cell development and regeneration. *Stem Cell Res. Ther.* 8:240. doi: 10.1186/s13287-017-0694-z

16

The Relationship of Tinnitus Distress with Personality Traits

Juliëtte J. C. M. van Munster[1,2*†], *Wouter H. van der Valk*[1†], *Inge Stegeman*[3,4], *Arno F. Lieftink*[3] *and Adriana L. Smit*[3,4]

[1] *Department of Otorhinolaryngology and Head & Neck Surgery, Leiden University Medical Center, Leiden University, Leiden, Netherlands,* [2] *Department of Neurosurgery, Leiden University Medical Center, Leiden University, Leiden, Netherlands,* [3] *Department of Otorhinolaryngology and Head & Neck Surgery, University Medical Center Utrecht, Utrecht, Netherlands,* [4] *Brain Center Rudolf Magnus, University Medical Center Utrecht, Utrecht, Netherlands*

***Correspondence:**
Juliëtte J. C. M. van Munster
j.j.c.m.van_munster@lumc.nl

† These authors have contributed equally to this work

Objectives: An association between tinnitus distress with anxiety and depression is described in literature. A similar relationship might exist between tinnitus distress and personality traits, especially since associations between personality traits and other chronic diseases are already revealed. In this systematic review, we aim to investigate whether personality is a risk factor for tinnitus distress.

Design: We searched PubMed and EMBASE databases from inception up to December 31, 2018 for articles on the association between tinnitus distress and personality. Two researchers screened titles, abstracts, and full texts for eligibility. Directness of evidence and risk of bias were assessed. From the included studies, study characteristics and outcome data of tinnitus distress and personality traits were extracted.

Results: A total of 323 unique articles were screened of which 11 cross-sectional studies were eligible for critical appraisal and were used for data extraction. Including study populations were heterogenous, and studies scored high to moderate risk of bias. Nine out of 11 articles showed an association between tinnitus distress and the personality of neuroticism.

Conclusions: By limitations in the methodology of included studies, the evidence on specific personality traits as a risk factor for tinnitus distress is inconclusive. Some evidence on a positive association with neuroticism is identified. To draw conclusions about causal relations, these further studies should be of longitudinal design in a cohort setting. These studies should assess tinnitus distress using validated questionnaires with multiple personality dimensions and validated questionnaires to assess personality traits.

Keywords: tinnitus, tinnitus distress, personality traits, five-factor model, neuroticism

INTRODUCTION

Tinnitus is the presence of a buzzing or tinkling sound in one or both ears without an acoustic external source to the head and can be associated with a reduction in health-related quality of life (1–3). Growing evidence shows that many cases of tinnitus are associated with de-afferentation of the central auditory structures due to aging, noise exposure, otologic injury, or other causes. The prevalence of tinnitus varies widely, depending on the used methodology, selected population, and definition of tinnitus. For that reason, the prevalence of the adult population experiencing tinnitus is estimated to be 10–25% (4). Where only 1–7% of the adult tinnitus population seems to struggle with bothersome tinnitus, others experience this symptom without any difficulties, which underlines the heterogeneity of the experienced disease (4). This heterogeneity is not only the experienced diversity in the tinnitus itself (e.g., lateralization, temporal course, sound characteristics) but also due to differences in tinnitus-related problems such as sleep and concentration difficulties and accompanying co-morbidities. Tinnitus-related distress is diverse and can be described as a complex phenomenon associated with negative appraisal, selective attention, safety behaviors, beliefs, and a distorted perception of tinnitus (5, 6). Thereby, it is not surprising that the individual needs of patients for tinnitus-related healthcare are various (4, 7).

So far, it is unclear to what extent psychopathological disorders are predisposing to tinnitus complaints, do aggravate symptoms, or refrain patients from tinnitus relief by diverse tinnitus therapies (8–10). The same might be argued for possible influences of personality traits (10) whereby personality can be defined as the characteristic pattern of thinking, feeling, and behaving of an individual (11). Early appearance of personality after birth indicates that personality is partly genetic determined (12, 13). Many studies have investigated the association between personality and diseases, for instance, between personality and the development of cardiovascular disease and cancer (14–17). A similar relationship could exist between personality characteristics and tinnitus. In the cognitive tinnitus model, it is assumed that tinnitus provokes distress in persons who hold overly negatively thoughts about it, thereby motivating maintaining factors. Subsequently, patients gain a distorted perception of their tinnitus. In 2014, Mucci et al. analyzed the relationship between tinnitus and personality by reviewing the literature from 1968 to 2012 (5, 18). They concluded that tinnitus is associated with several personality characteristics, especially on neuroticism, though a clear distinction between tinnitus perception and tinnitus distress was not made and the quality of data was not assessed. Personality characteristics in patients with more distress might differ from others without high distress levels. A scoping review by Durai et al. in 2016 found associations between tinnitus distress and multiple personality traits such as high neuroticism and low extraversion (19). Still, this review has important limitations due to the scoping method: relevant studies may not have been identified, and a quality assessment was not performed.

To measure personality traits, a wide range of questionnaires can be used. Some questionnaires focus on specific personality traits (19) where other questionnaires are based on models dividing personality into dimensions, for instance, three (Eysenck's theory) or five dimensions [the five-factor model (FFM): the "Big Five"] (19, 20). The variance between factors in the FFM is substantial compared to the variance of other personality inventories (21), and thereby, the FFM adopted a prominent position in the field of personality assessment (22). Assessing personality traits by a validated instrument in tinnitus patients might contribute to a better understanding about the relationship between both. As differences in personality traits can influence tinnitus-related distress and the response on different tinnitus treatments, which is especially important for tinnitus patients with severe complaints of tinnitus, this insight might be of benefit to understand the disease and treatment outcome. Therefore, we aim to investigate whether personality is a risk factor for tinnitus distress by a systematic review of the literature.

TABLE 1 | Eligibility criteria.

Inclusion criteria
Studies that correlated tinnitus distress with personality characteristics
Participants ≥18 years of age
Exclusion criteria
Studies that correlated tinnitus with psychiatric disease or pathological personality
Studies on personality characteristics in patients with hearing loss, dizziness, or chronic disease
Validation studies of a questionnaire
Reviews or case reports
Studies investigating a therapy for tinnitus

MATERIALS AND METHODS

Search Strategy

We searched PubMed and Embase to access records, which analyzed the relationship between tinnitus distress and personality up to December 2018. PubMed was searched by entering the following search criteria in PubMed: [personal*(Title/Abstract)] AND {[tinnitus (MeSH Terms)] OR tinnitus (Title/Abstract)}. A similar search strategy was used to search Embase. The Preferred Reporting Items for Systematic Reviews and Meta-analysis (PRISMA) was used as a writing guideline (23).

Study Selection

After removal of duplicates, two researchers (JM and WV) independently screened titles and abstracts of searched articles. Eligible full text articles were retrieved through the databases and by emailing the authors. Full text eligibility was determined by the in- and exclusion criteria listed in **Table 1**. We included studies if they included adults with tinnitus that correlated tinnitus distress with personality characteristics. With tinnitus distress, terms such as tinnitus loudness, annoyance, and handicap were also included. When there was a different opinion on eligibility, the two reviewers tried to reach consensus. Studies investigating a therapy for tinnitus were excluded since interventions can change personality traits (24). The third and fifth author (IS and AS) were consulted if no unanimity was achieved.

Data Collection

Two researchers (JM and WV) extracted data regarding study design, study population, group size, setting, questionnaires

TABLE 2 | Correlation between non-FFM personality questionnaires and the FFM personality traits based on the literature.

Questionnaire	FFM neuroticism	FFM extraversion	FFM openness	FFM agreeableness	FFM conscientiousness	References
EPI-Neuroticism	Neuroticism	–	–	–	–	(35)
EPQ	Neuroticism	Extraversion	–	Psychoticism (R)	Psychoticism (R)	(35)
FMPS	Mistakes, standards, parent criticism	–	Parent criticism, doubts	Parent expectations (R)	Standards (R), doubts, organization	(33)
FPI-R	Life satisfaction (R) Excitability Strain Somatic complaints Emotionality	Inhibitedness (R) Extraversion Achievement orientation Aggressiveness	Openness	Social orientation Aggressiveness (R)	Need for achievement	(36)
MMPI	Hypochondriasis Depression Psychasthenia	Social introversion (R)	Masculine/feminine (R)	Paranoia (R)	Psychopathic deviate (R)	(37)
MPQ	PEM (R), NEM	PEM (R)	Constraint (R)	NEM (R)	PEM, constraint	(26)
TCI	Harm avoidance Self-directedness (R)	Harm avoidance (R) Persistence	Self-transcendence	Cooperativeness Reward Dependence	Self-directedness Persistence Novelty Seeking (R)	(28, 31)

Different personality questionnaires and their domains were compared and correlated to the personality traits of the FFM. Reverse correlations are depicted by (R). EPI, Eysenck Personality Inventory; EPQ, Eysenck Personality Questionnaire; FMPS, Frost Multidimensional Perfectionism Scale; FPI-R, Freiburger Personlichkeitsinventar; MMPI, Minnesota Multiphasic Personality Inventory; MPQ, Multidimensional Personality Questionnaire; NEM, Negative Emotionality superfactor; TCI, Temperament and Character Inventory; PEM, Positive Emotionality superfactor.

regarding tinnitus distress and personality, and outcomes of the evaluation concerning tinnitus distress and personality. Primary outcome was the relationship between tinnitus distress and personality traits, as described by the FFM. The FFM is a taxonomy of five traits: neuroticism, extraversion, openness, agreeableness, and conscientiousness (25). The Big Five Personality Dimensions Scale, the NEO Five-Factor Inventory (NEO-FFI), and the Big Five Inventory (BFI) are based on the FFM. When included trials used personality trait questionnaires not based on the FFM categorization, these personality traits were matched to the FFM categories. For this, the literature was searched to find a correlation between the non-FFM personality trait category and the traits as defined and scored by the FFM (26–34). Those associations and stratifications between FFM personality traits and non-FFM traits are described in **Table 2**. Mean scores of the questionnaires including standard deviations and *P*-values were distracted from the articles when available. When a *t*-test was used, the *F*-ratio and *P*-value were documented.

Risk of Bias

Critical appraisal of selected studies regarding risk of bias (RoB) was performed by two researchers (WV and JM), using the Newcastle–Ottawa Quality Assessment Scale, using different assessment scales for cohort studies and for case-control studies (38). This instrument is divided into three subdomains concerning the bias in selection, comparability, and exposure. Each subdomain consists of one to four categories of potential bias. A study can be awarded one or two stars depending on each item within the categories. Selection can be awarded with a maximum of four stars, comparability with a maximum of two stars, and outcome with a maximum of three stars. The more stars were earned, the lower the risk of bias of the study was rated.

RESULTS

Study Selection

Our flow chart of the study selection, including reasons for exclusion of articles, is shown in **Figure 1**. After removal of duplicates, 323 unique records were identified. Of these, 255 articles were excluded based on title and abstract screening. After reading the full text of 68 articles, 11 articles were eligible for critical appraisal.

Risk of Bias and Quality Assessment

Critical appraisal of the 11 articles is outlined in **Table 3**. None of the studies were awarded with the maximal amount of nine stars; the range is between three and six stars. The majority used a selected group of tinnitus patients by including them from outpatient clinics (40, 41, 43, 44, 46–49). Furthermore, none of the case-control studies did provide information about non-respondents, and all cohort studies were of cross-sectional study design hindering the assessment of adequate follow-up. In addition, the majority of studies did not correctly control for confounding factors (40, 41, 43–49). Together, this limits the number of stars awarded for all subdomains. Only two studies used a representative cohort of patients with tinnitus out of the general population; however, these studies used a single question of tinnitus distress in contrast to validated multi-item questionnaires (45, 50).

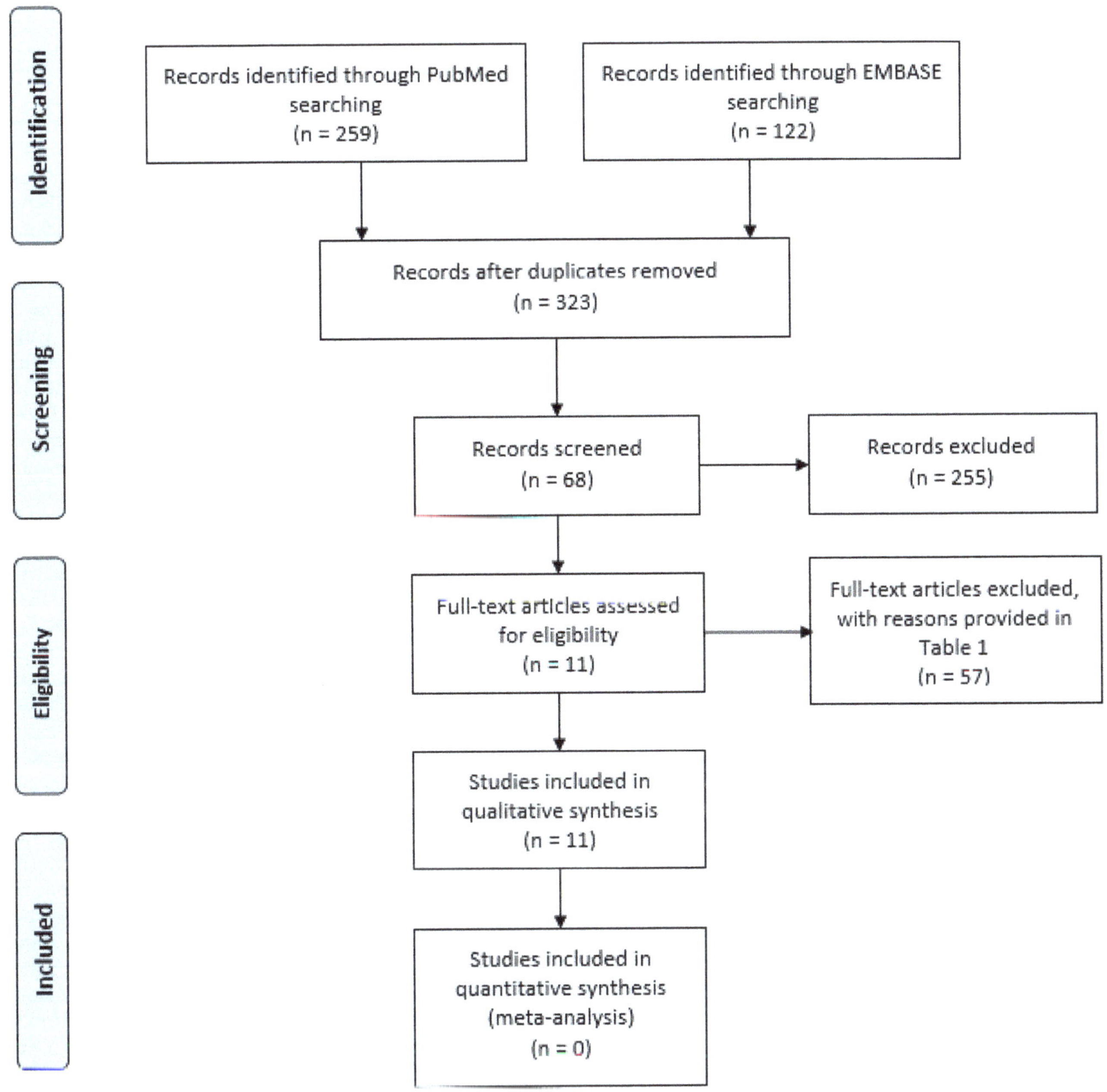

FIGURE 1 | The Preferred Reporting Items for Systematic Reviews and Meta-Analyses (PRISMA) Flow Diagram of Study Selection (39).

Characteristics of Studies

There was a large heterogeneity in tinnitus questionnaires and personality questionnaires to measure tinnitus distress and personality traits, respectively, in the included studies. Because of this heterogeneity, no meta-analysis could be performed. Therefore, a descriptive analysis of the included articles is provided. All but three (42, 45, 50) studies included patients who visited the tinnitus department or Ear-, Nose-, Throat (ENT), which leads to a specific patient selection. The two cohort studies included patients from large-population studies in Dunedin (New Zealand) and the United Kingdom (UK) (45, 50) and assessed personality traits in a cross-sectional manner.

Synthesis of the Results

Extensive descriptions of the articles and outcomes are presented in **Table 4**.

Tinnitus Distress and Personality Traits

A majority (9 out of 11 studies) of the included studies showed one or more associations (both positive and negative) between

TABLE 3 | Risk of bias assessment using the Newcastle–Ottawa Quality Assessment Scale.

References	Selection (Max. ****)	Comparability (Max. **)	Outcome (Max. ***)	Total number of stars[b]
Adami Dehkordi et al. (40)[a]	***		**	*****
Andersson et al. (41)	**		*	***
Durai et al. (42)[a]	***	**	*	******
Gerber et al. (43)	*		**	***
Langguth et al. (44)	**		*	***
McCormack et al. (45)	***			***
Meric et al. (46)	**	**	*	*****
Salviati et al. (47)	**		*	***
Strumila et al. (48)	**		*	***
Weber et al. (49)	**		*	***
Welch and Dawes (50)	***	**		*****

[a]*Newcastle–Ottawa Quality Assessment Scale for case-control studies was used.*
[b]*A maximum of nine stars could be earned in total and implies the lowest Risk of Bias.*

tinnitus distress and personality (41, 44–47, 49, 50). Two out of 11 articles studied the association between tinnitus distress and the FFM personality traits by usage of the NEO five-factor inventory (44) or a short version of the Big Five Personality dimensions scale (48). Of those, Langguth et al. did find a negative association between scores on the Tinnitus Handicap Inventory (THI) and consciousness (correlation coefficient $= -0.367$, $p = 0.003$), and a positive association between tinnitus distress on the Tinnitus Questionnaire (TQ) and neuroticism (correlation coefficient $= 0.276$, $p = 0.028$) (44). Furthermore Strumila et al. (48) stated that high THI scores did not predict high scores on any of the personality traits, but neuroticism did influence distress of tinnitus perception ($p < 0.001$, standardized coefficient 0.38).

The other nine studies used non-FFM-based questionnaires to assess personality traits in similar domains to the FFM division (40–43, 45–47, 49, 50). To be able to make a comparison, we converted these outcomes of personality traits to the FFM personality traits when a comparison between both was described in literature, as stated previously (**Tables 2**, **5**). One study found a positive association between bothersome tinnitus and neuroticism [odds ratio (95% CI) $= 4.11$ (3.69–4.58), $p < 0.001$] using the EPI-neuroticism questionnaire (45). Eight of nine non-FFM-based studies indicated a positive correlation between neuroticism and increased tinnitus distress, including the New Zealand study, which represents a sample of the general population (**Table 5**) (40–42, 45–47, 49, 50). For the other categories of personality traits (extraversion, openness, agreeableness, and consciousness), we found no conclusive results about an association with tinnitus distress.

DISCUSSION

In the present review, we studied personality traits as a risk factor for tinnitus distress, in which 11 cross-sectional studies with a high degree of heterogeneity in methods and outcomes were included. Owing to heterogeneity in the reported personality traits, it was not possible to perform a meta-analysis. Of the FFM, neuroticism was the only trait with a positive relationship with tinnitus distress in multiple studies. The association between neuroticism and tinnitus distress is in line with previous findings about emotional health and tinnitus: tinnitus distress shows close relationships with factors related to emotional health, and emotional health may be prognostic for the development of tinnitus distress (51, 52). One could argue that patients with more severe complaints of tinnitus are indeed more likely to have a neurotic personality, since neuroticism is described as the tendency to experience negative emotions. However, neuroticism is also associated with psychopathological symptoms of depression and anxiety (53), which complicates the causality of this association, since anxiety and depression are more prevalent among tinnitus patients (8, 19, 54). Moreover, both tinnitus and personality are potentially influenced by genetic factors (55, 56). Interestingly, of the FFM traits, the strongest associations were revealed between genetic variants and neuroticism (56–58). One of these studies used the same prospective cohort in the United Kingdom as the study of McCormack et al. (45) of which results were included in this systematic review. Indeed, this study found a positive association between neuroticism and tinnitus.

Several major limitations of this systematic review must be mentioned. Most of the studies included a selected population of tinnitus patients visiting an ENT department, audiological clinic, or tinnitus clinics and, thus, are not necessarily representative of the general population. For instance, headache-prone individuals have found to differ in personality profiles when comparing institutionalized patients to non-institutionalized controls from outside the clinic (59). Potentially, help-seeking tinnitus patients might differ in personality from non-help-seeking tinnitus patients. Owing to the selected sample of tinnitus patients used in the included studies in our review, generalization of outcomes is hindered. Moreover, most studies are prone to bias as scored by the Newcastle–Ottawa Quality Assessment Scale. For instance, confounders in the relation between personality traits and tinnitus distress exist, but not all studies described or analyzed these potential confounding factors such as gender (41, 48, 50). Additionally, as many different questionnaires were used to assess the personality traits, we used previously described correlations to convert the personality domains out of these questionnaires into the FFM categorization, to be able to compare outcomes of different studies. To our knowledge, however, this method is not validated nor described previously.

For all these reasons, the evidence we present in this systematic review about the relationship between personality and tinnitus is inconclusive. The aim of our review was to assess personality as a risk factor for tinnitus distress. Longitudinal cohort studies are needed to assess the causality of personality in tinnitus, address the limitations, and reveal additional potential confounders in this relationship.

TABLE 4 | Summary of studies on personality characteristics in tinnitus patients according to tinnitus distress.

References	Questionnaires (personality, tinnitus)	Study design	Study population	Sample number (Tinnitus number)	Outcomes
Andersson et al. (41)	HADS, ISI, FMPS TRQ	Case series Cross-sectional	Tinnitus patients visiting the Audiology Department	256 (256)	Severity of tinnitus was correlated with Concern over Mistakes, Personal Standards, Parental Expectations, Parental Criticism, Doubts about Action and Organization ($p < 0.05$)
Adami Dehkordi et al. (40)	EPQ TET, TSI	Case control Cross-sectional	Patients with idiopathic tinnitus from the ENT Department and matched, healthy non-tinnitus volunteers from patients' family	66 (33)	No associations between the TSI, the 1–10 Tinnitus Scale Score and any of the personality traits were found
Durai et al. (42)	MPQ TFI	Case control Cross-sectional	Tinnitus sufferers recruited from the University of Auckland Tinnitus Research Volunteer Database Non-tinnitus sufferers recruited via the University of Auckland Hearing and Tinnitus database, posters, and social media	215 (61)	Within tinnitus sufferers, stress reaction scores were negatively correlated with constraint ($r = -0.365$, $p = 0.004$) and social closeness/positive emotionality ($r = -0.296$, $p = 0.02$) and positively correlated with alienation scores/negative emotionality ($r = 0.406$, $p = 0.001$) Total TFI scores was significantly negatively correlated with social closeness ($r = -0.312$, $p < 0.001$) The tinnitus group had lower levels of self-control scores (mean = 12.70, SD = 4.15) and social closeness scores (mean = 8.46, SD = 3.57) than controls (respectively, mean = 13.76, SD = 3.26; mean = 10.11, SD = 4.06) and higher alienation scores (mean = 3.48, SD = 3.87) than controls (mean = 10.11, SD = 4.06)
Gerber et al. (43)	MMPI, scaling method to assess severity of stress events by Homes and Rahe 26-item questionnaire designed to obtain a subjective measure of tinnitus severity (not validated)	Case series Cross-sectional	Male tinnitus patients referred to the Audiology Clinic with subjective tinnitus as a primary complaint	45 (45)	Severity of tinnitus was not related to stress events or differences on the MMPI profile
Langguth et al. (44)	NEO-FFI, BDI THI, TQ	Case series Cross-sectional	Patients with tinnitus for at least 6 months, visiting the Tinnitus Clinic	72 (72)	High tinnitus handicap was correlated with low agreeableness ($p = 0.003$), but not with neuroticism, extraversion, openness, and conscientiousness High tinnitus severity was correlated with high neuroticism ($p = 0.028$), but not with extraversion, openness, agreeableness, and conscientiousness
McCormack et al. (45)	EPI-Neuroticism Single question concerning tinnitus annoyance	Cohort Cross-sectional	Tinnitus, and non-tinnitus participants, aged 40 to 69 years, recruited from the UK Biobank Dataset	172.621 (27.964)	Neuroticism had a stronger association with bothersome tinnitus [4.11 (OR 95% CI 3.69–4.58); $p < 0.001$] than tinnitus presence [OR 2.11 (95% CI 2.00–2.22); $p < 0.001$]
Meric et al. (46)	French short MMPI TRQ, THQ, STSS scale	Case series Cross-sectional	Tinnitus patients visiting the ENT Department	281 (281)	Increasing tinnitus impact and handicap were correlated with paranoia, psychasthenia, schizophrenia, and hypochondriasis ($p < 0.0001$). No association was present for mania
Salviati et al. (47)	VRS, SCL90-R, TCI THI	Case series Cross-sectional	Tinnitus patients from the Tinnitus Center of the Department of Sense Organs	239 (239)	Tinnitus handicap was associated with all psychopathological dimensions (somatization, obsessive–compulsive, anxiety, depression, sensitivity, hostility, phobic anxiety, paranoid ideation, psychoticism; $p < 0.001$) Harm avoidance and self-directedness were also correlated with tinnitus handicap ($p < 0.004$), but not with reward dependence ($p = 0.88$), novelty seeking ($p = 0.90$), persistence ($p = 0.70$), cooperativeness ($p = 0.32$), and self-transcendence ($p = 0.21$)

(Continued)

TABLE 4 | Continued

References	Questionnaires (personality, tinnitus)	Study design	Study population	Sample number (Tinnitus number)	Outcomes
Strumila et al. (48)	HADS, short version of Big Five Personality Dimensions Scale and sociodemographic questions THI, VAS of tinnitus severity	Case series Cross-sectional	Tinnitus sufferer recruited via internet	212 (212)	Tinnitus severity was not correlated with personality traits [in mean (SD)]: - Extraversion mean 26.49 (5.13) - Agreeableness 26.46 (5.13) - Consciousness 26.33 (4.02) - Neuroticism 18.55 (5.45) - Openness 21.39 (5.32)
Weber et al. (49)	FPI-R, BDI TQ	Case series Cross-sectional	Adult, tinnitus patients visiting the ENT Department	121 (121)	Based on tinnitus severity, patients differed in - Life satisfaction (F = 5.497; p = 0.001), lower if increasing severity - Excitability (F = 5.151; p = 0.002), higher if increasing severity - Aggressiveness (F = 3.483; p = 0.018), higher if increasing severity - Stress (F = 10.846; p < 0.001), higher if increasing severity - Physical complaints (F = 12.876; p < 0.001), higher if increasing severity - Health concerns (F = 3.610; p = 0.015), higher if increasing severity - Emotionality (F = 12.708; p < 0.001), higher if increasing severity
Welch and Dawes (50)	MPQ Single question concerning tinnitus annoyance	Cohort Cross-sectional	Tinnitus and non-tinnitus participants born between April 1972 and March 1973 from a birth cohort of Dunedin (New Zealand's South Island)	970 (437)	Based on amount of tinnitus, personality differed significantly: Positive emotionality [$F_{(2.946)} = 3.675$; $p = 0.026$] - Social closeness lower in groups with more tinnitus [$F_{(2.946)} = 13.242$; $p < 0.001$] - Well-being, social potency, and achievement did not differ Negative emotionality [$F_{(2.946)} = 12.810$; $p < 0.001$] - Stress reaction [$F_{(2.946)} = 9.144$, $p < 0.001$] higher in groups with more tinnitus - Alienation higher in groups with more tinnitus (Wald = 12.206; p<0.001) - Aggression did not differ Constraint [$F_{(2.946)} = 5.516$; $p = 0.004$] - Self-control lower in groups with more tinnitus [$F(2.946) = 4.752$; $p = 0.009$] - Harm avoidance or Traditionalism did not differ Based on the annoyance of tinnitus, personality differed significantly: Positive emotionality [$F_{(2.424)} = 3.010$, $p = 0.050$] - Social closeness lower in patients more tinnitus distress [$F_{(2.424)} = 3.471$; $p = 0.032$] - Well-being lower in groups with more annoyance (Wald = 6.579, p = 0.010) - Social potency or achievement did not differ Negative emotionality [$F_{(2,424)} = 6.039$, $p = 0.003$) higher in groups with more annoyance. Annoyance was not related to constraint [$F_{(2.424)} = 1.722$, $p = 0.180$].

Secondary outcome on tinnitus distress, annoyance, or severity on personality characteristics in tinnitus patients per publication (first author, year of publication). Per publication, the used tinnitus and personality questionnaires used are depicted; if underlined, they assessed personality traits. Study design and information on the included populations are shown. The outcomes show results of tinnitus distress in relation to personality traits in tinnitus patients. BDI, Beck Depression Inventory; EPI, Eysenck Personality Inventory; EPQ, Eysenck Personality Questionnaire; FMPS, Frost Multidimensional Perfectionism Scale; FPI-R, Freiburger Personlichkeitsinventar; HADS, Hospital Anxiety and Depression Scale; ISI, Insomnia Severity Index; MMPI, Minnesota Multiphasic Personality Inventory; MPQ, Multidimensional Personality Questionnaire; NEO-FFI, NEO Five-Factor Inventory; SCL-90-R, Symptom Checklist-90-Revised; STSS, Subjective Tinnitus Severity Scale; TCI, Temperament and Character Inventory; TET, Tinnitus Evaluation Test; TFI, Tinnitus Functional Index; THI, Tinnitus Handicap Inventory; THQ, Tinnitus Handicap Questionnaire; TQ, Tinnitus Questionnaire; TRQ, Tinnitus Reaction Questionnaire; TSI, Tinnitus Severity Index; VAS, Visual Analog Scale; VRS, Stress-Related Vulnerability Scale.

TABLE 5 | Association of personality trait outcomes to tinnitus distress.

FFM	**Association between tinnitus distress and personality**		
	Positive association	**Negative association**	**No association found**
Neuroticism	Neuroticism (44)*(45) Positive emotionality (42, 50) Negative emotionality (42) Parental criticism (41) Concerns over mistakes (41) Hypochondriasis (46) Depression (46) Psychasthenia (46) Harm avoidance (47) Self-directedness (47) Life satisfaction (49) Excitability (49) Strain (49) Somatic complaints (49) Emotionality (49)		Neuroticism (48)* Neuroticism (40) Hypochondria (43) Depression (43) Psychasthenia (43)
Extraversion	Aggressiveness (49)	Social introversion (46) Social closeness (50) Positive emotionality (42, 50)	Extraversion (44, 48)* Extraversion (40) Social introversion (43) Wellbeing, social potency, achievement (50)
Openness	Constraint (50) Parental criticism (41) Doubts about Action (41)	Masculinity/Femininity (46)	Openness (44, 48)* Harm avoidance and traditionalism (50) Masculine/feminine (43)
Agreeableness	Parental expectations (41)	Agreeableness (48)* Negative emotionality (42)	Psychoticism (40) Agreeableness (44)* Negative emotionality Paranoia (46) Aggressiveness (49) Paranoia (43)
Consciousness	Personal standards (41) Doubts about action (41)	Consciousness (44, 48)* Constraint (42) Positive emotionality (42) Self-control (50)	Psychoticism (40) Positive emotionality (50) Harm avoidance and traditionalism (50) Psychopathic deviate (43, 46)

Personality traits as measured using the FFM personality traits. Other personality traits are "translated" according to **Table 2 and clustered under the corresponding FFM personality traits.*

The potential relationship of tinnitus distress with neuroticism may affect the success of specific tinnitus treatments, making the execution of high-quality studies on this topic of eminent importance. For example, cognitive behavioral treatment (CBT) targets the emotional reactivity and (dysfunctional) behavioral mechanisms. Studies assessing tinnitus outcome after CBT treatment show a reduction in disease-related distress and increased daily life functioning in individuals with subjective tinnitus (60–62). Interestingly, FFM personality can affect the tinnitus outcome after CBT treatment as demonstrated by Kleinstauber et al. in a clinical trial (63). Therefore, one should not only consider tinnitus distress (64) but also individual characteristics as personality traits to tailor tinnitus treatment for this heterogenous group of patients.

CONCLUSION

We endeavored to present the evidence on the relationship between tinnitus distress and personality traits in this systematic review. Owing to limitations in the methodology of included studies, the evidence on specific personality traits as a risk factor for tinnitus distress is inconclusive. Some evidence on a positive association with neuroticism is identified. To draw conclusions about causal relations, future studies should be of longitudinal design in a cohort setting. These studies should assess tinnitus distress using validated questionnaires with multiple personality dimensions and validated questionnaires to assess personality traits.

AUTHOR CONTRIBUTIONS

This study was conceived and designed by JM, WV, IS, and AS. All authors contributed to acquisition, analysis, and interpretation of data. The drafting of the manuscripts was performed by JM and WV. Critical revision of the manuscript for important intellectual content as well as study supervision was performed by AS, IS, and AL.

REFERENCES

1. Henry JA, Dennis KC, Schechter MA. General review of tinnitus: prevalence, mechanisms, effects, and management. *J Speech Lang Hear Res.* (2005) 48:1204–35. doi: 10.1044/1092-4388(2005/084)
2. Nondahl DM, Cruickshanks KJ, Dalton DS, Klein BE, Klein R, Schubert CR, et al. The impact of tinnitus on quality of life in older adults. *J Am Acad Audiol.* (2007) 18:257–66. doi: 10.3766/jaaa.18.3.7
3. Prestes R, Daniela G. Impact of tinnitus on quality of life, loudness and pitch match, and high-frequency audiometry. *Int Tinnitus J.* (2009) 15:134–8.
4. Bauer CA. Tinnitus. *N Engl J Med.* (2018) 378:1224–31. doi: 10.1056/NEJMcp1506631
5. Mckenna L, Handscomb L, Hoare DJ, Hall DA. A scientific cognitive-behavioral model of tinnitus: novel conceptualizations of tinnitus distress. *Front Neurol.* (2014) 5:196. doi: 10.3389/fneur.2014.00196
6. Brüggemann P, Szczepek AJ, Rose M, Mckenna L, Olze H, Mazurek B. Impact of multiple factors on the degree of tinnitus distress. *Front Hum Neurosci.* (2016) 10:341. doi: 10.3389/fnhum.2016.00341
7. Nemholt SS, Schmidt JH, Wedderkopp N, Baguley DM. Prevalence of tinnitus and/or hyperacusis in children and adolescents: study protocol for a systematic review. *BMJ Open.* (2015) 5:e006649. doi: 10.1136/bmjopen-2014-006649
8. Geocze L, Mucci S, Abranches DC, Marco MA, Penido Nde O. Systematic review on the evidences of an association between tinnitus and depression. *Braz J Otorhinolaryngol.* (2013) 79:106–11. doi: 10.5935/1808-8694.20130018
9. Pinto PC, Marcelos CM, Mezzasalma MA, Osterne FJ, De Melo Tavares De Lima MA, Nardi AE. Tinnitus and its association with psychiatric disorders: systematic review. *J Laryngol Otol.* (2014) 128:660–4. doi: 10.1017/S0022215114001030
10. Trevis KJ, Mclachlan NM, Wilson SJ. A systematic review and meta-analysis of psychological functioning in chronic tinnitus. *Clin Psychol Rev.* (2018) 60:62–86. doi: 10.1016/j.cpr.2017.12.006
11. Andersen AM, Bienvenu OJ. Personality and psychopathology. *Int Rev Psychiatr.* (2011) 23:234–47. doi: 10.3109/09540261.2011.588692
12. Thomas A, Chess S, Zrull JP, Chairman DO. Temperament and development. *J Am Acad Child Psychiatr.* (1978) 17:732–3. doi: 10.1016/S0002-7138(09)61026-8
13. Cloninger CR, Svrakic DM, Przybeck TR. A psychobiological model of temperament and character. *Arch Gen Psychiatr.* (1993) 50:975–90. doi: 10.1001/archpsyc.1993.01820240059008
14. Eysenck HJ. Personality, cancer and cardiovascular disease: a causal analysis. *Personal Individual Differ.* (1985) 6:535–56. doi: 10.1016/0191-8869(85)90003-0
15. Eysenck HJ. Psychosocial factors, cancer, and ischaemic heart disease. *BMJ.* (1992) 305:457–9. doi: 10.1136/bmj.305.6851.457
16. Eysenck HJ. Prediction of cancer and coronary heart disease mortality by means of a personality inventory: results of a 15-year follow-up study. *Psychol Rep.* (1993) 72:499–516. doi: 10.2466/pr0.1993.72.2.499
17. Eysenck HJ. Personality and coronary heart disease. *Br J Hosp Med.* (1994) 52:120.
18. Mucci S, Geocze L, Abranches DC, Antunez AE, Penido Nde O. [Systematic review of evidence on the association between personality and tinnitus]. *Braz J Otorhinolaryngol.* (2014) 80:441–7. doi: 10.1016/j.bjorl.2014.05.031
19. Durai M, Searchfield G. Anxiety and depression, personality traits relevant to tinnitus: a scoping review. *Int J Audiol.* (2016) 55:605–15. doi: 10.1080/14992027.2016.1198966
20. Vorkapić ST. The significance of preschool teacher's personality in early childhood education: analysis of eysenck's and big five dimensions of personality. *Int J Psychol Behav Sci.* (2012) 2:28–37. doi: 10.5923/j.ijpbs.20120202.05
21. O'connor BP. A quantitative review of the comprehensiveness of the five-factor model in relation to popular personality inventories. *Assessment.* (2002) 9:188–203. doi: 10.1177/10791102009002010
22. Hoekstra H, Ormel J, Fruyt F. *NEO-PI-R/NEO-FFI Big Five Persoonlijkheidsvragenlijst.* Amsterdam: Hogrefe Publishing (2007).
23. Moher D, Liberati A, Tetzlaff J, Altman DG. Preferred reporting items for systematic reviews and meta-analyses: the PRISMA statement. *BMJ.* (2009) 339:b2535. doi: 10.1136/bmj.b2535
24. Roberts BW, Luo J, Briley DA, Chow PI, Su R, Hill PL. A systematic review of personality trait change through intervention. *Psychol Bull.* (2017) 143:117–41. doi: 10.1037/bul0000088
25. McCrae RR, John OP. An introduction to the five-factor model and its applications. *J Pers.* (1992) 60:175–215. doi: 10.1111/j.1467-6494.1992.tb00970.x
26. Church AT. Relating the tellegen and five-factor models of personality structure. *J Pers Soc Psychol.* (1994) 67:898–909. doi: 10.1037/0022-3514.67.5.898
27. Eysenck HJ. *Five-Factor Model.* (2001) Available online at: http://www.personalityresearch.org/bigfive/eysenck.html (accessed Febuary 18, 2020).
28. MacDonald DA, Holland D. Examination of relations between the NEO personality inventory-revised and the temperament and character inventory. *Psychol Rep.* (2002) 91:921–30. doi: 10.2466/pr0.2002.91.3.921
29. Hoekstra H, Ormel J, Fruyt F. *Handleiding NEO-PI-R en NEO-FFI Persoonlijkheidsvragenlijsten* Amsterdam: Hogrefe Publishing (2007).
30. Rushton JP, Irwing P. A general factor of personality (GFP) from the multidimensional personality questionnaire. *Personal Indivi Differ.* (2009) 47:571–6. doi: 10.1016/j.paid.2009.05.011
31. Capanna C, Struglia F, Riccardi I, Daneluzzo E, Stratta P, Rossi A. Temperament and character inventory-R (TCI-R) and big five questionnaire (BFQ): convergence and divergence. *Psychol Rep.* (2012) 110:1002–6. doi: 10.2466/02.03.09.PR0.110.3.1002-1006
32. Howard S, Hughes BM. Construct, concurrent and discriminant validity of type D personality in the general population: associations with anxiety, depression, stress and cardiac output. *Psychol Health.* (2012) 27:242–58. doi: 10.1080/08870446.2011.603423
33. Briley DA, Domiteaux M, Tucker-Drob EM. Achievement-relevant personality: relations with the big five and validation of an efficient instrument. *Learn Individ Differ.* (2014) 32:26–39. doi: 10.1016/j.lindif.2014.03.010
34. Lars. *Das Freiburger Persönlichkeitsinventar.* (2015) Available online at: http://www.typentest.de/blog/2015/11/das-freiburger-personlichkeitsinventar/ (accessed Febuary 18, 2020).
35. Costa PT, McCrae RR. Four ways five factors are basic. *Personal Individ Differ.* (1992) 13:653–65. doi: 10.1016/0191-8869(92)90236-I
36. Borkenau P, Ostendorf F. Untersuchungen zum fünf-faktoren-modell der persönlichkeit und seiner diagnostischen erfassung. [Investigations of the five-factor model of personality and its assessment]. *Zeitschrift Differ Diagnosti Psychol.* (1989) 10:239–51.
37. Cortina JM, Doherty ML, Schmitt N, Kaufman G, Smith RG. The big five personality factors in the IPI and MMPI: predictors of police performance. *Person Psychol.* (1992) 45:119–40. doi: 10.1111/j.1744-6570.1992.tb00847.x
38. Wells G, O'Connell D, Peterson J, Welch V, Losos M, Tugwell P, et al. *The Newcastle-Ottawa Scale (NOS) For Assessing the Quality of Nonrandomised Studies in Meta-analyses.* (2000) Available: http://www.ohri.ca/programs/clinical_epidemiology/oxford.asp
39. Moher D, Liberati A, Tetzlaff J, Altman DG, The PRISMA Group. Preferred reporting items for systematic reviews and meta-analyses: the PRISMA statement. *PLoS Med.* (2009) 6:e1000097. doi: 10.1371/journal.pmed1000097
40. Adami Dehkordi M, Javanbakht M, Sarfarazi Moghadam S, Meshkat M, Abolbashari S. Personality traits in patients with subjective idiopathic tinnitus. *Iran J Otorhinolaryngol.* (2015) 27:369–75. doi: 10.22038/IJORL.2015.4791
41. Andersson G, Airikka M-L, Buhrman M, Kaldo V. Dimensions of perfectionism and tinnitus distress. *Psychol Health Med.* (2005) 10:78–87. doi: 10.1080/13548500512331315389
42. Durai M, O'Keeffe MG, Searchfield GD. The personality profile of tinnitus sufferers and a nontinnitus control group. *J Am Acad Audiol.* (2017) 28:271–82. doi: 10.3766/jaaa.15103
43. Gerber KE, Nehemkis AM, Charter RA, Jones HC. Is tinnitus a psychological disorder? *Int J Psychiatr Med.* (1985) 15:81–7. doi: 10.2190/E59L-2PRU-GPAE-VJ8B
44. Langguth B, Kleinjung T, Fischer B, Hajak G, Eichhammer P, Sand PG. Tinnitus severity, depression, and the big five personality traits. *Prog Brain Res.* (2007) 166:221–5. doi: 10.1016/S0079-6123(07)66020-8
45. McCormack A, Edmondson-Jones M, Fortnum H, Dawes P, Middleton H, Munro KJ, et al. The prevalence of tinnitus and the relationship with

neuroticism in a middle-aged UK population. *J Psychosom Res.* (2014) 76:56–60. doi: 10.1016/j.jpsychores.2013.08.018
46. Meric C, Gartner M, Collet L, Chery-Croze S. Psychopathological profile of tinnitus sufferers: evidence concerning the relationship between tinnitus features and impact on life. *Audiol Neurootol.* (1998) 3:240–52. doi: 10.1159/000013796
47. Salviati M, Bersani FS, Terlizzi S, Melcore C, Panico R, Romano GF, et al. Tinnitus: clinical experience of the psychosomatic connection. *Neuropsychiatr Dis Treat.* (2014) 10:267–75. doi: 10.2147/NDT.S49425
48. Strumila R, Lengvenyte A, Vainutiene V, Lesinskas E. The role of questioning environment, personality traits, depressive and anxiety symptoms in tinnitus severity perception. *Psychiatr Q.* (2017) 88:865–77. doi: 10.1007/s11126-017-9502-2
49. Weber JH, Jagsch R, Hallas B. [The relationship between tinnitus, personality, and depression]. *Z Psychosom Med Psychother.* (2008) 54:227–40. doi: 10.13109/zptm.2008.54.3.227
50. Welch D, Dawes PJ. Personality and perception of tinnitus. *Ear Hear.* (2008) 29:684–92. doi: 10.1097/AUD.0b013e318177d9ac
51. D'Amelio R, Archonti C, Schol S, Falkai P, Plinkert PK, Delb W. [Psychological distress associated with acute tinnitus]. *Hno.* (2004) 52:599–603. doi: 10.1007/s00106-003-0944-5
52. Wallhausser-Franke E, Delb W, Balkenhol T, Hiller W, Hormann K. Tinnitus-related distress and the personality characteristic resilience. *Neural Plast.* (2014) 2014:370307. doi: 10.1155/2014/370307
53. Muris P, Roelofs J, Rassin E, Franken I, Mayer B. Mediating effects of rumination and worry on the links between neuroticism, anxiety and depression. *Personal Individ Differ.* (2005) 39:1105–11. doi: 10.1016/j.paid.2005.04.005
54. Pattyn T, Van Den Eede F, Vanneste S, Cassiers L, Veltman DJ, Van De Heyning P, et al. Tinnitus and anxiety disorders: a review. *Hear Res.* (2016) 333:255–65. doi: 10.1016/j.heares.2015.08.014
55. Lo MT, Hinds DA, Tung JY, Franz C, Fan CC, Wang Y, et al. Genome-wide analyses for personality traits identify six genomic loci and show correlations with psychiatric disorders. *Nat Genet.* (2017) 49:152–6. doi: 10.1038/ng.3736
56. Maas IL, Brüggemann P, Requena T, Bulla J, Edvall NK, Hjelmborg JVB, et al. Genetic susceptibility to bilateral tinnitus in a Swedish twin cohort. *Gene Med.* (2017) 19:1007–12. doi: 10.1038/gim.2017.4
57. Okbay A, Baselmans BM, De Neve JE, Turley P, Nivard MG, Fontana MA, et al. Genetic variants associated with subjective well-being, depressive symptoms, and neuroticism identified through genome-wide analyses. *Nat Genet.* (2016) 48:624–33. doi: 10.1038/ng.3552
58. Smith DJ, Escott-Price V, Davies G, Bailey ME, Colodro-Conde L, Ward J, et al. Genome-wide analysis of over 106 000 individuals identifies 9 neuroticism-associated loci. *Mol Psychiatr.* (2016) 21:749–57. doi: 10.1038/mp.2016.49
59. Ziegler DK, Paolo AM. Headache symptoms and psychological profile of headache-prone individuals: a comparison of clinic patients and controls. *Arch Neurol.* (1995) 52:602–6. doi: 10.1001/archneur.1995.00540300076016
60. Martinez-Devesa P, Perera R, Theodoulou M, Waddell A. Cognitive behavioural therapy for tinnitus. *Cochrane Database Syst Rev.* (2010) 9:Cd005233. doi: 10.1002/14651858.CD005233.pub3
61. Hesser H, Weise C, Westin VZ, Andersson G. A systematic review and meta analysis of randomized controlled trials of cognitive-behavioral therapy for tinnitus distress. *Clin Psychol Rev.* (2011) 31:545–53. doi: 10.1016/j.cpr.2010.12.006
62. Cima RFF, Mazurek B, Haider H, Kikidis D, Lapira A, Norena A, et al. A multidisciplinary European guideline for tinnitus: diagnostics, assessment, and treatment. *HNO.* (2019) 67:10–42. doi: 10.1007/s00106-019-0633-7
63. Kleinstauber M, Weise C, Andersson G, Probst T. Personality traits predict and moderate the outcome of Internet-based cognitive behavioural therapy for chronic tinnitus. *Int J Audiol.* (2018) 57:538–44. doi: 10.1080/14992027.2018.1432902
64. Van De Heyning P, Gilles A, Rabau S, Van Rompaey V. Subjective tinnitus assessment and treatment in clinical practice: the necessity of personalized medicine. *Curr Opin Otolaryngol Head Neck Surg.* (2015) 23:369–75. doi: 10.1097/MOO.0000000000000183

17

Computing Endolymph Hydrodynamics during Head Impulse Test on Normal and Hydropic Vestibular Labyrinth Models

Jorge Rey-Martinez[1†], Xabier Altuna[1†], Kai Cheng[2], Ann M. Burgess[2] and Ian S. Curthoys[2†]*

[1] Neurotology Unit, ENT Department, Hospital Universitario Donostia, San Sebastián - Donostia, Spain, [2] Vestibular Research Laboratory, School of Psychology, The University of Sydney, Sydney, NSW, Australia

Correspondence:
Jorge Rey-Martinez
bendermh@hotmail.com

Hypothesis: Build a biologic geometry based computational model to test the hypothesis that, in some circumstances, endolymphatic hydrops can mechanically cause enhanced eye velocity responses during clinical conditions of the head impulse test.

Background: Some recent clinical and experimental findings had suggested that enhanced eye velocity responses measured with the video head impulse test could not only be caused by recording artifacts or central disfunction but also could be directly caused by the mechanical effect of endolymphatic hydrops on horizontal semicircular canal receptor.

Methods: Data from clinical video head impulse test was computed in three biologic-based geometry models governed by Navier-Stokes equations; six head impulses of incrementally increasing peak head velocity were computed in each one of the three different geometric models, depending on absence, canal or utricular hydrops.

Results: For all computed head impulses an increased endolymphatic pressure was measured at the ampullar region of the horizontal semicircular canal on both canal and utricular hydrops models. The mean of aVOR gain was 1.01 $\pm$ 0.008 for the no-hydrops model, 1.14 $\pm$ 0.010 for the canal hydrops model was, and 1.10 $\pm$ 0.007 for the utricular hydrops model.

Conclusion: The results of the physical computation models support-the hypothesis that in endolymphatic hydrops conditions, which are affecting horizontal semicircular canal and utricular region on moderate dilatations, the eye velocity responses output-by the aVOR will be enhanced by a 1.14 factor and aVOR gain values will be enhanced by over 1.1 for impulses to the right side.

Keywords: menière disease, endolymphatic hydrops, vHIT, VOR, clinical sign, enhanced eye velocity, CFD

INTRODUCTION

The video head impulse test (vHIT) is a computer-quantified clinical test of semicircular canal function that has a wide clinical application for vestibular and central pathologies in which the angular vestibulo-ocular reflex (aVOR) is affected (1, 2). vHIT has two main quantified outputs that are used in clinical practice. The first is the quotient between eye and head velocity during the slow phase period (1) known as the gain of the aVOR (3) and the second is the timing, velocity and synchronicity of the saccadic eye responses produced during slow- or fast-phase periods (4).

About the gain of aVOR parameter it is also widely accepted that the presence of a lower value of aVOR gain—corresponding to situations where the slow-phase eye velocity is lower than head velocity most of the time—is a direct indicator of vestibular hypofunction (1), but recently published case reports have suggested that enhanced eye velocity responses during the head impulse test could be a quantified sign of endolymphatic hydrops (5). Enhanced aVOR responses are characterized by an enhanced eye velocity in response to head velocity. This enhanced eye velocity is reflected as a slight increase of the aVOR gain parameter, usually measured in a gain range between 1.1 and 1.3 (5). In this previously published case report we suggest that although enhanced eye velocity responses could be related with central vestibular disorders or vHIT goggle slippage due to an inadequate acquisition technique, there are some cases in which the most probable cause of the enhanced eye velocity responses is the endolymphatic hydrops.

Based on previous investigations (6), we suggest that the increase of volume and pressure on the horizontal semicircular canal will provoke an increased (transcupular) pressure on the cupula receptor that will also increase the vestibular afferent signal.

Because direct experimentation of this hypothesis on humans will cause loss of vestibular and auditive functions, researchers classically returned to experimental animal models to explore vestibular function tests (7) under different normal or pathologic biologic conditions. As an alternative to experiments, mathematical, and physical models supporting vestibular physiology do not cause any loss of biologic function, and they give strong evidence that modeled hypotheses are plausible from a physical and mathematical point of view. But these models are sometimes difficult to solve because of the complex mathematical methods required, making the physical-based predictions of the models very basic and imprecise.

Despite computer science has many outstanding figures who has significantly contributed to its development, it's probably since Alan Turing introduced the possibility of complex mathematical function computation by using recursive algorithms based on simple mathematical operations that could be automatically computed by a (theoretical) machine (8), that the use of computational models has grown significantly, with robust methods to develop realistic computer models to explain complex physical and biological phenomena. In the vestibular research field, these complex computational methods have recently been successfully used to model and predict vestibular caloric test responses in normal and endolymphatic hydrops on simplified anatomic models (9) or to reach a better understanding of the Tullio Phenomenon (10).

The main purpose of this research is to develop an anatomical model of the membranous vestibular labyrinth to compute and simulate endolymph hydrodynamics during real clinical head impulse test movement for models of both normal endolymph volume, and of endolymph volume increased by hydrops. With these models we will try to test the hypothesis that, in some circumstances, endolymphatic hydrops can mechanically cause enhanced eye velocity responses during head impulse testing in clinical conditions.

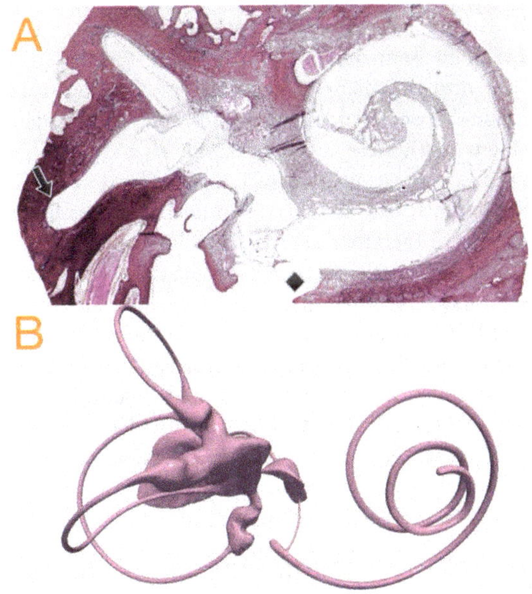

FIGURE 1 | (A) Temporal bone histologic (hematoxylin-eosin) preparation showing cochlear and vestibular structures on a parasagittal plane. The black arrow indicates the relation of endolymph horizontal duct inside the osseous space. The black diamond shows post mortom promontorial cochleostomy with endosteal layer injury and *scala tympani* traumatic penetration. **(B)** Micro-CT volumetric of the endolymphatic spaces of the membranous labyrinth reconstruction used in this study as original 3D model of the inner ear.

MATERIALS AND METHODS

Development of Geometric Models of the Vestibular Organ for Normal and Hydropic Endolymph Volumes

The anatomic model used in this study was obtained from an intact *ex vivo* temporal bone using micro-computer tomography (microCT) scan; a Skyscan 1,172 (Bruker, DKSH Management Ltd, Zurich, Switzerland) microCT desktop scanner device was used in this study. Multiple images obtained using x-ray transmission were saved as uncompressed True Image File Format (TIFF) files.

The TIFF image sequence of the temporal bone was then loaded, processed, combined and exported as a single file in Nearly Raw Raster Data (NRRD) file format. The NRRD file was loaded into 3D Slicer (https://www.slicer.org) reconstruction software where a final 3D reconstructed anatomic model surface of the endolymphatic spaces of the membranous labyrinth model was created as seen in **Figure 1B**. The reconstructed 3D model was finally exported as standard triangle language (STL) file format that was used in computations as the anatomic model, and was also used as the base model to develop the hydrops models.

To develop the hydrops model we considered as McGarvie et al. had previously published (11) that, in human anatomy, the horizontal semicircular duct can be expanded to six times its normal diameter, because of the relative space distribution between endolymph duct and semicircular bone canal (**Figure 1A**): these authors describe an endolymph duct of 0.23 mm inside a osseous canal of 1.53 mm.

Based on this, because our 3D model duct has a diameter of 0.45 mm, we therefore allowed it to be uniformly increased x3 to reach a plausible 1.3 mm hydropic diameter, that still fit inside the osseous canal frame. Because utricular hydrops is not so well-defined in the literature, we decided to develop the hydrops model with a uniform expansion similar to the model of canal hydrops. Normal, canal hydrops and utricular hydrops are presented in **Figure 2**. The two hydrops models were designed using 3D computer design software Blender 2.8 (Blender—a 3D modeling and rendering package, Blender Foundation, Amsterdam, Netherlands; www.blender.org).

Computer Fluid Dynamics Simulations

All developed 3D models were exported in STL file format to the computational fluid dynamics (CFD) software: fully licensed SimFlow 3.1 (SIMFLOW technologies, Warsaw, Poland; https://sim-flow.com) CFD software was used to perform the model simulations to explore the endolymph hydrodynamics during the head impulse test. Once the 3-D models were imported into SimFlow a high-resolution mesh was created using the STL geometric models, defining the outer surfaces of the volumetric model.

The next step in the computer simulation was to select the solver, the mathematic algorithms used to compute the fluid dynamics during head impulses. The transient state with dynamic mesh capability "*PimpleDyMFoam*" (OpenFOAM documentation, The OpenFOAM Foundation Ltd, London, England; https://www.openfoam.org) solver was used on parallel running for our head impulse test computations. "*PympleDyMFoam*" algorithm's governing equation is based on the Navier-Stokes equations (12) for incompressible fluids, considering the vestibular labyrinth as the rotating absolute velocity frame. According to the solver's algorithm developer (OpenFOAM documentation, The OpenFOAM Foundation Ltd, London, England; https://www.openfoam.org) these governing equations are:

$$\begin{cases} \nabla \bullet \left(\overrightarrow{u_{\mathcal{R}}} \otimes \overrightarrow{u_{\mathcal{I}}}\right) + \overrightarrow{\Omega} \times \overrightarrow{u_{\mathcal{I}}} = -\nabla\left(p/\rho\right) + \upsilon \nabla \bullet \nabla\left(\overrightarrow{u_{\mathcal{I}}}\right) \\ \nabla \bullet \overrightarrow{u_{\mathcal{I}}} = 0 \end{cases}$$

Where $\overrightarrow{\Omega}$ is the acceleration of the rotating frame, $\mathcal{I}$ is notation for inertial movement, $\mathcal{R}$ is notation for rotating movement, $\overrightarrow{u}$ is (endolymph) velocity vector, ρ is the endolymph viscosity and p is the pressure. The $\otimes$ operator is used to denote the tensor product between velocity vectors.

For the external (vestibular labyrinth) rotational head velocity input vector we used head velocity data from a video head impulse test database at Royal Prince Alfred Hospital, Sydney. These impulses were all from the same participant and testing session and operator, and were selected to have values of peak head velocity ranging from 102.62°/s to 249.47°/s (**Appendix Figure 1**). The head impulses were recorded with a prototype ICS Impulse (GN Otometrics, Taastrup, Denmark) vHIT device with a sampling time of 0.004 s per frame, i.e., with an acquisition frequency of 250 Hz. The total duration recorded for each head impulse was 0.7 s.

The recorded head velocity data of the six impulses were lowpass-filtered and exported to the SimFlow software to be computed each one with so that each impulse could be applied to all of the three 3D models: normal, canal hydrops and utricular hydrops. For initial conditions endolymph and vestibular organ rotation velocities were set to 0 °/s, and the thermodynamic properties of endolymph were directly extrapolated from water thermodynamic properties: for the present research endolymph kinematic viscosity was 1 e-06 m^2/s.

All computation step was recorded, step duration was set to 0.004 s and simulation total time was set to 0.7, to exactly agree with vHIT sampling frequency and impulse recording duration.

Accordingly, a total of eighteen head impulses were computed in three geometric biologic-based models governed by Navier-Stokes equations; six incremental peak velocity head impulses were computed in each one of the three different geometric models depending on absence, canal or utricular hydrops. CSV head impulse velocity data, STL vestibular geometric models and CFD configuration files for each geometric model are available at **Appendix Datasheet 1–5**.

Computer Fluid Dynamics Simulations Postprocessing and Analysis

Computed head impulses were analyzed and postprocessed with Paraview 5.7.0 (Sandia National Laboratories, Albuquerque & Kitware Inc, New York, USA; https://www.paraview.org) software. Pressure and velocity 3D spaces and endolymph steam lines were the main outputs measured and visualized using Paraview; **Appendix Videos 1–3** supplementary files shows the Paraview exported videos of the normal and canal hydrops models for the head impulse test VI. The main pressure outcome was measured by selecting as pressure receptors the middle and superior points of the internal wall of the ampullar region; the mean pressure measures over time were exported to be analyzed using MATLAB R2019B (The MathWorks, Inc, Natick, Massachusetts, USA; https://www.mathworks.com).

As was described by Grant and Curthoys, the ampullar crista receptor was considered as an highly overdamped pressure—accelerometer sensor that directly responds to endolymph displacement velocity (13) that is directly proportional to angular head velocity (14) and according to Ramat (15), the neural discharge of vestibular afferents for high frequency head movements, in the range of physiological movements, is also a transduction of head angular velocity.

But in our developed geometric model the cupula was modeled as a rigid wall and it was not possible to directly measure the cupula deflection that occurs on biological semicircular canal. As an approach, cupular volume displacement can be estimated from the variation over time of transcupular pressure, that was the main variable measured in our CFD model.

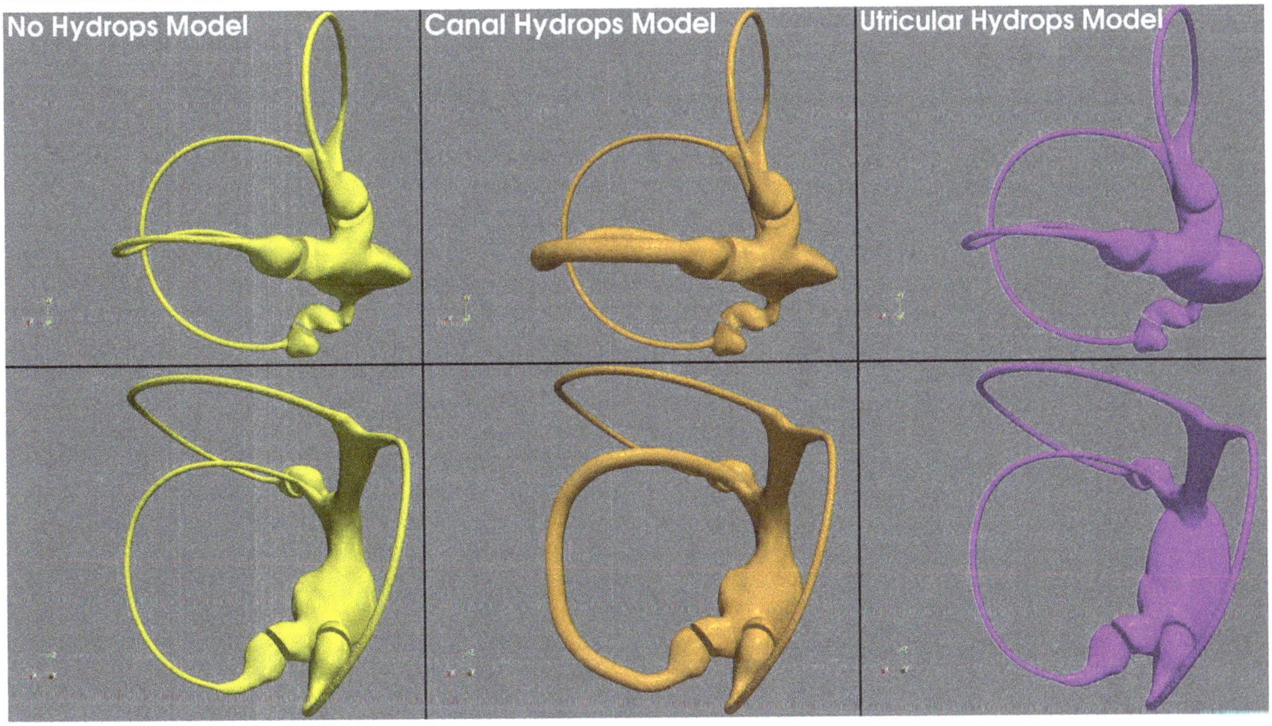

FIGURE 2 | 3D geometric models used in this research. The no hydrops model **(left)** obtained with conservative postprocessing from micro-CT scan, the canal hydrops model **(center)** with a uniform x3 horizontal endolymph duct dilatation, and the utricular hydrops model **(right)** with a similar to canal hydrops model expansion applied to the utricular region.

According to Squires et al. cupular volume displacement $V_c(t)$ is in relation to the applied pressure variation $\Delta P_c(t')$ by the equation (16):

$$V_c(t) = \frac{1}{\gamma}\int_{-\infty}^{t} \Delta P_c(t')\, e^{\frac{-(t-t')}{\tau_c}}\, dt'$$

Where τ_c, cupular time constant, is given by the equation (16):

$$\tau_c = \frac{8\mu\beta_d R}{\pi b_d^4 K}$$

And γ is given by the equation (16):

$$\gamma = \frac{8\mu\beta_d R}{\pi b_d^4}$$

Where μ is the endolymph viscosity, β_d is the angle subtended by semicircular duct, R is the major radius of semicircular canal, b_d is the duct radius and K the cupular elastic constant.

Finally, head movement Ω_0 is related with cupular volume displacement V_c by the expression, for human beings (16):

$$\frac{\Omega_0}{V_c} \approx 5.6 \times 10^{-2}\left(\frac{\circ}{pL\, s}\right)$$

With the computed cupular displacement V_c approximated from the measured ΔP_c on the CFD simulations for each (hydropic and not hydropic) models we obtained the theoretical head movement measured by the cupula in both normal and hydropic semicircular canal for each one of the six head impulses. Assuming that because the unique perturbation introduced in our models was the hydrops of the duct or utricle regions, keeping intact all the other structures from cupula to eye that participates on the aVOR response, we predicted the eye responses by applying a (normofunctional) aVOR gain of $\sim$1 between eye and head responses. Using this approach, we predicted the final eye response based on the obtained head velocity by computing the measured ΔP_c.

To calculate the gain of the aVOR response on the computer simulation results, the obtained eye velocity values for each head impulse computation area under curve value were divided by the area under the curve of the head impulse velocity data for the corresponding simulation. To measure the area under the curve from both real head velocity and computed eye velocity, the HITCal (4) open source calculus tool (https://github.com/bendermh/HITCal/releases) was used under a MATLAB computational environment.

RESULTS

Vestibular model computations with CFD software were successfully performed with a residuals level under 0.01 during the head impulse movement for all cases. None of the variables, grouped by geometric model, showed statistical differences from a normal distribution on Kolmogorov-Smirnov normality test ($p > 0.5$).

TABLE 1 | Main outputs of the model's computation.

Impulse	Hydrops model	Increment of ampular pressure (Pa)	Predicted eye velocity peak (°/s)	Head velocity peak (°/s)
I	No Hydrops	0.054	102.33	102.62
II	No Hydrops	0.081	137.06	137.46
III	No Hydrops	0.089	141.22	140.50
IV	No Hydrops	0.100	173.22	173.81
V	No Hydrops	0.126	210.97	209.11
VI	No Hydrops	0.125	248.06	249.47
I	Canal Hydrops	0.061	115.79	102.62
II	Canal Hydrops	0.091	155.16	137.46
III	Canal Hydrops	0.101	159.74	140.50
IV	Canal Hydrops	0.113	195.53	173.81
V	Canal Hydrops	0.142	238.64	209.11
VI	Canal Hydrops	0.137	282.98	249.47
I	Utricular Hydrops	0.058	111.40	102.62
II	Utricular Hydrops	0.088	148.58	137.46
III	Utricular Hydrops	0.097	152.82	140.50
IV	Utricular Hydrops	0.109	184.43	173.81
V	Utricular Hydrops	0.136	229.01	209.11
VI	Utricular Hydrops	0.131	272.03	249.47

Computationally measured increment of pressure on the internal wall of the ampulla, and predicted eye velocity values according to measured pressure levels for all the six head impulses on each three anatomical hydrops models.

The main results of computations are presented in **Table 1** and are also plotted in **Figure 3**. For measured ampullar pressure values (**Table 1, Figure 3A** and **Appendix Figure 2**) higher peak pressure was measured in canal hydrops model with a mean pressure between impulses of 0.107 ± 0.030 Pa, followed by utricular hydrops model with a mean pressure of 0.103 ± 0.028 Pa. Lowest peak pressure levels were measured in no-hydrops model with a mean pressure of 0.095 ± 0.027.

Predicted eye velocity peak values (**Table 1, Figure 3B** and **Appendix Figure 3**) were also highest in canal hydrops model, with a mean peak eye velocity of 191.355 ± 61.10 °/s, followed by peak velocity values from utricular hydrops model of 183.61 ± 58.79 °/s. Lowest peak eye velocity values were also measured in no-hydrops model with a mean velocity of 168.82 ± 53.51 °/s.

For all models highest peak pressure and peak eye velocity were measured on V and VI impulses (209.11 °/s and 249.47 °/s head peak velocity values, respectively) while lowest predicted peak eye velocity and peak pressure vales were measured on impulse I (102.62 °/s).

The computed aVOR gain values using area under the curve method (**Table 2, Figure 4**) did show a mean aVOR gain of 1.01 ± 0.008 for the no-hydrops model, a mean gain of 1.14 ± 0.014 for the canal hydrops model, and a mean gain of 1.10 ± 0.007 for the utricular hydrops model.

DISCUSSION

In this study we predicted the endolymph hydrodynamics in geometric models of both normal and hydropic vestibular membranous labyrinths, using computer fluid dynamics software during the movement condition of the head impulse test.

Probably the most important question before discussing the computations performed in this research itself is about the actual evidence of the presence of vestibular hydrops affecting utriculus and semicircular canals in Menière disease and near spectrum human pathologies.

Although there are published cases of utricular and canal hydrops observation on 3 Tesla magnetic resonance imaging (MRI) with specific endolymph sequences (17), most actual imaging sequences of Menière disease and endolymphatic hydrops show cochlear and saccular hydrops, but not utricular or canal hydrops, which are rare findings in the published literature. It is not clear if this absence of MRI hydrops is related to a real lack of hydrops in these structures or other factors could be underlie these "anecdotal" cases of hydrops location. Probably, as suggested by Lopez-Escamez on a recent systematic review of the published papers on hydrops detection on 3 Tesla MRI sequences, actual MRI methods to adequate evaluate the endolymphatic hydrops are too novel and heterogenous to be considered as mature and reproducible techniques, especially in patients with early Menière disease (18).

On the other hand, despite the fact that most histologic published papers are focused on cochlear hydrops there are some histologic studies that strongly support the idea that utricular and canal hydrops may be also (relatively) frequent in the Menière disease population. Okuno and Sando (19) described the histopathological findings in 22 temporal bones from Menière's disease patients. Regarding vestibular organ hydrops, these authors found that saccular hydrops was present in 19 of 22 (86%) temporal bones, but also 11 of 22 (50%) temporal bones showed evident hydrops signals in the utricle region and 5–8 (23–36%) showed hydrops on at least one of the semicircular canals, the posterior canal being the most often affected (8/22) 36%. Concerning the severity of hydrops, these authors also described that saccular hydrops is less conservative with the original vestibular organ anatomy than utricular and semicircular canal hydrops are. Considering the histologic evidences published by Okuno and Sando, utricular hydrops could not be considered as infrequent, because it was present in 50% of temporal bones; also, canal hydrops should not be considered as a rare event, with a 23–35% of prevalence on temporal bones from Menière's disease patients.

The lack of an actual descriptive geometric model of the vestibular organ hydrops developed from radiological or histological findings forced us to develop a hydrops models based on McGarvie (11) descriptions but also inside the real measurements published by Okundo and Sando (19). Unfortunately, at the present moment, we were not able to find a more precise source to develop our vestibular hydrops models. This limitation in our models could be solved with future histological and radiological data or performing new CFD simulations, based on the here presented, where the hydrops geometry will be the main parameter to be tested.

In the developed models we only considered one volumetric dilatation ratio for each model. The effect of other dilatation ratios and its influence on VOR gain values should be evaluated

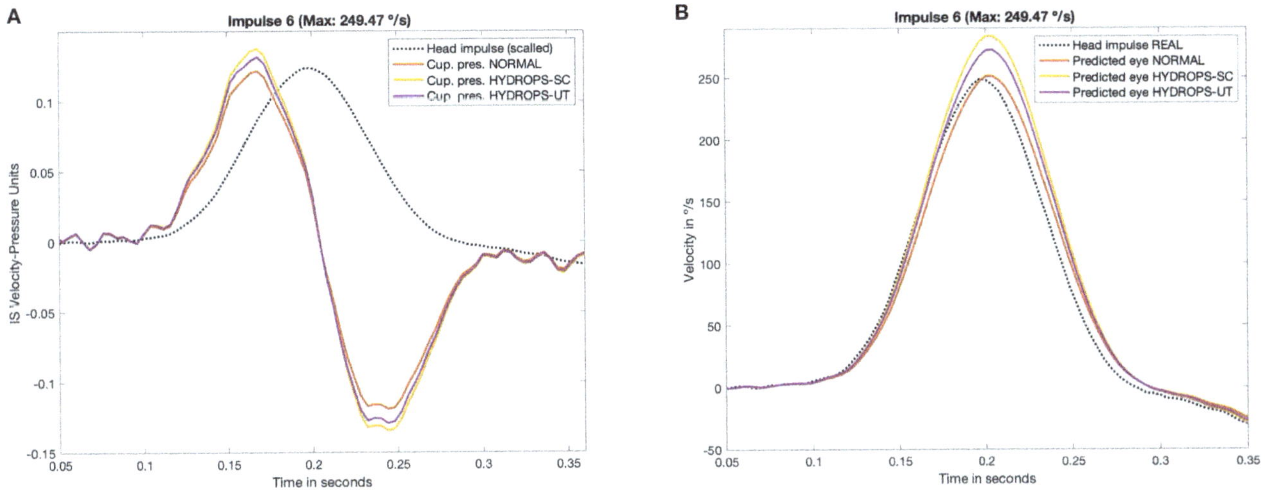

FIGURE 3 | Measured pressure **(A)** on CFD simulation and predicted eye velocity responses **(B)** of the three hydrops models (non-hydrops, utricular hydrops and semicircular canal hydrops), for the head impulse with the highest peak velocity included in this study (249.47 °/s). The pressure and velocity plots obtained from all the others impulses included in this study are available in **Appendix Figures 2, 3**.

on further studies, this will be of particular interest to determine how will be the eye velocity enhancement at different Menière disease clinical stages.

Obviously, despite computer simulations being plausible from a physical point of view, they are not the strongest scientific evidence and also have limitations. In our computations we used anatomic 3D models from microCT reconstruction (**Figure 1B**), that have never before been used with this purpose in vestibular physiopathology research. In our model we considered the membranous labyrinth to consist of rigid walls, when really, they are elastic, and this elasticity could influence the endolymph flow during the head impulse test (20).

In our model cupula region was represented as a rigid wall. Goyens et al. (21) has recently evaluated the effect of different cupula designs and its biophysical effects on main variables that could affect to the VOR responses, concluding that the use of simplified models where the cupula is represented as a rigid wall, the same as we used in our model, are also adequate and valid models to evaluate the vestibular system biomechanics. Also, other vestibular models, like the model developed by Grieser et al. (6) that includes an elastic cupula in a simplified vestibular model has outputted similar enhancement of eye velocity responses reported by here.

The evidence of the concordance between models supports the mathematical approach used in our model to predict the (hypothetical) cupula deflection from a given variation of transcupular pressure over time which appears to be an acceptable approximation to overcome the lack of an anatomical and elastic cupula in our model. Other limitation about this research is that we build a model where only the information of ipsilateral afference vestibular signal was computed and the contralateral vestibular organ was not included on our model. To reach a better understanding of hydrops effect on vestibular system a more complete vestibular model, including contralateral vestibular organ signal should be considered on further researches.

TABLE 2 | Gain (aVOR) values computed using area-under-curve method for predicted eye velocity values and real measured head velocity values for the six head impulse tests included and the three hydrops models included in this study.

Impulse	Hydrops Model	Predicted aVOR gain
I	No Hydrops	1.014
II	No Hydrops	1.010
III	No Hydrops	1.024
IV	No Hydrops	1.000
V	No Hydrops	1.019
VI	No Hydrops	1.019
I	Canal Hydrops	1.149
II	Canal Hydrops	1.148
III	Canal Hydrops	1.158
IV	Canal Hydrops	1.122
V	Canal Hydrops	1.159
VI	Canal Hydrops	1.149
I	Utricular Hydrops	1.104
II	Utricular Hydrops	1.095
III	Utricular Hydrops	1.109
IV	Utricular Hydrops	1.091
V	Utricular Hydrops	1.104
VI	Utricular Hydrops	1.111

Also, although microCT reconstruction of the vestibular labyrinth has a high resolution, the anatomic details of the ampullar receptor were not included in our models, and the cupula region was modeled as a simple wall, not including other geometric and elastic details. With the obtained computations we suggest that micro-CT geometric models using CFD software to

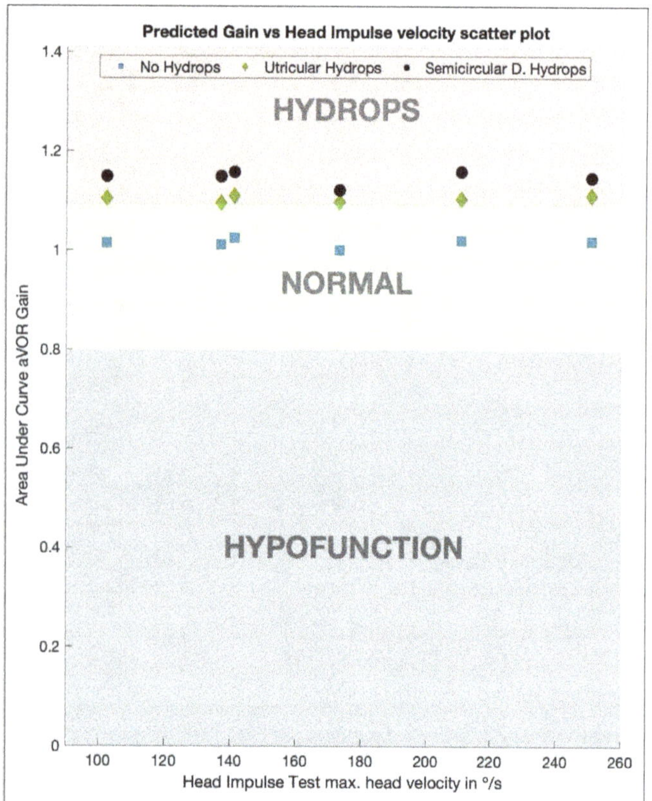

FIGURE 4 | Predicted values of aVOR gain for normal, utricular and canal hydrops models. For both (utricular and canal) hydrops models aVOR gains were always >1.09 on all the tested head impulse velocities. Gains for the utricular model were slightly lower than for the canal model, but always over 0.1 more than the normal model gain values, which had gain value of 1.

predict endolymph flow appear to be a very strong experimental method that could be applied to other vestibular function tests and other models of vestibular pathology.

As similar experimental research that partially supports the results obtained in this study, Yamauchi et al. (22) found that in animal models of horizontal canal hydrops that afferent vestibular nerve discharge is increased by the experimental induction of a hydropic environment, for both during static conditions and during sinusoidal (not impulsive) head movements. Nevertheless, Yamauchi et al. (22) describes that the static increase of discharge is adapted by the system along time and the dynamic (sinusoidal) response is variable depending on stimulus frequency. A very interesting point in this research is that Yamauchi et al. also describes that the increased vestibular discharges observed due the hydrops are not sustained over time. To explain this, the authors suggests that the vestibular system adaptation circuits will decrease these increased responses along time. If this vestibular adaptation mechanism is also applied to our human vestibular model it is probable that the enhanced eye responses will be more evident on the nearest time to the hydrops attack and probably will be decreased (due vestibular system adaptation) over time.

In this research results, we found that for head impulses of all head velocities, the velocities of the eye response are amplified by a 1.14 factor; for the canal hydrops model this was also in concordance with the aVOR gain values obtained in the canal hydrops model (**Figure 4**). With a slightly lower magnitude, aVOR gain was also significantly enhanced in the utricular hydrops model. These predicted enhanced eye velocities and aVOR gains were observed in the same proportion on all the head impulses included in this study. Because we obtained a 1.01 mean value for aVOR gain on non-hydrops models, the gain enhancement predicted by this study can be only directly extrapolated to right-side head impulse tests, in which the vHIT camera records responses of the right eye. This is because a gain value of 1 is only observed on the right side impulses of vHIT device with right-side mounted camera, and left-side impulses have a slightly lower than 1 aVOR gain value (23). But probably x1.14 enhancement of velocity data could be applied to left-side impulses.

Histopathological findings have also pointed a possible vestibular labyrinth structural alteration that, owing to the effect of hydrops, could affect to the pressure on ampullar receptors of horizontal semicircular canal. In the temporal bone series presented by Okuno and Sando (19) severe saccular hydrops had caused in 7 of 22 (31%) temporal bones a herniation of part of the saccular dilated structure into non-ampullar side of the horizontal side of this semicircular canal. Although our models did not compute the effect on ampullar pressure of this saccular herniation into the posterior region of the horizontal canal, it is probable that this herniation will also provoke an enhanced eye velocity response, probably greater than the observed in our models.

From a more hypothetical point of view, but based on findings of this study and the actual evidence of utricular or semicircular hydrops incidence in Menière disease patients (17–19), the enhanced eye velocity sign should appear in no more than half of Menière's disease patients, according to the described prevalence of canal and utricular hydrops (19). But there is a second factor that should be considered in addition to hydrops location: the time of evolution of the Menière disease. It has been described that for longstanding Menière disease patients type II hair cell vestibular receptors number is decreased and also an even more significant loss of cells on Scarpa's ganglion (24). These two histopathological findings present in patient with well-defined Menière disease could predict that the (related to hydrops) enhanced eye velocity will decrease to a normal or reduced eye velocity response due to the loss of sensitivity of vestibular receptors. Because this cellular damage depends on the time of evolution of the Menière disease, the initial prevalence of enhanced eye responses will also decrease with time. Considering these factors, it is probable that enhanced eye velocities will be only observed only in a fraction of Menière disease patients, and should be more prevalent in patients in the (relatively) early stage of the disease.

This theoretical prevalence of enhanced eye velocity responses in early Menière patients could suggest that enhanced velocity on head impulse test will be a very specific sign for early stages of Menière disease, but with a limited clinical sensibility due to the relatively low incidence of utricular or semicircular hydrops.

We conclude that, with the described limitations, the results of our physical computation model support the hypothesis that in endolymphatic hydrops conditions, when they are affecting horizontal semicircular canal and utricular region on moderate dilatations, the eye velocity responses output by the aVOR will be enhanced by an 1.14 factor, and aVOR gain values will be over 1.1 for right-sided impulses. These predictions must be confirmed by clinical trials, but should be considered in clinical practice, especially when cases of early Menière disease are suspected.

ETHICS STATEMENT

This study was designed and performed in accordance with the ethical guidelines of the 1975 Declaration of Helsinki.

AUTHOR CONTRIBUTIONS

JR-M designed the computation model, performed the computer simulations and redacted the manuscript. XA co-designed the computation model and redacted the manuscript. KC developed the 3D geometric model and redacted the manuscript. AB submitted the clinical data, reviewed and redacted the manuscript. IC co-designed the computation model, redacted the manuscript and reviewed and supervised this research.

FUNDING

IC was receipt of a conjoint grant from the Garnett Passe and Rodney Williams Memorial Foundation; that grant pays the salary of AB.

ACKNOWLEDGMENTS

First author wants to thank to Michal Sajkowski and SIMFLOW Technologies (www.sim-flow.com) that very kindly contributed to this research by giving a full license of SimFlow computational fluid dynamics software. We thank L. A. McGarvie of Royal Prince Alfred Hospital, Sydney, for the data for six head impulses.

SUPPLEMENTARY MATERIAL

Appendix Videos 1–3 | Paraview software exported videos of the normal (**Video S1**), canal hydrops (**Video S2**) and utricular hydrops (**Video S3**) models for the raw head impulse test VI.

Appendix Figure 1 | Video head impulse tests used in the simulations. Traces of head velocity versus time for the set 6 head impulses, obtained from a real vHIT measurement database after lowpass filter postprocess, with peak head velocity varying in approximately equal steps from 102.62 °/s to 249.47 °/s.

Appendix Figure 2 | Increase of ampullar pressure during the head impulse test for the six progressive velocity head impulses computed on the three hydrops models. Higher pressure values were measured in both the models of canal hydrops, and those of utricular hydrops.

Appendix Figure 3 | Predicted eye velocity values during head impulse test for the six progressive velocity head impulses computed on the four hydrops models, showing the pressure values measured, assuming semicircular receptors to be highly overdamped accelerometer sensors. Higher velocity values were measured in both the models of canal hydrops, and those of utricular hydrops.

Appendix Simulation Files (Datasheet 1–5) | Compressed in this folder the reader can find: The anatomic 3D models folder, where the STL files used in this research can be found, these models are also automatically incorporated to the simulations folders. The head impulses folder, where the CSV files containing the head velocity real data used in this research can be found, these files are ready to be imported to the simulation software. In the "Dynamic mesh" section of the software, reader should select rigid type and rotating motion with omega from table, selecting the impulse of interest to be used as simulated head impulse and also setting the origin on movement to a medial point of the utricular region. In the Hydrops_SC, Hydrops_UC and NoHydrops folders configuration files ready to be open by the SimFlow 3.1 version simulation software are provided for each 3D STL model of the vestibular labyrinth. See methods section for detailed info about simulation software reference.

REFERENCES

1. Halmagyi G, Chen L, MacDougall H, Weber K, McGarvie L, Curthoys I. The video head impulse test. *Front Neurol.* (2017) 8:258. doi: 10.3389/fneur.2017.00258
2. Curthoys I, Halmagyi G. What does head impulse testing really test? *JAMA Otolaryngol Head Neck Surg.* (2019) 145:1080–1. doi: 10.1001/jamaoto.2019.2779
3. Aw S, Haslwanter T, Halmagyi G, Curthoys I, Yavor R, Todd M. Three dimensional vector analysis of the human vestibuloocular reflex in response to high-acceleration head rotations. I. responses in normal subjects. *J Neurophysiol.* (1996) 76: 4009–20. doi: 10.1152/jn.1996.76.6.4021
4. Rey-Martinez J, Batuecas-Caletrio A, Matiño E, Perez Fernandez N. HITCal: a software tool for analysis of video head impulse test responses. *Acta Otolaryngol.* (2015) 135:886–94. doi: 10.3109/00016489.2015.1035401
5. Rey-Martinez J, Burgess A, Curthoys I. Enhanced vestibulo-ocular reflex responses on vHIT. is it a casual finding or a sign of vestibular dysfunction? *Front Neurol.* (2018) 15:866. doi: 10.3389/fneur.2018.00866
6. Grieser B, McGarvie L, Kleiser L, Manzari L, Obrist D, Curthoys I. Numerical investigations of the effects of endolymphatic hydrops on the VOR response. Presented as poster presentation P-Q-4 at XXVIII bárány society meeting. buenos aires, Argentina. *J Vestib Res.* (2014) 24:219. doi: 10.3233/VES-140517
7. Valli P, Buizza A, Botta L, Zucca G, Ghezzi L, Valli S. Convection, buoyancy or endolymph expansion: what is the actual mechanism responsible for the caloric response of semi- circular canals? *J Vestib Res.* (2002) 12:155–65.
8. Turing AM. On Computable numbers, with an application to the entscheidungsproblem. *Proc Lond Math Soc.* (1937) s2–42:230–65. doi: 10.1112/plms/s2-42.1.230
9. Rey-Martinez J, McGarvie L, Perez-Fernandez N. Computing simulated endolymphatic flow thermodynamics during the caloric test using normal and hydropic duct models. *Acta*

Otolaryngol. (2017) 137:270–4. doi: 10.1080/00016489.2016.1242775
10. Grieser B, Kleiser L, Obrist D. Identifying mechanisms behind the tullio phenomenon: a computational study based on first principles. *J Assoc Res Otolaryngol.* (2016) 17:103–18. doi: 10.1007/s10162-016-0553-0
11. McGarvie L, Curthoys I, MacDougall H, Halmagyi G. What does the dissociation between the results of video head impulse versus caloric testing reveal about the vestibular dysfunction in Ménière's disease? *Acta Otolaryngol.* (2015) 135:859–65. doi: 10.3109/00016489.2015.1015606
12. Wesseling P. *Principles of Computational Fluid Dynamics.* Berlin, Heidelberg: Springer-Verlag (2001). doi: 10.1007/978-3-642-05146-3
13. Grant W, Curthoys I. Otoliths - accelerometer and seismometer; implications in Vestibular Evoked Myogenic Potential (VEMP). *Hear Res.* (2017) 253:26–35. doi: 10.1016/j.heares.2017.07.012
14. Wilson VJ, Jones GM. Biophysics of the peripheral end organs. In: VJ. Wilson, ed *Mammalian Vestibular Physiology.* Boston: Springer (1979). doi: 10.1007/978-1-4757-5702-6_3
15. Ramat S. Understanding the rotational vestibular ocular reflex: from differential equations to laplace transforms. *Prog Brain Res.* (2019) 248:29–44. doi: 10.1016/bs.pbr.2019.04.030
16. Squires T, Weidman M, Hain T, Stone H. A mathematical model for top-shelf vertigo: the role of sedimenting otoconia in BPPV. *J Biomech.* (2004) 37:1137–46. doi: 10.1016/j.jbiomech.2003.12.014
17. Gürkov R, Flatz W, Ertl-Wagner B, Krause E. Endolymphatic hydrops in the horizontal semicircular canal: a morphologic correlate for canal paresis in Ménière's disease. *Laryngoscope.* (2012) 123:503–6. doi: 10.1002/lary.23395
18. Lopez-Escamez J, Attyé A. Systematic review of magnetic resonance imaging for diagnosis of meniere disease. *J Vestib Res.* (2019) 29:121–9. doi: 10.3233/VES-180646
19. Okuno T, Sando I. Localization, frequency, and severity of endolymphatic hydrops and the pathology of the labyrinthine membrane in Menière's disease. *Ann Otol Rhinol Laryngol.* (1987) 96:438–45. doi: 10.1177/000348948709600418
20. Rabbitt R. Semicircular canal biomechanics in health and disease. *J Neurophysiol.* (2019) 121:732–55. doi: 10.1152/jn.00708.2018
21. Goyens J, Pourquie M, Poelma C, Westerweel J. Asymmetric cupula displacement due to endolymph vortex in the human semicircular canal. *Biomech Model Mechanobiol.* (2019) 18:1577–90. doi: 10.1007/s10237-019-01160-2
22. Yamauchi A, Rabbitt R, Boyle R, Highstein S. Relationship between inner-ear fluid pressure and semicircular canal afferent nerve discharge. *J Assoc Res Otolaryngol.* (2002) 3:26–44. doi: 10.1007/s1016200 10088
23. Rey-Martinez J, Thomas-Arrizabalaga I, Espinosa-Sanchez J, Batuecas-Caletrio A, Trinidad-Ruiz G, Matiño-Soler E, et al. Vestibulo-ocular reflex gain values in the suppression head impulse test of healthy subjects. *Laryngoscope.* (2018) 128:2383–9. doi: 10.1002/lary.27107
24. Tsuji K, Velázquez-Villaseñor L, Rauch S, Glynn R, Wall C III, Merchant S. Temporal bone studies of the human peripheral vestibular system. Meniere's disease. *Ann Otol Rhinol Laryngol Suppl.* (2000) 181:26–31. doi: 10.1177/00034894001090S505

18

Applications of Multivariate Statistical and Data Mining Analyses to the Search for Biomarkers of Sensorineural Hearing Loss, Tinnitus and Vestibular Dysfunction

Paul F. Smith[1,2,3*] *and Yiwen Zheng*[1,2,3]

[1] *Department of Pharmacology and Toxicology, Brain Health Research Centre, School of Biomedical Sciences, University of Otago, Dunedin, New Zealand,* [2] *Brain Research New Zealand Centre of Research Excellence, University of Auckland, Auckland, New Zealand,* [3] *The Eisdell Moore Centre for Hearing and Balance Research, University of Auckland, Auckland, New Zealand*

Correspondence:
Paul F. Smith
paul.smith@otago.ac.nz

Disorders of sensory systems, as with most disorders of the nervous system, usually involve the interaction of multiple variables to cause some change, and yet often basic sensory neuroscience data are analyzed using univariate statistical analyses only. The exclusive use of univariate statistical procedures, analyzing one variable at a time, may limit the potential of studies to determine how interactions between variables may, as a network, determine a particular result. The use of multivariate statistical and data mining methods provides the opportunity to analyse many variables together, in order to appreciate how they may function as a system of interacting variables, and how this system or network may change as a result of sensory disorders such as sensorineural hearing loss, tinnitus or different types of vestibular dysfunction. Here we provide an overview of the potential applications of multivariate statistical and data mining techniques, such as principal component and factor analysis, cluster analysis, multiple linear regression, random forest regression, linear discriminant analysis, support vector machines, random forest classification, Bayesian classification, and orthogonal partial least squares discriminant analysis, to the study of auditory and vestibular dysfunction, with an emphasis on classification analytic methods that may be used in the search for biomarkers of disease.

Keywords: multivariate statistical analysis, data mining, orthogonal partial least squares discriminant analysis, hearing loss, tinnitus, vestibular dysfunction

INTRODUCTION

Experimental phenomena in neuroscience often involve the complex, sometimes non-linear interaction, of multiple variables. In the context of sensorineural hearing loss (SNHL), tinnitus or vestibular disorders, a number of independent variables may interact with one another, such as age, sex, drug use, and genetic predispositions; similarly, many biochemical systems may interact with one another to cause such disorders (see **Figure 1** for an example in the context of age-related neurochemical changes in the brainstem vestibular nucleus and cerebellum). Despite this, the majority of statistical analyses in basic auditory and vestibular neuroscience have tended

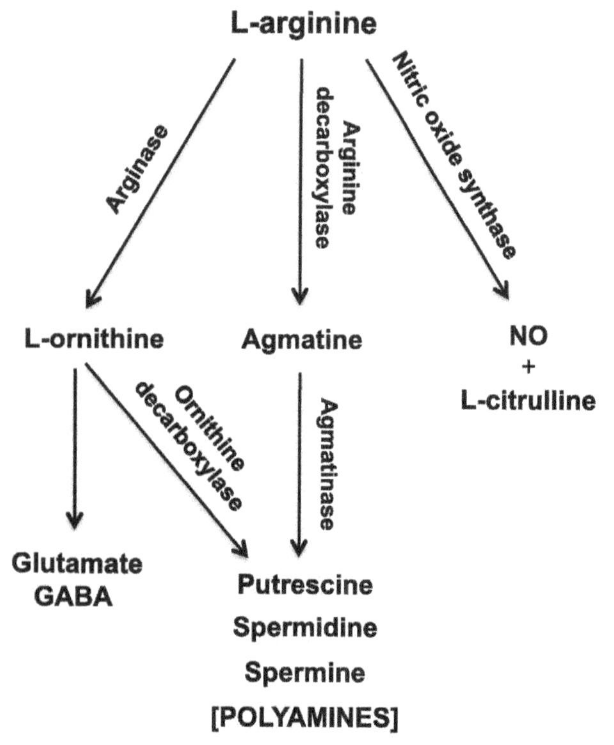

FIGURE 1 | Schematic diagram of the L-arginine metabolic pathways in the vestibular nucleus and cerebellum, which change during the brain aging process. NO, nitric oxide; GABA, γ-aminobutyric acid. From Liu et al. (4) with permission.

to focus on comparisons between treatment groups, analyzing one variable at a time. In many areas of sensory neuroscience in general, univariate statistical analyses have been used almost exclusively. This approach neglects the fact that changes may occur at the level of the interaction within a network or system of variables, that cannot be detected in any individual variable alone (1–6) (see **Figure 1** for an example). In addition, the use of multiple univariate statistical analyses may inflate the type 1 error rate, or the probability of rejecting the null hypothesis when it is true, as a result of a large number of individual analyses (1, 2, 7) (**Figure 2**). In situations in which there are a large number of variables, for example, gene microarray, proteomic and metabolomic data, and more recently, medical diagnostics, multivariate statistical analyses and data mining approaches have been increasingly employed in order to understand the complex interactions that can occur between systems of variables, as well as to avoid increasing the type I error rate [e.g., (6, 8–30)].

Multivariate statistical analyses (MVAs) and data mining analyses can be broadly divided into those that are "supervised" and those that are "unsupervised". A "supervised" method of analysis is directed at a specific dependent variable, in order to determine the relationship between a set of independent variables and one or more dependent variables, (e.g., to make a prediction; e.g., multiple linear regression). By contrast, in "unsupervised" methods, there is no specific dependent variable; instead, the objective is to explore associations between variables (e.g., cluster analyses) (see **Table 1**). Furthermore, some MVAs and data mining methods are concerned with predicting categorical variables ("classification," e.g., linear discriminant analysis), and some concerned with predicting continuous variables ("regression," e.g., multiple linear regression). Some of these methods involve only one dependent variable, e.g., multiple linear regression, while others may involve multiple dependent variables, e.g., canonical correlation analysis; however, for the purposes of this paper, MVAs will be defined as a collection of methods that involve *multiple variables*, either independent or dependent, or both. Clearly, regression methods such as multiple linear regression can be extended to include more than one dependent variable [e.g., multivariate multiple regression; (1, 2)].

Some unsupervised MVAs are not focussed on a specific dependent variable or the implication of causality, but more the degree of co-variation amongst multiple variables, as an indicator of association. For example, cluster analyses could be used to investigate the degree to which different variables related to SNHL co-vary with one another. Cluster analyses have been used extensively in genomics and proteomics research as a means of exploring the association between variables. Still other MVAs are concerned with investigating the way that groups of variables with different weightings, explain most of the variation in a system of variables (e.g., **Figure 1**; e.g., principal component analysis). Data mining analyses are related to MVAs; however, some have arisen out of computer science rather than conventional statistics. Data mining analyses include procedures such as random forest regression, random forest classification and support vector machines.

The aim of this paper is to provide a succinct guide to some MVAs and data mining analytic methods that can be applied to auditory and vestibular neuroscience data related to SNHL, tinnitus, and vestibular dysfunction, at both the basic experimental and clinical levels. Particular emphasis will be placed on "classification methods" that are relevant to the search for biomarkers of auditory and vestibular dysfunction, i.e., linear discriminant analysis, support vector machines, random forest classification, Bayesian classification, and orthogonal partial least squares discriminant analysis. However, classification and regression methods are related statistically, and for this reason, regression methods, in which there is no categorical dependent variable, will also be addressed. The review is intended to exemplify the application of MVA and data mining methods to problems in vestibular and auditory neuroscience, and is not meant to be exhaustive in terms of the specific methods described; procedures such as artificial neural network modeling (ANN), structural equation modeling, multivariate regression, canonical correlation analysis and many others, are also important, but are outside the scope of this review.

Abbreviations: GC/MS, gas chromatography/mass spectrometry; MVA, multivariate statistical analysis; OLPSDA, orthogonal partial least squares discriminant analysis; SNHL, sensorineural hearing loss.

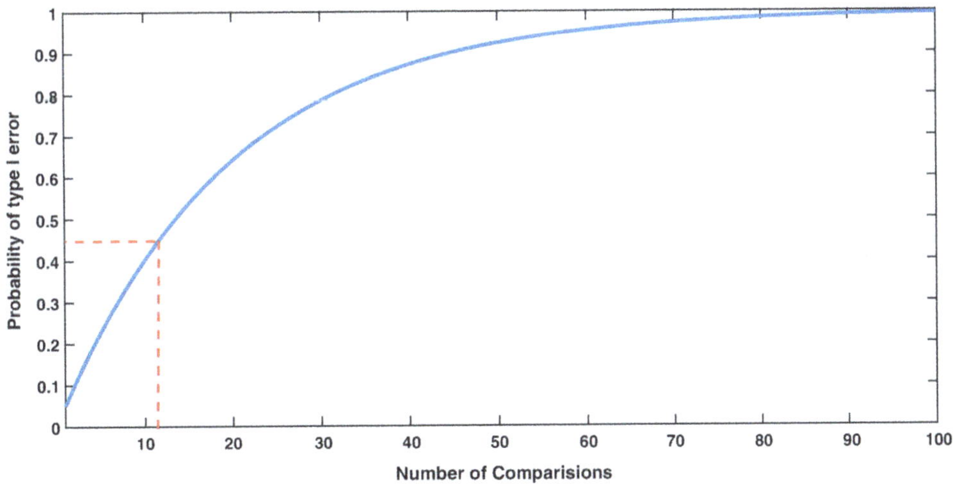

FIGURE 2 | The Type I error rate (False Alarm rate) strongly depends on the number of comparisons. For example, with 12 comparisons (red dashed lines), the probability of making at least one False Alarm is 0.46, i.e., much increased compared to 0.05 with only 1 comparison. From Herzog et al. (7) with permission.

UNSUPERVISED METHODS

Principal Component Analysis and Factor Analysis

Principal Component Analysis (PCA) attempts to explain variation in data using linear combinations of variables. It is a "dimension reduction" procedure, often used to reduce the number of variables to a smaller number of "components," which account for most of the variation in the data. In contexts such as metabolomics, where hundreds of metabolites may be investigated for their relationship to some disease state, it can be difficult to conceptualize their role just because of their sheer number. PCA looks for underlying latent components or factors, which represent linear combinations of variables, but without predicting a dependent variable. The objective is to find linear combinations of variables that explain most of the variation in the data, in the process reducing the number of separate variables in the data ("reducing dimensionality") (1, 32–34). These components or factors are expressed as "eigenvalues," which in PCA are represented as linear combinations of the original variables, each with a coefficient or "eigenvector" that indicates the "direction" of that particular variable for each component. An important attribute is that the different PCs are uncorrelated or "orthogonal" (32–34), and this property means that they can be used in other statistical techniques such as discriminant analysis, where correlation between independent variables can be a problem (see orthogonal partial least squares discriminant analysis below in Orthogonal Partial-Least Squares Discriminant Analysis).

For each PC, each of the original independent variables is expressed in a linear equation with specific coefficients that represent the "weighting" of the variable in that component. The number of PCs, which can be large, is usually displayed in decreasing order of importance in explaining the variability in the data matrix, often shown graphically as a "Scree plot." PCA is often performed using the correlation matrix for the data, in which case the data have to be standardized, i.e., each value subtracted from the mean for that variable and divided by the standard deviation (i.e., "z scores"). This prevents extreme differences in variance, e.g., due to different measurement scales, disproportionately affecting the analysis. While PCA is an exploratory method that does not make very many assumptions, the related method, Factor Analysis, has a formal statistical model, and assumptions such as multivariate normality (see below in Linear Discriminant Analysis) become important.

The interpretation of the PCs relies on the magnitude of the eigenvalues, and the contrasts between the eigenvectors for the variables relating to that eigenvalue. There is no specific criterion for how many PCs should be used; however, ideally, there should be a small number of PCs that explain most of the variation of the data. Loading plots, which represent the variance or magnitude of the variables within a PC, are often used to compare the different variables in the first two or three components. Because the interpretation of the PCs relies on the loadings, sometimes "rotations" are used to maximize the contrasts between them while maintaining the relationship between the variables in the components. Examples include "varimax" and "quartimax" rotations (1, 32–34).

Whether PCA is of any use in the analysis of multiple variables, depends on whether considering the different variables together, as a component, makes sense in the context of the research question, and also on what meaning can be attributed to the differences between the loadings. For example, if changes in free radicals are related to SNHL, does it make sense to reduce chemicals related to free radical generation to single components that combine the individual variables, or does this lose information? This problem of interpretability, which undermines many MVAs, will be addressed in a later section (see section Data pre-processing and imputation, overfitting

TABLE 1 | Different types of MVA and Data Mining Methods categorized according to whether they involve a categorical or continuous (quantitative) dependent variable and whether they specify a dependent variable (i.e., Supervised) or not (i.e., Unsupervised).

Supervised
Qualitative or categorical variables
Linear discriminant analysis
Logistic regression
Partial least squares discriminant analysis
Structural equation modeling
Support vector machines (DM)
Random forest classification (DM)
Neural networks (DM)
K nearest neighbors
Quantitative variables
Multiple linear regression
Canonical correlation analysis
Multivariate multiple regression
Structural equation modeling
Random forest regression (DM)
Gradient boosted decision trees (DM)
Neural networks (DM)
K nearest neighbors
Unsupervised
Qualitative or categorical variables
Correspondence analysis
Quantitative variables
Principal component analysis
Factor analysis
Cluster analysis
Multidimensional scaling
Ordination

"DM" denotes those methods that emerged out of dating mining research in computer science. From Smith (31) with permission.

and the problem of interpretability). PCA is often useful in a context where there are hundreds of variables, e.g., genomics, metabolomics, where it is useful to determine whether there is a change in the overall pattern of genes or metabolites [e.g., (35)].

Cluster Analysis

Another MVA method that has not been used extensively in the context of auditory or vestibular neuroscience, is cluster analysis. Cluster analyses are a type of non-parametric statistical analysis that is used to explore the natural groupings of variables in a data set (1). Therefore, assumptions such as multivariate normality and equality of the variance-covariance matrices (see below in Linear Discriminant Analysis) are not required (1, 36). Different measurements of the distance between the variables, such as squared Euclidean or Mahalanobis distance, are used to relate them to one another, and specific algorithms (e.g., Ward Minimal Variance Linkage) are used to determine the clusters (36). As with PCA, the standardized data (i.e., z scores) are usually used in order to prevent bias introduced by differences in scales of measurement. The results are usually displayed using a "dendrogram." Some cluster analysis algorithms, such as single linkage, are susceptible to producing long strings of clusters ("chaining") (1, 36). Ward's Minimal Variance Linkage method, based on the objective of obtaining the smallest within-cluster sum of squares (the "minimal variance principle"), is often a good option (1, 36). The results of PCA and cluster analysis are often related, and it can be observed that many of the original independent variables that co-vary closely together in the dendrogram, also appear to have similar eigenvectors in the dominant PCs. In this way, PCA and cluster analysis provide similar information regarding which variables "work together," but in different ways.

K-Nearest Neighbors Algorithm

The K-Nearest Neighbors ("*k*-NN") Algorithm can be used for regression or classification purposes. It is a non-parametric procedure in which either a category (in the case of classification) or a continuous variable value (in the case of regression) is estimated on the basis of its "nearest neighbours," where "*k*" is usually a small positive integer (2, 37). The data are usually standardized (see above) before the analysis is performed. The main challenges of this method include determining the appropriate value for *k* (i.e., how many neighbors?) and how the distance between neighbors should be quantified [see (37) for a discussion]. It is possible to use the *k*-NN algorithm in unsupervised or supervised forms.

SUPERVISED METHODS

Regression

Multiple Linear Regression

Another statistical method that has been under-employed in auditory and vestibular neuroscience is multiple linear regression (MLR). MLR is a part of the general linear model (GLM), that is useful for determining whether one continuous variable can be predicted from a combination of other variables. Simple linear regression can be expanded to include more than one predictor variable to become MLR, which has the general form: $Y = \beta_0 + \beta_1 X_1 + \beta_2 X_2 + ... \beta_p X_p + \varepsilon$, where Y = the continuous dependent variable; $X_1, X_2,...X_p$ are independent variables; $\beta_1, \beta_2... \beta_p$ are coefficients; β_0 is the intercept and ε is the error term (2, 36–41).

Canonical correlation analysis is an extension of MLR in which multiple Y variables are related to multiple X variables (1).

Formal statistical hypothesis tests for MLR, like those for simple linear regression, make assumptions regarding the distribution of the data, which cannot always be fulfilled (see section Data pre-processing and imputation, overfitting and the problem of interpretability). These assumptions are the same as those for other methods that are part of the GLM, such as analysis of variance (ANOVA): that the residuals are normally distributed, with homogeneity of variance, and that they are independent of one another (e.g., not autocorrelated) (31, 36–43). Furthermore, the predictor variables should be numerical, although indicator variables can be used in order to include nominal variables (e.g., binary coding to represent male and female). The violation of the assumption of normality can sometimes be redressed using data transformation, which may also correct heterogeneity of variance, but other issues such as autocorrelation, are not easily dealt with and may require methods such as time series regression (31, 36–43).

Unlike simple linear regression, MLR is more complicated in terms of avoiding potential artifacts. Because the coefficient of determination, the R^2, which indicates as a percentage or fraction, how much of the variation in the dependent variable is explained by the independent variables, will increase as more independent variables are incorporated into the regression model, an "adjusted R^2" must be used in order to compensate for the number of variables included. The adjusted R^2 = [R^2-(k/n−1)][(n−1)(n−(k + 1))]. For k = 1 variables, the R^2 and adjusted R^2 are approximately equal.

There are various forms of MLR: forward regression, backward regression, stepwise regression and best subsets regression. In forward regression, predictors are added into the model one at a time (if α is set to 1.0, then all of them will be included, in ascending order of significance). In backward regression, predictors are taken out one at a time (if α is set to 0, all of them will be taken out, in descending order of significance). Backward regression tends to be preferred over forward regression because it allows examination of the interaction between variables (31, 36–43). In stepwise regression, the program stops at each step and checks whether the variables, either in the model or not, are the best combination for that step. The adjusted R^2 will change as different variables are included in a model and an ANOVA can be done at each step to determine whether it has made a significant difference. Best subsets regression, however, computes all possible MLR models from which the researcher must choose the best, based on the adjusted R^2 and various diagnostic information regarding the validity of the regression model (31, 36–43). One of the greatest problems in MLR is "over-fitting" and "multicollinearity" (31, 36–39, 44–46). If the regression variables are highly intercorrelated, multicollinearity occurs. This inflates the variance of the least square estimates and therefore the coefficients will be inaccurate, which can lead to the situation in which the ANOVA for the regression is significant without any single t-test for an individual variable being significant. In this case, one or more of the highly correlated variables needs to be removed from the regression model. One way of controlling for multicollinearity is using an index such as the Mallow's Cp index. The adjusted R^2 should be high but the Mallow's Cp index [= (the sum of squares for the error at the current step/mean square error for the full regression)−(n−2p), where n = total number of observations and p = number of estimated coefficients], should be as small as possible. Ideally, it should be one more than the number of parameters in the current step. Other indices of multicollinearity include the variance inflation factor and tolerance (1/variance inflation factor) (36–39, 45, 46). Different software packages (e.g., SPSS and Minitab) offer different options. Autocorrelation in the data can be tested using the Durban-Watson statistic (36–39, 45, 46). Like most other multivariate statistical procedures, MLR is prone to artifacts and researchers need to be cautious when using it [see (44) for a rigorous discussion of this issue].

Random Forest Regression

Although modeling using regression trees has been used for over 25 years, its use in auditory and vestibular neuroscience has been very limited. In regression tree modeling, a flow-like series of questions is asked about each variable ("recursive partitioning"), subdividing a sample into groups that are as homogeneous as possible by minimizing the within-group variance, in order to determine a numerical response variable (47, 48). The predictor variables can be continuous variables also, or they can be categorical. By contrast with MLR, which makes assumptions about the distribution of the data, regression trees make no distributional assumptions. The data are sometimes split into training and test data sets (e.g., 70:30) and the mean square error between the model based on the training data and the test data, is calculated as a measure of the model's success. Variables are chosen to split the data based on the reduction in the mean square error achieved after a split (i.e., the information gained). Unlike MLR, interactions between different predictor variables are automatically incorporated into the regression tree model and variable selection is unnecessary because irrelevant predictors are excluded from the model. This makes complex, non-linear interactions between variables easier to accommodate than in linear regression modeling (47, 48). Breiman et al. (48) extended the concept of regression trees by exploiting the power of computers to simultaneously generate hundreds of trees ("bagging"), known as "random forests," which were based on a random selection of a subset of data from the training set. The various regression tree solutions are averaged in order to predict the target variable with the smallest mean square error (47–52). An alternative form of cross-validation of the random forest model, which does not require splitting the data set and therefore is particularly useful in the context of small sample sizes, is the leave-one-out ("LOO") procedure. Here, each subject is removed from the sample, in turn, and the model based on the remaining data is used to predict for that subject; then, another subject is removed, and the procedure repeated, until the entire data set has been cross-validated (47–51).

Gradient boosted decision trees (GBDTs) are an alternative to the random forest procedure in which learning algorithms are combined ("boosting") so that each decision tree tries to minimize the error of the previous tree (37, 52).

Classification

Logistic Regression

Logistic regression is similar to linear regression but applied to the prediction of a binary outcome (37, 39). Rather than fitting a linear function to the prediction of a continuous dependent variable, logistic regression employs the logistic function, logistic(η) = 1/(1 + exp(-η)), to generate an outcome between 0 and 1. The logistic function is then incorporated into the probability function, $P(y^{(i)} = 1) = 1/(1 + exp(-(\beta_0 + \beta_1 x_1^{(i)} + \ldots. \beta_p x_p^{(i)})))$, where P is a probability, x are predictor variables, the β's represent coefficients and β_0 is the intercept (37). The output of this function is then a probability of classification to one of two groups, although logistic regression can also be extended to multinomial regression (39).

Linear Discriminant Analysis

Linear discriminant analysis is a statistical method that is often used to predict the membership of two or more groups from a linear combination of independent variables (1, 2). A linear discriminant function (LDF) has the general form: $Z = a_1X_1 + a_2X_2 + ...a_pX_p$, where Z refers to the group, X, X_2,...X_p are independent variables, and a_1, a_2,...a_p are coefficients (1). Linear discriminant analysis is similar in aim, but different in approach, to logistic regression, in which the dependent variable is binary (0/1) and consists of positive (a "success") and negative responses (a "failure") only (1). An example in the context of auditory neuroscience might be the prediction of SNHL by a linear combination of neurochemical variables in the peripheral or central auditory systems [e.g., (35)]. The statistical significance of the LDF can be assessed using statistics such as Wilk's λ and its success in separating the groups can be evaluated using cross-validation (e.g., a LOO procedure), in which the linear equation is used to classify the data, one observation at a time, without knowledge of the actual group membership. It is possible to use a stepwise linear discriminant analysis. However, some authors [e.g., (1, 45, 46)] suggest that stepwise methods can result in suppressor effects and an increase in type II error. Linear discriminant analysis is readily available in programs such as SPSS and Minitab. It is part of the GLM, and therefore makes similar assumptions to MLR, but other forms of discriminant analysis, which do not make all of these assumptions, include quadratic discriminant analysis, where the data are assumed to be normally distributed but the variance-covariance matrices need not be identical. Orthogonal partial least squares discriminant analysis is another type of discriminant analysis in which the discriminant function consists of PCs from a PCA (see below in Orthogonal Partial-Least Squares Discriminant Analysis).

As mentioned, MVA methods that are part of the GLM, such as linear discriminant analysis, do make assumptions. The first is that, for formal tests of statistical significance to be valid, the data within groups should have a multivariate normal distribution (1). Unlike univariate statistical analyses such as ANOVA, linear discriminant analysis is quite sensitive to the violation of the assumption of multivariate normality (1, 2, 36, 53). It is difficult to test for multivariate normality, because most programs such as SPSS do not offer such an assumption test (1). Because univariate normality, i.e., the normality of the individual variables, is necessary but not sufficient for multivariate normality, it is possible for each individual variable to be normally distributed without the multivariate distribution being normally distributed. Stevens (2) points out that because a multivariate normal distribution entails that all subsets of variables have normal distributions, one way to assess multivariate normality is to determine whether all pairs of variables are bivariate normal. Box's test for the homogeneity of the covariance matrices (see below) is sensitive to violation of multivariate normality; therefore, in order to obtain results from that test that are valid, whether the assumption of multivariate normality is fulfilled, must be of concern (2). However, there is a multivariate formulation of the central limit theorem and sample sizes of 10–20 per group appear to be sufficient to afford protection against the consequences of violating multivariate normality (2, 45, 46). It should be noted that linear discriminant analysis may still discriminate between groups even if the assumption of multivariate normality does not hold. On the other hand, multivariate normality does not necessarily mean that it will effectively discriminate between the groups.

A second assumption of linear discriminant analysis, but not quadratic discriminant analysis, is that the population covariance matrices are equal for all groups, usually tested using Box's M-test (1, 36). If this assumption is violated, a quadratic discriminant analysis, can be used instead. In a review of several Monte Carlo studies, Stevens (2) concluded that, provided that the sample sizes are equal, even moderate heterogeneity of the covariances does not substantially affect type I error. Unequal sample sizes, on the other hand, are potentially very problematic if the covariances are unequal (2). While Box's M-test is often used, its null hypothesis may be rejected only because the multivariate normality assumption is violated (2). Therefore, it is important to determine whether this is the reason for a significant Box's M-test. Box's M-test is also very sensitive to departure from homogeneity of the covariances (45, 46). Both Stevens (2), Field (45), and Field et al. (46) suggest that even if Box's M-test is significant, the type I error rate will be only slightly affected provided that there are equal sample sizes, although the power may be somewhat reduced.

One of the common problems in many MVAs is the sample size for each variable, n, relative to the number of variables, p. While unequal sample sizes can be problematic, as described above, when p is greater than n, statistical analyses such as linear discriminant analysis can become invalid. Stevens (2), Field (45), and Field et al. (46) suggest that, unless the n is large, $p \leq 10$. Monte Carlo studies have shown that if the sample size is not large compared to the number of variables, the standardized discriminant function coefficients and correlations obtained in a linear discriminant analysis, are unstable (2). By "large," Stevens (2) suggests a ratio of n (total sample size):p (number of variables) of 20:1. He further cautions that a small n:p ratio (i.e., ≤ 5) can be problematic for stepwise linear discriminant analysis in particular, because the significance tests are used to determine which variables are included in the solution (2).

These methods, and others related to them such as orthogonal partial least squares discriminant analysis, should be applicable to many situations in auditory and vestibular neuroscience in which multiple variables interact to determine a categorical dependent variable, e.g., SNHL, tinnitus, Meniere's Disease, vestibular neuritis, and benign paroxysmal positional vertigo, provided that the sample sizes are sufficient and the cross-validations demonstrate the predictive accuracy of the LDFs. Given that Box's M-test of the equality of the covariance matrices assumes multivariate normality, one way to proceed is to determine whether all pairs of variables appear to be bivariate normal. If so, Box's M-test can be used as a guide to whether the assumption of the equality of the covariance matrices is fulfilled. However, the cross-validation procedure can be used as the ultimate arbiter of the effectiveness of the LDF (31).

Random Forest Classification

The random forest method that is used for regression, can also be used for classification purposes, in which case the solution is based on the number of "votes" from the different trees for a particular category (48, 49). The effect of variable removal on

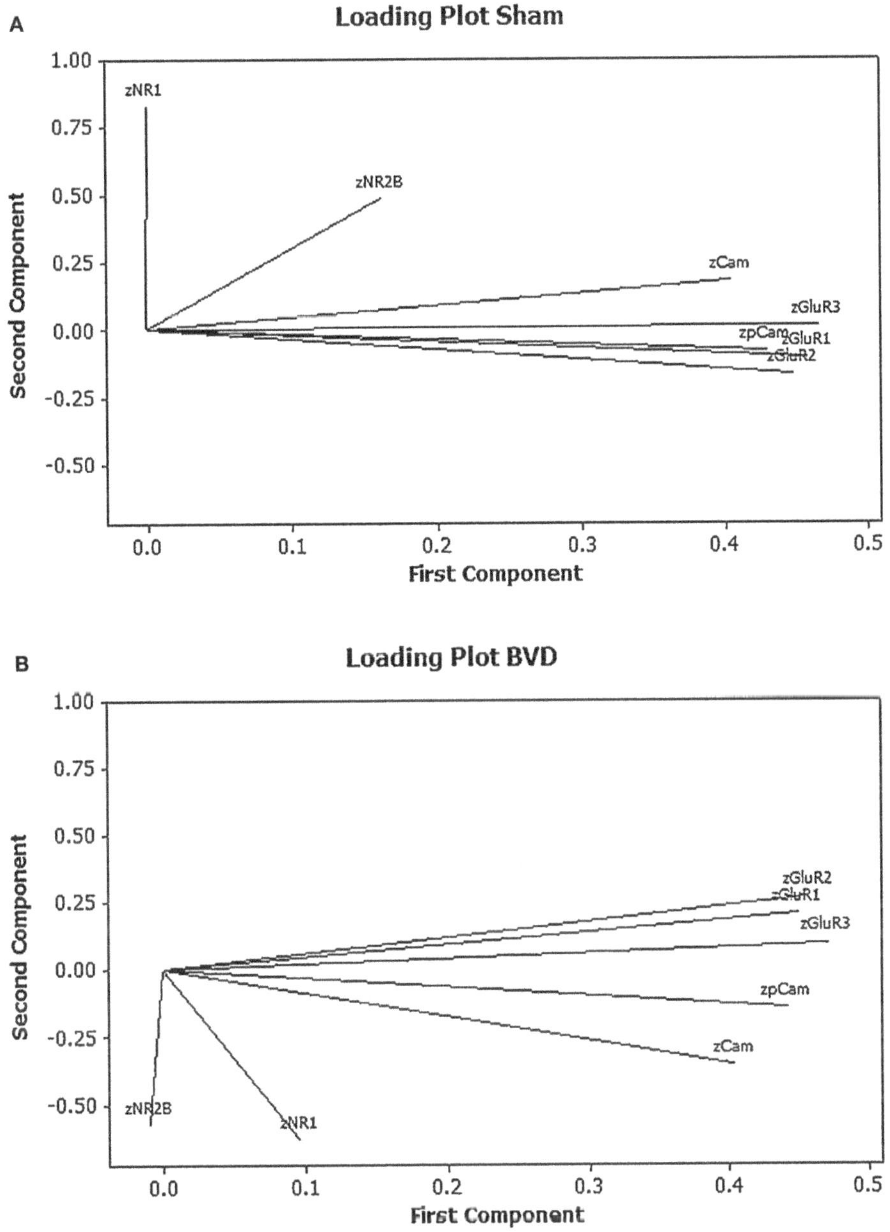

FIGURE 3 | Loading plots for the first 2 principal components for the mean normalized density of expression of NR1, NR2B, GluR1, GluR2, GluR3, CaMKII, and pCaMKII in the CA1, CA2/3, and dentate gyrus (DG) regions of the hippocampus at 6 months following sham **(A)** or BVD **(B)** surgery. Note the inverted pattern of loadings for the BVD group compared to the sham group. From Smith and Zheng (6) with permission.

the mean decrease in accuracy, the "out of bag" ("OOB") error, and the overall classification matrix error ("confusion matrix error"), are used to evaluate the success of the classification. The OOB error is the error based on the observations that were excluded from the subset of the training data (the "bag") used to generate the decision tree (47, 48). Unlike linear discriminant analysis, random forest classification makes no distributional assumptions and therefore can be applied to situations in which the sample sizes are small relative to the number of variables (47, 48). Random forest classification, along with support vector machines, can be carried out using specific packages in the statistics program, R (47, 54–57). For those who do not wish to use code in R, there is a data mining graphics user interface available, called "Rattle," which is menu-driven and easy to use (55).

Support Vector Machines

Support vector machines are an alternative method for classification, which employ "support vectors," observations that form the spatial boundary between different classes (47–49, 54).

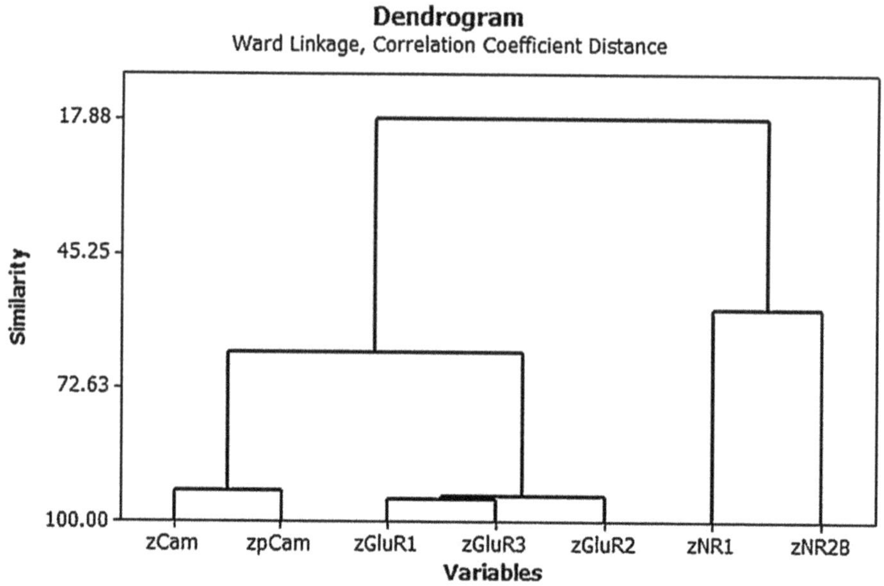

FIGURE 4 | Ward's minimal variance cluster analysis on the correlation coefficient distance for the mean normalized density of expression of NR1, NR2B, GluR1, GluR2, GluR3, CaMKII, and pCaMKII in the CA1, CA2/3, and dentate gyrus (DG) regions of the hippocampus at 6 months following BVD or sham surgery (i.e., both groups shown together). The *y* axis shows degrees of similarity, where 100.00 is the highest similarity and 17.88 is the lowest. Note that the NMDA receptor subunits vary together, as do the AMPA receptor subunits, as well as the CaMKII isoforms. From Smith and Zheng (6) with permission.

TABLE 2 | Results of the multiple linear regression analysis of the data from Smith et al. (51), showing the adjusted R^2-values, the residual standard errors (RSEs) and the significant input variables.

	GABA	put	spd	spm	arg	glut	agm	orn	cit
R^2	0.811	0.675	0.861	0.938	0.936	0.698	0.796	0.623	0.958
MSE	846.57	0.23	203.29	34.89	225.48	50064.54	0.12	189.54	119.52
Significant predictor variables	cit***	ag***	spm***	spd***	cit***	GABA***	put***	age***	arg***
	glut***	orn*	age***	cit***	orn*	spm***	cit***	cit***	GABA**
	spd*		orn**	glut***		orn**	age***	glut**	age**
			glut*					spd**	spm**
								enrich*	orn**

$^{***}P \leq 0.0001$, $^{**}P \leq 0.001$, $^{*}P \leq 0.05$. From Smith et al. (51) with permission.

These support vectors are then used to determine a hyperplane that defines the boundary between the classes (46–54). Support vector machines can employ a variety of functions, such as radial kernel and Laplace functions, to remap the data and generate new variables that can separate the different categories (47–54). The data are usually split into training and test data sets (e.g., 70:30) and the difference between the model based on the support vectors in the training data set, and the test data set, is calculated as a measure of the model's success. As with linear discriminant analysis, classification error matrices can be used to evaluate the success of the classification, as well as receiver operating characteristic ("ROC") curves, that quantify the relationship between the true positive rate of classification ("sensitivity") and the false positive rate of classification ("1—the specificity") (47).

One of the major advantages of support vector machines is that they do not make distributional assumptions like linear discriminant analysis, other than that the data are independent and identically distributed. Wilson (54) suggests that for this reason, even small sample sizes can provide accurate estimates of prediction error when there are a large number of variables.

Bayesian Classifiers

Bayesian classification methods are based on Bayes' Theorem, which relates a posterior probability of an event to a prior probability: $P(H/X) = P(X/H)(P(H)/P(X)$, where X represents the data and H represents the hypothesis; $P(H/X)$ = the probability of H given X (the posterior probability), $P(X/H)$ = the probability of X given H, $P(H)$ = the probability of H (the prior probability), and $P(X)$ = the probability of X, which cannot = zero. $P(H/X)$ and $P(X/H)$ are known as "conditional probabilities" and $P(X)$ and $P(H)$ as "marginal probabilities"

TABLE 3 | Results of the random forest regression models of the data from Smith et al. (51), showing the proportion of variance explained values, the residual standard errors (RSEs) and the input variables chosen using the stepwise process.

	GABA	put	spd	spm	arg	glut	agm	orn	cit
R^2	0.939	0.868	0.947	0.989	0.986	0.914	0.910	0.861	0.983
MSE	271.63	0.09	77.38	6.14	47.96	14,285.84	0.05	69.75	48.63
Most important predictor variables	cit	agm	spm	arg	cit	spm	arg	age	arg
	glut	arg	arg	cit	spm	GABA	put	glut	spm
	arg		agm	agm		cit	spm	cit	agm
			cit					GABA	GABA
								arg	spd

From Smith et al. (51) with permission.

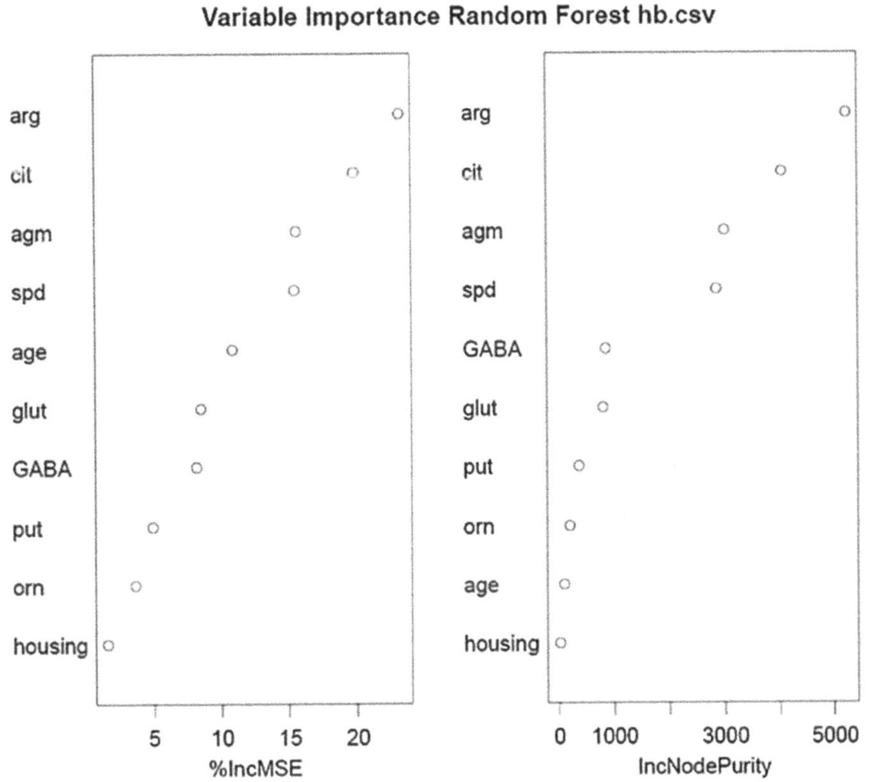

FIGURE 5 | Variables in order of importance for the random forest regression analysis for spermine, which had the highest proportion of variance explained (0.94). From Smith et al. (51) with permission.

(58–61). In simple terms, Bayes' Theorem relates the degree of belief in an hypothesis before accounting for the data, to that after accounting for the data, so that the probability of the hypothesis being true given the data, equals (the probability of obtaining the data given that the hypothesis is true, multiplied by the probability that the hypothesis is true), divided by the probability of obtaining the data (58–61). The calculation of the conditional and marginal probabilities can be used to generate a Bayesian Network, which can be displayed in graphical form such as directed acyclic graphs (61).

Orthogonal Partial-Least Squares Discriminant Analysis

Also known as orthogonal projection to latent structures discriminant analysis, orthogonal partial-least squares discriminant analysis (OPLS-DA) is a method of discriminant analysis that cleverly combines PCA with discriminant analysis and partial least squares regression, in order to classify subjects (62). Therefore, it can be seen as an alternative to methods such as linear discriminant analysis, support vector machines and random forest classification. OPLS-DA is an ideal method to use in the search for biomarkers

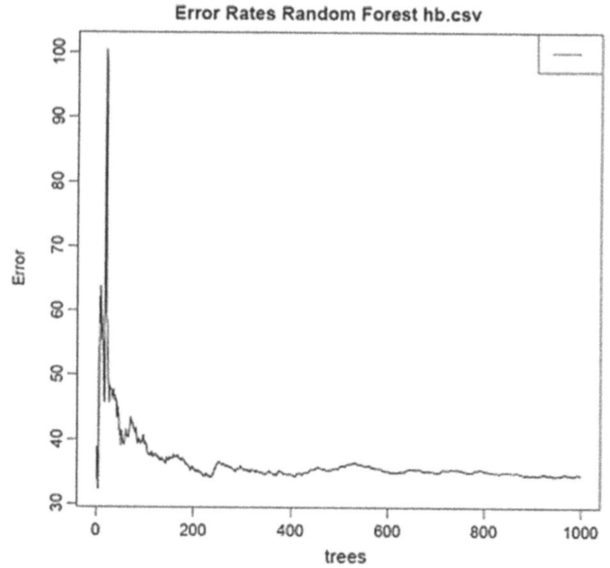

FIGURE 6 | Decrease in error as a function of the number of trees for the random forest regression model for spermine, which had the highest proportion of variance explained (0.94). From Smith et al. (51) with permission.

of SNHL, tinnitus or vestibular disorders, for e.g., using metabolomic data from animals or humans with those conditions. In partial least squares regression, which is an extension of MLR, factors are extracted from the $Y'XX'Y$ matrix in order to generate prediction functions, only in the case of partial least squares discriminant analysis, the dependent variable is categorical. One major advantage of partial least squares discriminant analysis is that it is minimally restrictive because it allows for fewer observations than variables (i.e., less n than p), a problem that is significant for linear discriminant analysis (62). As with PCA and cluster analysis, the data would normally be standardized to z scores before proceeding.

In OPLS-DA, the X variables are latent variables that maximize the separation between the groups, ranked according to how much variation in Y that they explain. OPLS-DA separates the systematic variation in X into 2 parts: (1) that which is linearly related to Y; and (2) that which is unrelated or "orthogonal" to Y (62). The OPLS method uses a modification of the non-linear iterative partial least squares algorithm (62). An orthogonal signal correction procedure, developed by Trygg and Wold (62), employs an iterative process to find orthogonal components in the X matrix. For this it depends on a starting vector, which can use PCs from a PCA. The main problem with discriminant analysis is over-fitting, particularly where the $p >$ the n, so that the model works well on the training data but not on new data, and where there is multicollinearity. However, this possibility can be addressed using permutation testing (63). In permutation testing, variables are assigned randomly to the different samples, and new models are generated many times, e.g., 2,000. A null distribution of classifications is created, which is expected to be non-significant. The results obtained from the original data should be outside the 95 or 99% confidence intervals for the null distribution, in order to be statistically significant, i.e., not part of the null distribution (63).

Biplots can be used to show some of the results of an OPLS-DA, where the x axis is labeled "t[1]," which are the X scores predictive of Y, and the y axis is labeled "to[2]," which are the X scores that are not predictive of Y. Therefore, the x axis represents the between group variation and the y axis represents the within group variation. OPLS-DA calculates various indices of the success of the model. R^2X (cum) is the sum of the predictive and orthogonal variation in X that is explained by the model, which can be split into the predictive and orthogonal components. R^2Y (cum) is the total sum of variation in Y explained by the model. Q^2 is the effectiveness of the prediction, based on the OPLS-DA equation, using cross-validation, e.g., using a LOO procedure, where 0.9 would be excellent.

S plots are often used to help interpret the OPLS-DA results. In the S plot, the x axis "p[1]" is the magnitude of each variable in the x axis. The y axis "p(corr)[1]" is the reliability (obtained with confidence intervals using jack-knifing and cross-validation). Values close to zero on both axes are close to noise, i.e., they have almost zero magnitude and reliability. OPLS-DA can be carried out in R, or using the programs Metaboanalyst and Metscape 3.1 (35, 64).

Pathway impact analyses can also be carried out on the OPLS-DA. Using the prior knowledge of pathways, these methods look for over-representation of specific pathways in the data. They calculate the sum of the importance measures of the matched metabolites normalized by the sum of the importance measures of all metabolites in each pathway. Over-representation analysis, quantitative enrichment analysis, and single sample profiling are three different types of pathway analysis that can be used in the program Cytoscape 3.30 (35, 64, 65).

DATA PRE-PROCESSING AND IMPUTATION, OVERFITTING, AND THE PROBLEM OF INTERPRETABILITY

When using MVA and data mining methods to analyse data, some pre-processing of the data is often necessary. In the case of MVA, methods that are part of the General Linear Model (GLM), such as multiple linear regression, multivariate multiple linear regression, linear discriminant analysis, structural equation modeling, and canonical correlation analysis, require that the assumption of multivariate normality be met (see section Linear Discriminant Analysis). Therefore, data need to be checked to determine whether they are normally distributed or even whether they have a multivariate normal distribution (see Linear Discriminant Analysis). Normality (Q–Q) plots and plots of residuals vs. fitted values usually need to be obtained and formal assumption tests conducted, such as the Anderson-Darling, Shapiro-Wilk or Kolmogorov-Smirnov tests for univariate normality, and Bartlett's or Levene's tests for homogeneity of variance. If these tests are statistically significant (i.e., $P \leq 0.05$), a decision may be made to transform variables in order to achieve fulfillment of the normality and homogeneity of

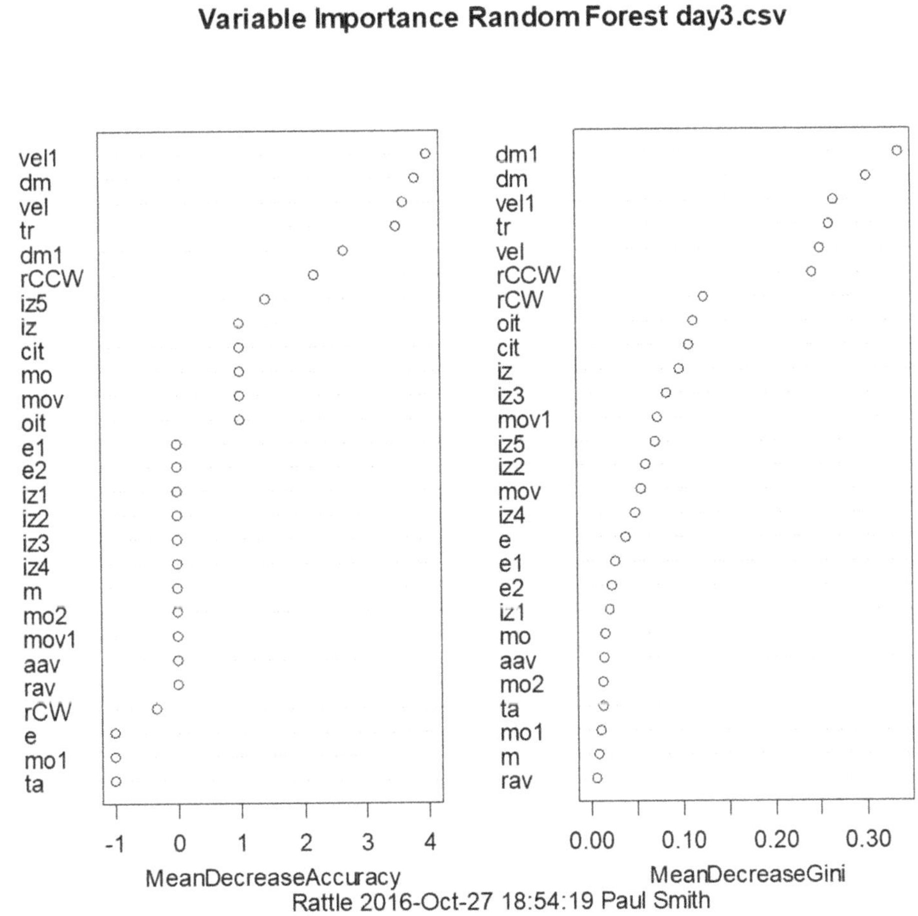

FIGURE 7 | Order of variable importance for the random forest classification for day 3 following BVD, showing the decrease in the accuracy of the prediction as the variables are removed. The mean decrease in Gini coefficient is an indication of the extent to which each variable contributes to the homogeneity of the nodes and leaves in the random forest. dm, distance moved nose-point; dm1, distance moved center-point; e, contracted; e1, elongation normal; e2, elongation stretched; iz, in zone outer zone, nose-point; iz1, in zone inner zone, nose-point; iz2, in zone mid zone, nose-point; iz3, in zone outer zone center-point; iz4, in zone inner zone center-point; iz5, in zone mid zone center-point; m, meander center-point; cit, center inter-transition center-point; mo, mobility immobile; mo1, mobility mobile; mo2, mobility highly mobile; mov, movement center-point/moving; mov1, movement center-point/not moving; rCCW, rotation counter-clockwise center-nose; rCW, rotation clockwise center-nose; ta, turn angle center-point; vel, velocity nose-point; vel1, velocity center-point; aav, absolute angular velocity center-point; oit, outer inter-transition center-point; rav, relative angular velocity; tr, total rotations. From Aitken et al. (72) with permission.

variance assumptions; however, great care needs to be taken in transforming non-linear dependent variables into linear ones, as in Scatchard plots, because of the way that it can distort the error around the line of best fit (66). For receptor binding data, non-linear regression is now considered preferable to linear regression following transformation (66). In the case of other methods such as PCA, OPLS-DA and cluster analysis, pre-processing may involve standardizing the data (see Principal Component Analysis and Factor Analysis), in order to ensure that differences in measurement scales do not bias the analysis.

Even for univariate statistical analyses, many statistical programs delete experimental subjects if they have missing data for procedures such as repeated measures ANOVAs (43, 45). Many animal studies in auditory and vestibular neuroscience already have small and unequal sample sizes; therefore, simply deleting data in the case of missing values will result in lower statistical power and may bias the results (67). For alternatives to repeated measures ANOVAs such as linear mixed model analysis, "imputation" procedures are employed in order to estimate the missing values ("Missing Values Analysis or MVA") (43, 67, 68). A maximum likelihood (ML) and expectation-maximization (EM) approach (a combination of imputation and ML) can be used (68). However, only some programs (e.g., SPSS) offer the EM algorithm and for the ML and EM methods to be used, the missing data must be "missing at random" (MAR, i.e., the probability that an observation is missing must not depend on the unobserved missing value but may depend on the group to which it would have belonged) or "missing completely at random" (MCAR, i.e., the probability that an observation is missing must not depend on the observed or missing values) (67, 68). In other words, there can be no bias to the way that data are missing, a condition that is sometimes difficult to satisfy. The

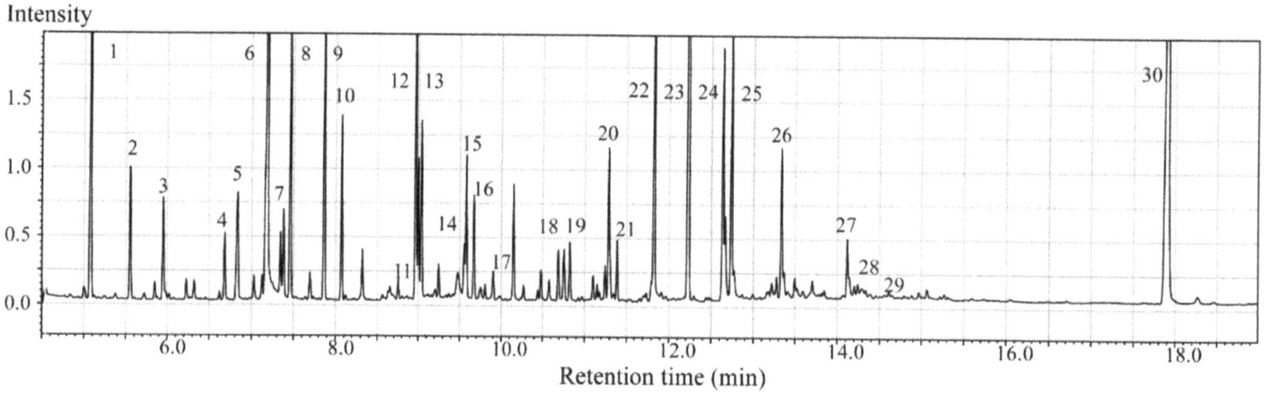

FIGURE 8 | Typical GC/MS chromatograms of extracts from brain tissue of a sham animal. The compounds were identified as: 1. Lactic Acid, 2. Alanine, 3. Oxalic acid, 4. Valine, 5. Urea, 6. Phosphoric acid, 7. Proline, 8. Glycine, 9. Serine, 10. Threonine, 11. Malic acid, 12. Aspartic acid, 13. γ-Aminobutanoic acid, 14. Creatinine, 15. Glutamic acid, 16. Phenylalanine, 17. N-Acetylaspartic acid, 18. Hypoxanthine, 19. Citric acid, 20. Lysine, 21. Tyrosine, 22. Palmitic acid, 23. Myo-Inositol, 24. Oleic acid, 25. Stearic acid, 26. Arachidonic acid, 27. Docosahexaenoic acid, 28. Inosine, 29. Glycerol monostearate, 30. Cholesterol. From He et al. (35) with permission.

K-NN algorithm discussed in K-Nearest Neighbors Algorithm can be used for imputation and there is a variety of multivariate imputation procedures [see (69) for a review].

"Overfitting" is an enormous problem in MVA and data mining methods which involve regression modeling. Overfitting occurs when a model for prediction is based so closely on a particular data set that it has little predictive value for other, similar data sets, often a result of including too many parameters in the model (44). As a result, a regression model based on a training data set may have no predictive value for the test data set. Although the problem is well-recognized in MLR (44), Breiman et al. (48) have suggested that random forest methods do not overfit, a view that has been challenged (70). Solutions to overfitting include collecting more data so that there is a larger n for each predictor variable, *p*, combining predictors in order to reduce correlation between them and the use of "shrinkage and penalization" procedures (44). The adjusted R^2 in MLR is one type of shrinkage estimator because it takes into account the number of predictor variables. "Lasso" regression ("least absolute shrinkage and selection operator") is a method that generates a linear regression model with greater "sparsity" [see (37) for a review].

One of the advantages of univariate statistical methods is that they are relatively easy to understand and this is partly why they are so popular. Researchers turn to multivariate statistical and data mining (or machine learning) methods because they have to deal with many variables, sometimes hundreds or thousands, but in the process of using such procedures, they sacrifice simplicity and interpretability. Molnar (37) has written extensively about the problem of "interpretability" with MVA and data mining methods, which involve complex modeling. Even if they provide good predictive value, they may be difficult to understand. Simpler models, by definition, such as shorter decision trees, are more easily interpreted than longer ones. Molnar (37) has suggested that "model agnostic interpretation methods" be used for machine learning in preference to "model-specific ones." These are methods that can be applied to any machine learning model, are not restricted to a certain form of explanation (e.g., a linear formula vs. a graphic representation) and should have flexibility in the way that the explanation is represented. Examples include partial dependence plots (PDP), feature importance and Shapley values [see (37) for a review].

EXAMPLES OF APPLICATIONS OF MULTIVARIATE STATISTICAL AND DATA MINING METHODS TO THE ANALYSIS OF OTOLOGICAL DATA

Principal Component Analysis and Cluster Analysis

One of our research interests has been the role of neurochemical changes in the hippocampus in the cognitive deficits that occur following peripheral bilateral vestibular damage. In this process we have used western blotting to analyse the expression of various glutamate receptor subtypes in the rat hippocampus, given the importance of glutamate receptors to memory processes such as long-term potentiation [see (71) for a review]. Due to the fact that we quantified 5 different glutamate receptor subunit subtypes (GluR1, GluR2, GluR3, NR1, and NR2) and 2 forms of calmodulin kinase II (CaMII and phosphorylated CaMII), related to glutamate receptor activation, we decided to use PCA and cluster analysis to analyse the results, particularly so that we could understand the co-variation and interactions of any changes in the expression of the proteins. Using univariate statistical analysis, there were no significant differences in the expression of any individual protein between the bilateral vestibular deafferentation (BVD) group and the sham controls (15); however, PCA suggested that when the 1st and 2nd components were plotted against one another using a loading plot, the relationship between the expression of the different proteins had changed [see **Figure 3**; (6)]. Although the meaning

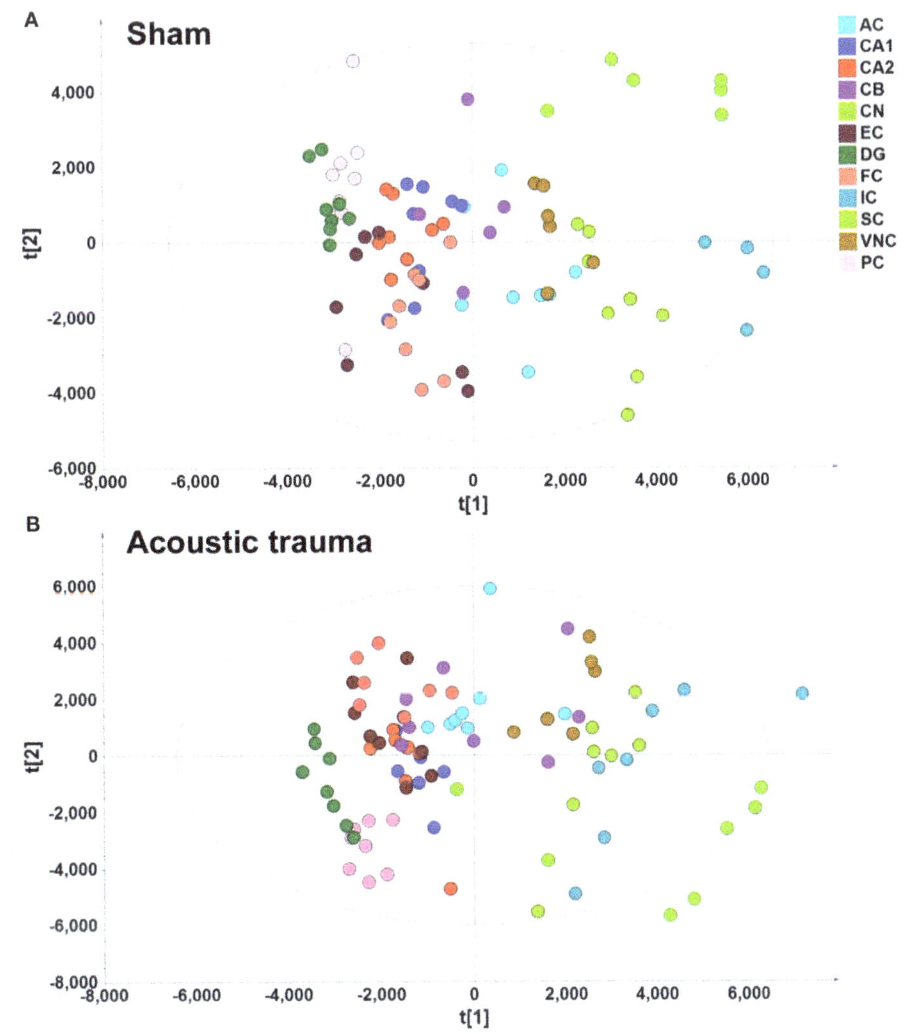

FIGURE 9 | PLS-DA score plot of different brain regions from sham **(A)** and acoustic trauma **(B)** groups. **(A)** sham [PC1: *R2X* = 0.344, *R2Y* = 0.0842, Q^2 =0.0726; PC2: *R2X* = 0.249, *R2Y* = 0.0525, Q^2 = 0.0373; All 6 PCs: *R2X* (cum) = 0.84, *R2Y* (cum) = 0.381, Q^2 (cum) = 0.286]; **(B)** acoustic trauma [PC1: *R2X* = 0.336, *R2Y* = 0.0759, Q^2 = 0.0683; PC2: *R2X* = 0.307, *R2Y* = 0.0513, Q^2 = 0.0407; All 6 PCs: *R2X* (cum) = 0.875, *R2Y* (cum) = 0. 384, Q^2 (cum) = 0.325]. AC, auditory cortex; CB, cerebellum; IC, inferior colliculus; CN, cochlear nucleus; VNC, vestibular nucleus complex; SC, superior colliculus; CA1 and CA2 of the hippocampus; DG, dentate gyrus; FC, frontal cortex; PC, perirhinal cortex; EC, entorhinal cortex. From He et al. (35) with permission.

of this shift is not easy to interpret—one of the perennial problems of PCA—this MVA revealed a change in the pattern of interaction between the different proteins which the univariate analysis could not. Note that all of the data were transformed to z scores.

Cluster analysis of the individual protein variables showed that they co-varied in a predictable way [see **Figure 4**; (15)]. Note again the use of z scores and the fact that the AMPA (GluR1, 2, and 3) and NMDA (NR1 and 2) receptor subunits tended to co-vary closely with one another.

Multiple Linear Regression

Another area of interest for us has been the L-arginine cycle and its role in producing nitric oxide synthase, polyamines and glutamate in the brainstem vestibular nucleus and cerebellum (**Figure 1**). This complex pathway is involved in brain aging in the central vestibular system and has been the target for drug treatments aimed at interfering with neurodegenerative diseases such as Alzheimer's Disease (3, 4). Because these neurochemicals interact in a network, it is important to understand how each part of the system affects the other parts. We have used MLR in an attempt to predict different neurochemicals in this pathway from one another, with adjusted R^2 values ranging from 0.50 (ornithine) to 0.95 (citrulline) (51). The best predictions were for citrulline (0.95), spermine (0.93) and arginine (0.92) (see **Table 2**). Assumptions were tested using normal Q-Q plots and residuals vs. fitted values plots, and were fulfilled. In this study, MLR was compared directly with random forest regression on the same data set (51) (see below).

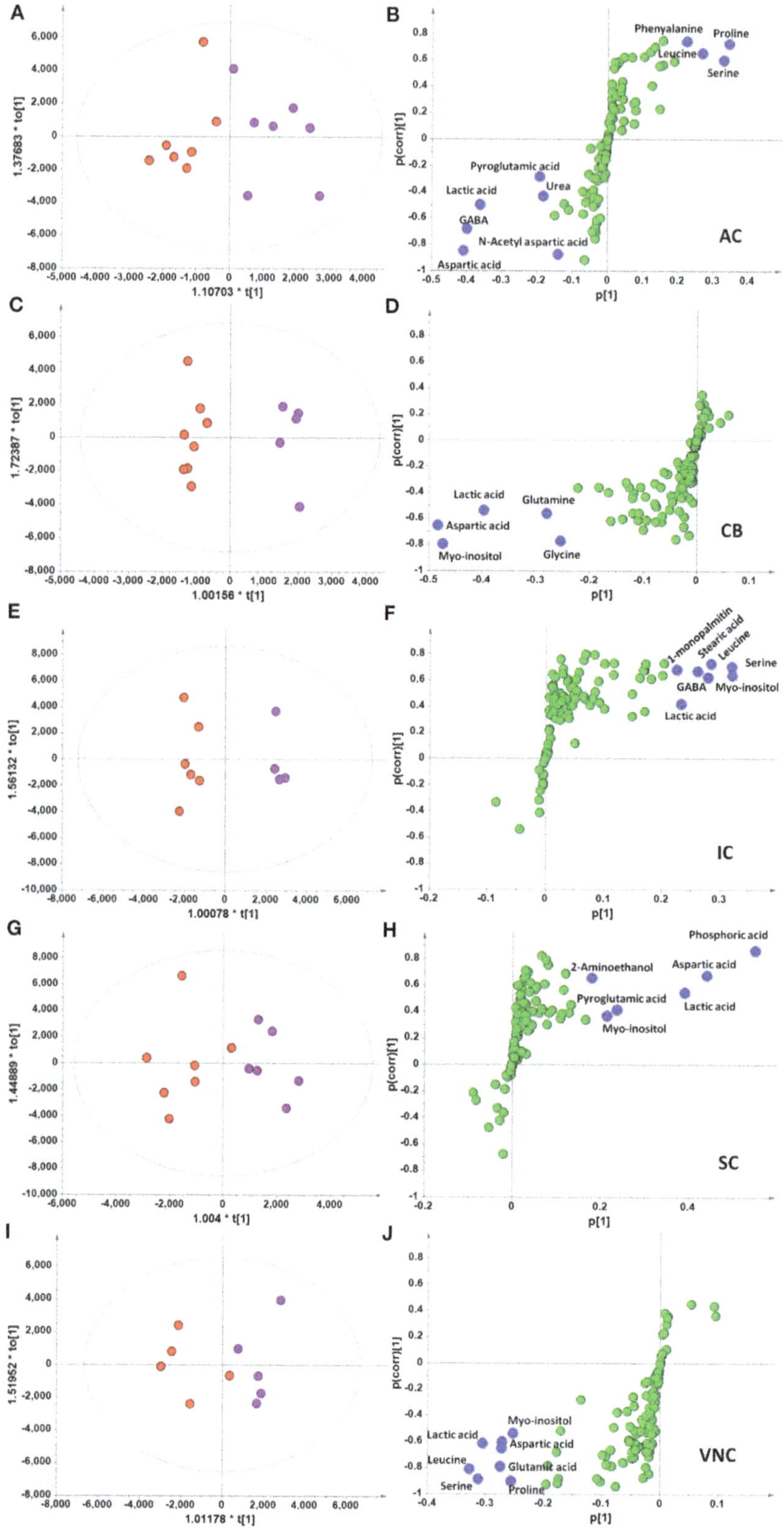

FIGURE 10 | OPLS-DA and S-plot analysis comparing the OPLSDA scores between sham and acoustic trauma animals in different brain regions. Left panel, OPLSDA scores plots, red dots: Sham, purple dots: Acoustic trauma; Right panel, S-plots. **(A,B)** AC [Predictive component: $R2X = 0.194$, $R2Y = 0.76$, $Q^2 = 0.45$;

(Continued)

FIGURE 10 | Orthogonal component 1: $R2X = 0.446$; All components: $R2X$ (cum) $= 0.64$]; **(C,D)** CB [Predictive component: $R2X = 0.152$, $R2Y = 0.973$, $Q^2 = 0.68$; Orthogonal component 1: $R2X = 0.364$; All components: $R2X$ (cum) $= 0.927$]; **(E,F)** IC [Predictive component: $R2X = 0.293$, $R2Y = 0.978$, $Q^2 = 0.702$; Orthogonal component 1: $R2X = 0.417$; All components: $R2X$ (cum) $= 0.905$]; **(G,H)** SC [Predictive component: $R2X = 0.238$, $R2Y = 0.791$, $Q^2 = 0.691$; Orthogonal component: $R2X = 0.562$; All components: $R2X$ (cum) $= 0.8$]; **(I,J)** VNC [Predictive component: $R2X = 0.403$, $R2Y = 0.779$, $Q^2 = 0.445$; Orthogonal component: $R2X = 0.389$; All components: $R2X$ (cum) $= 0.792$]. In the right panel, the blue dots show variables with high negative magnitude and reliability scores (everything is scaled and relative) or high positive magnitude and reliability scores, i.e., potential biomarkers. AC, auditory cortex; CB, cerebellum; IC, inferior colliculus; CN, cochlear nucleus; VCN, vestibular nucleus complex. From He et al. (35) with permission.

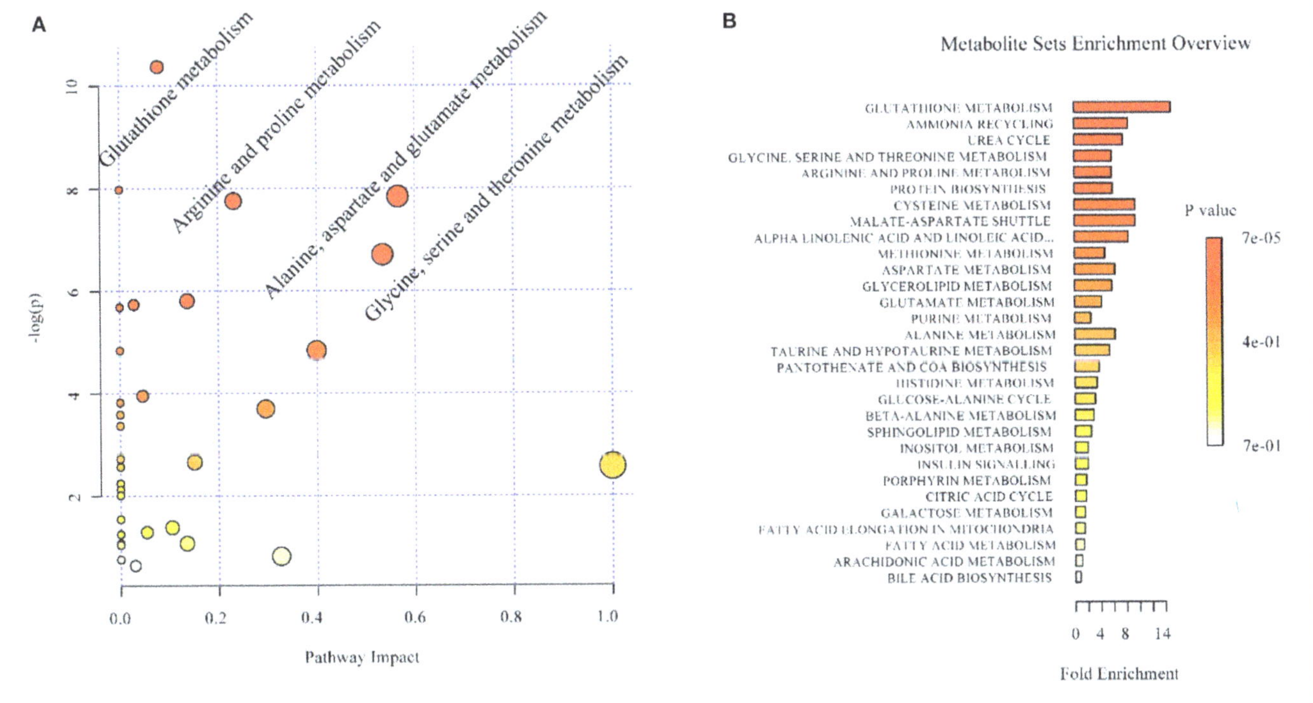

FIGURE 11 | Overview of the impact of acoustic trauma on brain metabolites. **(A)** The pathway impact of acoustic trauma on metabolites. The y axis shows the p-values and the x axis, the pathway impact values; the node color is based on its p-value and the node size reflects the pathway impact values. **(B)** The enrichment overview of the pathway-associated metabolite sets perturbed by acoustic trauma. From He et al. (35) with permission.

Random Forest Regression

Using the same data set, we found that random forest regression was also successful in predicting the neurochemical concentrations in the L-arginine pathway, with the best values for the proportion of variance explained, 0.94 (spermine), 0.92 (arginine), and 0.90 (citrulline) [see **Table 3**; (51)] However, for this data set, random forest regression was somewhat less successful than MLR in predicting some of the variables (e.g., 0.27 for ornithine; see **Table 3**). Variable importance plots (VIPs) were obtained and **Figure 5** shows the variables in order of importance for the prediction of spermine, where arginine and citrulline were clearly the most important variables (51). **Figure 6** shows the degree of error in the prediction of spermine as a function of the number of trees generated. It can be seen that the error decreases rapidly after the first 150–200 trees (51).

Linear Discriminant Analysis

We have also used linear discriminant analysis to predict the age of animals based on the concentrations of neurochemicals in the L-arginine pathway (**Figure 1**). This research is directly applicable to the identification of biomarkers that might be used to predict pathological changes that occur in brain aging in vestibular areas of the brain. In Liu et al. (3), we identified an LDF that could predict whether rats were young (4 months old) or aged (24 months old). The LDF based on putrescine, spermidine, spermine, citrulline, glutamate and GABA in the vestibular nucleus (note the z transformation), could predict age with 100% accuracy using cross-validation ($P = 0.000$, Wilks'λ). Using the cerebellum, age could be predicted with 93% accuracy ($P = 0.000$, Wilks'λ), using only spermine and spermidine. Similar results were reported by Liu et al. (4), who found 90% accuracy in classifying animals to the aged group based on neurochemicals in the vestibular nucleus and 80% accuracy in classifying them based on neurochemicals in the cerebellum. We have also applied linear discriminant analysis to the prediction of whether rats have had a BVD or a sham procedure based on a combination of their behavioral symptoms, such as unsupported rearing, locomotor activity in the inner vs. outer zones of the open field maze and performance in the spatial alternation in a T maze task, and found that whether the animals had received a BVD could be predicted with 100% accuracy ($P = 0.000$, Wilks'λ) (5). These kinds of methods may be applicable to the differential diagnosis of vestibular and auditory disorders.

Random Forest Classification

With a similar aim to the use of linear discriminant analysis to predict whether animals have BVD on the basis of their behavioral symptoms, we have also employed random forest classification using a range of symptoms measured using the Ethovision tracking system (72). For days 3 and 23 post-BVD, we found that random forest classification could predict which rats had received BVD and which were sham animals with 100% accuracy. **Figure 7** shows the variables in order of importance for day 3 and indicates that the most important variables were the animals' locomotor velocity (hyperactivity is a common symptom of BVD in rats), distance moved and rotation (72).

Ahmadi et al. (26, 27) have recently used logistic regression and random forest classification, as well as artificial neural networks, to support differential diagnosis of peripheral and central vestibular disorders in humans. In general, they observed that machine learning methods outperformed univariate scores. Karmali et al. (28) also used logistic regression to predict the probability of falling based on age and thresholds for the perception of 0.2 Hz roll head tilt.

OPLS-DA

In the context of auditory neuroscience, we have used OPLS-DA on metabolomics data from brain samples to successfully predict whether rats have been exposed to acoustic trauma or a sham procedure (35, 65). The ultimate aim here is to use metabolomic analysis of blood samples to predict whether humans might develop tinnitus or whether they might respond to particular tinnitus treatments (65). In what we believe to be the first study of its kind, we analyzed brain samples from 12 different brain regions in rats that had been exposed to either acoustic trauma or a sham procedure, and used GC-MS to isolate a total of 107 distinct peaks in the chromatogram, with 88 authentically identified as amino acids, small organic acids, carbohydrates, fatty acids, lipids and amines (see **Figure 8**). PCA and OPLS-DA were performed on the data. In **Figure 9**, each dot represents the summarized information from the 88 authentically identified molecules for a particular brain region. The distance between the dots indicates the similarity of the metabolic composition of the samples. Brain regions with similar functions appeared to have a similar metabolic composition in both sham and acoustic-trauma exposed animals. However, OPLS-DA in specific brain regions such as the auditory cortex, cerebellum, inferior colliculus, superior colliculus and vestibular nucleus, showed that the metabolic profile was separated for the sham and acoustic-trauma-exposed animals (35). This suggested that a shift in the metabolic pattern had occurred in these brain regions in the animals exposed to acoustic trauma. The associated S plots (**Figure 10**) indicated that potential biomarkers of acoustic trauma in these brain regions included urea, amino acids, fatty acids, sugar acids, nucleosides and organic acids, in a region-specific fashion. For example, GABA was significantly increased only in the auditory cortex. The overall impact of the acoustic trauma on brain metabolites is summarized in a pathway analysis in **Figure 11** (35).

SUMMARY

Phenomena in vestibular and auditory neuroscience, as in other areas of neuroscience, almost always involve the complex interaction of multiple variables, and yet many areas of basic vestibular and auditory neuroscience, in particular, employ univariate statistical analyses almost exclusively. This may limit the ability of studies to reveal how the interactions between different variables may determine a particular outcome. We have used MVAs and data mining methods to explore the way that combinations of variables can account for neurochemical and behavioral changes following the loss of vestibular function (3–6, 15, 72, 73) and auditory function [e.g., (35, 65)]. In clinical neuroscience research, MVAs and data mining methods have been used to predict the progression of patients from one neurological disorder to another [e.g., (9, 12)] and the probability that the early adolescent use of *Cannabis* can lead to the development of psychotic symptoms in later life [e.g., (74)]. These methods are now in routine use in areas such as genomics, proteomics, metabolomics (10, 11), and the analysis of fMRI data [e.g., (75)]. Electrophysiological research in neuroscience is increasingly moving to the use of multi-electrode arrays using dozens or more micro-electrodes simultaneously, and in this situation one of the main objectives is to determine how different brain regions change in relation to one another, which requires MVA [e.g., (76, 77)].

MVAs and data mining methods can be applied to every aspect of vestibular and auditory neuroscience in order to gain a better understanding of the way in which networks or systems of variables affect otological function. In the search for biomarkers of SNHL, tinnitus and vestibular dysfunction, classification methods such as linear discriminant analysis, support vector machines, random forest classification, Bayesian classifiers and OPLS-DA, can be applied to behavioral, neurophysiological and neurochemical data to predict the probability of a disease or disorder developing, in order to intervene and provide treatments that will prevent or impede the pathological changes. In the context of metabolomics, MVAs and data mining methods have already been proven to be useful in the prediction of disease [e.g., (8, 9, 11–13, 78–80)]. OPLS-DA is an example of an MVA that has successfully been applied to metabolomic data in order to predict hearing loss in rats (35, 65) and may be particularly useful in the search for biomarkers of SNHL, tinnitus, and vestibular dysfunction [e.g., (81)].

AUTHOR CONTRIBUTIONS

PS and YZ: conceptualization and writing—review and editing. PS: writing—original draft preparation.

ACKNOWLEDGMENTS

The content of this manuscript has been published in part as part of the MApplStat thesis of Smith (73).

REFERENCES

1. Manly BFJ. *Multivariate Statistical Analyses. A Primer.* 3rd ed. London: Chapman and Hall/CRC (2005).
2. Stevens, J.P. *Applied Multivariate Statistics for the Social Sciences.* 5th ed. Hillsdale NJ, Lawrence Erlbaum (2009).
3. Liu P, Zhang H, Devaraj R, Ganesalingam G, Smith PF. A multivariate analysis of the effects of aging on glutamate, GABA and arginine metabolites in the rat vestibular nucleus. *Hear Res.* (2010) 269:122–33. doi: 10.1016/j.heares.2010.06.019
4. Liu P, Gupta N, Jing Y, Collie ND, Zhang H, Smith PF. Further studies of age-related changes in arginine metabolites in the rat vestibular nucleus and cerebellum. *Neuroscience.* (2017) 348:273–87. doi: 10.1016/j.neuroscience.2017.02.033
5. Smith PF, Haslett SJ, Zheng, Y. A multivariate statistical and data mining analysis of spatial memory-related behaviour following bilateral vestibular deafferentation in the rat. *Behav Brain Res.* (2013) 246:15–23. doi: 10.1016/j.bbr.2013.02.033
6. Smith PF, Zheng, Y. Principal component analysis suggests subtle changes in glutamate receptor subunit expression in the rat hippocampus following bilateral vestibular deafferentation in the rat. *Neurosci Lett.* (2013) 548:265–8. doi: 10.1016/j.neulet.2013.05.036
7. Herzog MH, Francis G, Clarke A (editors). The multiple testing problem. In: Understanding Statistics and Experimental Design. Learning Materials in Biosciences. Cham: Springer (2009). doi: 10.1007/978-3-030-03499-3_5
8. Pang H, Lin A, Holford M, Enerson BE, Lu B, Lawton MP, et al. Pathway analysis using random forests classification and regression. *Bioinformatics.* (2006) 22:2028–36. doi: 10.1093/bioinformatics/btl344
9. Krafczyk S, Tietze S, Swoboda W, Valkovic P, Brandt, T. Artificial neural network: A new diagnostic posturographic tool for disorders of stance. *Clin Neurophysiol.* (2006) 117:1692–8. doi: 10.1016/j.clinph.2006.04.022
10. Dziuda DM. *Data Mining for Genomics and Proteomics.* Hoboken, NJ: Wiley (2010).
11. Ryan M, Mason-Parker SE, Tate WP, Abraham WC, Williams, JM. Rapidly induced gene networks following induction of long-term potentiation at perforant synapses *in vivo. Hippocampus.* (2011) 21:541–53. doi: 10.1002/hipo.20770
12. Brandt T, Strupp M, Novozhilov S, Krafczyk, S. Artificial neural network posturography detects the transition of vestibular neuritis to phobic postural vertigo. *J Neurol.* (2012) 259:182–4. doi: 10.1007/s00415-011-6124-8
13. Prochazka A, Vysata O, Valis M, Tupa, O, Schatz M, Marík V, et al. Bayesian classification and analysis of gait disorders using image and depth sensors of Microsoft Kinect. *Digital Signal Proc.* (2015) 47:169–77. doi: 10.1016/j.dsp.2015.05.011
14. Smith PF. Statistical analysis in pharmacology is not always BO. *Trends Pharmacol Sci.* (2012) 33:565–6. doi: 10.1016/j.tips.2012.08.006
15. Zheng Y, Wilson G, Stiles L, Smith PF. Glutamate receptor subunit and calmodulin kinase II expression in the rat hippocampus, with and without T maze experience, following bilateral vestibular deafferentation. *PLOS ONE.* (2013) 8:e54527. doi: 10.1371/journal.pone.0054527
16. Agrawal Y, Carey JP, Della Santina CC, Schubert MC, Minor LB. Diabetes, vestibular dysfunction, and falls: analyses from the National Health and Nutrition Examination Survey. *Otol Neurotol.* (2010) 31:1445–50. doi: 10.1097/MAO.0b013e3181f2f035
17. Semenov YR, Bigelow RT, Xue QL, du Lac S, Agrawal Y. Association between vestibular and cognitive function in U.S. Adults: data from the national health and nutrition examination survey. *J Gerontol A Biol Sci Med Sci.* (2016) 71:243–50. doi: 10.1093/gerona/glv069
18. Düwel P, Ilgner J, Engelke JC, Westhofen M. Subclassification of vestibular disorders by means of statistical analysis in caloric labyrinth testing. *Acta Otolaryngol.* (2004) 124:595–602. doi: 10.1080/00016480310015182
19. Dimitri PS, Wall C 3rd, Oas JG, Rauch SD. Application of multivariate statistics to vestibular testing: discriminating between Menière's disease and migraine associated dizziness. *J Vestib Res.* (2001) 11:53–65.
20. Dimitri PS, Wall C III, Oas JG. Classification of human rotation test results using parametric modeling and multivariate statistics. *Acta Otolaryngol.* (1996) 116:497–506. doi: 10.3109/00016489609137880
21. Chien WW, Janky K, Minor LB, Carey JP. Superior canal dehiscence size: multivariate assessment of clinical impact. *Otol Neurotol.* (2012) 33:810–5. doi: 10.1097/MAO.0b013e318248eac4
22. Rossi-Izquierdo M, Basta D, Rubio-Rodríguez JP, Santos-Pérez S, Ernst A, Sesar-Ignacio Á, et al. Is posturography able to identify fallers in patients with Parkinson's disease? *Gait Posture.* (2014) 40:53–7 doi: 10.1016/j.gaitpost.2014.02.003
23. Gabelić T, Krbot Skorić M, Adamec I, Barun B, Zadro I, Habek M. The vestibular evoked myogenic potentials (VEMP) score: a promising tool for evaluation of brainstem involvement in multiple sclerosis. *Eur J Neurol.* (2015) 22:261–9. doi: 10.1111/ene.12557
24. Abouzari M, Goshtasbi K, Sarna B, Khosravi P, Reutershan T, Mostaghni N, et al. Prediction of vestibular schwannoma recurrence using artificial neural network. *Laryngoscope Investig Otolaryngol.* (2020) 5:278–85. doi: 10.1002/lio2.362
25. Vibert N, Hoang T, Gilchrist DP, MacDougall HG, Burgess AM, Roberts RD, et al. Psychophysiological correlates of the inter-individual variability of head movement control in seated humans. *Gait Posture.* (2006) 23:355–63. doi: 10.1016/j.gaitpost.2005.04.006
26. Ahmadi SA, Vivar G, Navab N, Möhwald K, Maier A, Hadzhikolev H, et al. Modern machine-learning can support diagnostic differentiation of central and peripheral acute vestibular disorders. *J. Neurol.* (2020) 267:143–52. doi: 10.1007/s00415-020-09931-z
27. Ahmadi SA, Vivar G, Frei J, Nowoshilow S, Bardins S, Brandt T, et al. Towards computerized diagnosis of neurological stance disorders: data mining and machine learning of posturography and sway. *J Neurol.* (2019) 266 (Suppl. 1):108–17. doi: 10.1007/s00415-019-09458-y
28. Karmali F, Bermudez MC, Clark TK, Wang W, Merfeld DM. Multivariate analyses of balance test performance, vestibular thresholds, and age. *Front Neurol.* (2017) 8:578. doi: 10.3389/fneur.2017.00578
29. Molina ME, Perez A, Valente JP. Classification of auditory brainstem responses through symbolic pattern recovery. *Artif Intell Med.* (2016) 70:12–30. doi: 10.1016/j.artmed.2016.05.001
30. Exarchos TP, Rigas G, Bibas A, Kikidis D, Nikitas C, Wuyts FL, et al. Mining balance disorders' data for the development of diagnostic decision support systems. *Comput Biol Med.* (2016) 77:240–8. doi: 10.1016/j.compbiomed.2016.08.016
31. Smith PF. On the application of multivariate statistical and data mining analyses to data in neuroscience. *J Undergrad Neurosci Educ.* (2018) 16:R20–32.
32. Kline P. *An Easy Guide to Factor Analysis.* London: Routledge (2002).
33. Lattin J, Carroll JD, Green PE. *Analyzing Multivariate Data.* Pacific Grove, CA: Duxbury (2003).
34. Jolliffe, I.T. *Principal Component Analysis.* 2nd ed. New York, NY: Springer (2004).
35. He J, Zhu Y, Aa J, Smith PF, De Ridder D, Wang G, et al. Brain metabolic changes in rats following acoustic trauma. *Front. Neurosci.* (2017) 11:148. doi: 10.3389/fnins.2017.00148

36. Marcoulides GA, Hershberger SL. *Multivariate Statistical Methods. A First Course.* Mahwah, NJ: Lawrence Erlbaum Associatio (1997).
37. Molnar, C. *Interpretable Machine Learning. A Guide for Making Black Box Models Explainable.* Victoria, BC: Lean Publishing (2019).
38. Brook RJ, Arnold GC. *Applied Regression Analysis and Experimental Design.* Boca Raton, FL: Chapman and Hall/CRC (1985).
39. Ryan TP. *Modern Regression Methods.* New Jersey, NY: Wiley (2009). doi: 10.1002/9780470382806
40. Rutherford, A. *Introducing ANOVA and ANCOVA. A GLM Approach.* London: Sage Publications (2001).
41. Vittinghoff E, Glidden DV, Shiboski SC, McCulloch CE. *Regression Methods in Statistics: Linear, Logistic, Survival and Repeated Measures Models.* New York, NY: Springer (2005).
42. Doncaster CP, Davey AJH. *Analysis of Variance and Covariance.* Cambridge: Cambridge University Press (2007).
43. Gamst G, Meyers LS, Guarino, A.J. *Analysis of Variance Designs. A Conceptual and Computational Approach with SPSS and SAS.* New York, NY: Cambridge University Press (2008). doi: 10.1017/CBO9780511801648
44. Babayak MA. What you see may not be what you get: a brief, non-technical introduction to over-fitting in regression-type models. *Psychosomat Med.* (2004) 66:411–21. doi: 10.1097/00006842-200405000-00021
45. Field A. *Discovering Statistics Using SPSS.* Los Angeles, CA: Sage (2011).
46. Field A, Miles J, Field Z. *Discovering Statistics Using R.* Los Angeles, CA: Sage (2012).
47. Hastie T, Tibshirani R, Friedman, J. *Elements of Statistical Learning: Data Mining, Inference and Prediction.* 2nd ed. Heidelberg: Springer Verlag (2009).
48. Breiman L, Friedman J, Stone CJ, Olshen RA. *Classification and Regression Trees.* 1st ed. Boca Raton, FL: CRC Press (1984).
49. Marsland, S. *Machine Learning. An Algorithmic Perspective.* Boca Raton, FL: CRC Press (2019).
50. Williams, G.J. *Data Mining With Rattle And R.* New York, NY: Springer (2011). doi: 10.1007/978-1-4419-9890-3
51. Smith PF, Ganesh S, Liu P. A comparison of random forest regression and multiple linear regression for prediction in neuroscience. *J Neurosci Methods.* (2013) 220:85–91. doi: 10.1016/j.jneumeth.2013.08.024
52. Friedman JH. Greedy function approximation: a gradient boosting machine. *Ann. Stats.* (2001) 29:1189–232. doi: 10.1214/aos/1013203451
53. Tabachnick BG, Fidell LS. *Using Multivariate Statistics.* 5th ed. Boston, MA: Pearson Education Inc (2007).
54. Wilson MD. Support vector machines. In: Jorgensen SE, Fath BD, editors. Encyclopedia of Ecology. New York, NY: Elsevier (2008). p. 3431–7. doi: 10.1016/B978-008045405-4.00168-3
55. Williams GJ. Rattle: a data mining GUI for R. *R J.* (2009) 1/2:45–55. doi: 10.32614/RJ-2009-016
56. Crawley MJ. *The R Book.* Chichester: Wiley (2007). doi: 10.1002/9780470515075
57. Davies TM. *The Book of R.* San Francisco, CA: No Starch Press (2017).
58. Bolstad WM. *Introduction to Bayesian Statistics.* 2nd ed. New York, NY: Wiley (2007).
59. Lesaffre E, Lawson LB. *Bayesian Biostatistics.* New York, NY: Wiley (2012). doi: 10.1002/9781119942412
60. Link WA, Barker RJ. *Bayesian Inference.* New York, NY: Elsevier (2010).
61. Junker BH, Koschutzki D, Schreiber F. Exploration of biological network centralities with CentiBiN. *BMC Bioinform.* (2006) 7:219. doi: 10.1186/1471-2105-7-219
62. Trygg T, Wold S. (2002) Orthogonal projections to latent structures (O-PLS). *J Chemomet.* (2002) 16:119–28. doi: 10.1002/cem.695
63. Westerhuis JA, Hoefslott HCJ, Smit S, Vis DJ, Smilde AK, van Velzen EJJ, et al. Assessment of PLSDA cross validation. *Metabolom.* (2008) 4:81–9. doi: 10.1007/s11306-007-0099-6
64. Chong J, Wishard DS, Xia J. Using metaboanalyst 4.0 for comprehensive and integrative metabolics data analysis. *Curr Protoc Bioinform.* (2019) 68:e86. doi: 10.1002/cpbi.86
65. He J, Aa J, Sun J, Smith PF, De Ridder D, Wang G, et al. Metabolic changes in the blood and brain following acoustic trauma, tinnitus and hyperacusis. *Prog Brain Res.* (2021) (in press). doi: 10.1016/bs.pbr.2020.09.002
66. Motulsky H. *Intuitive Biostatistics.* Oxford: Oxford University Press (1995).
67. Smith PF. A guerrilla guide to common problems in 'neurostatistics': essential statistical topics in neuroscience. *J Undergrad Neurosci Educ.* (2017) 16:R1–12.
68. Quinn GP, Keough MJ. *Experimental Design and Data Analysis for Biologists.* Cambridge: Cambridge University Press (2002). doi: 10.1017/CBO9780511806384
69. De Waale T, Pannekoek J, Scholtus S. Multivariate imputation. In: *Handbook of Statistical Data Editing and Imputation.* New York, NY: Wiley (2011). doi: 10.1002/9780470904848
70. Cueto-Lopez N, Garcia-Ordas MT, Davila-Batista V, Moreno V, Aragones N, Alaiz-Rodríguez R, et al. A comparative study of feature selection for a risk prediction model for colorectal cancer. *Comput Methods Programs Biomed.* (2019) 177:219–29. doi: 10.1016/j.cmpb.2019.06.001
71. Smith PF, Truchet B, Challain F, Zheng Y, Besnard S. Vestibular modulation of long-term potentiation and NMDA receptor expression in the hippocampus. *Front Mol Neurosci.* (2020) 13:140. doi: 10.3389/fnmol.2020.00140
72. Aitken P, Zheng Y, Smith P.F. Ethovision^{TM} analysis of open field behaviour in rats following bilateral vestibular loss. *J Vestib Res.* (2017) 27:89–101. doi: 10.3233/VES-170612
73. Smith PF. *A Multivariate Analysis of Vestibular Loss.* (MApplStat. Thesis), Massey University, Palmerston North, New Zealand (2014).
74. Caspi A, Moffitt TE, Cannon M, McClay J, Murray R, Harrington H, et al. Moderation of the effect of adolescent-onset cannabis use on adult psychosis by a functional polymorphism in the catechol-O-methyltransferase gene: longitudinal evidence of a gene X environment interaction. *Biol Psychiat.* (2005) 57:1117–27. doi: 10.1016/j.biopsych.2005.01.026
75. Chen H, Cao G, Cohen RA. Multivariate semiparametric spatial methods for imaging data. *Biostatistics.* (2017) 18:386–401. doi: 10.1093/biostatistics/kxw052
76. Staude B, Rotter S, Grün S. CuBIC: cumulant based inference of higher-order correlations in massively parallel spike trains. *J Comput Neurosci.* (2010) 29:327–50. doi: 10.1007/s10827-009-0195-x
77. Hitier M, Zhang Y, Sato G, Besnard S, Zheng Y, Smith PF. Effects of selective electrical stimulation of the rat cochlea on hippocampal field potentials. *Hear Res.* (2020) 395:108023. doi: 10.1016/j.heares.2020.108023
78. Sun L, Diao X, Gang X, Lv Y, Zhao X, Yang S, et al. Risk factors for cognitive impairment in patients with Type 2 Diabetes. *J Diabetes Res.* (2020) 2020:4591938. doi: 10.1155/2020/4591938
79. Hong X, Zhang B, Liang L, Zhang Y, Ji Y, Wang G, et al. Postpartum plasma metabolomic profile among women with preeclampsia and preterm delivery: implications for long-term health. *BMC Med.* (2020) 18:277. doi: 10.1186/s12916-020-01741-4
80. Wang J, Zheng J, Ren X, Wang S, Wang G, Hu, et al. Integrative analysis of hepatic metabolomic and transcriptomic data reveals potential mechanism of non-alcoholic steatohepatitis in high-fat diet-fed mice. *J Diabetes.* (2020) (in press). doi: 10.1111/1753-0407.13120
81. Gomaa NA, Jimoh Z, Campbell S, Zenke JJ, Szczepek AJ. Biomarkers for inner ear disorders: scoping review on the role of biomarkers in hearing and balance disorders. *Diagnostics.* (2020) 11:E42. doi: 10.3390/diagnostics11010042

19

Exergaming with Integrated Head Turn Tasks Improves Compensatory Saccade Pattern in Some Patients with Chronic Peripheral Unilateral Vestibular Hypofunction

Jaap Swanenburg[1,2], *Fabienne Büchi*[1], *Dominik Straumann*[3], *Konrad P. Weber*[3,4] *and Eling D. de Bruin*[5,6*]

[1] Physiotherapy and Occupational Therapy Research Center, Directorate of Research and Education, University Hospital Zurich, University of Zurich, Zurich, Switzerland, [2] Department of Chiropractic Medicine, Integrative Spinal Research ISR, Balgrist University Hospital, Zurich, Switzerland, [3] Department of Neurology, University Hospital Zurich, University of Zurich, Zurich, Switzerland, [4] Department of Ophthalmology, University Hospital Zurich, University of Zurich, Zurich, Switzerland, [5] Department Health Sciences and Technology, Institute of Human Movement Sciences and Sport, ETH Zurich, Zurich, Switzerland, [6] Division of Physiotherapy, Department of Neurobiology, Care Sciences and Society, Karolinska Institute, Stockholm, Sweden

***Correspondence:**
Eling D. de Bruin
eling.debruin@hest.ethz.ch

Background: This study aimed to determine whether vestibular rehabilitation using active video games (Exergames), including promoted head turns and unsupported locomotion, may facilitate vestibular compensation and gait in subjects with one-sided chronic peripheral vestibular hypofunction (cPVH).

Methods: 12 patients with cPVH (mean age of 65 ± 12 years, 8 male) were recruited for this study. The study consisted of a four-week baseline control period T1-T2 followed by a four-week intervention period T2-T3. The intervention included exergames that required physical tasks such as steps, weight shifts or balance control to cognitive challenges, in a virtual environment to play the game. The subjects participated in a total of 176 min of exergaming in eight sessions. Because of the changing projection direction of the game to the wall, the subjects had to turn their heads constantly while playing the game. Dynamic visual acuity (DVA) was assessed. Vestibulo-Ocular reflex (VOR) gain deficit and cumulative overt saccade amplitude (COSA) were measured with the video head-impulse test. Additionally, the functional gait assessment (FGA), Extended Timed Get-Up-and-Go (ETGUG), and the Dizziness handicap inventory (DHI), were assessed.

Results: DVA showed no significant group level change ($p = 0.475$, $z = -0.714$, $d = 0.295$) with a small effect size and improvements in five out of 12 subjects. Ipsilesional VOR gain did not improve ($p = 0.157$, $z = -1.414$, $d = 0.481$) on group level while there was an intermediate effect size and improvements in six out of 12 subjects. COSA got significant smaller ($p = 0.006$, $z = -2.746$, $d = 1.354$) with improvements in seven out of 12 subjects. The contralesional sides did not change. The FGA for the group significantly improved with an intermediate effect size ($p < 0.001$, $z = -3.08$, $d = 1.617$) and five individuals showed clinically relevant improvements. The ETGUG group value improved significantly with a strong effect size ($p < 0.001$, $z = -2.67$, $d = 1.030$), with seven individuals contributing to this change. The DHI showed no change ($p = 0.172$, z $= -1.381$, d $= 0.592$) neither on the group nor on the individuals' level. The game scores of the subjects improved during the intervention period of the intervention for every game.

Conclusion: The results of this study demonstrate that exergaming with promoted head turns facilitates vestibular compensation in some subjects with cPVH. This is the first study that shows an improvement in cumulative overt saccade amplitude after exergaming in chronic vestibular subjects.

Keywords: vestibular loss, exergaming, head turns, dynamic visual acuity, saccades

INTRODUCTION

Vestibular disorders are either assessed through cardinal symptoms of vestibular dysfunction, through balance testing or through diagnosing of specific vestibular disorders (1). Subjects with vestibular disorders often experience symptoms like vertigo, dizziness, visual disturbance, and imbalance (2, 3). The lifetime prevalence of vertigo alone in adults aged 18–79 years was 7.4% (4). Furthermore, subjects experience anxiety and distress of depression. Many patients suffer from cognitive impairments, problems with spatial memory and attention (5–7) and sustain repeated falls (8). Having vestibular disorders, hence, relates to reduced quality of life and it negatively affects many aspects of daily living (3).

Non-pharmacological vestibular rehabilitation is thus far the only effective method for improving symptoms related to many chronical vestibular disorders (3) and two recent systematic reviews partly confirm some of this beneficial effects of exercise-based rehabilitation (9, 10). However, both reviews point out the necessity of further non-pharmacological studies into determining the optimal protocol and effect for newly developed therapies, as also reflected in clinical guidelines (11). Therefore, the further development of non-pharmacological approaches for the treatment of vestibular disorders is warranted.

Perceptual and cognitive decline in individuals with vestibular disorders can be counteracted through sustained practice of a martial art or through exposing individuals to a virtual reality environment. Both approaches relate to improved symptoms of vestibular disorders (1, 12, 13). To reduce their sensation of dizziness, patients often move their head as little as possible while moving around (14); e.g., while walking, a strategy associated with negative effects on postural balance and walking behavior on stairs (15, 16) and on community ambulation (17). Therefore, improving gait is an important goal of vestibular rehabilitation (1, 18) and this goal may be achieved by specifically including head movements into the exercise programs (19). Gaze stabilization rehabilitation may lead to some improvements in visual acuity and vestibulo-ocular reflex in these patients (20, 21), especially when applied in early disease stages (22). Next to gaze stabilization, balance training, and walking exercise for endurance, habituation exercise is one of four main exercise categories that can be used for rehabilitation (11). Habituation exercises are used to treat symptoms of dizziness produced by self-motion or that are produced by visual stimuli and are referred to as "the reduction in a behavioral response to repeated exposure to a provocative stimulus, with the goal of reducing symptoms related to the vestibular system (11)."

Neurophysiologically, individuals should in their therapy program be provided with a series of performance tasks that require using the eyes while at the same time moving the head and body (23). A proof-of-concept study from our group showed improved functional gait following training in a virtual environment that integrated visual observation and head turning movements while physically playing the Exergames. This theory-based intervention facilitated gaze stability during head movements in older adults as measured by the computerized dynamic visual acuity (DVA) test (24). The results of this study led to the hypothesis that also chronic subjects with vestibular disorders would be able to train and improve their vestibular functioning.

Video-games that require whole-body physical activity to play the game combine motor and cognitive exercises and are labeled Exergames (25). Exergames provide a motivational and entertaining way to be physically active for patients (12, 26), and recent studies demonstrated a positive effect of virtual reality-based interventions on patients with vestibular hypofunction (27–29). This form of training theoretically allows addressing all four important exercise components for vestibular subjects (11) into one exercise program: gaze stability exercises and habituation exercises (24), balance and gait exercises (30, 31), and endurance (32).

The purpose of this pilot study is to further develop the theory-based exergame intervention and describe its effects on vestibular compensation in multiple subjects with one-sided chronic peripheral vestibular hypofunction (cPVH). We hypothesized that, similar to older adults, individual patient symptoms could be influenced based on the current available evidence (11) for, and the ecological validity of, the training content.

METHODS

Participants

For this pilot study, 12 outpatients with one-sided cPVH were recruited in the Departments of Neurology and Otorhinolaryngology at the University Hospital Zurich (USZ). A senior neurologist identified patients with one-sided cPVH at baseline. A horizontal video head-impulse test (video HIT) to both sides was used to identify cPVH at T1. A video HIT gain (eye velocity divided by head velocity at peak head acceleration) below 0.7 was considered pathological. Exclusion criteria were; (1) walking disability (independent walking <10 meters), (2) acute pain, (3) medication reducing postural balance (4) weakness resulting from neurological problems, (5), uncontrolled cardiovascular disease (e.g.,: uncontrolled blood pressure) (6) gait disorders putatively attributed to other than primarily vestibular causes, (7) uncorrected severe visual impairment. Additionally, patients with Menière's disease or with benign paroxysmal positional vertigo were excluded. All measurements and exergame sessions took place at the University Hospital Zurich. The measurement assistants were blinded. All subjects provided written informed consent before partaking in the therapy sessions and the study was approved by the ethics committee of the Canton of Zurich under BASEC 2018-00337. Trial registration was done at ClinicalTrials.gov Identifier; NCT03536533.

Design

Subjects were included and primarily assessed using an A-B study design (33). Vestibular function was tested on three separate test sessions T1, T2, and T3 at intervals of one month. The first month served as control period (A) between T1 and T2 whereas, the second month functioned as intervention period (B) between T2 and T3. DVA and VOR gain were used to test for chronicity (T1-T2-T3) of the clinical presentation of symptoms and functional impairment in enrolled subjects with cPVH.

Intervention

Purpose-developed games were used in the study that are targeting to improve cognitive functions such as divided attention, working memory, inhibition, and attention shifting. Physical functions, such as balance and gait, are trained because the games are played through whole body movements in standing position and, preferably, without support from a handrail. By changing the orientation of the projection during the game-play (see Video Exergame) participants need to turn their head to successfully play the games. Additionally, in every session one game had to be played while the participant stood rotated 90° to the left or right and with head turned toward the projection. The detailed exercise protocol is described in detail elsewhere (24). During the intervention, the subjects received one-on-one supervision from the research assistant. In total, eight exergaming sessions were accomplished for each patient over the 4-week intervention period T2–T3. The training principles of progression and overload were applied (31). Each session lasted for 40 min, with an actual exercise duration of 22 min. The total cumulative intervention exercise time of 176 min slightly exceeded the recommended time (150 min) for an efficient virtual reality intervention (12, 24). The certified medical device exercise system Senso (dividat, Schindellegi, Switzerland), a pressure-sensitive plate, was used for the training (24). The Senso pad provided the participants with real-time visual and auditory feedback. The visual angle of the projected game was ±81° in width and ±54°in height. To promote head movements during the exercises the projector was either rotated ±45 degrees horizontally or ±15 degrees vertically. A remote-controlled power panner (Maxwell MPR–202) was used to move the projector with 6° per second horizontally and 2° per second vertically. Misery Score (MISC) was used to determine whether the training could be continued in a given level. The MISC is a simple scale to gather nausea symptoms. It is categorized in 1 = no nausea, 2 = initial symptoms, but no nausea, 3 = mild nausea, 4 = moderate nausea, 5 = severe nausea, and 6 = vomiting. In the present study, MISC 1-3 was accepted during training. A MISC score 4 and more would have led to a training stop (27) or to lowering the exercise level of difficulty. The exercise set-up is shown in a **Video 1** (see Video Exergame).

Games

Four different games were used during the intervention session. As a warm-up, the game "Simple" was used. This game trains focused attention. Thereafter the game "targets" was played. This game trains goal-oriented reacting. Cognitive flexibility was trained with the third game "flexi." The final game was the game "snake," which focuses on visual processing. The difficulty of all games was progressively adapted by speeding up the game according to the performance of the player, or in the fourth game "snake" the length of the snake increased progressively (24) screen images of all games in the **Supplementary File 1**.

Measurements

DVA

DVA measures visual acuity during head movement relative to baseline static visual acuity (SVA) (34, 35). Passive head impulses were performed using a DVA testing system that consisted of a personal computer with a 19-inch monitor (1280 × 1024 pixels, 75 Hz) and a Sparkfun velocity sensor (Sparkfun Electronics, Boulder, Colorado), which was fixed on a headset to the participant's head (36, 37). The test gives information on the vestibulo-ocular reflex (VOR) performance, mainly of the semicircular canal function (36) and has change in visual acuity, when moving the head compared to static acuity, as output (38). For horizontal testing, the head rotation was assessed in both left and right directions, for each patient. (39). One of two experienced examiners conducted testing.

VOR Gain

The video head-impulse-test measurements (vHIT) were used to assess the VOR gain (40, 41). This test gives information about the function of the six semicircular canals individually by measuring the eye rotation response to an abrupt head rotation in the plane of the canal (41). The measurement protocol is described in detail in previous studies (41, 42). An ICS Impulse, Natus Medical Inc., Taastrup, Denmark was used to measure the horizontal canals. One of two experienced examiners conducted testing.

Cumulative Overt Saccades Amplitudes (COSA)

The characteristic saccade pattern responses are highly effective in distinguishing patients with unilateral vestibular loss compared to controls (43). OtosuiteV 2.0 (GN Otometrics) was used to re-analyse VOR gains. To qualify corrective saccades we used a custom-written MATLAB (The MathWorks,

Natick, MA, USA) routine. This provided cumulative overt saccade amplitudes (44–46). Saccades that occurred after the head-impulse are defined as "overt" (46).

Functional Gait Assessment (FGA)

FGA is used to measure disturbances in balance and gait (47) and includes the following 10 items (48): (1) Gait on level surface, (2) Change in gait speed, (3) Gait with horizontal head turns, (4) Gait with vertical head turns, (5) Gait and pivot turn, (6) Step over obstacle, (7) Gait with narrow base of support, (8) Gait with eyes closed, (9) Ambulating backwards, (10) Steps. Each item was scored on a 4-point ordinal scale with scores of 0, 1, 2, and 3 (Maximum total score = 30). Higher scores represented better balance and gait capacity (47). The minimal detectable change is 6 points for the FGA (49) and was used to assess change on individual level.

Extended Timed Get-Up-And-Go (ETGUG)

The ETGUG test (50) measures times in seconds to complete a series of functionally important tasks and the overall time needed (seconds) to complete the test with a multimemory stopwatch. ETGUG test included the following tasks: (1) Rising from a chair, (2) Initiating gait, (3) Walking 6 meters straight, (4) Turning around, (5) Walking back, (6) Sitting down again. The time measured during each task and the overall time depicted the functional mobility of the participant (51). With an ICC of 0.97 for the test-retest reliability the test exhibits excellent reliability in vestibular patients (52). For the minimal detectable change we used the 4 seconds difference between patients with both-sided vestibular loss and healthy controls reported in literature (52).

Dizziness Handicap Inventory (DHI)

The DHI German version is a validated, 25-item-self-report questionnaire to evaluate the self-perceived handicapping effects caused by dizziness (53). The DHI is categorized in three domains; functional (9 questions, 36 points), emotional (9 questions, 36 points), and physical (7 questions, 28 points). Subjects answer the questions with no (0 points), sometimes (2 points), and yes (4 points) (54). The higher the score, the greater the handicap caused by dizziness. The cut-off value of clinical relevance is 9 points (53).

Simulator Sickness Questionnaire (SSQ)

The SSQ questionnaire was used to assess virtual reality users' level of sickness symptoms (55). It contains 16 items which had to be weighed by the participants in terms of severity on a 4-level scale with the options including "none," "slight," "moderate," and "severe."(56). (Minimum score = 0, Maximum total score = 48). After each exercise session and a few hours later the same day, the subjects completed the SSQ.

Game Scores

Game scores and therapy attendance of the exercise sessions were recorded to monitor progression and adherence to the training plan.

Statistical Analysis

Descriptive statistics were used to describe the community dweller's characteristics. Normality of data distribution was tested using the Shapiro-Wilk test. In case of non-normal distribution, the Wilcoxon test was chosen to test the differences between measurement time points. Additionally, for the effect size, Cohen's d (d) values were calculated. Cohen (1988) reports the following intervals for d: 0.1 to 0.3: small effect; 0.3 to 0.5: intermediate effect; 0.5 and higher: strong effect. For sub analysis of FGA and ETGUG tasks a Bonferroni correction was used. Game scores and SSQ were described with descriptive statistics. Additionally a scatterplot with VOR gain and COSA before and after intervention with associated linear regression line was plotted.

IBM SPSS Statistics 25 for Windows (Inc; Chicago, Illinois) was used for all the statistical analyses.

RESULTS

The scores of 12 (mean age of 64.9 ± 11.7 years, 8 male) subjects with one-sided cPVH were analyzed. The mean weight of the subjects was 69.6 ± 10.3 kg and the mean height 168.0 ± 7.7 cm. Two DVA measurements at T1 could not be executed due to technical failure of the measurement device (PT 7 and PT 12). Four subjects received physiotherapy whereof one patient received cervical physiotherapy before the intervention program (PT 3) and the other three subjects were treated for lower extremity issues. Assessed by the MISC no exercise session had to be stopped. There were no adverse events.

Control Period T1–T2

During the control period T1–T2 the DVA lesion side (p = 0.646, z = −0.459, d = 0.188) and the contralateral side (p = 0.944, z = −0.070, d = 0.029) were stable and showed no significant change. A similar result was found with the vHit gain, assessed with the head impulse paradigm, of the affected (p = 0.694, z = −0.393, d = 0.161) and the contralateral side (p = 0.695, z = −0.393, d = 0.161) both showing no significant change.

Intervention Period T2–T3

Vestibular Compensation

DVA showed no significant change (p = 0.475, z = −0.714, d = 0.295) with a small effect size and improvements in five out of 12 subjects. In addition, VOR gain at the ipsilesional side did not improve (p = 0.157, z = −1.414, d = 0.481) on group level and there was an intermediate effect size and improvements in six out of 12 subjects. COSA got significant smaller (p = 0.006, z = −2.746, d = 1.354) with improvements in seven out of 12 subjects. The contralesional sides did not change. A graphical plot example of an impulse test can be seen in **Figure 1**. All data of vestibular compensation can be found in **Table 1**. Results and changes of each individual participant can be found in **Table 2** and **Figures 2–4**.

Scatterplots between DVA and COSA before and after intervention with associated linear regression lines are shown in

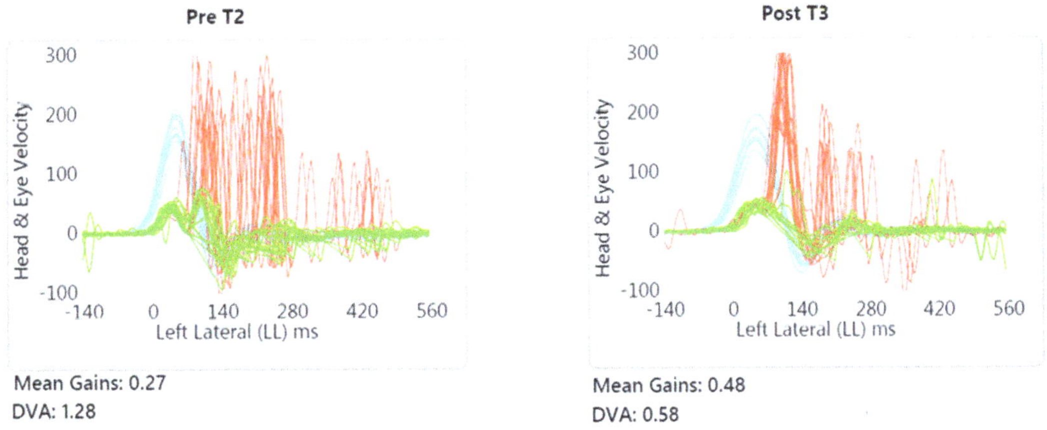

FIGURE 1 | Typical example (patient no. 9) of improved VOR gain and reduced compensatory saccade variability. Blue, head velocity; Green, eye velocity; Red, compensatory saccades.

TABLE 1 | Results of the Vestibular compensation pre and post intervention (T2–T3).

	DVA (logMAR)				VOR Gain				COSA			
	Lesion side		Contralateral side		Lesion side		Contralateral side		Lesion side		Contralateral side	
	T2	T3	T2	T3	T2	T3	T2	T3	T2	T3	T2	T3
Mean	0.630	0.633	0.470	0.439	0.518	0.667	0.911	0.933	3.502	2.543	0.546	0.623
SD	0.367	0.2.80	0.147	0.140	0.213	0.162	0.148	0.078	1.301	1.040	0.666	0.380
Z	−0.714		−0.512		−1.414		−1.070		−2.746		−0.941	
p	0.475		0.609		0.157		0.347		0.006*		0.941	

*SD, standard deviation; Range, min/max; Z, p, Wilcoxon Signed Rank Test; *p < 0.05 significant.*

Figure 5. A scatterplot with VOR gain and COSA before and after intervention with associated linear regression line is shown in **Figure 6**.

Gait Function

The FGA showed significant group-level improvement with a large concomitant Effect Size ($p < 0.001$, $z = -3.08$, $d = 1.617$). The total points improved from 19.58 at T2 to 26.17 points at T3. Five subjects who improved more than the minimal detectable change of six points drove this change. For the sub-tasks gait with horizontal head turns ($p < 0.001$), gait with eyes closed ($p < 0.001$), and ambulating backward ($p < 0.001$) significantly improved. All results of all FGA tasks can be found in **Supplementary Table 1**.

The ETGUG improved significantly on the group level with a strong effect size ($p < 0.001$, $z = -2.67$, $d = 1.030$). The total time decreased from 19.95 s at T2 to 15.61 s at T3. Seven subjects improved more than 4 seconds. The ETGUG sixth task "slow down, stop, turnaround, and sit down" significantly ($p < 0.001$) improved for the group of twelve individuals. All results of all individual ETGUG component tasks can be found in the **Supplementary Table 2**.

Dizziness

There was a non-significant decrease in DHI after the intervention session albeit there was a strong effect size ($p = 0.172$, $z = -1.381$, $d = 0.592$). The total points were 32.83 at T2 and 29.48 points at T3. Four subjects improved more than nine points. All DHI results can be found in **Supplementary Table 3**.

Simulator Sickness

The SSQ showed a decrease immediately following each intervention session. The total points improved from 7.4 at the first session to 4.2 points at the last session. They mainly recorded "fullness of the head" and "sweating during the exercise." Some noted general discomfort or moderate dizziness. During the evening hours of the same day, none of the participants experienced any symptom(s). The mean results of all SSQ measurements after each intervention session are presented in **Supplementary Table 4**.

Game Scores

The subjects' game high scores showed in the beginning continuous improvement in game performance. About half of the course of the intervention period there was a leveling off

TABLE 2 | Individual descriptive data.

Nr	Age range	Diagnosis	Lesion side	Medication	Additional non-vestibular therapy*	DVA	VOR gain	COSA	FGA	ETGUG	DHI
						Change ± 0.05	Change ± 0.05	Change ± 0.1°	Change ± 6 points	Change ± 4 s	Change ± 9 points
1	55-60	cPVH	Right	None	None	+	~	+	~	+	~
2	60-65	cPVH	Left	Aspirin Cardio	None	+	–	~	~	~	~
3	50-55	cPVH	Right	None	Physiotherapy cervical	~	+	–	~	+	+
4	45-50	cPVH	Right	Insulin	None	+	+	~	+	+	~
5	55-60	cPVH	Left	Cholesterol-lowering	Physiotherapy lower extremity	–	~	+	~	+	~
6	60-65	cPVH	Right	Aspirin Cardio, Antihypertensive	None	~	+	+	~	~	~
7	80-85	cPVH	Right	Aspirin Cardio Antihypertensive, Cholesterol-lowering, rare: temesta	Physiotherapy lower extremity	+	+	+	+	~	~
8	65-70	cPVH	Left	Aspirin Cardio, Cholesterol-lowering	None	~	~	–	~	~	+
9	80-85	chronic dizziness under stress	Left	Antihypertensive drug, Aspirin Cardio	None	+	+	+	+	+	~
10	75-80	cPVH	Left	Antihypertensive drug	Physiotherapy lower extremity	–	~	–	+	+	~
11	60-65	cPVH	Left	Aspirin Cardio	None	~	–	+	+	+	+
12	55-60	chronic neuritis vestibularis	Left	None	None	–	+	+	~	~	+

+, improvement, –, deterioration, ~, no change by minimal detectable values or by clinical judgment in case of VOR gain.
**Additional non-vestibular complaints related therapy received during this study.*

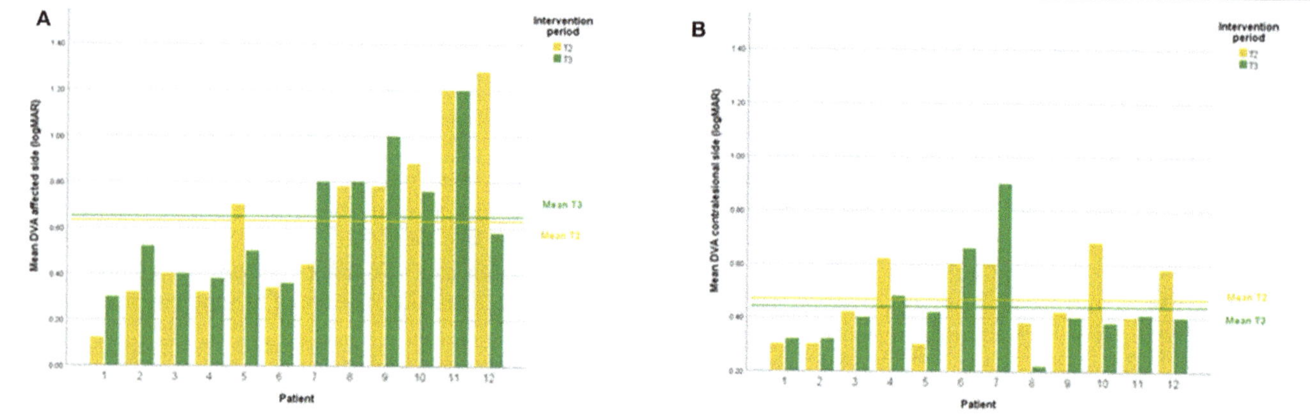

FIGURE 2 | (A) Individual DVA results lesion side at T2 and T3. **(B)** Individual DVA results contralesional side at T2 and T3.

in performance increments. The game scores can be found **Supplementary Figures 1A–H.**

DISCUSSION

Vestibular Compensation

The goal of this study was to evaluate the effects of a purpose-designed Exergaming rehabilitation program, including challenging conditions such as combined visual observation, head turns and unsupported stepping movements, on the vestibular compensation in subjects with cPVH. Based on the combined group and individual patient level assessment using an A-B research design there was clinically relevant improvement in some of the chronic subjects following the Exergame intervention phase. This might indicate that processes underlying central vestibular compensation were activated following the exergaming therapy in subjects with cPVH as opposed to non-observable change in the control phase. We found significantly smaller cumulative overt saccades amplitudes in more than half of the subjects. However, there was no change in VOR gain. A similar

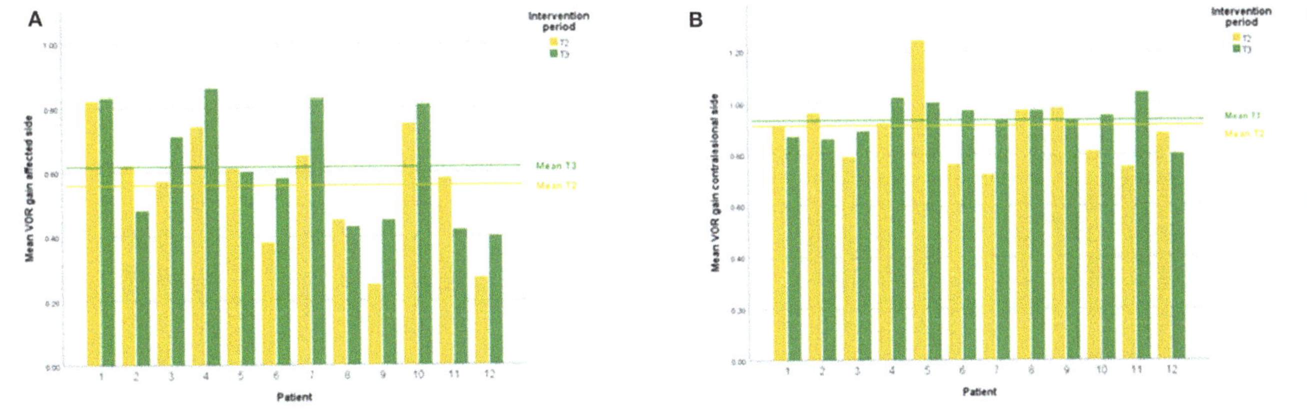

FIGURE 3 | (A) Individual VOR gain results lesion side at T2 and T3. **(B)** Individual VOR gain results contralesional side at T2 and T3.

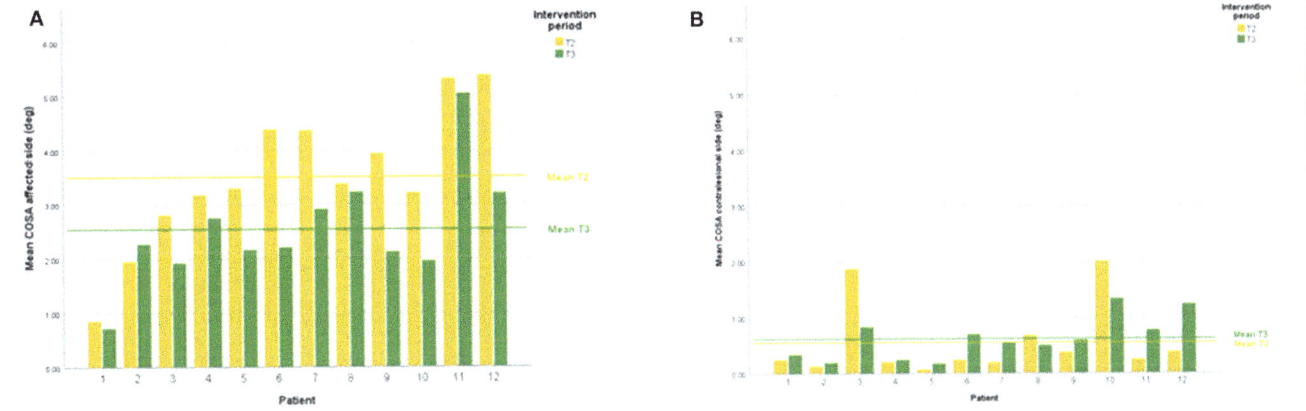

FIGURE 4 | (A) Individual COSA results lesion side at T2 and T3. **(B)** Individual COSA results contralesional side at T2 and T3.

result was recently reported by Millar et al. (57). In their study, a progressive vestibular rehabilitation program was conducted with subjects after unilateral vestibular deafferentation surgery. Their subjects clinically and statistically improved despite absent change in VOR gain (57). The interventions compared to this study were different. The vestibular physical therapy used in the study by Millar et al. was five times longer (total of 945 min over five weeks) than the exergaming performed in this study (total of 176 min over four weeks).

The COSA in this study positively correlated with DVA. Thus, smaller COSA mean better visual acuity.

After the intervention, the correlation between COSA and VOR gains was no longer significant, suggesting that the patients were able to compensate their VOR deficit with covert saccades during the head impulses, which are not accounted for in the COSA measure.

Gait Function

The subjects' gait function showed significant improvements. The FGA improved significantly and five subjects improved their FGA scores by at least nine points, which lies well above the minimal detectable change value for this measure (49). This makes the chance of a measurement error less likely as possible alternative explanation. When the training principle of specificity applies, the improved FGA task "gait with horizontal head turns" might be caused by the training content of provoked head turns while exergaming. The exergaming led to a safer locomotion. It is important to stress that the individuals partaking in our program were all chronic subjects from whom further treatment effects were expected being more difficult to achieve (22) based on their chronicity status. Seeing an improvement in half of the chronic patients in our sample is encouraging for the relevance of exergaming as a novel intervention and important on an individual subjects' daily living level. Finally, subjects' game scores showed continuous improvement in game performance meaning they could play the Exergames better and faster over the intervention course.

Study Limitations

The approach for the data analysis we used may be seen as a limitation of our study. The combination of group- and individual-level data analysis has intuitive appeal allowing

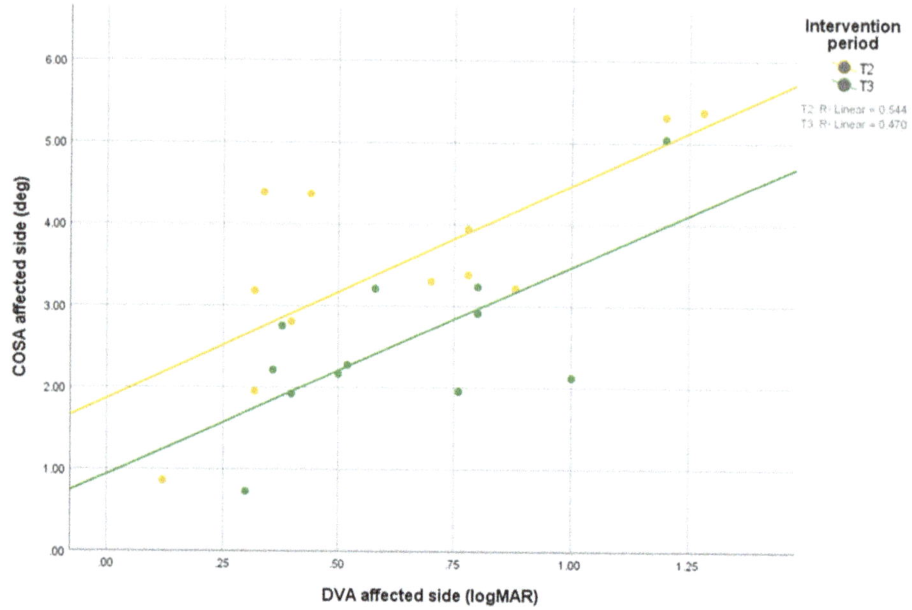

FIGURE 5 | Relationship between DVA and overt saccade amplitude before and after intervention with associated linear regression line.

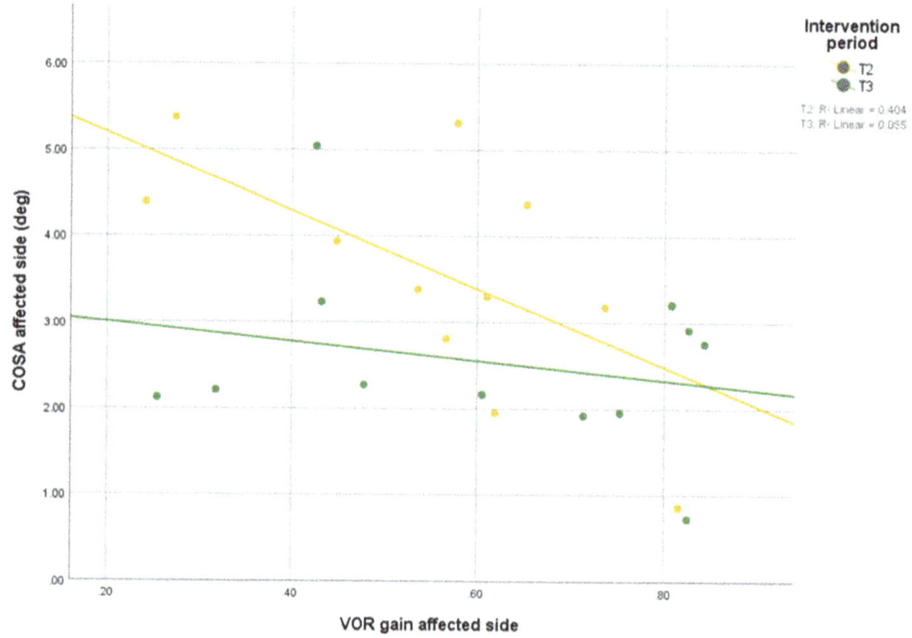

FIGURE 6 | Relationship between VOR gain and overt saccade amplitude before and after intervention with associated linear regression line.

individual-level associations through the mechanisms of bias control (AB design), the separation of contextual within and between-group effects, and the repeated checking of the treatment underlying model (58). However, such an approach theoretically necessitates knowledge about previous rehabilitation programs which each individual experienced as these may effect on the observable treatment effects of individuals (59). Gathering such detailed information for our participants was beyond the means of our study. A further limitation of the present study is the rather small sample size of 12 subjects that led to a weak statement regarding the population level, thus, limiting the generalizability of our treatment. However, in the current stage of intervention development we were mainly interested in individual patient responses to the intervention, since the expectation for these individuals to improve were rather low based on the chronicity of their symptoms and the years of previous therapy these individuals had undergone.

CONCLUSION

The results of the present study demonstrate that exergaming with promoted head turns facilitates vestibular compensation in some subjects with cPVH. This is the first study that shows an improvement in cumulative overt saccade amplitude after exergaming in several chronic vestibular subjects. The findings of this study warrant further research in which more complex research designs in larger samples should be employed.

ETHICS STATEMENT

The studies involving human participants were reviewed and approved by Ethics committee of the Canton of Zurich under BASEC 2018-00337. Trial registration was done at ClinicalTrials.gov Identifier; NCT03536533. The patients/participants provided their written informed consent to participate in this study.

AUTHOR CONTRIBUTIONS

JS developed the research question. The concept and design part were established by FB and JS. FB executed the intervention. FB, JS, and KW did the analysis of the results. KW, DS, and JS did the interpretation of the results. JS and FB produced an early version of the manuscript. EB, KW, and DS critically revised the manuscript to bring it to its current version. All authors have read and approved the final manuscript.

REFERENCES

1. Agrawal Y, Ward BK, Minor LB. Vestibular dysfunction: prevalence, impact and need for targeted treatment. *J Vestib Res.* (2013) 23:113–7. doi: 10.3233/VES-130498
2. Swanenburg J, Babler E, Adelsberger R, Straumann D, de Bruin ED. Patients with chronic peripheral vestibular hypofunction compared to healthy subjects exhibit differences in gaze and gait behaviour when walking on stairs and ramps. *PLoS ONE.* (2017) 12:e0189037. doi: 10.1371/journal.pone.0189037
3. McDonnell MN, Hillier SL. Vestibular rehabilitation for unilateral peripheral vestibular dysfunction. *Cochrane Database Syst Rev.* (2015) 1:CD005397. doi: 10.1002/14651858.CD005397.pub4
4. Neuhauser HK, von Brevern M, Radtke A, Lezius F, Feldmann M, Ziese T, et al. Epidemiology of vestibular vertigo: a neurotologic survey of the general population. *Neurology.* (2005) 65:898–904. doi: 10.1212/01.wnl.0000175987.59991.3d
5. Monzani D, Casolari L, Guidetti G, Rigatelli M. Psychological distress and disability in patients with vertigo. *J Psychosom Res.* (2001) 50:319–23. doi: 10.1016/S0022-3999(01)00208-2
6. Gufoni M, Guidetti G, Nuti D, Pagnini P, Vicini C, Tinelli C, et al. [The relationship between cognitive impairment, anxiety-depression symptoms and balance and spatial orientation complaints in the elderly]. *Acta Otorhinolaryngol Ital.* (2005) 25:12–21.
7. Smith PF, Zheng Y, Horii A, Darlington CL. Does vestibular damage cause cognitive dysfunction in humans? *J Vestib Res.* (2005) 15:1–9.
8. Agrawal Y, Carey JP, Della Santina CC, Schubert MC, Minor LB. Diabetes, vestibular dysfunction, and falls: analyses from the national health and nutrition examination survey. *Otol Neurotol.* (2010) 31:1445–50. doi: 10.1097/MAO.0b013e3181f2f035
9. Kendall JC, Hartvigsen J, Azari MF, French SD. Effects of nonpharmacological interventions for dizziness in older people: systematic review. *Phys Ther.* (2016) 96:641–9. doi: 10.2522/ptj.20150349
10. Kundakci B, Sultana A, Taylor AJ, Alshehri MA. The effectiveness of exercise-based vestibular rehabilitation in adult patients with chronic dizziness: a systematic review. *F1000Res.* (2018) 7:276. doi: 10.12688/f1000research.14089.1
11. Hall CD, Herdman SJ, Whitney SL, Cass SP, Clendaniel RA, Fife TD, et al. Vestibular rehabilitation for peripheral vestibular hypofunction: an evidence-Based clinical practice guideline: from the american physical therapy association neurology section. *J Neurol Phys Ther.* (2016) 40:124–55. doi: 10.1097/NPT.0000000000000120
12. Bergeron M, Lortie CL, Guitton MJ. Use of virtual reality tools for vestibular disorders rehabilitation: a Comprehensive analysis. *Adv Med.* (2015) 2015:916735. doi: 10.1155/2015/916735
13. Muinos M, Ballesteros S. Sports can protect dynamic visual acuity from aging: a study with young and older judo and karate martial arts athletes. *Atten Percept Psycho.* (2015) 77:2061–73. doi: 10.3758/s13414-015-0901-x
14. Whitney SL, Alghwiri AA, Alghadir A. An overview of vestibular rehabilitation. *Handb Clin Neurol.* (2016) 137:187–205. doi: 10.1016/B978-0-444-63437-5.00013-3
15. Cromwell R, Wellmon R. Sagittal plane head stabilization during level walking and ambulation on stairs. *Physiother Res Int.* (2001) 6:179–92. doi: 10.1002/pri.226
16. Swanenburg J, Zurbrugg A, Straumann D, Hegemann SCA, Palla A, de Bruin ED. A pilot study investigating the association between chronic bilateral vestibulopathy and components of a clinical functional assessment tool. *Physiother Theory Pract.* (2017) 33:454–61. doi: 10.1080/09593985.2017.1323362
17. Paul SS, Dibble LE, Walther RG, Shelton C, Gurgel RK, Lester ME. Reduced purposeful head movements during community ambulation following unilateral vestibular loss. *Neurorehabil Neural Repair.* (2018) 32:309–16. doi: 10.1177/1545968318770271
18. Han BI, Song HS, Kim JS. Vestibular rehabilitation therapy: review of indications, mechanisms, key exercises. *J Clin Neurol.* (2011) 7:184–96. doi: 10.3988/jcn.2011.7.4.184
19. Sulway S, Whitney SL. Advances in vestibular rehabilitation. *Adv Otorhinolaryngol.* (2019) 82:164–9. doi: 10.1159/000490285
20. Scherer M, Migliaccio AA, Schubert MC. Effect of vestibular rehabilitation on passive dynamic visual acuity. *J Vestib Res.* (2008) 18:147–57.
21. Schubert MC, Migliaccio AA, Clendaniel RA, Allak A, Carey JP. Mechanism of dynamic visual acuity recovery with vestibular rehabilitation.

Arch Phys Med Rehabil. (2008) 89:500–7. doi: 10.1016/j.apmr.2007.11.010
22. Michel L, Laurent T, Alain T. Rehabilitation of dynamic visual acuity in patients with unilateral vestibular hypofunction: earlier is better. *Eur Arch Otorhinolaryngol.* (2020) 277:103–13. doi: 10.1007/s00405-019-05690-4
23. Hain TC. Neurophysiology of vestibular rehabilitation. *NeuroRehabilitation.* (2011) 29:127–41. doi: 10.3233/NRE-2011-0687
24. Swanenburg J, Wild K, Straumann D, de Bruin ED. Exergaming in a moving virtual world to train vestibular functions and gait; a proof-of-Concept-Study with older adults. *Front Physiol.* (2018) 9:988. doi: 10.3389/fphys.2018.00988
25. McCaskey MA, Schattin A, Martin-Niedecken AL, de Bruin ED. Making more of iT: enabling intensive motor cognitive rehabilitation exercises in geriatrics using information technology solutions. *Biomed Res Int.* (2018) 2018:4856146. doi: 10.1155/2018/4856146
26. Meldrum D, Herdman S, Vance R, Murray D, Malone K, Duffy D, et al. Effectiveness of conventional versus virtual reality-based balance exercises in vestibular rehabilitation for unilateral peripheral vestibular loss: results of a randomized controlled trial. *Arch Phys Med Rehabil.* (2015) 96:1319–28 e1. doi: 10.1016/j.apmr.2015.02.032
27. Hondebrink MS, Mert A, van der Lint R, de Ru JA, van der Wurff P. Motion-based equilibrium reprocessing therapy a novel treatment method for chronic peripheral vestibulopathies: a pilot study. *Medicine (Baltimore).* (2017) 96:e7128. doi: 10.1097/MD.0000000000007128
28. Hsu SY, Fang TY, Yeh SC, Su MC, Wang PC, Wang VY. Three-dimensional, virtual reality vestibular rehabilitation for chronic imbalance problem caused by meniere's disease: a pilot study<sup/>. *Disabil Rehabil.* (2017) 39:1601–6. doi: 10.1080/09638288.2016.1203027
29. Viziano A, Micarelli A, Augimeri I, Micarelli D, Alessandrini M. Long-term effects of vestibular rehabilitation and head-mounted gaming task procedure in unilateral vestibular hypofunction: a 12-month follow-up of a randomized controlled trial. *Clin Rehabil.* (2019) 33:24–33. doi: 10.1177/0269215518788598
30. Eggenberger P, Wolf M, Schumann M, de Bruin ED. Exergame and balance training modulate prefrontal brain activity during walking and enhance executive function in older adults. *Front Aging Neurosci.* (2016) 8:66. doi: 10.3389/fnagi.2016.00066
31. Schattin A, Arner R, Gennaro F, de Bruin ED. Adaptations of prefrontal brain activity, executive functions, and gait in healthy elderly following exergame and balance training: a Randomized-Controlled study. *Front Aging Neurosci.* (2016) 8:278. doi: 10.3389/fnagi.2016.00278
32. Rebsamen S, Knols RH, Pfister PB, de Bruin ED. Exergame-Driven high-Intensity interval training in untrained community dwelling older adults: a Formative one group quasi- experimental feasibility trial. *Front Physiol.* (2019) 10:1019. doi: 10.3389/fphys.2019.01019
33. Tate RL, Perdices M, Rosenkoetter U, Shadish W, Vohra S, Barlow DH, et al. The single-Case reporting guideline in bEhavioural interventions (SCRIBE) 2016 statement. *Phys Ther.* (2016) 96:e1–e10. doi: 10.2522/ptj.2016.96.7.e1
34. Schubert MC, Migliaccio AA, Della Santina CC. Dynamic visual acuity during passive head thrusts in canal planes. *J Assoc Res Otolaryngol.* (2006) 7:329–38. doi: 10.1007/s10162-006-0047-6
35. Herdman SJ, Tusa RJ, Blatt P, Suzuki A, Venuto PJ, Roberts D. Computerized dynamic visual acuity test in the assessment of vestibular deficits. *Am J Otol.* (1998) 19:790–6.
36. Vital D, Hegemann SC, Straumann D, Bergamin O, Bockisch CJ, Angehrn D, et al. A new dynamic visual acuity test to assess peripheral vestibular function. *Arch Otolaryngol Head Neck Surg.* (2010) 136:686–91. doi: 10.1001/archoto.2010.99
37. Wettstein VG, Weber KP, Bockisch CJ, Hegemann SC. Compensatory saccades in head impulse testing influence the dynamic visual acuity of patients with unilateral peripheral vestibulopathy1. *J Vestib Res.* (2016) 26:395–402. doi: 10.3233/VES-160591
38. Mohammad MT, Whitney SL, Marchetti GF, Sparto PJ, Ward BK, Furman JM. The reliability and response stability of dynamic testing of the vestibulo-ocular reflex in patients with vestibular disease. *J Vestib Res.* (2011) 21:277–88. doi: 10.3233/VES-2011-0430
39. Petersen JA, Straumann D, Weber KP. Clinical diagnosis of bilateral vestibular loss: three simple bedside tests. *Ther Adv Neurol Disord.* (2013) 6:41–5. doi: 10.1177/1756285612465920
40. Eza-Nunez P, Farinas-Alvarez C, Fernandez NP. Comparison of three diagnostic tests in detecting vestibular deficit in patients with peripheral vestibulopathy. *J Laryngol Otol.* (2016) 130:145–50. doi: 10.1017/S0022215115003114
41. Weber KP, MacDougall HG, Halmagyi GM, Curthoys IS. Impulsive testing of semicircular-canal function using video-oculography. *Ann Ny Acad Sci.* (2009) 1164:486–91. doi: 10.1111/j.1749-6632.2008.03730.x
42. Curthoys IS, MacDougall HG, Manzari L, Burgess AM, Bradshaw AP, McGarvie L, et al. Clinical application of a new objective test of semicircular canal dynamic function-the video head impulse test (vHIT). A safe, simple, and fast clinical vestibular test. In: *Vertigo-Kontroverses und Bewährtes 8. Hennig Symposium*, New York, NY: SpringerWien (2011). p. 53–64. doi: 10.1007/978-3-7091-0736-2_6
43. MacDougall ML, Halmagyi GM. Anti-compensatory saccades as an indicator of peripheral vestibular function in a new complementary video head impulse test paradigm. *Eur J Neurol.* (2015) 22.
44. Weber KP, Aw ST, Todd MJ, McGarvie LA, Curthoys IS, Halmagyi GM. Head impulse test in unilateral vestibular loss: vestibulo-ocular reflex and catch-up saccades. *Neurology.* (2008) 70:454–63. doi: 10.1212/01.wnl.0000299117.48935.2e
45. Weber KP, Aw ST, Todd MJ, McGarvie LA, Curthoys IS, Halmagyi GM. Horizontal head impulse test detects gentamicin vestibulotoxicity. *Neurology.* (2009) 72:1417–24. doi: 10.1212/WNL.0b013e3181a18652
46. Tarnutzer AA, Bockisch CJ, Buffone E, Weiler S, Bachmann LM, Weber KP. Disease-specific sparing of the anterior semicircular canals in bilateral vestibulopathy. *Clin Neurophysiol.* (2016) 127:2791–801. doi: 10.1016/j.clinph.2016.05.005
47. Wrisley DM, Marchetti GF, Kuharsky DK, Whitney SL. Reliability, internal consistency, and validity of data obtained with the functional gait assessment. *Phys Ther.* (2004) 84:906–18. doi: 10.1093/ptj/84.10.906
48. Walker ML, Austin AG, Banke GM, Foxx SR, Gaetano L, Gardner LA, et al. Reference group data for the functional gait assessment. *Phys Ther.* (2007) 87:1468–77. doi: 10.2522/ptj.20060344
49. Marchetti GF, Lin CC, Alghadir A, Whitney SL. Responsiveness and minimal detectable change of the dynamic gait index and functional gait index in persons with balance and vestibular disorders. *J Neurol Phys Ther.* (2014) 38:119–24. doi: 10.1097/NPT.0000000000000015
50. Wall JC, Bell C, Campbell S, Davis J. The timed get-up-and-Go test revisited: measurement of the component tasks. *J Rehabil Res Dev.* (2000) 37:109–13.
51. Swanenburg J, Humphreys K, Langenfeld A, Brunner F, Wirth B. Validity and reliability of a german version of the neck disability index (NDI-G). *Man Ther.* (2014) 19:52–8. doi: 10.1016/j.math.2013.07.004
52. Swanenburg J, Hegemann SC, Zurbrugg A, Palla A, de Bruin ED. Reliability and validity of the extended timed-get-up-and-go test in patients with bilateral vestibular loss. *NeuroRehabilitation.* (2014) 34:799–807. doi: 10.3233/NRE-141083
53. Kurre Annette BCH, van Gool Christel JAW, Gloor-Juzi T, De Bruin Eling D, Straumann D. Exploratory factor analysis of the dizziness handicap inventory (German version). *BMC Ear, Nose Throat Disorders.* (2010) 10:3. doi: 10.1186/1472-6815-10-3
54. Jacobson GP, Newman CW. The development of the Dizziness Handicap Inventory. *Arch Otolaryngol Head Neck Surg.* (1990) 116:424–7. doi: 10.1001/archotol.1990.01870040046011
55. Keshavarz B, Hecht H. Validating an efficient method to quantify motion sickness. *Hum Factors.* (2011) 53:415–26. doi: 10.1177/0018720811403736

56. Kennedy RS, Lane NE, Berbaum KS, Lilienthal MG. Simulator sickness questionnaire: an enhanced method for quantifying simulator sickness. *Int J Avi Psychol.* (1993) 3:203–20. doi: 10.1207/s15327108ijap0303_3
57. Millar JL, Gimmon Y, Roberts D, Schubert MC. Improvement after vestibular rehabilitation not explained by improved passive vOR gain. *Front Neurol.* (2020) 11:79. doi: 10.3389/fneur.2020.00079
58. Haneuse S, Bartell S. Designs for the combination of group- and individual-level data. *Epidemiology.* (2011) 22:382–9. doi: 10.1097/EDE.0b013e3182125cff
59. Wirtz MA. [Multilevel analysis as a tool to analyze research questions in rehabilitation science]. *Rehabilitation (Stuttg).* (2019) 58:274–81. doi: 10.1055/s-0043-124334

20

From Acute to Chronic Tinnitus: Pilot Data on Predictors and Progression

Veronika Vielsmeier[1]*, Ryan Santiago Stiel[2], Pingling Kwok[1], Berthold Langguth[3] and Martin Schecklmann[3]

[1] Department of Otorhinolaryngology, University of Regensburg, Regensburg, Germany, [2] Department of Otorhinolaryngology, Klinikum St. Elisabeth Straubing GmbH, Straubing, Germany, [3] Department of Psychiatry and Psychotherapy, University of Regensburg, Regensburg, Germany

***Correspondence:**
Veronika Vielsmeier
veronika.vielsmeier@ukr.de

Little is known about the transition from acute tinnitus to chronic tinnitus. By means of this study, we are attempting to close this gap by presenting prospective pilot data of patients with acute tinnitus, followed by tracking their condition's trajectory over a period of 6 months. Forty-nine patients presenting with acute tinnitus (duration < 28 days) were recruited in two clinics. We recorded demographic and clinical tinnitus-related data as well as data on personality, health, treatments, and life-style, during patients' first appearance in the clinic and again three and 6 months thereafter. Standard audiograms were performed at the first and the second visit. Nine (18.4%) patients showed full remission of their tinnitus. These patients differed from patients with a chronic course of tinnitus by shorter tinnitus duration, lower fear-related hyperacusis, higher proportion of female gender, increased ear pressure, and lower levels of alcohol consumption. Among the patients with a chronification of tinnitus, there was no change in tinnitus characteristics. However, their tinnitus distress improved moderately over time. These preliminary data are in line with earlier studies that have shown that only a small proportion of those patients presenting in the clinic with acute tinnitus experience a full remission. The results of this study can be of service in deducing hypotheses for the transition from acute to chronic tinnitus and in developing designs for interventional studies.

Keywords: acute tinnitus, chronic tinnitus, questionnaire, causes for progression, predictors

INTRODUCTION

Subjective chronic tinnitus has a high prevalence, affecting 10–15% of adults worldwide (1, 2), and is responsible for high costs for health care systems (3). Research on chronic tinnitus has been growing during the last decade.

Several hypotheses about risk factors for developing chronic or decompensated tinnitus exist. Hearing impairment can be found in almost all patients with chronic tinnitus (4, 5). However, not every patient with hearing difficulty has tinnitus, meaning that hearing impairment may be a required but not sufficient risk factor. For example, Muhlmeier et al. published a study including 113 patients with acute idiopathic sudden sensorineural hearing loss. Here, tinnitus loudness decreased rapidly in cases of mild-moderate hearing loss and tinnitus had completely resolved in two-thirds of the patients after 3 months. In contrast, when tinnitus is associated with severe-profound hearing loss, it improved significantly less (6). Also, temporomandibular joint or neck pathologies are discussed as moderators for tinnitus (7).

Additional comorbidities such as depression (8), anxiety (8), hyperacusis (9), and personality traits such as neuroticism (10), are discussed as determining factors for the development of decompensated tinnitus, resulting in patients seeking for help. Anxiety disorders in tinnitus patients seem to be associated with more psychosocial stress (11). Other studies could show that low resilience is associated with low emotional health and distressing tinnitus (12). D'Amelio et al. described a high correlation between the degree of depression on one side and the dysfunctional coping with stress and emotional distress caused by tinnitus on the other side, frequently present in acute tinnitus cases (13).

Most findings on risk factors for chronic or decompensated tinnitus are based on cross-sectional and retrospective datasets or specific populations. Up to now, prospective and longitudinal studies are sparse. Overall, the transition and progression from acute to chronic tinnitus has not been sufficiently addressed.

We were only able to identify two studies investigating the course of acute tinnitus. One study followed the trajectory of tinnitus over 6 months (14). There, 10 out of 44 patients showed full recovery. Tinnitus-attributed sleep disturbance, anxiety, and life satisfaction, each assessed at first investigation, independently predicted tinnitus distress at the second assessment 6 months later in patients with a chronic course of tinnitus. These three variables together predicted 56% of the variance of tinnitus distress at the time of the second assessment. This is in accordance with a follow-up study of patients with tinnitus after 2 years, showing that severe tinnitus suffering was associated with a higher likelihood of anxiety disorders, more psychosocial stress and lower global assessment of function scores (11).

The second observational study on the development of acute tinnitus over time showed that almost 90% of participants developed chronic tinnitus, only five out of 41 patients showed complete remission after 6 months (15). Aspects of mental health like level of depression and anxiety at the beginning of tinnitus seem to be predicting a higher level of tinnitus decompensation after 6 months (15).

The prevalence data of these two prospective studies are in contrast to a retrospective study by Forti et al. of 269 patients who were treated with Tinnitus Retraining Therapy and sound generators, 26% did not use the sound generator in a mean time of 49 (± 16,89) months of follow-up, because their tinnitus apparently was no longer a problem (16).

In sum, data on the progression of acute tinnitus are limited, and the focus seems to be on the prediction of tinnitus worsening and not on predictors for tinnitus remission; or studies are based on a specific sub-group of patients with sudden hearing loss. Thus, we performed a two-center observational survey to evaluate possible predictors for tinnitus remission and investigate the transition from acute to chronic tinnitus during a time interval of 6 months after onset.

MATERIALS AND METHODS

We included 50 patients presenting in either one of two clinics of Otorhinolaryngology in Eastern Bavaria (Regensburg, Straubing), beginning from October 2013, with a duration of acute tinnitus of up to 28 days. For this work, acute tinnitus was defined by a tinnitus duration below 28 days, with the intention of investigating the transition from acute to chronic tinnitus. There is heterogeneity of definition of acute (<3 months), sub-acute (<6 months), and chronic tinnitus (>6 months but also >3 months) in the literature (15, 17). However, as we were interested in the transition from one stage to the other, we restricted our inclusion criteria to the very acute duration of tinnitus and decided to conduct the follow-up visits 3 and 6 months after the first consultation.

All patients gave written informed consent to the study which was approved by the ethics committee of the University of Regensburg (13-101-0160).

All patients presented twice in the hospital—for the first consultation and a first follow-up 3 months thereafter. The first contact took place in emergency settings. Three months after the second visit, patients received questionnaires by mail. We recorded different categories of data (i.e., demographic, tinnitus-related, audiology, psychopathological, health-related, treatment and life-style data). Most of the data were ratings or subjective reported variables. Audiology was recorded by the investigator team (pure tone audiogram; frequencies 125 Hz, 250 Hz, 500 Hz, 1 kHz, 2 kHz, 3 kHz, 4 kHz, 6 kHz, and 8 kHz). Standardized ratings included the Tinnitus Sample Case History Questionnaire (18) for tinnitus characteristics, numeric ratings scales for different aspects of tinnitus (19), the Mini Tinnitus Questionnaire (20) for measurement of tinnitus distress, the Big-Five-Inventory-10 (21) for measurement of five personality traits, the Life Orientation Test (LOT-R) (22) for measurement of optimism and pessimism, and the Generalized Anxiety Disorder 7 (GAD-7) of the Patient Health Questionnaire (PHQ) (23).

For group comparisons of categorial variables we used chi-square tests of independence, and of metric variables Student *t*-tests. Longitudinal analyses were done with Student *t*-test for dependent samples or, in the case of three observations, with analyses of variance with the within-subjects factor time. Significance threshold was set to 5%. Analyses were done with SPSS 24 (IBM SPSS Statistics).

RESULTS

Sample Description

Fifty patients presented from October 2013 to December 2016 with a tinnitus onset of up to 28 days. Due to a high number of missing values, one patient had to be excluded from the study. The analysis sample consisted of 49 patients presenting in either one of two clinics for Otorhinolaryngology in Eastern Bavaria (Regensburg: $n = 14$; Straubing: $n = 35$). The recruitment time interval was from October 2013 to December 2016.

Demographics

Twenty-one out of these 49 patients were females. Mean age was 46 ± 14 years (range: 21–81 years). Seventeen reported A-levels or equivalently high education. Thirty-one were married, seven with and 11 without partnership. Mean height was 1.73 ± 0.76 m and mean weight was 79 ± 14 kg. The mean number of alcoholic drinks per week was 2.8 ± 3.6. Eight patients reported regular smoking. Mean hearing (dB HL) loss was 27 ± 29 on the right and 24 ± 22 on the left side.

Tinnitus Characteristics

Tinnitus duration was 8.5 ± 5.3 days (range: 1–25 days), tinnitus loudness was 44 ± 25, tinnitus awareness 61 ± 31, and tinnitus annoyance 54 ± 34 (all three variables with a scale from 0 to 100). Numeric ratings showed values for severity of 3.2 ± 1.1 (on a scale from 0 to 5). Numeric ratings with a scale from 0 to 10 showed 4.3 ± 2.7 for loudness, 5.1 ± 3.0 for discomfort, 5.3 ± 3.2 for annoyance, 5.5 ± 3.4 for ignorability, and 5.2 ± 3.1 for unpleasantness. The Mini Tinnitus Questionnaire showed a mean value of 11.6 ± 6.5 (range 0–23) indicating moderate distress in average. Eighteen (37%) patients reported tinnitus in relatives, 12 reported a gradual and 37 a sudden beginning of tinnitus. All patients experienced non-pulsatile tinnitus. Nineteen (39%) reported fluctuations of their tinnitus over time. Twenty patients had tinnitus purely on the right, 18 purely on the left side. Three reported a right-dominant tinnitus, five a left-dominant, and three patients equal distributed tinnitus over both ears. Most patients reported a tonal tinnitus ($n = 39$), two noise-like, one crickets-like, and seven other sounds. With respect to pitch, tinnitus was rated very high in six, high in 24, middle in 14, and low in five patients. Thirty-one reported maskability of tinnitus by sounds, 10 patients reported it not maskable, and eight were unable to answer this question. Modulation of tinnitus by somatic maneuvers was possible in 16 (33%) patients.

Comorbidities

Half of patients ($n = 23$; 46.9%) reported worsening of tinnitus by stress and the remaining patients reported no impact of stress on their tinnitus. Only one patient was equipped with hearing aids. Thirteen patients reported painful hyperacusis, 27 had no hyperacusis, and nine patients did not answer this question. Fear-related hyperacusis was 2.8 ± 1.0 on a scale from 1 to 5.

Headache was prevalent in 14 patients, temporomandibular joint problems in 11 patients, neck pain in 22 patients, and general pain in six patients. Two patients reported concomitant psychiatric treatment.

With respect to putative tinnitus-causing factors, five patients reported to have a noisy hobby, 29 reported stress in the last weeks, five an acute and two long lasting noise exposition. Ear infections in the previous weeks were present in three patients, a common cold in nine patients, a recent hearing loss in 18 and a long-lasting hearing loss in eight patients. Ear pressure was prevalent in 28 patients and vertigo in 12 patients. Two patients reported a diving accident, six patients ear surgery, one patient acute and six patients earlier cervical spine injury. One patient reported head injury in the last weeks before tinnitus onset and two in the past.

With respect to diseases, we asked for diabetes ($n = 2$), stroke ($n = 1$), heart attack ($n = 1$), hypertension ($n = 16$), hypotension ($n = 2$), diseases of the immune system ($n = 4$), high cholesterol ($n = 11$), and gout ($n = 3$). No patient had any kidney disease or an infectious disease.

TABLE 1 | Significant differences in patients with full remission vs. patients with chronic course of tinnitus.

	Remitted tinnitus ($n = 9$)	Chronic tinnitus ($n = 40$)	
Sex (female/male)	7/2	14/26	$\chi^2 = 5.490$; df = 1; $p = 0.019$
Tinnitus duration (days)	4.78 ± 12.74	9.38 ± 5.36	$T = 2.501$; df = 47; $p = 0.016$
Loudness hyperacusis (never/rarely/sometimes/usually/always)	2.00 ± 1.00	2.98 ± 0.95	$T = 2.764$; df = 47; $p = 0.008$
Drinks per week (500 ml beer or 250 ml wine)	0.44 ± 0.88	3.33 ± 3.85	$T = 2.217$; df = 47; $p = 0.032$
Ear pressure (yes/no)	8/1	20/20	$\chi^2 = 4.537$; df = 1; $p = 0.033$

Concerning regular medication, five patients took anticoagulants, four diuretics, 15 blood pressure medication, eight antibiotics, and three contraceptives. No patient was undergoing chemotherapy.

Treatment

During the observation period 30 patients (61.2%) received tinnitus treatment. Nineteen received steroid hormones (cortisone, prednisolone, and dexamethasone), five local anesthetics (lidocaine, procaine, and novocaine), six antihistamines (betahistine, dimenhydrinate), eight cardiac medication (several different medications), and nine herbal drugs (different herbal drugs and vitamines). Eleven underwent physiotherapy, two psychosomatic interventions (rehabilitation, autogenic training), one hyperbaric oxygen therapy. No ear surgery was reported. Four patients could not specify the treatment they received.

Psychological Measures

The evaluation of personality traits with the Big-Five Personality Inventory (scale from 1 to 5), revealed extraversion to be 3.4 ± 1.0, neuroticism 3.2 ± 0.9, openness 3.5 ± 0.9, conscientiousness 4.3 ± 0.6, and agreeableness 3.1 ± 0.8. Pessimism was 11.1 ± 2.2 and optimism 6.6 ± 2.4, both measured on a scale from 1 to 15. Depressivity on a scale from 0 to 2 was 0.7 ± 0.9, and anxiety on a scale from 0 to 15 was 6.5 ± 4.4.

Predictor Analysis

Nine out of 49 patients (18.4%) showed a full remission of tinnitus after 3 and 6 months. All measured variables were tested for group differences. Patients with full remission differed from patients with "chronic tinnitus" with respect to tinnitus duration, fear-related hyperacusis, drinks per week, gender, and ear pressure (i.e., tinnitus remission was associated with the following characteristics at baseline: shorter tinnitus duration, lower fear-related hyperacusis, lower consumption of alcoholic drinks, higher incidence of increased ear pressure and a higher proportion of women). For statistical values see **Table 1**. All other variables turned out not to differ significantly between groups.

TABLE 2 | Course of tinnitus related variables over time in patients with chronic tinnitus.

	Visit 1	Visit 2 (3 months)	Visit 3 (6 months)	Statistics
Tinnitus loudness (0–100)	46.6 ± 25.0	43.7 ± 25.7	46.5 ± 23.7	$F = 0.545$; df = 2,70; $p = 0.582$
Tinnitus loudness (0–10)	4.6 ± 2.9	3.9 ± 2.9	3.9 ± 2.9	$F = 2.581$; df = 2,68; $p = 0.083$
Tinnitus awareness (0–100)	62.8 ± 30.1	50.0 ± 32.3	76.5 ± 140.8	$F = 0.872$; df = 2,70; $p = 0.423$
Tinnitus annoyance (0–100)	57.4 ± 32.9	49.1 ± 35.5	43.8 ± 31.0	$F = 4.981$; df = 2,68; $p = 0.010$
Tinnitus severity (0–5)	3.3 ± 1.1	2.7 ± 1.1	2.5 ± 1.1	$F = 18.964$; df = 2,68; $p < 0.001$
Tinnitus discomfort (0–10)	5.4 ± 3.0	4.4 ± 3.2	4.3 ± 3.2	$F = 3.547$; df = 2,68; $p = 0.034$
Tinnitus annoyance (0–10)	5.7 ± 3.2	4.1 ± 3.4	3.9 ± 3.2	$F = 10.214$; df = 2,68; $p < 0.001$
Tinnitus ignorability (0–10)	6.2 ± 3.4	4.8 ± 3.5	4.1 ± 3.2	$F = 11.032$; df = 2,68; $p < 0.001$
Tinnitus unpleasantness (0–10)	5.7 ± 3.1	4.3 ± 3.2	3.8 ± 3.2	$F = 10.693$; df = 2,68; $p < 0.001$
Mini tinnitus questionnaire (0-24; distress)	12.5 ± 6.5	10.3 ± 6.3	9.3 ± 6.3	$F = 11.816$; df = 2,66; $p < 0.001$
Tinnitus laterality (right/left/ left>right/right>left/ equal)	16/13/4/2/2	14/10/5/6/2	n.a.	$\chi^2 = 34.585$; $p < 0.001$
Tinnitus laterality (right/left/ left>right/right>left/ equal/inside head)	15/13/3/2/2	n.a.	9/11/4/4/5/2	$\chi^2 = 40.558$; $p < 0.001$
Tinnitus type (tone/noise/ crickets/other)	28/2/1/6	29/1/4/3	n.a.	$\chi^2 = 17.196$; $p = 0.047$
Tinnitus type (tone/noise/ crickets/other)	27/2/1/6	n.a.	29/3/1/3	$\chi^2 = 17.200$; $p = 0.053$
Tinnitus frequency (very high/high/middle/low)	5/17/10/5	9/16/9/3	n.a.	$\chi^2 = 16.355$; $p = 0.016$
Tinnitus frequency (very high/high/middle/low)	4/17/10/5	n.a.	5/20/8/3	$\chi^2 = 18.147$; $p = 0.005$
Mean hearing right (dB HL)	32 ± 32	28 ± 29	n.a.	$T = 3.855$; df = 33; $p = 0.001$
Mean hearing left (dB HL)	27 ± 25	23 ± 23	n.a.	$T = 2.890$; df = 33; $p = 0.007$

Please note that for χ^2 statistics statistical significance means that there is no change over time.

Longitudinal Analysis

For 37 out of the 40 patients with chronic tinnitus complete data sets of both follow-up visits were available. These patients showed no significant changes over time for tinnitus loudness or tinnitus awareness, but for tinnitus annoyance, discomfort, ignorability, unpleasantness, and distress. The reduction of the Mini TQ score over the observation period of 6 months was in the range of a medium effect size (Cohen's d(?) 0.691). Tinnitus laterality, type, and subjective reported frequency were similar for both visits as indicated by (near) significant chi-square tests. For details see **Table 2**. Hearing functions improved from visit 1 to visit 2, but there was no significant correlation between changes in hearing and changes in annoyance, discomfort, ignorability, unpleasantness, and distress. Correlations analyses were not significant (all $r < 0.296$; all $p > 0.094$).

DISCUSSION

Discussion of Our Results

The aim of our study was to observe the transition from acute to chronic tinnitus and to identify predictors for the remission and trajectory of tinnitus. Our main results are (1) that among patients who present with a tinnitus duration of <4 weeks at the clinic only a small amount (18%) lose their tinnitus and show full remission, (2) that putative predictors for remission may be shorter tinnitus duration, female sex, lower consumption of alcoholic drinks, lower fear-related hyperacusis, and increased subjective ear pressure, and (3) that among those patients who develop chronic tinnitus, the perceptual tinnitus characteristics remain unchanged, whereas tinnitus distress improves over time.

To our knowledge, two studies with a comparable approach exist (14, 15). Particularly similar was the investigation by Wallhausser-Franke. Patients were also recruited between 2013 and 2016, the sample size and inclusion criteria (tinnitus onset below 4 weeks) were similar, the observation period equally was 6 months, and some rating instruments were identical. Our findings confirm the main findings of the two previous publications. Both studies indicate a high heterogeneity with respect to tinnitus etiology and applied treatments, both suggest remission rates below 20% and both converge in the observation that tinnitus characteristics (localization, sound quality) tend to stay stable, whereas the average tinnitus distress improves moderately over time. Predictor analysis was done with respect to variables of tinnitus distress as an outcome variable and not with respect to the complete remission of tinnitus. By this means, higher tinnitus distress and depressivity in the acute phase of tinnitus were identified as predictors for a worsening of tinnitus over time.

Limitations

These three small studies highlight the need for further investigations of larger samples. The design of these investigations should consider the experiences and the limitations of the available studies. One lesson from previous undertakings is the need of a uniform definition of variables. For example, Wallhausser-Franke and colleagues find changes in tinnitus awareness over time that we weren't able to, which may be related to the operationalisation of this variable (15). Wallhausser-Franke coded this variable as "permanent" and "intermittent," and we asked for percentage values (0–100%).

Another limitation of the available studies is the heterogeneity of performed interventions. These studies investigating the natural course of tinnitus over time should be complemented by interventional research. Even if we gathered data prospectively, it is not possible to draw causal conclusions as long as treatments are not controlled and randomized. For example, we can only speculate if a therapeutic intervention targeting the identified risk factors will improve the course of tinnitus. For example, consumption of alcoholic drinks was identified as one predictor. Only an interventional study could tell whether a corresponding intervention (e.g., decrease of alcohol consumption may help to increase the chance of remission or whether alcohol consumption is not a cause, but rather the consequence of a more affected chronic and decompensated tinnitus). Another limitation is the short period of a 6 months of follow-up and a missing question for thyroid disease.

Perspective for Future Studies

In the future, increasing the validity of data by collecting a highly operationalized case history, interview, and diagnosis of patients as well as medical records, instead of relying solely on subjective reports as has been done in the present study, should be considered. In order to avoid a selection bias, one should aim not only to recruit from hospital clinics but also from ENT- and GP-practices. Moreover, one should aim at an early assessment of tinnitus patients as soon as possible after tinnitus onset. As heterogeneity of etiology and treatment is high, large-scale multi-center trials will be necessary to create a sufficiently large data basis.

The remission rate for acute tinnitus in our study is quite low. It is not clear whether the results are representative. One might assume a selection bias, as those patients in which the tinnitus did disappear spontaneously a few days after tinnitus onset did not present in the clinic. This selection bias is particularly relevant for those patients who present at a later timepoint after tinnitus onset. Accordingly, we observed that a longer tinnitus duration at presentation in the clinic was a predictor for a chronic manifestation of tinnitus.

The remission rate identified in our study and in comparable previous investigations (14, 15) was lower than remission rates for conditions such as sudden hearing loss and acoustic trauma [for overview see (15)]. Even if hearing recovery is a predictor for tinnitus improvement (6), our finding of a lower remission rate of tinnitus when compared to hearing recovery after sudden hearing loss suggests that the chances for hearing recovery after acute hearing loss are higher than the chances for tinnitus disappearance after acute tinnitus onset. Indeed, in clinical practice patients frequently report about good hearing recovery but ongoing tinnitus after sudden hearing loss.

These preliminary data will help in deducing hypotheses about which aspects might be relevant for the chronification of tinnitus. The finding that female sex is associated with a higher chance for tinnitus disappearance might explain why chronic tinnitus is more prevalent in men. Hyperacusis was speculated to be a precursor for tinnitus (9). It might be necessary to screen for hyperacusis in acute tinnitus patients and to find out which aspects of hyperacusis are relevant (in our sample this was fear-related, even if general anxiety did not predict remission). Interestingly, we did no see a significant effect of personality or anxiety even if there is evidence that these variables are involved in decompensated tinnitus (24, 25). It would be highly interesting to see whether ear pressure could be validated by means of diagnostic tests. One could speculate that the subjectively reported increased ear pressure might be an indicator of endolymphatic hydrops, which in turn might characterize a subtype of tinnitus with more fluctuations (26). For this purpose, a more exact definition of ear pressure is also necessary.

In conclusion, acute tinnitus is a highly heterogeneous phenomenon with up to 20% full recovery after 6 months and is taking a moderately positive trajectory in terms of tinnitus distress over time, despite unchanged tinnitus characteristics.

ETHICS STATEMENT

The studies involving human participants were reviewed and approved by University of Regensburg, Germany. The patients/participants provided their written informed consent to participate in this study.

AUTHOR CONTRIBUTIONS

VV study concept, patient recruitment, manuscript, and statistics. RS patient recruitment. PK study concept and manuscript. BL study concept, patient recruitment, and manuscript. MS study concept, manuscript, and statistics. All authors contributed to the article and approved the submitted version.

REFERENCES

1. Langguth B. Treatment of tinnitus. *Curr Opin Otolaryngol Head Neck Surg.* (2015) 23:361–8. doi: 10.1097/MOO.0000000000000185
2. Henry JA, Reavis KM, Griest SE, Thielman EJ, Theodoroff SM, Grush LD, et al. Tinnitus: an epidemiologic perspective. *Otolaryngol Clin North Am.* (2020) 53:481–99. doi: 10.1016/j.otc.2020.03.002
3. Maes IH, Cima RF, Vlaeyen JW, Anteunis LJ, Joore MA. Tinnitus: a cost study. *Ear Hear.* (2013) 34:508–14. doi: 10.1097/AUD.0b013e31827d113a
4. Schaette R, Kempter R. Development of tinnitus-related neuronal hyperactivity through homeostatic plasticity after hearing loss: a computational model. *Eur J Neurosci.* (2006) 23:3124–38. doi: 10.1111/j.1460-9568.2006.04774.x

5. Gopinath B, McMahon CM, Rochtchina E, Karpa MJ, Mitchell P. Risk factors and impacts of incident tinnitus in older adults. *Ann Epidemiol.* (2010) 20:129–35. doi: 10.1016/j.annepidem.2009.09.002
6. Muhlmeier G, Baguley D, Cox T, Suckfull M, Meyer T. Characteristics and spontaneous recovery of tinnitus related to idiopathic sudden sensorineural hearing loss. *Otol Neurotol.* (2016) 37:634–41. doi: 10.1097/MAO.0000000000001081
7. Sanchez TG, Rocha CB. Diagnosis and management of somatosensory tinnitus: review article. *Clinics.* (2011) 66:1089–94. doi: 10.1590/S1807-59322011000600028
8. Park E, Kim H, Choi IH, Han HM, Han K, Jung HH, et al. Psychiatric distress as a common risk factor for tinnitus and joint pain: a National Population-Based Survey. *Clin Exp Otorhinolaryngol.* (2019) 13:234–40. doi: 10.21053/ceo.2019.00563
9. Schecklmann M, Landgrebe M, Langguth B, T.R.I.Group DS. Phenotypic characteristics of hyperacusis in tinnitus. *PLoS ONE.* (2014) 9:e86944. doi: 10.1371/journal.pone.0086944
10. Langguth B, Kleinjung T, Fischer B, Hajak G, Eichhammer P, Sand PG. Tinnitus severity, depression, and the big five personality traits. *Prog Brain Res.* (2007) 166:221–5. doi: 10.1016/S0079-6123(07)66020-8
11. Holgers SZKM, Svedlund K. Predictive factors for development of severe tinnitus suffering-further characterisation. *Int J Audiol.* (2005) 44:584–92. doi: 10.1080/14992020500190235
12. Wallhausser-Franke E, Delb W, Balkenhol T, Hiller W, Hormann K. Tinnitus-related distress and the personality characteristic resilience. *Neural Plast.* (2014) 2014:370307. doi: 10.1155/2014/370307
13. D'Amelio CAR, Scholz S, Falkai P, Plinkert PK, Delb W. Psychological distress associated with acute tinnitus. *HNO.* (2004) 52:599–603. doi: 10.1007/s00106-003-0944-5
14. Olderog M, Langenbach M, Michel O, Brusis T, Kohle K. Predictors and mechanisms of tinnitus distress—a longitudinal analysis. *Laryngorhinootologie.* (2004) 83:5–13. doi: 10.1055/s-2004-814235
15. Wallhausser-Franke E, D'Amelio R, Glauner A, Delb W, Servais JJ, Hormann K, et al. Transition from acute to chronic tinnitus: predictors for the development of chronic distressing tinnitus. *Front Neurol.* (2017) 8:605. doi: 10.3389/fneur.2017.00605
16. Forti S, Ambrosetti U, Crocetti A, Del Bo L. Tinnitus patients lost to follow-up. *Int J Audiol.* (2010) 49:877–80. doi: 10.3109/14992027.2010.505583
17. Cima RFF, Mazurek B, Haider H, Kikidis D, Lapira A, Norena A, et al. A multidisciplinary European guideline for tinnitus: diagnostics, assessment, and treatment. *HNO.* (2019) 67:10–42. doi: 10.1007/s00106-019-0633-7
18. Landgrebe M, Zeman F, Koller M, Eberl Y, Mohr M, Reiter J, et al. The Tinnitus Research Initiative (TRI) database: a new approach for delineation of tinnitus subtypes and generation of predictors for treatment outcome. *BMC Med Inform Decis Mak.* (2010) 10:42. doi: 10.1186/1472-6947-10-42
19. Manning C, Grush L, Thielman E, Roberts L, Henry JA. Comparison of tinnitus loudness measures: matching, rating, and scaling. *Am J Audiol.* (2019) 28:137–43. doi: 10.1044/2018_AJA-17-0115
20. Hesse G. *Tinnitus.* Stuttgart, KG: Georg Thieme Verlag (2008).
21. Rammstedt KCJB, Klein MC, Beierlein C, Kovaleva A. *Eine kurze Skala zur Messung der fünf Dimensionen der Persönlichkeit: Big-Five-Inventory-10 (BFI-10); GESIS-Working Papers 2012|22.* Köln/Mannheim: GESIS-Leibniz-Institut für Sozialwissenschaften (2012).
22. Glaesmer HJH, Klotsche J, Herzberg PJ. *Deutsche Version der Revision des Life-Orientation-Tests (LOT-R).* Heft: Zeitschrift für Gesundheitspsychologie (2008).
23. Spitzer KMR, Williams J, Löwe B. A brief measure for assessing generalized anxiety disorder: the GAD-7. *Archiv Internal Med.* (2006) 166:1092–7. doi: 10.1001/archinte.166.10.1092
24. Fuller TE, Cima RFF, Van den Bussche E, Vlaeyen JWS. The fear of tinnitus questionnaire: toward a reliable and valid means of assessing fear in adults with tinnitus. *Ear Hear.* (2019) 40:1467–77. doi: 10.1097/AUD.0000000000000728
25. Simoes J, Schlee W, Schecklmann M, Langguth B, Farahmand D, Neff P. Big five personality traits are associated with tinnitus improvement over time. *Sci Rep.* (2019) 9:18234. doi: 10.1038/s41598-019-53845-4
26. De Luca P, Cassandro C, Ralli M, Gioacchini FM, Turchetta R, Orlando MP, et al. Dietary restriction for the treatment of Meniere's disease. *Transl Med UniSa.* (2020) 22:5–9.

Permissions

All chapters in this book were first published by Frontiers; hereby published with permission under the Creative Commons Attribution License or equivalent. Every chapter published in this book has been scrutinized by our experts. Their significance has been extensively debated. The topics covered herein carry significant findings which will fuel the growth of the discipline. They may even be implemented as practical applications or may be referred to as a beginning point for another development.

The contributors of this book come from diverse backgrounds, making this book a truly international effort. This book will bring forth new frontiers with its revolutionizing research information and detailed analysis of the nascent developments around the world.

We would like to thank all the contributing authors for lending their expertise to make the book truly unique. They have played a crucial role in the development of this book. Without their invaluable contributions this book wouldn't have been possible. They have made vital efforts to compile up to date information on the varied aspects of this subject to make this book a valuable addition to the collection of many professionals and students.

This book was conceptualized with the vision of imparting up-to-date information and advanced data in this field. To ensure the same, a matchless editorial board was set up. Every individual on the board went through rigorous rounds of assessment to prove their worth. After which they invested a large part of their time researching and compiling the most relevant data for our readers.

The editorial board has been involved in producing this book since its inception. They have spent rigorous hours researching and exploring the diverse topics which have resulted in the successful publishing of this book. They have passed on their knowledge of decades through this book. To expedite this challenging task, the publisher supported the team at every step. A small team of assistant editors was also appointed to further simplify the editing procedure and attain best results for the readers.

Apart from the editorial board, the designing team has also invested a significant amount of their time in understanding the subject and creating the most relevant covers. They scrutinized every image to scout for the most suitable representation of the subject and create an appropriate cover for the book.

The publishing team has been an ardent support to the editorial, designing and production team. Their endless efforts to recruit the best for this project, has resulted in the accomplishment of this book. They are a veteran in the field of academics and their pool of knowledge is as vast as their experience in printing. Their expertise and guidance has proved useful at every step. Their uncompromising quality standards have made this book an exceptional effort. Their encouragement from time to time has been an inspiration for everyone.

The publisher and the editorial board hope that this book will prove to be a valuable piece of knowledge for researchers, students, practitioners and scholars across the globe.

List of Contributors

Angela Schrader
Department of Otolaryngology, Washington University School of Medicine, St. Louis, MO, United States

Mark E. Warchol
Department of Otolaryngology, Washington University School of Medicine, St. Louis, MO, United States
Department of Neuroscience, Washington University School of Medicine, St. Louis, MO, United States

Lavinia Sheets
Department of Otolaryngology, Washington University School of Medicine, St. Louis, MO, United States
Department of Developmental Biology, Washington University School of Medicine, St. Louis, MO, United States

Lisa Kabara, Catherine Martin, Ariane Kanicki, David C. Kohrman and David F. Dolan
Kresge Hearing Research Institute, Department of Otolaryngology, Head and Neck Surgery, University of Michigan, Ann Arbor, MI, United States

Courtney E. Stewart
Kresge Hearing Research Institute, Department of Otolaryngology, Head and Neck Surgery, University of Michigan, Ann Arbor, MI, United States
VA Ann Arbor Health Care System, Ann Arbor, MI, United States

Richard A. Altschuler
Kresge Hearing Research Institute, Department of Otolaryngology, Head and Neck Surgery, University of Michigan, Ann Arbor, MI, United States
VA Ann Arbor Health Care System, Ann Arbor, MI, United States
Department of Cell and Developmental Biology, University of Michigan, Ann Arbor, MI, United States

Isabel Varela-Nieto, Silvia Murillo-Cuesta and Lourdes Rodríguez-de la Rosa
Institute for Biomedical Research "Alberto Sols," Spanish National Research Council (CSIC)-Autonomous University of Madrid, Madrid, Spain
Biomedical Research Networking Center on Rare Diseases (CIBERER), Institute of Health Carlos III, Madrid, Spain
Hospital La Paz Institute for Health Research, Madrid, Spain

María Jesús Oset-Gasque
Department of Biochemistry and Molecular Biology, School of Pharmacy, Complutense University of Madrid, Madrid, Spain
Institute of Neurochemistry Research, Complutense University of Madrid, Madrid, Spain

José Marco-Contelles
Laboratory of Medicinal Chemistry, Institute of General Organic Chemistry, CSIC, Madrid, Spain

Juan Carlos Alvarado and Verónica Fuentes-Santamaría
Facultad de Medicina, Instituto de Investigación en Discapacidades, Neurológicas (IDINE), Universidad de Castilla-La Mancha, Albacete, Spain

José M. Juiz
Facultad de Medicina, Instituto de Investigación en Discapacidades, Neurológicas (IDINE), Universidad de Castilla-La Mancha, Albacete, Spain
Department of Otolaryngology, Hannover Medical School, NIFE-VIANNA, Cluster of Excellence Hearing4all-German Research Foundation, Hannover, Germany

Wei Liu, Hao Li and Helge Rask-Andersen
Section of Otolaryngology, Department of Surgical Sciences, Head and Neck Surgery, Uppsala University Hospital, Uppsala, Sweden

Maria Luque, Anneliese Schrott-Fischer and Rudolf Glueckert
Department of Otorhinolaryngology, Medical University of Innsbruck, Innsbruck, Austria

Sven Tylstedt
Department of Olaryngology, Västerviks Hospital, Västervik, Sweden

Gunesh Rajan
Department of Otolaryngology, Head & Neck Surgery, Luzerner Kantonsspital, Luzern, Switzerland
Department of Otolaryngology, Head & Neck Surgery, Division of Surgery, Medical School, University of Western Australia, Perth, WA, Australia

Hanif Ladak
Department of Otolaryngology-Head and Neck Surgery, Department of Medical Biophysics and Department of Electrical and Computer Engineering, Western University, London, ON, Canada

Sumit Agrawal
Department of Otolaryngology-Head and Neck Surgery, Western University, London, ON, Canada

Teresa Nicolson
Department of Otolaryngology, Stanford University, Stanford, CA, United States

Igor Majewski and Martin Durisin
Clinic for Otolaryngology–Head & Neck Surgery, Hanover Medical School, Hanover, Germany

Athanasia Warnecke and Jennifer Harre
Clinic for Otolaryngology–Head & Neck Surgery, Hanover Medical School, Hanover, Germany
Cluster of Excellence "Hearing4all" of the German Research Foundation (EXC 2177/1), Oldenburg, Germany

Matthew Shew
Department of Otolaryngology–Head & Neck Surgery, Washington University School of Medicine in St. Louis, St. Louis, MO, United States

Adam J. Mellott
Ronawk Inc., Olathe, KS, United States

Hinrich Staecker
Department of Otolaryngology–Head & Neck Surgery, University of Kansas School of Medicine, Kansas City, KS, United States

Yutaka Koizumi, Tsukasa Ito and Seiji Kakehata
Department of Otolaryngology-Head and Neck Surgery, Faculty of Medicine, Yamagata University, Yamagata, Japan

Kunio Mizutari
Department of Otolaryngology-Head and Neck Surgery, National Defense Medical College, Saitama, Japan

Li Gao, Tomoko Kita, Tatsuya Katsuno, Norio Yamamoto, Koichi Omori and Takayuki Nakagawa
Department of Otolaryngology, Head and Neck Surgery, Graduate School of Medicine, Kyoto University, Kyoto, Japan

Andrea Zhang, Richard Kuang, Ryan Lu, Albert S. Edge and David H. Jung
Department of Otolaryngology, Massachusetts Eye and Ear Infirmary, Harvard Medical School, Boston, MA, United States

Judith S. Kempfle
Department of Otolaryngology, Massachusetts Eye and Ear Infirmary, Harvard Medical School, Boston, MA, United States
Department of Otolaryngology, University Medical Center Tübingen, Tübingen, Germany

Marlon V. Duro, Carolina D. Amador, Boris A. Kashemirov and Charles E. McKenna
Department of Chemistry, University of Southern California, Los Angeles, CA, United States

Thomas Parzefall, Martin Koenighofer, Julia Eckl-Dorna, Wolfgang Gstoettner and Klemens Frei
Department of Otorhinolaryngology, Head and Neck Surgery, Medical University of Vienna, Vienna, Austria

Alexandra Frohne
Department of Otorhinolaryngology, Head and Neck Surgery, Medical University of Vienna, Vienna, Austria
Department for Cell and Developmental Biology, Orphan Disease Genetics Group, Center for Anatomy and Cell Biology, Medical University of Vienna, Vienna, Austria

Christian Schoefer and Trevor Lucas
Department for Cell and Developmental Biology, Orphan Disease Genetics Group, Center for Anatomy and Cell Biology, Medical University of Vienna, Vienna, Austria

Juergen Neesen and Franco Laccone
Institute of Medical Genetics, Center for Pathobiochemistry and Genetics, Medical University of Vienna, Vienna, Austria

Jonathan J. Waters and Emma Ashton
Rare and Inherited Disease Laboratory, London North Genomic Laboratory Hub, Great Ormond Street Hospital for Children NHS Foundation Trust, London, United Kingdom

Markus Schreiner
Department of Biomedical Imaging and Image-Guided Therapy, Medical University of Vienna, Vienna, Austria

Sami Samir Amr
Laboratory for Molecular Medicine, Partners Healthcare Personalized Medicine, Cambridge, MA, United States
Department of Pathology, Brigham and Women's Hospital and Harvard Medical School, Boston, MA, United States

Toru Miwa
Department of Otolaryngology and Head and Neck Surgery, Kitano Hospital, Tazuke Kofukai Medical Research Institute, Osaka, Japan
Department of Otolaryngology and Head and Neck Surgery, Graduate of School of Medicine, Kyoto University, Kyoto, Japan

German Nacher-Soler, Marta Coelho and Francis Rousset
The Inner Ear and Olfaction Lab, Department of Pathology and Immunology, Faculty of Medicine, University of Geneva, Geneva, Switzerland

Sébastien Lenglet
Forensic Toxicology and Chemistry Unit, University Centre for Legal Medicine, Geneva University Hospital, Geneva, Switzerland

Aurélien Thomas
Forensic Toxicology and Chemistry Unit, University Centre for Legal Medicine, Geneva University Hospital, Geneva, Switzerland
Faculty Unit of Toxicology, University Centre of Legal Medicine, Lausanne University Hospital, Lausanne, Switzerland

François Voruz and Pascal Senn
The Inner Ear and Olfaction Lab, Department of Pathology and Immunology, Faculty of Medicine, University of Geneva, Geneva, Switzerland
Department of Clinical Neurosciences, Service of ORL & Head and Neck Surgery, University Hospital of Geneva, Geneva, Switzerland

Karl-Heinz Krause
Department of Pathology and Immunology, Faculty of Medicine, University of Geneva, Geneva, Switzerland

Mami Matsunaga, Ryosuke Yamamoto and Takayuki Okano
Department of Otolaryngology, Head and Neck Surgery, Graduate School of Medicine, Kyoto University, Kyoto, Japan

Satoko Sakamoto
Medical Innovation Center, Kyoto University, Kyoto, Japan

Amrita A. Iyer
Department of Molecular and Human Genetics, Baylor College of Medicine, Houston, TX, United States
Program in Genetics & Genomics, Houston, TX, United States

Andrew K. Groves
Department of Molecular and Human Genetics, Baylor College of Medicine, Houston, TX, United States
Program in Genetics & Genomics, Houston, TX, United States
Department of Neuroscience, Baylor College of Medicine, Houston, TX, United States

Wouter H. van der Valk
Department of Otorhinolaryngology and Head & Neck Surgery, Leiden University Medical Center, Leiden University, Leiden, Netherlands

Juliëtte J. C. M. van Munster
Department of Otorhinolaryngology and Head & Neck Surgery, Leiden University Medical Center, Leiden University, Leiden, Netherlands
Department of Neurosurgery, Leiden University Medical Center, Leiden University, Leiden, Netherlands

Arno F. Lieftink
Department of Otorhinolaryngology and Head & Neck Surgery, University Medical Center Utrecht, Utrecht, Netherlands

Inge Stegeman and Adriana L. Smit
Department of Otorhinolaryngology and Head & Neck Surgery, University Medical Center Utrecht, Utrecht, Netherlands
Brain Center Rudolf Magnus, University Medical Center Utrecht, Utrecht, Netherlands

Jorge Rey-Martinez and Xabier Altuna
Neurotology Unit, ENT Department, Hospital Universitario Donostia, San Sebastián - Donostia, Spain

Kai Cheng, Ann M. Burgess and Ian S. Curthoys
Vestibular Research Laboratory, School of Psychology, The University of Sydney, Sydney, NSW, Australia

Paul F. Smith and Yiwen Zheng
Department of Pharmacology and Toxicology, Brain Health Research Centre, School of Biomedical Sciences, University of Otago, Dunedin, New Zealand
Brain Research New Zealand Centre of Research Excellence, University of Auckland, Auckland, New Zealand
The Eisdell Moore Centre for Hearing and Balance Research, University of Auckland, Auckland, New Zealand

Fabienne Büchi
Physiotherapy and Occupational Therapy Research Center, Directorate of Research and Education, University Hospital Zurich, University of Zurich, Zurich, Switzerland

Jaap Swanenburg
Physiotherapy and Occupational Therapy Research Center, Directorate of Research and Education, University Hospital Zurich, University of Zurich, Zurich, Switzerland
Department of Chiropractic Medicine, Integrative Spinal Research ISR, Balgrist University Hospital, Zurich, Switzerland

Dominik Straumann
Department of Neurology, University Hospital Zurich, University of Zurich, Zurich, Switzerland

Konrad P. Weber
Department of Neurology, University Hospital Zurich, University of Zurich, Zurich, Switzerland
Department of Ophthalmology, University Hospital Zurich, University of Zurich, Zurich, Switzerland

Eling D. de Bruin
Department Health Sciences and Technology, Institute of Human Movement Sciences and Sport, ETH Zurich, Zurich, Switzerland
Division of Physiotherapy, Department of Neurobiology, Care Sciences and Society, Karolinska Institute, Stockholm, Sweden

Veronika Vielsmeier and Pingling Kwok
Department of Otorhinolaryngology, University of Regensburg, Regensburg, Germany

Ryan Santiago Stiel
Department of Otorhinolaryngology, Klinikum St. Elisabeth Straubing GmbH, Straubing, Germany

Berthold Langguth and Martin Schecklmann
Department of Psychiatry and Psychotherapy, University of Regensburg, Regensburg, Germany

Index

www.ingramcontent.com/pod-product-compliance
Lightning Source LLC
Chambersburg PA
CBHW081215180926
51613CB00003B/246
9781639897643